Immuno-Psychiatry

Michael Berk • Marion Leboyer
Iris E. Sommer
Editors

Immuno-Psychiatry

Facts and Prospects

Springer

Editors
Michael Berk
Deakin University
IMPACT - The Institute for Mental and Physical Health and Clinical Translation, School of Medicine, Barwon Health
Geelong, VIC, Australia

Marion Leboyer
University Paris Est Créteil (UPEC)
Inserm, IMRB (Translational NeuroPsychiatry lab), AP-HP, DMU IMPACT, AP-HP, Fondation FondaMental
Créteil, France

Iris E. Sommer
UMC Groningen
Groningen, The Netherlands

ISBN 978-3-030-71228-0 ISBN 978-3-030-71229-7 (eBook)
https://doi.org/10.1007/978-3-030-71229-7

This Springer imprint is published by the registered company Springer Nature Switzerland AG
The registered company address is: Gewerbestrasse 11, 6330 Cham, Switzerland

Foreword

I am an ideal person to write this Foreword because *Immuno-Psychiatry* is the perfect solution for anyone wondering where the cutting edge of psychoneuroimmunology is now. Once upon a time, I fancied myself on that same cutting edge, but as the years have passed and other scientific pursuits have largely lured me away, I've felt increasingly out of touch, and diminished thereby. Like many of us in science who started out with time to read, write, and think, I now find myself consumed by far less interesting administrative duties. Agreeing to write the Foreword for *Immuno-Psychiatry* provided me with a "work-related" mandate to read the book, and I am happy to report that I now feel far less diminished.

It may seem hard to believe that not so long ago no one thought the brain and the immune system had anything to do with each other. I went to a leading medical school in the late 1980s specifically to be a psychiatrist. For that reason, I dozed through much of our immunology class. It was so patently unrelated to my interests. No big surprise that I didn't make the brain–immune connection. But in retrospect, it is surprising that so few scientists in those times realized how similar both systems were in terms of their evolutionary mandates. Both the central nervous system (CNS) and immune system evolved to maximize the ability of organisms to avoid risk and benefit from opportunity, and—crucially—both are the systems par excellence that learn from experience and remember the past to better cope with the future.

Then, of course, with the discovery that the brain could influence immune function, psychoneuroimmunology (PNI) was born. I remember writing a Foreword for an edition of *Psychoneuroimmunology* at the turn of the twenty-first century. While that large volume had some material on the impact of the immune system on the brain, the vast bulk of the text focused on the impact of the brain on immunity, a discovery still somewhat startling at that late date. We were just then discovering the impact of inflammation on brain and behavior and the notion of this type of powerful bottom-up causality was still a bit suspect.

How times have changed. *Immuno-Psychiatry* provides an update on the field's original top-down direction of influence in a chapter by Giacobbe et al. on the impact of prenatal and early life stress on immune system programing across the life span, especially as this programing relates to the risk for mental illness. But otherwise the focus of *Immuno-Psychiatry* is on the pathways by which the immune system influences the brain and the behavioral states that result from this influence.

Like an archeological dig, the various layers of this discovery are on display in *Immuno-Psychiatry*. Once animal models demonstrated that inflammatory cytokines produced a syndrome highly concordant with syndromes induced by stress, the search was on in the 1990s for evidence that something similar happened in humans. This led to repeated observations that patients with psychiatric conditions—especially major depressive disorder—demonstrated increased levels of cytokines and other immune modulators compared to healthy control subjects. These findings on peripheral biomarkers are updated and discussed in chapter 5 on "Cytokines as Biomarkers In psychiatric disorders: Methodological Issues" and "Complement Pathway in the Risk for Schizophrenia," as well as in chapters 13 to 21 discussing associations between inflammation and various neuropsychiatric conditions. Another implication of the inflammation-to-brain connection that was seized upon early in the field's development was the realization that this connection might account for the strong association between medical illness and psychiatric morbidity. This observation is admirably updated and mechanistically expanded in chapter 3 on "Immunity as a Common Risk Pathway for Psychiatric and Medical Comorbidity" by Rosenblatt and McIntyre and chapter 1 on "Auto-Immune Disorders and Infections as Risk Factors for Mental Disorders" by Sonja Orlovska Waast and Michael Benros.

It is a truism that association is not causation. Just showing that cytokines and other immune biomarkers are altered in psychiatric conditions does not prove that these alterations are causing the conditions. From various perspectives, much of the remainder of Immuno-Psychiatry is dedicated to demonstrating the biological pathways and factors by which immune signaling can change brain function and thus contribute to mental illness causation. As is so often the case, the evidence is stronger in animal models than in human animals, but all in all the book makes a compelling case that the immune system and brain really do form a unified biological system relevant to human mental health.

Two discoveries in the last decade have really brought this home for me. Much work was done in the 1990s and early 2000s on the question of how peripheral immune activity could signal across the blood–brain barrier (BBB). Neural and circulating routes were identified. Cytokines seemed perhaps able to cross at leaky areas of the BBB, but that was about it. We held onto the myth that brain and the peripheral immune system were neighbors, not family. Then came the discovery of a functional meningeal lymphatic system in humans that directly connects CNS and peripheral immunity in ways that defy a generation's worth of immune privilege.

I was also struck by discoveries discussed in a chapter I had a minor hand in writing, "Role of the T cell Network in Psychiatric Disorders." Much early work in PNI was directed toward understanding the impact of the brain in general—and stress in particular—on circulating T cell subsets. Nowhere has the subsequent reversal of causality been more impressive than in our growing realization that the balance of power between peripheral T cells and the brain favors the T cells. I find no discovery in PNI more astounding than the fact that these cells home to the brain and/or the meninges in the context of stress and from that position secret cytokines (e.g., interleukin-4) that are essential for adaptive stress responses. Truly the immune system, although mostly located outside the cranium, is a key player in perceptions of reality most essential for survival and reproduction.

I was pleased to see that *Immuno-Psychiatry* includes chapters that reflect developments on the cutting edge of immune physiology or that stray a bit from the straight and narrow in terms of subject matter. The chapter by Robert Dantzer and colleagues brilliantly describes the developing field of immunometabolism, which I applaud both for its direct relevance to cancer and for the fact that alone among the topics in this book it touches directly on the need for evolutionary, and not just proximal, understandings of why immune–brain interactions are the way they are.

I thought about evolutionary considerations repeatedly as I read the excellent chapter 19 that asks "Is Suicide a Systemic Disorder?" by Courtet and colleagues. As Dantzer et al. discuss in chapter 16, although no one likes to be sick, sickness behavior evolved as a strategy for surviving and/or avoiding infection. Unpleasant, but adaptive. We and others have argued that depression—which shares so many symptoms with sickness—may have evolved out of sickness and may have been adaptive for similar reasons. But what could possibly be adaptive about the fact that inflammation seems to drive suicide? Why would inflammatory processes promote a desire for death at a moment when the immune processes in the body are valiantly working to keep the person alive? This conundrum speaks to the need for including more evolutionary theory, not just in *Psycho-Immunology*, but the field of PNI as a whole.

In terms of straying off the straight and narrow, I was pleased to see chapters on diet and inflammation and exercise and inflammation, as well as two chapters addressing various aspects of the gut microbiome.

Finally, and most appropriately, *Immune-Psychiatry* ends with chapters on treatment implications of the immune–brain connection. Chapters examining the potential effects of immune modulators for depression and psychosis are generally even-handed and informative although perhaps a bit overly optimistic by my reading of the data in this area. I think many of us thought in the heady days of the 2000s that anti-inflammatory strategies would show themselves to be all-purpose antidepressants. However, all studies that have most rigorously tested this possibility have come up short, despite positive meta-analyses of non-steroidals and such. It now appears that only a subgroup of depressed individuals with chronically elevated inflammation will benefit from anti-inflammatory treatments, and indeed that many patients with MDD and lower levels of inflammation may actually be harmed—at least in comparison to placebo—by these same treatments.

With these thoughts I end this Foreword, and do so with some excitement to see what the next issue of *Immuno-Psychiatry* will bring. Certainly, we will learn things in the next decade that will greatly expand our current understanding. And one hopes this expansion will be especially fulsome in terms of translating knowledge of immune–brain interactions into new and effective therapies for the wide range of mental disorders in which the immune system is implicated.

Madison, WI, USA Charles L. Raison

Contents

Part I

Immune Mechanisms and Pathways Leading to Psychiatric Disorders

Autoimmune Diseases and Infections as Risk Factors for Mental Disorders

1

Sonja Orlovska-Waast and Michael Eriksen Benros

1.1 Introduction

With a lifetime prevalence of one-third [1, 2], mental disorders represent a major disease burden and understanding the etiology of mental disorders is crucial in order to improve treatment. Emerging evidence indicates that immunopathological mechanisms might play a role in the development of mental disorders in subgroups. Inflammation is inherent to autoimmune diseases, and infections and increased levels of inflammation have been found in a broad range of mental disorders. Studies have consistently shown associations between autoimmune disease and mental disorders as schizophrenia spectrum disorders [3–6], affective disorders [5, 7–9], eating disorders [10–12], ADHD [13], and PTSD [14]. Large epidemiological studies have consistently shown associations between a broad range of infections with most mental disorders [15] including both affective disorders [7, 16, 17] and schizophrenia spectrum disorders [3, 17].

Elevated levels of particularly peripheral blood markers of inflammation [18] and also increased permeability of the blood–brain barrier (BBB) [19] have been found in schizophrenia, major depressive disorder, and bipolar disorder. Moreover, elevated levels of cerebrospinal fluid (CSF) IL-6 and IL-8 have been shown to be increased in psychosis suggesting elevated levels of neuroinflammation [19]. Of particular interest is that anti-inflammatory treatment has shown beneficial effects on depression [20, 21] and schizophrenia [22–24] which holds clinical utility of identifying individuals with immunological contribution to their psychiatric symptoms that would be more likely to benefit from additional treatment targeting the immune response.

S. Orlovska-Waast · M. E. Benros (✉)
Biological and Precision Psychiatry, Copenhagen Research Center for Mental Health (CORE), Mental Health Centre Copenhagen, Copenhagen University Hospital, Copenhagen, Denmark

Department of Immunology and Microbiology, Faculty of Health and Medical Sciences, University of Copenhagen, Copenhagen, Denmark
e-mail: sonja.orlovska-waast@regionh.dk; benros@dadlnet.dk

M. Berk et al. (eds.), *Immuno-Psychiatry*, https://doi.org/10.1007/978-3-030-71229-7_1

The purpose of this review is to give an overview of key findings from relevant studies investigating autoimmune diseases and infections as risk factors for mental disorders.

1.2 Linkage Between Autoimmune Diseases and Mental Disorders

1.2.1 Autoimmune Diseases and Schizophrenia Spectrum Disorders

The temporal association between schizophrenia and autoimmune diseases has in several large-scale epidemiological studies been shown to be bidirectional [3–6, 9]. A Danish register-based study including 39,076 persons with a new schizophrenia spectrum disorder diagnosis found a 45% increased risk of schizophrenia in persons with a hospital contact for an autoimmune disease [3]. Another Danish epidemiological study based on 20,317 cases with schizophrenia found that the risk of schizophrenia was increased by 40% within the first 4 years after the diagnosis of the autoimmune disease and by 30% following the first 4 years suggesting that the association cannot only be explained by ascertainment bias [5]. An epidemiological study based on Taiwanese data with 10,811 persons with schizophrenia found the incidence of schizophrenia following a diagnosis of an autoimmune disease to be increased by 72% compared to persons without an autoimmune disease [6]. Conversely, a Danish nationwide register-based study based on 39,364 persons with schizophrenia spectrum disorders found an increased risk of the subsequent development of one or more autoimmune diseases by 53% [9]. Other epidemiological studies based on, respectively, Taiwanese registers including 10,811 in-patients with schizophrenia [4] and Swedish registers with 5278 persons with schizophrenia [25] also found the risk of several autoimmune diseases to be increased compared to controls. A recent meta-analysis found similar results with an increased risk of psychosis by 1.43 in persons with nonneurological autoimmune diseases and a risk for non-neurological autoimmune diseases of 1.55 in persons with psychosis [26]. The meta-analysis found significant positive associations for pernicious anemia, pemphigoid, psoriasis, celiac disease and Graves' disease and significant negative associations for ankylosing spondylitis and rheumatoid arthritis [26].

A higher risk of schizophrenia spectrum disorders has been found in persons with thyrotoxicosis [3, 5] and autoimmune thyroiditis [6], while an increased risk of Graves' disease was also found in persons with schizophrenia [4] and the prevalence of hypothyroidism was higher in persons with schizophrenia compared to controls [25]. Several studies found bidirectional associations between psoriasis vulgaris and schizophrenia spectrum disorders [3–5, 27–29]. Furthermore, persons with psoriasis and comorbid cerebrovascular and chronic pulmonary disease have been shown to have a further increased risk for schizophrenia compared to persons with psoriasis without this comorbidity suggesting that a higher inflammatory burden might contribute to the development of schizophrenia [27].

Moreover, studies have both found a significantly elevated [3, 5] and decreased [30] risk of schizophrenia spectrum disorders in persons with type 1 diabetes. However, other studies did not find a significant association in any direction [6, 25, 31]. Celiac disease has been found to increase the risk of schizophrenia spectrum disorders [3] and nonschizophrenic psychosis [32], and the risk of celiac disease has also been shown to be increased after the diagnosis of schizophrenia [4]. Interestingly, a systematic review on the effects of a gluten-free diet in persons with schizophrenia showed that 6 of the 9 included studies found improvement of functioning and symptom severity [33]. However, other studies did not find celiac disease to increase the risk of schizophrenia [32, 34]. Varying results have also been found for other autoimmune gastrointestinal diseases where one study found an increased risk of schizophrenia in persons with Crohn's disease [5], while others did not find an increased risk for schizophrenia in persons with Crohn's disease or ulcerative colitis [34].

Rheumatoid arthritis is one of the only autoimmune diseases where a large amount of studies have found a significant negative bidirectional association with schizophrenia [4, 9, 35, 36], confirmed by a meta-analysis with the finding of an overall negative association between psychosis and rheumatoid arthritis [26]. A decreased risk of nonautoimmune musculoskeletal disorders has also been found in persons with schizophrenia [35, 36] suggesting that underreporting of somatic symptoms in persons with schizophrenia might explain the finding of a negative association. Nonetheless, one study found a significantly elevated risk of the subsequent development of schizophrenia in persons with rheumatoid arthritis [6], while others did not find a significant association [3, 5, 25, 37].

1.2.2 Autoimmune Diseases and Affective Disorders

Several epidemiological studies have found the risk of developing an affective disorder to be increased by 20–98% in persons with autoimmune diseases [5, 7, 38]. A large Danish epidemiological study including 91,637 persons with a new-onset diagnosis of affective disorders found a 46% increase in the risk of unipolar depression and 25% for bipolar disorder in persons with autoimmune disease [7]. Moreover, a study based on Taiwanese registers including 936 cases of new-onset bipolar disorder found a 98% increase in the likelihood of developing bipolar disorder in individuals with systemic autoimmune diseases [38]. Another study found that the risk of bipolar disorder was increased by 70% within the first 4 years after the diagnosis of the autoimmune disease and by 20% following the first 4 years indicating that it is unlikely that the association is only due to ascertainment bias [5]. However, as with schizophrenia, studies have indicated a bidirectional association between affective disorders and autoimmune disease. Hence, large-scale Danish register-based studies have found the risk of developing an autoimmune disease to be increased by 25% in persons with unipolar depression ($N = 145{,}217$) [8] and by 71% in persons with bipolar disorder [9]; the risk was still significantly elevated more than 11 years following the diagnosis of unipolar depression [8].

Epidemiological studies have both found evidence of an increased risk of unipolar depression and bipolar disorder in persons with SLE [7, 38, 39] but also of an increased risk of SLE in persons with unipolar depression [8], even though a Swedish register-based study did not find a higher prevalence of SLE in persons with bipolar disorder [25]. A clinical study following 326 female persons with SLE found a lifetime prevalence of 47% for major depressive disorder (MDD) and 6% for bipolar 1 disorder [40]; the SLE diagnosis had preceded the MDD diagnosis in 61.1% of the persons, while this percentage was 44.4% for bipolar 1 disorder [40]. Regarding rheumatoid arthritis, a Taiwanese register-based study found a bidirectional association between rheumatoid arthritis and depression [41]. Other epidemiological studies have found that the risk of bipolar disorder [38, 39] and unipolar depression [39] was increased in persons with rheumatoid arthritis confirmed by a meta-analysis showing that depression was more common in persons with rheumatoid arthritis than in healthy individuals [42]. The prevalence of rheumatoid arthritis has also been shown to be increased in persons with bipolar disorder [25]. Moreover, the risk of unipolar depression and bipolar disorder has been shown to be increased in persons with thyrotoxicosis and Graves' disease [7], while a higher prevalence of hyperthyroidism was also found in persons with bipolar disorder compared to healthy controls [25]. Moreover, in a clinical study based on 71 persons, the authors found autoimmune thyroiditis in 38.5% of the persons with unipolar depression, 30.8% in persons with BD, and 10.5% in persons with schizophrenia [43]. Also, a significantly higher proportion of the patients with mood disorders had pathologically increased levels of anti-TPO compared with the persons with schizophrenia [43]. Nevertheless, a survey based on 30,175 participants with assays of thyroid function did not find an association between the presence of serum anti-TPO and the prevalence of self-reported depression [44]. Celiac disease has been found to increase the risk of unipolar depression and bipolar disorder in an epidemiological study [7]. Furthermore, a meta-analysis including 18 studies found that depression was more common in persons with celiac disease compared with healthy controls, even though there was no difference when compared with persons with other somatic illnesses [45]. The risk of unipolar depression [7] and bipolar disorder [7, 38] has in epidemiological studies been shown to be increased in persons with Crohn's disease even though the reverse association between unipolar depression and Crohn's disease has also been found [8]. Furthermore, studies found that persons with unipolar depression had an increased risk of developing type 1 DM, MS, psoriasis vulgaris, and primary adrenocortical insufficiency [8], while the risk of unipolar depression and bipolar disorder was also found to be increased in persons with the mentioned autoimmune diseases [7].

1.2.3 Autoimmune Diseases and Other Mental Disorders

Regarding eating disorders, epidemiological studies based on Swedish ($N = 26{,}454$ persons with eating disorders) [10], English ($N = 14{,}454$) [12], and Danish ($N = 3914$) [11] registers have found a bidirectional association with autoimmune disease, even though the risk of autoimmune disease following eating disorders primarily was increased in females in one study [10]. A study based on the Finnish registers found the risk for having an autoimmune disease to be increased 2.13-fold in persons with eating disorders ($n = 2342$) before the initiation of the psychiatric treatment, while the risk for having an autoimmune disease after the start of the treatment for an eating disorder was not significant [46].

Regarding ADHD, a Danish register study found an increased risk of ADHD ($N = 23{,}645$) following the diagnosis of an autoimmune disease [47]. Norwegian ($N = 63{,}721$ persons with ADHD) [13] and Taiwanese ($N = 8201$) [48] epidemiological studies found an increased risk for the comorbidity between ADHD and psoriasis [13], ankylosing spondylitis, autoimmune thyroid disease, and ulcerative colitis [48]. In the Norwegian study, the risk for ulcerative colitis and Crohn's disease was only significantly increased in females and the risk for Crohn's disease was found to be significantly decreased in males [13].

A study investigating 203,766 veterans diagnosed with PTSD found an increased risk of a subsequent diagnosis of an autoimmune disease [14]. Interestingly, the relationship did not seem to be bidirectional since in the veterans with autoimmune diseases, the study found a significantly decreased risk of subsequently developing PTSD [14].

1.3 Linkage Between Infections and Mental Disorders

1.3.1 Infections and Schizophrenia Spectrum Disorders

Infections have also been associated with schizophrenia spectrum disorders in several epidemiological studies [3, 9, 17, 49, 50]. A large Danish register study found hospital contact for infections to increase the risk of schizophrenia by 60% with the highest risk being observed after sepsis and hepatitis infections [3]. The number of infections increased the risk in a dose–response manner, and in individuals with autoimmune disease and three or more infections, the risk of schizophrenia was increased by 3.4 times [3]. A Swedish study found that childhood hospital admission for infections increased the risk of later development of nonaffective psychosis with bacterial and CNS infections during preadolescence giving the largest risk [49]. A preceding meta-analysis found childhood CNS viral (but not bacterial) infections to increase the risk of developing adult schizophrenia by 2.12, even though some heterogeneity was found between the studies [51].

A meta-analysis including both studies based on analyses of blood, CSF, and brain tissue found significant associations between schizophrenia and infections with Human herpes virus 2, Borna disease virus, Human endogenous retrovirus W, Chlamydophila pneumoniae, Chlamydophila psittaci, and Toxoplasma gondii [52]; several other meta-analyses have confirmed the association with Toxoplasma gondii [53–56]. A meta-analysis including studies with healthy controls found a significantly higher risk of signs of Toxoplasma gondii infection in recent-onset schizophrenia compared with chronic schizophrenia [53], while another meta-analysis did not find this difference [55]. One study reported increased levels of Cytomegalovirus IgG in both serum and the CSF of 38 antipsychotic naïve persons with recent-onset schizophrenia compared with 73 healthy controls [57]. However, a review reported that results have been varying regarding Cytomegalovirus serum and CSF studies and that only one of nine studies of postmortem brain tissue from persons with schizophrenia found signs of Cytomegalovirus DNA in the brain [58]. A meta-analysis did not find evidence for an association between Herpes simplex virus 1 or Human herpes virus 6 detected in serum or brain tissue and schizophrenia [56]. In thread with these findings, a systematic review reported Herpes simplex virus 1 or 2 antibodies in the CSF of up to 69% of cases, but in studies comparing with various control groups, there was no difference between cases and controls [19].

Interestingly, a Danish study demonstrated multiplicative interaction between having a diagnosis of schizophrenia and hospital contact for infections on the risk of developing an autoimmune disease [9] indicating that infections could represent a common risk factor for autoimmune disease and schizophrenia.

1.3.2 Infections and Affective Disorders

In a large Danish epidemiological study with 93,637 new-onset cases of mood disorders, hospital contact for infections increased the risk of developing unipolar depression by 63% and bipolar disorder by 61% with the highest risk after hepatitis infection, sepsis, and urogenital infections [7]. There was a dose–response relationship with the number of infections and a synergistic effect of having both infection and autoimmune disease on the risk of mood disorders [7]. Another study with 1285 children found that infection during the first year of life increased the OR of developing major depression in youth by 3.9 [59], even though the study design was based on parent report and comprised a risk of recall bias.

Meta-analyses have not found association between Toxoplasma gondii and MDD [53, 60], while the risk of Toxoplasma gondii has been found to be increased in bipolar disorder [53, 61]. A Taiwanese register study investigated 48,010 persons with enterovirus infection before the age of 18 years and found an increased risk of subsequent unipolar depression, although the results were only significant for enterovirus infections specifically involving the CNS [62]. Small studies based on blood samples have both reported increased frequency of Borna disease virus in persons with mood disorders [63], while others did not find significant signs of Borna disease virus compared with controls [64–66]. A register study based on primary care contacts in the UK including 103,307 persons with MDD found that previous contacts for infections with influenza virus increased the risk of developing depression by 30% [67]. Another study measured antibody titers against influenza and corona virus and found significantly higher levels in persons with mood disorders than in healthy controls [68]. The risk of depression in persons with hepatitis C infection has in a meta-analysis been found to be increased by 2.30 times [69]. This association might be due to interferon therapy for the treatment of hepatitis C [70] or alcohol and substance abuse; however, a study adjusting for these factors still found an increased risk of recurrent brief depression in persons with chronic hepatitis C infection [71].

Conversely, a large Danish epidemiological study based on 142,169 persons with depression showed an increased risk of 61% for subsequent hospital contact with infections [16]; however, there was no temporal effect and the risk was increased throughout the first 11 years after the depression diagnosis [16]. Also, a study based on registers from Denmark and the UK found that the risk of having a previous diagnosis of depression in persons with herpes zoster was significantly increased compared with healthy controls [72]. Moreover, it has been shown that individuals with both autoimmune disease and hospital contacts for infections seem to have an additive risk increase for bipolar disorder [9].

1.4 Streptococcal Infection and the Risk of Mental Disorders—The PANDAS Hypothesis

The hypothesis regarding Pediatric Autoimmune Neuropsychiatric Disorders Associated with Streptococcal infections (PANDAS) remains controversial and debated [73]. The hypothesis suggests that in a subgroup of children with obsessive-compulsive disorder (OCD) and tic disorders the symptoms are caused by a preceding throat infection with group A β-hemolytic streptococcal bacteria [73]. The association is suggested to be caused by molecular mimicry where antibodies produced to attack the streptococcal bacteria cross-react with the basal ganglia of the brain resulting in neuropsychiatric symptoms [74]. This is supported by studies finding autoantibodies directed against the basal ganglia in the serum of some children suggested to have PANDAS [75, 76] even though other studies were not able to replicate these findings [77–79]. A large-scale Danish epidemiological study including 638,265 persons tested for streptococcal throat infection found that both streptococcal and nonstreptococcal throat infections increased the risk of all mental disorders including OCD and tic disorders, with the risk of OCD and a combined group of all mental disorders being more elevated after a streptococcal infection than after a nonstreptococcal throat infection [80]. Other studies have found that both the onset and worsening of OCD and tic disorders can be associated with nonstreptococcal infections [81–84]. However, a recent meta-analysis including some of the hitherto most robust prospective studies investigating PANDAS was not able to confirm the core criterion of PANDAS which is a higher rate of temporally associated streptococcal infections and neuropsychiatric exacerbations in PANDAS cases [85]. In the meta-analysis, PANDAS cases in general had more neuropsychiatric exacerbations than controls with OCD or tic disorders or healthy controls, suggesting that the PANDAS definition might represent a group of patients with more severe psychiatric illness [85]. These findings altogether might rather support the concept of Pediatric Acute-onset Neuropsychiatric Syndrome (PANS) [86], which is also considered to be a postinfectious condition but with broader diagnostic criteria without restriction to streptococcal infections.

1.5 Possible Pathophysiology

Infections have been shown to increase the permeability of the BBB [87] making the CNS susceptible to immune cells, pro-inflammatory cytokines, and other possibly harmful substances from the peripheral blood. Infections have also been shown to have the ability to penetrate and invade the CNS directly, possibly after reaching a certain threshold level [87]. These conditions might lead to an inflammatory state in the brain which has been suggested to play a role in the development of psychotic and affective disorders. In thread with these findings, a recent meta-analysis found signs of an increased permeability of the BBB in persons with psychosis and affective disorders and increased CSF levels of IL-6 and IL-8, even though the latter finding was not significant for affective disorders [19]. Moreover, infections are prime candidates for triggering autoimmunity, for example, through molecular mimicry with the production of autoantibodies directed against the body's own tissue [88]. In periods of BBB disruption, circulating autoantibodies might enter the CNS and cause or worsen inflammatory processes. Animal studies have also found that the presence of brain-reactive antibodies in the peripheral blood might induce neuropsychiatric symptoms when the permeability of the blood–CNS barrier is increased [89]. This might also explain the synergistic effect on the risk of developing schizophrenia spectrum disorders [3] and mood disorders [7] of having both an autoimmune disease and prior hospital contact for infections. In line with this, autoimmune diseases with suspected presence of brain-reactive antibodies have been found to be a larger risk factor for both schizophrenia spectrum disorders [3] and mood disorders [7] rather than autoimmune diseases without suspected presence of brain-reactive antibodies.

Moreover, the term sickness behavior refers to the typical behavior related to having a viral or bacterial infection resulting from the production of pro-inflammatory cytokines with symptoms of loss of interest, reduced energy and appetite, and affected sleep and cognition [90]. Since these symptoms represent an interesting overlap with some main symptoms of depression, it has been suggested that a prolonged sickness behavior due to infections can develop into depression in vulnerable individuals [90].

Several epidemiological studies have pointed toward possible underlying genetic mechanisms for the association between autoimmune disease and schizophrenia [5, 9, 91]. Some studies found a family history of schizophrenia, in persons with a personal history of schizophrenia, to increase the risk of developing an autoimmune disease [9, 91]. Conversely, others found that a family history of an autoimmune disease increased the risk of developing schizophrenia [5]. However, a GWAS study investigating shared genetic susceptibility loci between autoimmune disease and schizophrenia was not able to support a genetic overlap in common SNPs between the two disorders [92]. One study found that a family history of bipolar disease did not seem to increase the risk of autoimmune disease [9]. Other epidemiological studies found that a family history of autoimmune disease [93] and specifically maternal autoimmune disease showed significant association with ADHD in the offspring [47, 94]. A Danish study also found that maternal thyroid abnormalities increased the risk of ADHD and autism spectrum disorders in the offspring [95]; there was no association with paternal thyroid dysfunction, and the associations were only seen for maternal thyroid dysfunction diagnosed after birth as to prior to birth indicating that the child has been exposed to abnormal levels of thyroid hormone during pregnancy [95] with a possible disturbance of neurodevelopment. Others found that a maternal history of rheumatoid arthritis and celiac disease increased the risk of autism spectrum disorders in the offspring, while thyrotoxicosis decreased the risk [96]. Individuals with a family history of autoimmune or autoinflammatory disease had a risk of developing an eating disorder of up to 48% [11].

Furthermore, confounding factors such as BMI, smoking, and diet might also explain the found associations between autoimmune disease, infections, and mental disorders since these lifestyle factors could be common risk factors. However, very few studies investigating the association between inflammation and mental disorders take these aspects into account which is a limitation and should be considered in future studies.

1.6 Conclusion and Perspectives

A large amount of evidence points toward an association between autoimmune disorders and infections and schizophrenia spectrum disorders, affective disorders, and other mental disorders. Possible pathophysiological mechanisms might be an increased permeability of the BBB, circulating brain-reactive autoantibodies and neuroinflammation resulting in the development of psychiatric symptoms. The synergistic effect of having both an autoimmune disease and prior hospital contact for infections on the increased risk of developing both schizophrenia spectrum disorders [3] and mood disorders [7] speaks in favor of underlying biological mechanisms. Genetic aspects might also play a role. However, the association between autoimmune disorders and mental disorders is rather consistently shown to be bidirectional indicating that confounding factors, e.g. BMI and smoking, at least partly could explain the association. Future studies are needed in order to clarify if the association between infections and autoimmune disorders and mental disorders is causal or rather an epiphenomenon. Regardless, the knowledge we have so far clearly indicates that screening for somatic diseases and particularly autoimmune diseases and infections in psychiatry, preferably based on CSF in combination with serum, is essential in order to improve the health condition of persons with mental disorders. Continued research in the field is important to increase our understanding of the etiology of mental disorders, which can prompt a range of new treatment options in psychiatry. This would give the opportunity to identify a subgroup of persons with mental disorders with an abnormal and increased immunological response who would profit from targeted treatment.

References

1. Steel Z, Marnane C, Iranpour C, Chey T, Jackson JW, Patel V, et al. The global prevalence of common mental disorders: a systematic review and meta-analysis 1980–2013. Int J Epidemiol. 2014;43(2):476–93.
2. Pedersen CB, Mors O, Bertelsen A, Waltoft BL, Agerbo E, McGrath JJ, et al. A comprehensive nationwide study of the incidence rate and lifetime risk for treated mental disorders. JAMA Psychiat. 2014;71(5):573–81.
3. Benros ME, Nielsen PR, Nordentoft M, Eaton WW, Dalton SO, Mortensen PB. Autoimmune diseases and severe infections as risk factors for schizophrenia: a 30-year population-based register study. Am J Psychiatry. 2011;168(12):1303–10.
4. Chen SJ, Chao YL, Chen CY, Chang CM, Wu ECH, Wu CS, et al. Prevalence of autoimmune diseases in in-patients with schizophrenia: nationwide population-based study. Br J Psychiatry. 2012;200(5):374–80.
5. Eaton WW, Pedersen MG, Nielsen PR, Mortensen PB. Autoimmune diseases, bipolar disorder, and non-affective psychosis. Bipolar Disord. 2010;12(6):638–46.
6. Wang LY, Chen SF, Chiang JH, Hsu CY, Shen YC. Autoimmune diseases are associated with an increased risk of schizophrenia: a nationwide population-based cohort study. Schizophr Res. 2018;202:297–302.
7. Benros ME, Waltoft BL, Nordentoft M, Østergaard SD, Eaton WW, Krogh J, et al. Autoimmune diseases and severe infections as risk factors for mood disorders. JAMA Psychiat. 2013;70(8):812.
8. Andersson NW, Gustafsson LN, Okkels N, Taha F, Cole SW, Munk-Jorgensen P, et al. Depression and the risk of autoimmune disease: a nationally representative, prospective longitudinal study. Psychol Med. 2015;45(16):3559–69.
9. Benros ME, Pedersen MG, Rasmussen H, Eaton WW, Nordentoft M, Mortensen PB. A nationwide study on the risk of autoimmune diseases in individuals with a personal or a family history of schizophrenia and related psychosis. Am J Psychiatry. 2014;171(2):218–26.
10. Hedman A, Breithaupt L, Hübel C, Thornton LM, Tillander A, Norring C, et al. Bidirectional relationship between eating disorders and autoimmune diseases. J Child Psychol Psychiatry. 2019;60(7):803–12.
11. Zerwas S, Larsen JT, Petersen L, Thornton LM, Quaranta M, Koch SV, et al. Eating disorders, autoimmune, and autoinflammatory disease. Pediatrics. 2017;140(6):e20162089.
12. Wotton CJ, James A, Goldacre MJ. Coexistence of eating disorders and autoimmune diseases: record linkage cohort study, UK. Int J Eat Disord. 2016;49(7):663–72.
13. Hegvik TA, Instanes JT, Haavik J, Klungsøyr K, Engeland A. Associations between attention-deficit/hyperactivity disorder and autoimmune diseases are modified by sex: a population-based cross-sectional study. Eur Child Adolesc Psychiatry. 2018;27(5):663–75.
14. O'Donovan A, Cohen BE, Seal KH, Bertenthal D, Margaretten M, Nishimi K, et al. Elevated risk for autoimmune disorders in Iraq and Afghanistan veterans with posttraumatic stress disorder. Biol Psychiatry. 2015;77(4):365–74.
15. Köhler-Forsberg O, Petersen L, Gasse C, Mortensen PB, Dalsgaard S, Yolken RH, et al. A nationwide study in Denmark of the association between treated infections and the subsequent risk of treated mental disorders in children and adolescents. JAMA Psychiat. 2019;76(3):271–9.
16. Andersson NW, Goodwin RD, Okkels N, Gustafsson LN, Taha F, Cole SW, et al. Depression and the risk of severe infections: prospective analyses on a nationwide representative sample. Int J Epidemiol. 2016;45(1):131–9.
17. Köhler O, Petersen L, Mors O, Mortensen PB, Yolken RH, Gasse C, et al. Infections and exposure to anti-infective agents and the risk of severe mental disorders: a nationwide study. Acta Psychiatr Scand. 2017;135(2):97–105.
18. Goldsmith DR, Rapaport MH, Miller BJ. A meta-analysis of blood cytokine network alterations in psychiatric patients: comparisons between schizophrenia, bipolar disorder and depression. Mol Psychiatry. 2016;21:1696.

19. Orlovska-Waast S, Köhler-Forsberg O, Brix SW, Nordentoft M, Kondziella D, Krogh J, et al. Cerebrospinal fluid markers of inflammation and infections in schizophrenia and affective disorders: a systematic review and meta-analysis. Mol Psychiatry. 2019;24:869–87.
20. Köhler O, Benros ME, Nordentoft M, Farkouh ME, Iyengar RL, Mors O, et al. Effect of anti-inflammatory treatment on depression, depressive symptoms, and adverse effects: a systematic review and meta-analysis of randomized clinical trials. JAMA Psychiat. 2014;71(12):1381–91.
21. Köhler-Forsberg O, Lydholm CN, Hjorthøj C, Nordentoft M, Mors O, Benros ME. Efficacy of anti-inflammatory treatment on major depressive disorder or depressive symptoms: meta-analysis of clinical trials. Acta Psychiatr Scand. 2019;139(5):404–19.
22. Girgis RR, Ciarleglio A, Choo T, Haynes G, Bathon JM, Cremers S, et al. A randomized, double-blind, placebo controlled clinical trial of tocilizumab, an Interleukin-6 receptor antibody, for residual symptoms in schizophrenia. Neuropsychopharmacology. 2018;43(6):1317–23.
23. Sommer IE, De Witte L, Begemann M, Kahn RS. Nonsteroidal anti-inflammatory drugs in schizophrenia: ready for practice or a good start? A meta-analysis. J Clin Psychiatry. 2012;73(4):414–9.
24. Müller N, Ulmschneider M, Scheppach C, Schwarz MJ, Ackenheil M, Möller HJ, et al. COX-2 inhibition as a treatment approach in schizophrenia: immunological considerations and clinical effects of celecoxib add-on therapy. Eur Arch Psychiatry Clin Neurosci. 2004;254(1):14–22.
25. Cremaschi L, Kardell M, Johansson V, Isgren A, Sellgren CM, Altamura AC, et al. Prevalences of autoimmune diseases in schizophrenia, bipolar I and II disorder, and controls. Psychiatry Res. 2017;258:9–14.
26. Cullen AE, Holmes S, Pollak TA, Blackman G, Joyce DW, Kempton MJ, et al. Associations between non-neurological autoimmune disorders and psychosis: a meta-analysis. Biol Psychiatry. 2019;85(1):35–48.
27. Tu HP, Yu CL, Lan CCE, Yu S. Prevalence of schizophrenia in patients with psoriasis: a nationwide study. Dermatologica Sin. 2017;35(1):1–6.
28. Yu S, Yu CL, Huang YC, Tu HP, Lan CCE. Risk of developing psoriasis in patients with schizophrenia: a nationwide retrospective cohort study. J Eur Acad Dermatol Venereol. 2017;31(9):1497–504.
29. Yang Y-W, Lin H-C. Increased risk of psoriasis among patients with schizophrenia: a nationwide population-based study. Br J Dermatol. 2012;166(4):899–900.
30. Juvonen H, Reunanen A, Haukka J, Muhonen M, Suvisaari J, Arajärvi R, et al. Incidence of schizophrenia in a nationwide cohort of patients with type 1 diabetes mellitus. Arch Gen Psychiatry. 2007;64(8):894–9.
31. Dybdal D, Tolstrup JS, Sildorf SM, Boisen KA, Svensson J, Skovgaard AM, et al. Increasing risk of psychiatric morbidity after childhood onset type 1 diabetes: a population-based cohort study. Diabetologia. 2018;61(4):831–8.
32. Ludvigsson JF, Osby U, Ekbom A, Montgomery SM. Coeliac disease and risk of schizophrenia and other psychosis: a general population cohort study. Scand J Gastroenterol. 2007;42(2):179–85.
33. Levinta A, Mukovozov I, Tsoutsoulas C. Use of a gluten-free diet in schizophrenia: a systematic review. Adv Nutr. 2018;9(6):824–32.
34. West J, Logan RF, Hubbard RB, Card TR. Risk of schizophrenia in people with coeliac disease, ulcerative colitis and Crohn's disease: a general population-based study. Aliment Pharmacol Ther. 2006;23(1):71–4.
35. Mors O, Mortensen PB, Ewald H. A population-based register study of the association between schizophrenia and rheumatoid arthritis. Schizophr Res. 1999;40(1):67–74.
36. Sellgren C, Frisell T, Lichtenstein P, Landen M, Askling J. The association between schizophrenia and rheumatoid arthritis: a nationwide population-based Swedish study on intraindividual and familial risks. Schizophr Bull. 2014;40(6):1552–9.
37. Chen SF, Wang LY, Chiang JH, Hsu CY, Shen YC. Assessing whether the association between rheumatoid arthritis and schizophrenia is bidirectional: a nationwide population-based cohort study. Sci Rep. 2019;9(1):1–10.

38. Wang LY, Chiang JH, Chen SF, Shen YC. Systemic autoimmune diseases are associated with an increased risk of bipolar disorder: a nationwide population-based cohort study. J Affect Disord. 2018;227:31–7.
39. Sundquist K, Li X, Hemminki K, Sundquist J. Subsequent risk of hospitalization for neuropsychiatric disorders in patients with rheumatic diseases: a nationwide study from Sweden. Arch Gen Psychiatry. 2008;65(5):501–7.
40. Bachen EA, Chesney MA, Criswell LA. Prevalence of mood and anxiety disorders in women with systemic lupus erythematosus. Arthritis Care Res. 2009;61(6):822–9.
41. Lu M-C, Guo H-R, Lin M-C, Livneh H, Lai N-S, Tsai T-Y. Bidirectional associations between rheumatoid arthritis and depression: a nationwide longitudinal study. Sci Rep. 2016;6:20647.
42. Dickens C, McGowan L, Clark-Carter D, Creed F. Depression in RA—a systematic review of the literature with meta-analysis. Psychosom Med. 2002;64:52–60.
43. Degner D, Haust M, Meller J, Rüther E, Reulbach U. Association between autoimmune thyroiditis and depressive disorder in psychiatric outpatients. Eur Arch Psychiatry Clin Neurosci. 2015;265(1):67–72.
44. Engum A, Bjøro T, Mykletun A, Dahl AA. Thyroid autoimmunity, depression and anxiety; are there any connections? An epidemiological study of a large population. J Psychosom Res. 2005;59(5):263–8.
45. Smith DF, Gerdes LU. Meta-analysis on anxiety and depression in adult celiac disease. Acta Psychiatr Scand. 2012;125(3):189–93.
46. Raevuori A, Haukka J, Vaarala O, Suvisaari JM, Gissler M, Grainger M, et al. The increased risk for autoimmune diseases in patients with eating disorders. PLoS One. 2014;9(8):104845.
47. Nielsen PR, Benros ME, Dalsgaard S. Associations between autoimmune diseases and attention-deficit/hyperactivity disorder: a nationwide study. J Am Acad Child Adolesc Psychiatry. 2017;56(3):234–240.e1.
48. Chen MH, Su TP, Chen YS, Hsu JW, Huang KL, Chang WH, et al. Comorbidity of allergic and autoimmune diseases among patients with ADHD: a nationwide population-based study. J Atten Disord. 2017;21(3):219–27.
49. Blomström A, Karlsson H, Svensson A, Frisell T, Lee BK, Dal H, et al. Hospital admission with infection during childhood and risk for psychotic illness—a population-based cohort study. Schizophr Bull. 2014;40(6):1518–25.
50. Nielsen PR, Benros ME, Mortensen PB. Hospital contacts with infection and risk of schizophrenia: a population-based cohort study with linkage of Danish national registers. Schizophr Bull. 2014;40(6):1526–32.
51. Khandaker GM, Zimbron J, Dalman C, Lewis G, Jones PB. Childhood infection and adult schizophrenia: a meta-analysis of population-based studies. Schizophr Res. 2012;139(1–3):161–8.
52. Arias I, Sorlozano A, Villegas E, de Dios Luna J, McKenney K, Cervilla J, et al. Infectious agents associated with schizophrenia: a meta-analysis. Schizophr Res. 2012;136(1–3):128–36.
53. Sutterland AL, Fond G, Kuin A, Koeter MWJ, Lutter R, van Gool T, et al. Beyond the association. Toxoplasma gondii in schizophrenia, bipolar disorder, and addiction: systematic review and meta-analysis. Acta Psychiatr Scand. 2015;132(3):161–79.
54. Monroe JM, Buckley PF, Miller BJ. Meta-analysis of anti-Toxoplasma gondii IgM antibodies in acute psychosis. Schizophr Bull. 2015;41(4):989–98.
55. Torrey EF, Bartko JJ, Lun Z-R, Yolken RH. Antibodies to Toxoplasma gondii in patients with schizophrenia: a meta-analysis. Schizophr Bull. 2007 May;33(3):729–36.
56. Gutiérrez-Fernández J, de Dios Luna Del Castillo J, Mañanes-González S, Carrillo-Ávila JA, Gutiérrez B, Cervilla JA, et al. Different presence of chlamydia pneumoniae, herpes simplex virus type 1, human herpes virus 6, and toxoplasma gondii in schizophrenia: meta-analysis and analytical study. Neuropsychiatr Dis Treat. 2015;11:843–52.
57. Leweke FM, Gerth CW, Koethe D, Klosterkötter J, Ruslanova I, Krivogorsky B, et al. Antibodies to infectious agents in individuals with recent onset schizophrenia. Eur Arch Psychiatry Clin Neurosci. 2004;254(1):4–8.
58. Torrey EF, Leweke MF, Schwarz MJ, Mueller N, Bachmann S, Schroeder J, et al. Cytomegalovirus and schizophrenia. CNS Drugs. 2006;20(11):879–85.

59. Goodwin RD. Association between infection early in life and mental disorders among youth in the community: a cross-sectional study. BMC Public Health. 2011;11:878.
60. Chegeni TN, Sharif M, Sarvi S, Moosazadeh M, Montazeri M, Aghayan SA, et al. Is there any association between Toxoplasma gondii infection and depression? A systematic review and meta-analysis. PLoS One. 2019;14(6):e0218524.
61. de Barros JLVM, Barbosa IG, Salem H, Rocha NP, Kummer A, Okusaga OO, et al. Is there any association between toxoplasma gondii infection and bipolar disorder? A systematic review and meta-analysis. J Affect Disord. 2017;209:59–65.
62. Liao YT, Hsieh MH, Yang YH, Wang YC, Tsai CS, Chen VCH, et al. Association between depression and enterovirus infection. Medicine. 2017;96(5):e5983.
63. Terayama H, Nishino Y, Kishi M, Ikuta K, Itoh M, Iwahashi K. Detection of anti-Borna disease virus (BDV) antibodies from patients with schizophrenia and mood disorders in Japan. Psychiatry Res. 2003;120(2):201–6.
64. Zhang L, Xu MM, Zeng L, Liu S, Liu X, Wang X, et al. Evidence for Borna disease virus infection in neuropsychiatric patients in three western China provinces. Eur J Clin Microbiol Infect Dis. 2014;33(4):621–7.
65. Hornig M, Briese T, Licinio J, Khabbaz RF, Altshuler LL, Potkin SG, et al. Absence of evidence for Borna virus infection in schizophrenia, bipolar disorder and major depressive disorder. Mol Psychiatry. 2012;17(5):486–93.
66. Na KS, Tae SH, Song JW, Kim YK. Failure to detect Borna disease virus antibody and RNA from peripheral blood mononuclear cells of psychiatric patients. Psychiatry Investig. 2009;6(4):306–12.
67. Bornand D, Toovey S, Jick SS, Meier CR. The risk of new onset depression in association with influenza—a population-based observational study. Brain Behav Immun. 2016;53:131–7.
68. Okusaga O, Yolken RH, Langenberg P, Lapidus M, Arling TA, Dickerson FB, et al. Association of seropositivity for influenza and coronaviruses with history of mood disorders and suicide attempts. J Affect Disord. 2011;130(1–2):220–5.
69. Younossi Z, Park H, Henry L, Adeyemi A, Stepanova M. Extrahepatic manifestations of hepatitis C: a meta-analysis of prevalence, quality of life, and economic burden. Gastroenterology. 2016;150(7):1599–608.
70. Chiu WC, Su YP, Su KP, Chen PC. Recurrence of depressive disorders after interferon-induced depression. Transl Psychiatry. 2017;7(2):e1026.
71. Carta MG, Angst J, Moro MF, Mura G, Hardoy MC, Balestrieri C, et al. Association of chronic hepatitis C with recurrent brief depression. J Affect Disord. 2012;141(2–3):361–6.
72. Schmidt SAJ, Langan SM, Pedersen HS, Schønheyder HC, Thomas SL, Smeeth L, et al. Mood disorders and risk of herpes zoster in 2 population-based case-control studies in Denmark and the United Kingdom. Am J Epidemiol. 2018;187(5):1019–28.
73. Swedo SE, Leonard HL, Garvey M, Mittleman B, Allen AJ, Perlmutter S, et al. Pediatric autoimmune neuropsychiatric disorders associated with streptococcal infections: clinical description of the first 50 cases. Am J Psychiatry. 1998;155(February):264–71.
74. Pavone P, Parano E, Rizzo R, Trifiletti RR. Autoimmune neuropsychiatric disorders associated with streptococcal infection: Sydenham chorea, PANDAS, and PANDAS variants. J Child Neurol. 2006;21:727–37.
75. Pavone P, Bianchini R, Parano E, Incorpora G, Rizzo R, Mazzone L, et al. Anti-brain antibodies in PANDAS versus uncomplicated streptococcal infection. Pediatr Neurol. 2004;30(2):107–10.
76. Church AJ, Dale RC, Giovannoni G. Anti-basal ganglia antibodies: a possible diagnostic utility in idiopathic movement disorders? Arch Dis Child. 2004;89(7):611–4.
77. Singer HS, Hong JJ, Yoon DY, Williams PN. Serum autoantibodies do not differentiate PANDAS and Tourette syndrome from controls. Neurology. 2005;65(11):1701–7.
78. Brilot F, Merheb V, Ding A, Murphy T, Dale RC. Antibody binding to neuronal surface in Sydenham chorea, but not in PANDAS or Tourette syndrome. Neurology. 2011;76(17):1508–13.
79. Morris CM, Pardo-Villamizar C, Gause CD, Singer HS. Serum autoantibodies measured by immunofluorescence confirm a failure to differentiate PANDAS and Tourette syndrome from controls. J Neurol Sci. 2009;276(1–2):45–8.

80. Orlovska S, Vestergaard CH, Bech BH, Nordentoft M, Vestergaard M, Benros ME. Association of streptococcal throat infection with mental disorders. JAMA Psychiatry. 2017;74(7):740–6.
81. Leslie DL, Kozma L, Martin A, Landeros A, Katsovich L, King RA, et al. Neuropsychiatric disorders associated with streptococcal infection: a case-control study among privately insured children. J Am Acad Child Adolesc Psychiatry. 2008;47(10):1166–72.
82. Giulino L, Gammon P, Sullivan K, Franklin M, Foa E, Maid R, et al. Is parental report of upper respiratory infection at the onset of obsessive-compulsive disorder suggestive of pediatric autoimmune neuropsychiatric disorder associated with streptococcal infection? J Child Adolesc Psychopharmacol. 2002;12(2):157–64.
83. Murphy TK, Sajid M, Soto O, Shapira N, Edge P, Yang M, et al. Detecting pediatric autoimmune neuropsychiatric disorders associated with streptococcus in children with obsessive-compulsive disorder and tics. Biol Psychiatry. 2004;55(1):61–8.
84. Hoekstra PJ, Manson WL, Steenhuis M-P, Kallenberg CGM, Minderaa RB. Association of common cold with exacerbations in pediatric but not adult patients with tic disorder: a prospective longitudinal study. J Child Adolesc Psychopharmacol. 2005;15(2):285–92.
85. Nielsen M, Köhler-Forsberg O, Hjorthøj C, Benros ME, Nordentoft M, Orlovska-Waast S. Streptococcal infections and exacerbations in pandas: a systematic review and meta-analysis. Pediatr Infect Dis J. 2019;38(2):189–94.
86. Chang K, Frankovich J, Cooperstock M, Cunningham MW, Latimer ME, Murphy TK, et al. Clinical evaluation of youth with pediatric acute-onset neuropsychiatric syndrome (PANS): recommendations from the 2013 PANS consensus conference. J Child Adolesc Psychopharmacol. 2015;25(1):3–13.
87. Kim KS. Mechanisms of microbial traversal of the blood–brain barrier. Nat Rev Microbiol. 2008;6(8):625–34.
88. Getts DR, Chastain EML, Terry RL, Miller SD. Virus infection, antiviral immunity, and autoimmunity. Immunol Rev. 2013;255(1):197–209.
89. Kowal C, DeGiorgio LA, Nakaoka T, Hetherington H, Huerta PT, Diamond B, et al. Cognition and immunity: antibody impairs memory. Immunity. 2004;21(2):179–88.
90. Dantzer R, Connor JCO, Freund GG, Johnson RW, Kelley KW. From inflammation to sickness and depression: when the immune system subjugates the brain. Nat Rev Neurosci. 2008;9(1):46–56.
91. Eaton WW, Byrne M, Ewald H, Mors O, Chen CY, Agerbo E, et al. Association of schizophrenia and autoimmune diseases: linkage of Danish national registers. Am J Psychiatry. 2006;163(3):521–8.
92. Hoeffding LK, Rosengren A, Thygesen JH, Schmock H, Werge T, Hansen T. Evaluation of shared genetic susceptibility loci between autoimmune diseases and schizophrenia based on genome-wide association studies. Nord J Psychiatry. 2017;71(1):20–5.
93. Li X, Sjöstedt C, Sundquist J, Zöller B, Sundquist K. Familial association of attention-deficit hyperactivity disorder with autoimmune diseases in the population of Sweden. Psychiatr Genet. 2019;29:37–43.
94. Instanes JT, Halmøy A, Engeland A, Haavik J, Furu K, Klungsøyr K. Attention-deficit/hyperactivity disorder in offspring of mothers with inflammatory and immune system diseases. Biol Psychiatry. 2017;81(5):452–9.
95. Andersen SL, Laurberg P, Wu CS, Olsen J. Attention deficit hyperactivity disorder and autism spectrum disorder in children born to mothers with thyroid dysfunction: a Danish nationwide cohort study. BJOG An Int J Obstet Gynaecol. 2014;121(11):1365–74.
96. Atladóttir HÓ, Pedersen MG, Thorsen P, Mortensen PB, Deleuran B, Eaton WW, et al. Association of family history of autoimmune diseases and autism spectrum disorders. Pediatrics. 2009;124(2):687–94.

The Life-Long Consequences of Prenatal and Childhood Stress on the Innate and Adaptive Immune System

2

Juliette Giacobbe, Carmine M. Pariante, and Alessandra Borsini

2.1 Introduction

Stress is the natural response to a perceived physical or psychological threat, triggered in order to re-establish the homeostasis with the environment. Acute stress first results in the activation of the sympathetic nervous system (SNS) and the release of adrenaline and noradrenaline in the circulation, followed by the endocrine response of the hypothalamus–pituitary–adrenal (HPA) axis. Both of these have long been known to influence the regulation of the immune system [1]. While glucocorticoids produced by the HPA axis are commonly anti-inflammatory and dampen immune overactivation, repeated stress causes immune cells to mobilise to the possible site of injury to prepare for upcoming danger and to adopt a pro-inflammatory phenotype related to the development of glucocorticoid resistance [2, 3]. This is also observed in the context of social and psychological stressors, as illustrated by the increase of pro-inflammatory cytokines interleukin (IL)-6 [4] or IL-1β [5] measured in the periphery of participants upon exposure to a stressful event like the Trier social stress test (TSST). In this context, the release of glucocorticoids by the HPA axis and of noradrenaline by the SNS increases the transcription of pro-inflammatory factors and the consequent production of chemokines [6].

Importantly, the immunomodulatory effects of stress have consequences more widespread than simple changes in circulating cytokines levels [7]: glucocorticoids have been shown to affect haematopoiesis in the bone marrow, which receives nervous inputs from the SNS together with organs crucial for the maturation of immune cells like the spleen and lymph nodes [8]. Together, glucocorticoids and

J. Giacobbe · C. M. Pariante (✉) · A. Borsini
Stress, Psychiatry and Immunology Laboratory, Department of Psychological Medicine, Institute of Psychiatry, Psychology & Neuroscience, King's College London, London, UK
e-mail: juliette.giacobbe@kcl.ac.uk; carmine.pariante@kcl.ac.uk; alessandra.borsini@kcl.ac.uk

M. Berk et al. (eds.), *Immuno-Psychiatry*, https://doi.org/10.1007/978-3-030-71229-7_2

SNS-induced catecholamine secretion promote a shift towards myeloid lineage cells production [9, 10].

The immune system is divided into two arms, innate and adaptive, which accomplish different functions, and develops accordingly. The innate immune system represents the first line of defence against injury or infection and reacts to a very wide range of threats because it does not require previous exposure to them. It is composed of a variety of cells such as macrophages, mast cells and neutrophils, all of which originate from myeloid stem cells in the bone marrow [11]. For the most part, the development of these cells occurs *in utero* but their inflammatory response remains notably shifted towards a lower pro-inflammatory profile after birth and during the first few years of childhood before reaching maturation [12]. This phenomenon is a protective process to avoid a reaction against the mother's antigens and has been thought to maintain cytokines, IL-12 and interferon gamma (IFN-γ), for instance, at lower levels until adolescence [13].

Signals of the innate immune system, including cytokines and chemokines, and antigen-presenting cells trigger the adaptive immune system, which has the ability to eliminate and recognise extremely specific antigens. The main adaptive cells, B and T lymphocytes, both rise from the bone marrow, but the latter undergo an extensive maturation and selection process in the thymus [11]. Due to the necessity to encounter pathogens to acquire an immunological memory, characterised by the expression of antigen-specific receptors on the surface of lymphocytes, the number of adaptive immune cells peaks after birth and does not reach full maturation until adolescence [14].

Because of its sensitivity to external and environmental elements during the developmental period, the immune system could be affected by psychosocial factors such as prenatal or early life stress in a long-lasting manner. Many biological factors are already known to influence immune reactions: the transfer of maternal antibodies through the placenta provides antimicrobial protection but can also lead to autoimmune diseases [15, 16]. Epigenetic changes, for example, in the methylation of the glucocorticoid receptor, are observed in consequence of childhood trauma and might contribute to immune changes [17]. In turn, these play a role in psychiatric disorders, especially in the patients who present increased inflammation markers, namely cytokines IL-6 and IL-1β [18], and disruption of processes ranging from the HPA axis feedback loop [19] to neuroplasticity [20–22].

Unsurprisingly, prenatal stress and early life stress have been reported to have repercussions well into adulthood, notably on mental health [23]. Stress during pregnancy and childhood, including negative life events or trauma, has been associated with increased risk of developing disruptive behaviour disorder [24] schizophrenia [25], depression [26] or anxiety [27] and with their related biological correlates, such as cortisol response [28]. This indicates a role for psychosocial influence during those crucial periods of development. For instance, maternal mental illness has also been shown to increase the risk of developing psychopathological disorders for the child [29], via both immune system overactivation and physiological stress response [30, 31]. Because psychiatric disorders have widely been associated to alterations of the immune system [32], we will focus on psychosocial stress in the healthy population to disentangle its effects on the immune system from those of a pre-existing psychopathology.

Taken together, evidence strongly demonstrates the tight relationship existing between stress and the immune system. Nonetheless, their influence on the innate and adaptive immune systems needs to be further disentangled. Data tend to present the adaptive immune system as more sensitive to external factors due to its longer maturation period. But when mental disorders are considered, the innate immune system has been the most thoroughly investigated. We will thus compare the effects of prenatal and childhood stress, including changes in family structure, deaths, violence or abuse, on the innate and adaptive immune systems of general and healthy human populations over the course of the whole lifetime, excluding studies on participants suffering from psychopathological conditions (Table 2.1). In order to facilitate this comparison, the first part of each section will target molecules related to both the innate and adaptive immune systems, such as IL-1β or TNF-α. They are produced by cells across the whole immune system but are most often observed during an inflammatory state and have been referred to as monokines due to their association with monocytes of the innate immune system [33]. The second part of each section will focus on lymphocytes and molecules classically related to the adaptive immune system [34] (Fig. 2.1).

2.2 Prenatal Stress

2.2.1 Innate and Adaptive Immune System

Four studies measured the consequences of maternal stress on the activity of the innate and adaptive immune systems of infants at birth. In newborns, higher maternal prenatal perceived stress was associated with elevated levels of IL-6 and IL-8 in umbilical cord blood (UCB). In the same study, stressful life events during pregnancy related to the partner or health increased IL-1β and IL-6, or IL-8, respectively, but not TNF-α [35]. Cumulative stressful circumstances, including perceived community violence and neighbourhood conditions, over the whole course of pregnancy were also related to increased secretion of TNF-α and IL-8 and decreased production of IL-10 by UCB mononuclear cells upon *ex vivo* stimulation with various antigens, including peptidoglycan (PG) and lipopolysaccharide (LPS) [36]. In contrast, higher composite stress score, taking into account prenatal maternal stress, exposure to violence and prenatal negative life events, did not influence the methylation of the promoters of IL-8, IL-6 and TNF-α in UCB [37]. The mode of delivery, if linked to decreased endocrine stress response in mothers and newborns, such as caesarean section [38], decreased natural killer cells (NKC) in venous cord blood compared to vaginal delivery [39].

Four studies investigated changes related to prenatal stress lasting into childhood, and one investigated them into adulthood. In 6-month-old infants, prenatal maternal stress was found to correlate on a trend level with the concentration of serum IL-12 [40]. In 1-year-old boys but not girls, a major life stressor experienced

Table 2.1 Effects of prenatal and childhood stress on the innate and adaptive immune systems

		Prenatal stress			
Author	Type of stress	Stress time point	Measure of innate and adaptive immune system	Measure of adaptive immune system	Measure of immune system time point
Andersson (2016) [35]	• Prenatal perceived stress (PSS-14) • State and Trait Anxiety (STAI) • Stressful life events related to health or partner (Life Experience Interview)	Previous trimester of pregnancy	↗ IL-6, IL-8, IL-1β = TNF-α	↗ IL-4, IL-5 = IL-12	Birth
Wright (2010) [36]	• Difficult life circumstances (DLCS) • Neighbourhood conditions (CSQ) • Perceived community violence, housing worries, economic strain (Interview)	Any time during pregnancy	↗ TNF-α, IL-8, ↘ IL-10 after stimulation with PG, CpG, PIC, LPS or RSV	↘ IFN-γ after stimulation with phytohemagglutinin, cockroach and media control ↗ IL-13 after stimulation with dust mite antigen	Birth

Prenatal stress					
Wu (2018) [37]	Composite stress score: • Exposure to Violence (Exposure to Violence Questionnaire) • Prenatal Negative Life Events (Crisis in Family Systems–Revised Survey) • Postnatal Depression (Edinburgh Postnatal Depression Scale) • Anxiety (STAI)	Mainly second and third trimesters	= TNF-α, IL-8 and IL-6 promoter methylation		Birth
Duijts (2008) [39]	• Stressful mode of delivery Vaginal delivery or caesarean section (Standardised delivery registrations of midwives and obstetricians)	Birth	↗ NKC in vaginal delivery group ↘ NKC in caesarean section group	↗ CD3+/CD8+ T cells, CD3+/CD45RO+ memory T cells in vaginal delivery group ↘ CD3+/CD4+ helper T cells, CD3+/CD45RA+ naïve T cells in caesarean section group	Birth
O′Connor (2013) [40]	• Prenatal anxiety (PSWQ)	8–12 weeks, then 20–32 weeks		= IFN-γ, IL-2 or IL-4 in response to any antigen/mitogen at 2 m.o Trend neg. Correlation between prenatal anxiety and IL-12 ↗ IFN-γ, IL-4 to antigens at 6 m.o.	2 m.o. then 6 m.o.

(continued)

Table 2.1 (continued)

Author	Type of stress	Stress time point	Measure of innate and adaptive immune system	Measure of adaptive immune system	Measure of immune system time point
			Prenatal stress		
Brunwasser (2019) [41]	• Major Life Stress Separation, close death, financial problems, unemployment… (Interview)	Any time during pregnancy	↘ inflammation in boys = inflammation in girls With IL-6, TNF-α, IL-1β used as a composite for inflammation		1st year after birth
Veru (2015) [42]	• Objective stress after natural disaster Threat, loss, scope, changes due to disaster (Interview) • Subjective stress after natural disaster (IES-R)	Any time during pregnancy	Correlations: positive with TNF-α, IL-1β, IL-6, IL-10 ↗ LPS-induced TNF-α	Correlations: negative with total lymphocytes, CD4+, trend neg. With B cells; positive with Th2 cytokines ↘ CD4, total lymphocytes ↗ PHA-induced IL-4, IL-13	13 y.o. mean age
Entringer (2008) [44]	• Major negative life events Relationship conflicts, severe illness or close death, financial issues, etc. (Interview)	Any time during pregnancy	= NKC count	= total lymphocytes count, CD3+ T cells, CD4+ Th cells, CD8+ T cells count ↗ IL-4, IL-10, IL-6; ↘ IFN-γ/IL-4 ratio after PHA stimulation	25 y.o. mean age

Prenatal stress					
Slopen (2015) [43]	• Prenatal adversity Family structure, low SES • Childhood adversity Economic risk, family structure, close death, residential move	N/A	↗ CRP with high prenatal adversity = CRP with childhood adversity		42 y.o. mean age
Tyrka (2015) [45]	• Childhood maltreatment Physical abuse, sexual abuse, physical neglect and emotional maltreatment (System for Coding Subtype and Severity of Maltreatment in Child Protective Records) • Trauma Accident, attack, man-made or natural disasters, drowning, hospitalisation, etc. (DIPA) • Contextual stressors Death, separation, moving to a new house frequently, neighbourhood violence, etc. (Interview)	6 months prior (maltreatment) Lifetime (trauma and contextual stressors)	= IL-1β, CRP ↗ IL-1β at baseline in children with high number of traumas and high contextual stressors		4 y.o. mean age
Bielas (2012) [50]	• Childhood maltreatment Physical, sexual, psychological maltreatment, neglect (Interview following Arbeitsgruppe Kindesmisshandlung Guidelines)	N/A	= NKC and monocytes (CD14+/CD45+) count	↗ activated helper T cells (CD4+HLA-DR+/CD3+), activated cytotoxic T cells (CD8+HLA-DR+/CD3+) = absolute counts of lymphocytes, B cells (CD19+/CD45+), total T cells (CD3+/CD45+), helper (CD3+CD4+/CD45+) and cytotoxic (CD3+CD8+/CD45+) T cell populations, recent thymic emigrants (CD31+CD45RO+/CD4+)	9 y.o. mean age

(continued)

Table 2.1 (continued)

Author	Type of stress	Stress time point	Measure of innate and adaptive immune system	Measure of adaptive immune system	Measure of immune system time point
			Prenatal stress		
Copeland (2014) [46]	• Childhood bullying (Interview)	Recent: 3 months prior	↗ CRP when victim of bullying past/ cumulative but not recent		9–16 y.o.
Shirtcliff (2009) [70]	• Adoption (Interview) • Childhood adversity Physical abuse (CTS-PC or Child Protective Service reports)	N/A		↗ herpes simplex virus antibodies	11 y.o. mean age
Jonker (2017) [47]	• Childhood life events Separation, verbal, sexual, physical abuse (Interview)	Before 16 y.o.	= hsCRP (after correction)	= production of herpes simplex virus, Epstein–Barr virus or cytomegalovirus antibodies	16 y.o. mean age
Ehrlich (2016) [48]	• Early life adversity Familial disruption, low SES, parents with an affective disorder (Interview)	Before 15 y.o.	Creation of inflammatory cluster based on circulating IL-6 and GC sensitivity ↗ inflammatory cluster with ELA, which did not change over time		15–19 y.o., every 6 months for 2.5y

			Prenatal stress		
Walsh (2016) [49]	• Childhood abuse Physical, emotional or sexual abuse, physical or emotional neglect (CTQ)	Before 18 y.o.	= IL-6, CRP in abuse vs. no abuse ↗ IL-6 but not CRP in depression/abuse group		Pregnant adolescents: 17 y.o. mean age
Janusek (2017) [58]	• Childhood trauma Physical, emotional or sexual abuse, physical or emotional neglect (CTQ) • Community violence (SECV)	Before 18 y.o.	Higher rise and slower decline of IL-6 after TSST ↘ IL-6 promoter methylation		20 y.o. mean age
McDade (2013) [55]	• Childhood adversity Household income, household assets, absent parent for extended periods (Visits)	Before 11 y.o.	↗ CRP with parental absence, not economic adversity		21 y.o. mean age
Elwenspoek (2017) [51]	• Early life adversity Separation then adoption (Screening)	N/A		↗ CD57, especially in Th cells and overall T cells ↗ activation (GraB, perforin) in CD57+ cells Associated with high cytomegalovirus titres	22 y.o. mean age

(continued)

Table 2.1 (continued)

Author	Type of stress	Stress time point	Measure of innate and adaptive immune system	Measure of adaptive immune system	Measure of immune system time point
			Prenatal stress		
Elwenspoek (2017) [71]	• Early life adversity Separation then adoption (Screening)	N/A	= circulating CRP and IL-6 Trend ↘ monocyte count ↘ LPS-induced IL-6 in monocytes	= T and B cells proliferation, IFN-γ secretion after stimulation (PHA, PWM, PMA/ionomycin) = telomere length Trend ↘ Th17, ↗ CD4/CD25 ↘ CD8/CD69 ↗ HLA-DR+ on T cells ↘ IL-6 secretion by T and B cells after stimulation (PHA, PWM)	18–35 y.o. (6 times over 2.5 years)
Hantsoo (2019) [52]	• Childhood adversity Emotional, physical or sexual abuse, childhood neglect and household dysfunction (ACE-Q)	Before 18 y.o.	= IL-6, CRP, TNF-α in high vs. low childhood adversity group after TSST		27 y.o. mean age
Carpenter (2010) [57]	• Childhood maltreatment Physical, emotional or sexual abuse, physical or emotional neglect (CTQ)	Before 18 y.o.	Correlation with CTQ: positive with IL-6 change and max. IL-6 after TSST		27 y.o. mean age
Carpenter (2012) [54]	• Childhood maltreatment Physical, emotional or sexual abuse, physical or emotional neglect (CTQ)	Before 18 y.o.	= hsCRP		31 y.o. mean age

Prenatal stress					
Boeck (2018) [72]	• Childhood trauma Physical, emotional or sexual abuse, physical or emotional neglect (CTQ)	Before 18 y.o.	= monocytes, NKC	= B cells, T cells total, T cells subsets in PBMC ↘ reduction of telomere length in memory cytotoxic T cells only	32 y.o. mean age, assessed 3 m. postpartum
Danese (2009) [56]	• Childhood maltreatment Maternal rejection, physical or sexual abuse, harsh discipline, numerous changes of caregiver (Interview)	Before 11 y.o.	↗ hsCRP		32 y.o. mean age
Hartwell (2013) [53]	• Childhood trauma Physical, sexual, emotional, general traumas (ETI)	Before 18 y.o.	↗ IL-6, TNF-α, IL-1β = CRP		36 y.o. mean age
Taylor (2006) [59]	• Childhood adversity Psychological, physical or sexual abuse, household dysfunctions (RFQ)	Before 18 y.o.	= CRP correlation		40 y.o. mean age
Bertone-Johnson (2012) [60]	• Physical and sexual abuse (Interview)	Before 18 y.o.	↗ CRP, IL-6 with sexual abuse = CRP with physical abuse ↗ IL-6 with severe physical abuse		43 y.o. mean age

(continued)

Table 2.1 (continued)

Author	Type of stress	Stress time point	Measure of innate and adaptive immune system	Measure of adaptive immune system	Measure of immune system time point
			Prenatal stress		
Runsten (2014) [64]	• Childhood adversity Psychological, physical or sexual abuse, household dysfunctions (RFQ)	Before 18 y.o.	= CRP		43 y.o. mean age
Lacey (2013) [61]	• Childhood adversity Parental separation (Interview)	Before 16 y.o.	↗ CRP		44 y.o. mean age
Schwaiger (2016) [65]	• Childhood trauma Physical, emotional or sexual abuse, physical or emotional neglect (CTQ)	Before 18 y.o.	↗ pro-inflammatory TFs AP-1 and GATA in monocytes ↗ STAT1, CREB, GR, NFKB = CD16- transcript regulation ↗ CD16+ monocyte-genes after TSST		52 y.o. mean age
Rooks (2012) [62]	• Childhood trauma Physical, sexual, emotional, general traumas (ETI)	Before 18 y.o.	↗ CRP, IL-6		55 y.o. mean age

			Prenatal stress		
Slopen (2010) [63]	• Childhood adversity School failure, parental unemployment, parental drug or alcohol problems, verbal, physical or emotional abuse (Interview)	N/A	↗ sICAM-1 ↗ IL-6, E-selectin for African American subsample = CRP		55 y.o. mean age
Gouin (2012) [68]	• Childhood trauma Physical, emotional or sexual abuse, physical or emotional neglect (CTQ)	Before 18 y.o.	↗ IL-6 = hsCRP, TNF-α		65 y.o. mean age
Lin (2016) [67]	• Childhood adversity Repeat a year at school, physical abuse, parents drinking or using drugs • Adulthood trauma Major death, natural disaster, life-threatening event, etc. (Interviews)	Before or after 18 y.o.	↗ hsCRP with childhood trauma, not adulthood trauma		69 y.o. mean age
Kiecolt-Glaser (2011) [69]	• Childhood trauma Physical, emotional or sexual abuse, physical or emotional neglect (CTQ) • Childhood adversity Death of a parent, severe parental marital problems, immediate family member suffering from mental illness or abusing alcohol, etc. (Interview)	Before 18 y.o.	↗ IL-6 with childhood trauma and adversity ↗ TNF-α with childhood trauma	↘ telomere length with childhood adversity	72 y.o. mean age

(continued)

Table 2.1 (continued)

Author	Type of stress	Stress time point	Measure of innate and adaptive immune system	Measure of adaptive immune system	Measure of immune system time point
			Prenatal stress		
Norton (2017) [66]	• Childhood or adulthood trauma Family deaths (first-degree) in childhood or in adulthood	Before 18 y.o. or between 18 and 30 y.o.	↗ CRP childhood trauma, not adulthood trauma		80 y.o. mean age

Legend: ↗: increase, ↘: decrease, =: nonsignificant change, *ACE-Q* Adverse childhood experiences questionnaire, *AP-1* activator protein 1, *CpG* cytosine-phosphate-guanine dinucleotides, *CREB* c-AMP response element-binding protein, *CRP* C-reactive protein, *CSQ* community survey questionnaire, *CTQ* childhood trauma questionnaire, *CTS-PC* conflict tactics scale parent–child version, *DIPA* diagnostic infant and preschool assessment, *DLCS* difficult life circumstances scale, *EPI* epinephrine, *ETI* early trauma inventory, *GR* glucocorticoid receptor, *GraB* granzyme B, *hsCRP* high-sensitive C-reactive protein, *IES-R* impact of event scale—revised, *IFN-γ* interferon gamma, *IL* interleukin, *LPS* lipopolysaccharide, *MCP-1* monocyte chemoattractant protein 1, *NFKB* nuclear factor kappa light chain enhancer of activated B cells, *NKC* natural killer cell, *PBMC* peripheral blood mononuclear cells, *PG* peptidoglycan, *PHA* polyhydroxyalkanoates, *PIC* polyinosinic-polycytidylic acid, *PMA* phorbol 12-myristate 13-acetate, *PSS-14* perceived stress scale, *PSWQ* Penn State Worry Questionnaire, *PWM* pokeweed mitogen, *RFQ* risky families questionnaire, *RSV* respiratory syncytial virus, *SECV* survey of exposure to community violence, *SES* socio-economical status, *SLES* stressful life events schedule, *STAI* state-trait anxiety inventory, *STAT1* signal transducer and activator of transcription 1. *TF* transcription factor, *Th* T helper lymphocyte, *Th1* type 1 helper T lymphocyte, *Th17* T helper 17 lymphocyte, *Th2* type 2 helper T lymphocyte, *TNF-α* tumour necrosis factor alpha, *TSST* trier social stress test by their mother during pregnancy, such as a separation or the death of a close family member, authors found elevated the inflammation composite score, based on nasal wash IL-6, TNF-α and IL-1β concentrations [41]. In 13-year-old adolescents, a positive correlation was found between the level of hardship experienced as the consequence of a natural disaster during pregnancy and the cytokines IL-6, TNF-α and IL-1β in blood [42]. In middle-aged adults, the group whose mothers had experienced high prenatal adversity, such as death of a family member or low socio-economical status (SES), was found to have higher serum levels of the inflammatory C reactive protein (CRP) in comparison with the low and medium prenatal adversity groups [43].

2.2.2 Adaptive Immune System

Three studies measured the activity of the adaptive immune system at birth. In newborns, when comparing a mode of delivery associated with a lower endocrine stress response in mothers, such as caesarean section, with a vaginal delivery, T lymphocyte subsets were found to differ in UCB. Specifically, the caesarean section delivery group had lower UCB helper T lymphocytes, and naïve T lymphocytes were lower, whereas in the vaginal delivery group cytotoxic T lymphocytes and memory T lymphocytes were higher [39]. When mothers reported higher trait anxiety and more numerous stressful life events related to health while they were pregnant, UCB monocytes of newborns produced increased levels of IL-4 and IL-5, both secreted by type 2 helper T (Th2) lymphocytes [35]. In line with this, a group where mothers had experienced higher cumulative stressful circumstances, including difficult neighbourhood conditions or economic strain, had elevated Th2 IL-13 cytokine upon stimulation of UCB mononuclear cells with dust mite antigen. The secretion of type 1 helper T (Th1) IFN-γ cytokine was decreased after incubation of cells from the same infants with phytohemagglutinin (PHA) and control [36].

Regarding the influence of prenatal maternal stress on the adaptive immune system after birth, two studies focused on outcomes during childhood and one on outcomes in adulthood. In 6-month-old but not 2-month-old infants whose mother reported stress and worrying thoughts while they were pregnant, more IFN-γ and IL-4 were secreted by peripheral blood mononuclear cells (PBMCs) in response to hepatitis B and tetanus antigen stimulation, respectively [40]. In another study, the level of hardship experienced by mothers as the consequence of a natural disaster occurring during pregnancy correlated positively with the PHA-induced production of Th2 cytokines IL-4 and IL-13 in whole-blood cultures of 13-year-old adolescents. This correlation was not significant for Th1 cytokines, IL-2 and IFN-γ. The level of hardship was also negatively correlated with the total count of lymphocytes, as well as the number of CD4+ helper T lymphocytes, while only a trend was found with B lymphocytes [42]. In young adults with mothers having experienced stressful life events during pregnancy, such as relationship conflicts or severe illness of a close person, increased levels of IL-4, IL-10 and IL-6, as well as a decreased IFN-γ to IL-4 ratio, were produced after stimulation of PBMCs with PHA [44].

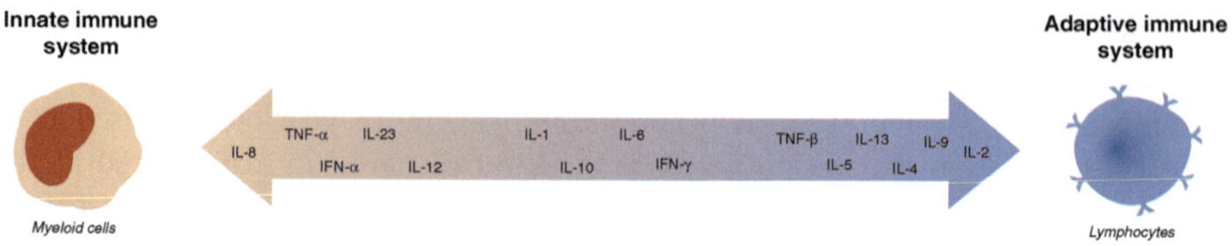

Fig. 2.1 Common cytokines associated and produced by the innate (left) and adaptive (right) immune systems. *IFN-α* interferon alpha, *IFN-γ* interferon gamma, *IL-10* interleukin 10, *IL-12* interleukin 12, *IL-13* interleukin 13, *IL-1β* interleukin 1 beta, *IL-2* interleukin 2, *IL-4* interleukin 4, *IL-5* interleukin 5, *IL-6* interleukin 6, *IL-8* interleukin 8, *IL-9* interleukin 9, *IL-23* interleukin 23, *TNF-α* tumour necrosis factor alpha, *TNF-β* tumour necrosis factor beta

2.3 Childhood Stress

2.3.1 Innate and Adaptive Immune System

Six studies investigated the consequences of childhood stress, including childhood trauma and maltreatment, on the innate and adaptive immune systems of children and adolescents. In 3–5-year-old children, a higher number of stressors and traumas, like family separation and severe accidents, but not maltreatment status were associated with increased level of saliva IL-1β, but not CRP [45]. However, in 9–16-year-old victims of bullying [46], and in 16-year-old victims of separation trauma and sexual abuse, there was a positive trend for an increase in high-sensitive CRP (hsCRP) in blood [47]. In 15–19-year-old adolescents, early life adversity, including low SES and family disruptions, was related to an increased inflammatory cluster score, composed of LPS-induced monocyte IL-6 secretion and glucocorticoid sensitivity [48]. In 17-year-old pregnant adolescents, neither childhood physical, emotional or sexual abuse, nor childhood neglect influenced blood IL-6 and CRP [49]. In 9-year-old children, having a history of physical, psychological or sexual maltreatment did not cause changes in NKC and CD14+/CD45+ monocyte count in PBMCs [50].

The effects of childhood stress on the activity of the innate immune system were examined by eight studies in young adults. Most studies did not find an association between physical, emotional or sexual abuse during childhood as well as early separation from parents and elevated CRP [51–53] or hsCRP [54] in plasma, serum or blood. However, when faced with household childhood adversity or maltreatment before the age of 11 years old, participants were found to have increased blood CRP and hsCRP [55, 56]. With respects to cytokines, childhood physical, emotional or sexual trauma was reported to elevate the plasma concentration of TNF-α in one study [53], while another did not observe any changes in serum TNF-α levels after the TSST [52]. Similarly, these types of trauma were associated with higher IL-6 in plasma [57] or saliva [58] but not serum [52] after the TSST and with decreased salivary IL-6 promoter methylation [58] and increased protein plasma concentration at baseline [53]. Early life adversity defined as separation from biological parents followed by adoption did in contrast not affect blood IL-6 but decreased LPS-induced IL-6 secretion in monocytes separated from the same sample population [51].

Seven studies investigated populations of middle-aged adults. In some but not all studies [59], various childhood traumas, including parental separation, sexual, physical, or emotional abuse, increased plasma CRP [60–62]. These traumas did not appear to influence serum nor blood CRP [63, 64]. However, plasma or serum IL-6 concentrations were consistently higher across these studies [60, 62] although an effect of ethnicity was reported [63]. Additionally, childhood trauma only increased the serum expression of the adhesion molecules sICAM-1 and E-selectin in the African American subgroup [63]. In participants having experienced physical, emotional or sexual trauma, the pro-inflammatory transcription factors activator protein 1 (AP-1), GATA, signal transducer and activator of transcription 1 (STAT1), c-AMP response element-binding protein (CREB) and glucocorticoid receptor (GR) showed a greater activity after the TSST. In the same group, genes characteristic to CD16+ monocytes also showed an increased expression after the TSST [65].

Four studies focused on elderly populations. Family deaths or difficult life circumstances, such as parents using drugs or repeating a year at school, were associated with elevated CRP and hsCRP in blood only if they had taken place in childhood but not adulthood [66, 67], while abuse did not affect hsCRP [68]. Childhood trauma, including physical, sexual or emotional abuse, was linked with higher serum levels of IL-6 in two studies [68, 69]. Serum TNF-α was also reported to be elevated in one study [69], but not the other [68].

2.3.2 Adaptive Immune System

Only three studies reported findings on the adaptive immune system in children who had a history of childhood stress. In a group of physically, emotionally or sexually abused 9-year-old children, PBMCs activated helper T lymphocytes and activated cytotoxic T lymphocytes were more numerous than in the control group. No difference was found with respect to the absolute lymphocyte count, nor in various CD45+ lymphocytes subtypes [50]. In 9–14-year-old children, being adopted or physically maltreated was associated with elevated saliva antibodies against the herpes simplex virus type 1 (HSV1) [70]. However, in 16-year-old adolescents, having experienced traumatic childhood life events, including separation or abuse, did not increase antibodies against HSV1, Epstein–Barr virus or cytomegalovirus in blood samples [47].

Three studies analysed the effects of childhood stress on the adult adaptive immune system of young adults. In adopted participants, less early activated cytotoxic T lymphocytes and more HLA-DR+ total T lymphocytes, cytotoxic and helper T lymphocytes were detected in PBMCs separated from the same sample population compared with controls. The CD25 marker, commonly upregulated upon T lymphocyte activation, was also found to be significantly elevated on cytotoxic T lymphocytes and marginally more present on helper T lymphocytes and total T lymphocytes. In contrast, there was no difference in the proliferation of T and B lymphocytes upon PHA or pokeweed mitogen (PWM) stimulation, nor in their IFN-γ secretion, although IL-6 production was lower [51]. Additionally, in a different subset of adopted participants from the same cohort, a trend was reported for a lower count of T helper 17 lymphocytes (Th17), which presented increased CD57 senescence marker and was associated with higher cytomegalovirus titres [71]. In a population of women, childhood abuse group was found to have a reduction in telomere length found in peripheral memory cytotoxic T lymphocytes at a follow-up 3-month postpartum [72].

One study investigated adaptive immune system changes in elderly. In a population with a history of childhood adversity, including death of a parent or severe marital problems, telomere length was reported to be reduced in PBMCs [69].

2.4 Discussion

In order to discuss the effects of stress on the immune system, this chapter gathered evidence on both innate and adaptive arms of the immune system after prenatal and childhood stress. Overall, prenatal stress most consistently increased IL-8 at birth, while it elevated the cytokines IL-6, IL-1β and TNF-α in studies measuring innate and adaptive immune activation later in life. Prenatal stress was also linked with the production of Th2 lymphocytes-associated cytokines, such as IL-4, IL-5 and IL-13 at birth. With regard to childhood stress, both the innate and adaptive immune systems were reported to have increased activation, although often in specific subgroups. Generally, IL-6 was increased and the most consistent changes in CRP after childhood trauma were observed in middle-aged and elderly populations. The adaptive immune system was generally reported to have a dampened activity, with more markers of T lymphocyte senescence and reduced levels of adaptive cytokines.

When stress occurred prenatally, the adaptive immune system was more consistently affected than the innate immune system. While acute innate cytokines were related to maternal stress in some studies [36, 42], they were not in all of them [37] which strongly contrasts with findings regarding the increase in Th2-related cytokines [35, 42, 44]. Nonetheless, these results support the observation that newborns naturally have an immune reaction shifted towards an anti-inflammatory profile [73] and suggest that that the activity of Th2 lymphocytes remain exacerbated later in life. Pro-inflammatory cytokines are produced by leucocytes and Th1 lymphocytes alike and are for this reason usually less present at birth and require interaction with antigens from the environment [73], which might explain the greater heterogeneity across studies when looking at individual molecules, although a generally increased activation is reported until adolescence.

Regardless of the time point at which immune activity was measured, it also appeared that major prenatal stressors that were more concrete or physical, such as the consequences of a natural catastrophe [42], a stressful delivery [39] or violence [36], were more predictive of immune overactivation than stress scores in general [37, 44]. A possible explanation to this is that the former is likely more closely related to the type of stress experienced in innate fear situations and the latter to the type of stress observed in states of anxiety. Furthermore, even though they are tightly associated, fear and anxiety are distinct concepts with respective neural activation patterns [74] and might therefore trigger different immune reactions. One study previously demonstrated that mice lacking mature T and B lymphocytes showed a more pronounced innate fear behaviour after predator odour exposure but did not express more anxiety in conditioning tasks [75]. This supports the existence of distinct relationships between the immune system and fear and anxiety and might need to be further investigated.

In children and adolescents with childhood trauma, individual cytokines were reported to be increased more often than the general inflammatory marker CRP [45, 49]. This seemingly weaker inflammatory activation could be due to the fact that the innate reactions have mainly reached maturity in childhood [14] and are less sensitive. It might thus be interesting to compare this against adaptive activation in this population since few studies report such data. Interestingly, the elevated innate immune system markers IL-6 and CRP were less present in young adults with a history of childhood trauma [51–53] but were in middle-aged [60, 62, 63] and older adults [66, 67]. This might indicate that childhood trauma does not affect innate immune reactions deeply and over time in the general population, which is in contradiction with results from a meta-analysis reporting that the impact of childhood trauma on CRP was significantly more pronounced in clinical populations [76]. These discrepancies could, however, be due to the meta-analysis using clinical and general samples, as well as the lack of age distinction. The commonly termed "inflamm-ageing" phenomenon might also affect the results in older participants and reflect natural changes of the immune system associated with age [77], rather than the trauma they endured as children.

A limitation of this chapter that must be taken into consideration and might also further explain these differences is the mental health of the participants. Childhood trauma is known to increase the risk of developing mental health disorders [26], which was partially reflected in the studies in this chapter. While the participants were part of the general population and were not clinically suffering from psychiatric disorders, it was nonetheless reported that some samples had significantly increased anxiety or depression symptom scores when comparing childhood stress and control groups. Only very few studies controlled for these scores in their analyses [46, 70] and reported an effect of childhood trauma that remained significant. However, it is difficult to fully exclude the influence of mental health on the results of the other studies and further emphasises the need to fully take this into account in order to obtain a clearer picture of the impact of childhood on the immune system.

Another notable trend in findings is that markers of senescence in T lymphocytes are more present in adults after childhood trauma or adversity, as, for example, with increased CD57 [71] and reduction in telomere length [72]. Senescence of cells is commonly observed with age, where more T lymphocytes become unable to proliferate and shift towards a low pro-inflammatory profile [78, 79], but more recently also in anxiety, where shorter leucocyte telomere length has been detected [80]. Whether stress during childhood could cause an accelerated senescence of immune cells remains to be determined, the link between anxiety and senescence has been demonstrated with obesity-induced senescence of glia causing anxiety-like behaviour in mice [81]. Given the well-established bidirectional relationship between stress and the immune system, it is conceivable to hypothesise that stress could reciprocally lead to senescence of T lymphocytes.

In summary, stress can impact both the innate and adaptive arms of the immune system, although differently depending on the stress time point. Overall, the production of cytokines associated with innate immune cells was more clearly affected by prenatal stress, but ageing of T lymphocytes was observed as a consequence of childhood stress. Nevertheless, it is difficult to draw a clear picture with respects to specific molecules even though stress has undeniable effects on the immune system. Indeed, the variety of makers is extremely wide, and most importantly, there is an evident interplay between the innate and adaptive immune systems. They influence each other constantly and can produce identical molecules, rendering their consequences extremely complex to disentangle. Thus, it is important that future studies replicate findings regarding particular cells or markers of the immune system and take into account its evolution throughout life. Better understanding of the presented differences could lead to improved predictions of the immune phenotype associated with specific types of stress and through this, more targeted identification of populations at risk for immunopsychiatric disorders.

References

1. Chrousos GP. Stress and disorders of the stress system. Nat Rev Endocrinol. 2009;5(7):374–81.
2. Horowitz MA, Zunszain PA, Anacker C, Musaelyan K, Pariante CM. Glucocorticoids and inflammation: a double-headed sword in depression? How do neuroendocrine and inflammatory pathways interact during stress to contribute to the pathogenesis of depression? Mod Trends Pharmacopsychiatry. Switzerland. 2013;28:127–43.
3. Pariante CM. Why are depressed patients inflamed? A reflection on 20 years of research on depression, glucocorticoid resistance and inflammation. Eur Neuropsychopharmacol. Netherlands. 2017;27:554–9.
4. Carroll JE, Low CA, Prather AA, Cohen S, Fury JM, Ross DC, et al. Negative affective responses to a speech task predict changes in interleukin (IL)-6. Brain Behav Immun. Netherlands. 2011;25:232–8.
5. Yamakawa K, Matsunaga M, Isowa T, Kimura K, Kasugai K, Yoneda M, et al. Transient responses of inflammatory cytokines in acute stress. Biol Psychol. Elsevier. 2009;82:25–32.
6. Slavich GM, Cole SW. The emerging field of human social genomics. Clin Psychol Sci A. J Assoc Psychol Sci. United States. 2013;1:331–48.
7. Borsini A, Zunszain PA, Thuret S, Pariante CM. The role of inflammatory cytokines as key modulators of neurogenesis. Trends Neurosci. 2015;38:145–57.
8. Katayama Y, Battista M, Kao W-M, Hidalgo A, Peired AJ, Thomas SA, et al. Signals from the sympathetic nervous system regulate hematopoietic stem cell egress from bone marrow. Cell. United States. 2006;124:407–21.
9. Wohleb ES, Franklin T, Iwata M, Duman RS. Integrating neuroimmune systems in the neurobiology of depression. Nat Rev Neurosci. 2016;17:497–511.
10. Trottier MD, Newsted MM, King LE, Fraker PJ. Natural glucocorticoids induce expansion of all developmental stages of murine bone marrow granulocytes without inhibiting function. Proc Natl Acad Sci U S A. United States. 2008;105:2028–33.

11. Delves PJ, Roitt IM. The immune system. N Engl J Med. Massachusetts Medical Society. 2000;343:37–49.
12. Kollmann TR, Crabtree J, Rein-Weston A, Blimkie D, Thommai F, Wang XY, et al. Neonatal innate TLR-mediated responses are distinct from those of adults. J Immunol. United States. 2009;183:7150–60.
13. Yerkovich ST, Wikstrom ME, Suriyaarachchi D, Prescott SL, Upham JW, Holt PG. Postnatal development of monocyte cytokine responses to bacterial lipopolysaccharide. Pediatr Res. United States. 2007;62:547–52.
14. Martin R, Nauta AJ, Ben Amor K, Knippels LMJ, Knol J, Garssen J. Early life: gut microbiota and immune development in infancy. Benef Microbes. 2010;1:367–82.
15. Ygberg S, Nilsson A. The developing immune system – From foetus to toddler. Acta Paediatr Int J Paediatr. 2012;101:120–7.
16. Di Benedetto MG, Bottanelli C, Cattaneo A, Pariante CM, Borsini A. Nutritional and immunological factors in breast milk: a role in the intergenerational transmission from maternal psychopathology to child development. Brain Behav Immun. Academic Press. 2020;85:57–68.
17. McGowan PO, Sasaki A, D'Alessio AC, Dymov S, Labonte B, Szyf M, et al. Epigenetic regulation of the glucocorticoid receptor in human brain associates with childhood abuse. Nat Neurosci. United States. 2009;12:342–8.
18. Bierhaus A, Wolf J, Andrassy M, Rohleder N, Humpert PM, Petrov D, et al. A mechanism converting psychosocial stress into mononuclear cell activation. Proc Natl Acad Sci U S A. 2003;100:1920–5.
19. Juruena MF, Cleare AJ, Papadopoulos AS, Poon L, Lightman S, Pariante CM. Different responses to dexamethasone and prednisolone in the same depressed patients. Psychopharmacology (Berl). Germany. 2006;189:225–35.
20. Borsini A, Alboni S, Horowitz MA, Tojo LM, Cannazza G, Su K-P, et al. Rescue of IL-1β-induced reduction of human neurogenesis by omega-3 fatty acids and antidepressants. Brain Behav Immun. 2017;65:230–8.
21. Borsini A, Cattaneo A, Malpighi C, Thuret S, Harrison NA, Zunszain PA, et al. Interferon-alpha reduces human hippocampal neurogenesis and increases apoptosis via activation of distinct STAT1-dependent mechanisms. Int J Neuropsychopharmacol. England. 2018;21:187–200.
22. Innes S, Pariante CM, Borsini A. Microglial-driven changes in synaptic plasticity: a possible role in major depressive disorder. Psychoneuroendocrinology. Elsevier. 2018;102:236–47.
23. Nettis MA, Pariante CM, Mondelli V. Early-life adversity, systemic inflammation and comorbid physical and psychiatric illnesses of adult life. Curr Top Behav Neurosci. Germany. 2020;44:207–25.
24. Plant DT, Pawlby S, Pariante CM, Jones FW. When one childhood meets another—maternal childhood trauma and offspring child psychopathology: a systematic review. Clin Child Psychol Psychiatry. England. 2018;23:483–500.
25. Cullen AE, Fisher HL, Roberts RE, Pariante CM, Laurens KR. Daily stressors and negative life events in children at elevated risk of developing schizophrenia. Br J Psychiatry. England. 2014;204:354–60.
26. Huh HJ, Kim KH, Lee H-K, Chae J-H. The relationship between childhood trauma and the severity of adulthood depression and anxiety symptoms in a clinical sample: the mediating role of cognitive emotion regulation strategies. J Affect Disord. Netherlands. 2017;213:44–50.
27. Salari A-A, Fatehi-Gharehlar L, Motayagheni N, Homberg JR. Fluoxetine normalizes the effects of prenatal maternal stress on depression- and anxiety-like behaviors in mouse dams and male offspring. Behav Brain Res. Netherlands. 2016;311:354–67.
28. Ouellet-Morin I, Wong CCY, Danese A, Pariante CM, Papadopoulos AS, Mill J, et al. Increased serotonin transporter gene (SERT) DNA methylation is associated with bullying victimization and blunted cortisol response to stress in childhood: a longitudinal study of discordant monozygotic twins. Psychol Med. Cambridge University Press. 2013;43:1813–23.
29. Pawlby S, Hay D, Sharp D, Waters CS, Pariante CM. Antenatal depression and offspring psychopathology: the influence of childhood maltreatment. Br J Psychiatry. England. 2011;199:106–12.

30. Plant DT, Pawlby S, Sharp D, Zunszain PA, Pariante CM. Prenatal maternal depression is associated with offspring inflammation at 25 years: a prospective longitudinal cohort study. Transl Psychiatry. United States. 2016;6:e936.
31. Osborne S, Biaggi A, Chua TE, Du Preez A, Hazelgrove K, Nikkheslat N, et al. Antenatal depression programs cortisol stress reactivity in offspring through increased maternal inflammation and cortisol in pregnancy: The Psychiatry Research and Motherhood—Depression (PRAM-D) Study. Psychoneuroendocrinology. England. 2018;98:211–21.
32. Baumeister D, Russell A, Pariante CM, Mondelli V. Inflammatory biomarker profiles of mental disorders and their relation to clinical, social and lifestyle factors. Soc Psychiatry Psychiatr Epidemiol. 2014;49:841–9.
33. Liles WC, Review VVWC. Nomenclature and biologic significance of cytokines involved in inflammation and the host immune response. J Infect Dis. 1995;172:1573–80.
34. Owen JA, Punt J, Stranford SA, Jones PP. Receptors and signaling: cytokines and chemokines. Kuby Immunol: W.H. Freeman; 2013. p. 113.
35. Andersson NW, Li Q, Mills CW, Ly J, Nomura Y, Chen J. Influence of prenatal maternal stress on umbilical cord blood cytokine levels. Arch Womens Ment Health. 2016;19:761–7.
36. Wright RJ, Visness CM, Calatroni A, Grayson MH, Gold DR, Sandel MT, et al. Prenatal maternal stress and cord blood innate and adaptive cytokine responses in an inner-city cohort. Am J Respir Crit Care Med. 2010;182:25–33.
37. Wu S, Gennings C, Wright RJ, Wilson A, Burris HH, Just AC, et al. Prenatal stress, methylation in inflammation-related genes, and adiposity measures in early childhood: the programming research in obesity, growth environment and social stress cohort study. Psychosom Med. 2018;80:34–41.
38. Vogl SE, Worda C, Egarter C, Bieglmayer C, Szekeres T, Huber J, et al. Mode of delivery is associated with maternal and fetal endocrine stress response. BJOG. England. 2006;113:441–5.
39. Duijts L, Bakker-Jonges LE, Labout JAM, Jaddoe VWV, Hofman A, Steegers EAP, et al. Perinatal stress influences lymphocyte subset counts in neonates. The generation R study. Pediatr Res. United States. 2008;63:292–8.
40. O'Connor TG, Winter MA, Hunn J, Carnahan J, Pressman EK, Glover V, et al. Prenatal maternal anxiety predicts reduced adaptive immunity in infants. Brain Behav Immun. Elsevier Inc. 2013;32:21–8.
41. Brunwasser SM, Slavich GM, Newcomb DC, Gebretsadik T, Turi KN, Stone C, et al. Sex-specific association between prenatal life stress exposure and infant pro-inflammatory cytokine levels during acute respiratory infection. Brain Behav Immun. Elsevier. 2019;76:275–9.
42. Veru F, Dancause K, Laplante DP, King S, Luheshi G. Prenatal maternal stress predicts reductions in CD4+ lymphocytes, increases in innate-derived cytokines, and a Th2 shift in adolescents: Project Ice Storm. Physiol Behav. Elsevier B.V. 2015;144:137–45.
43. Slopen N, Loucks EB, Appleton AA, Kawachi I, Kubzansky LD, Non AL, et al. Early origins of inflammation: an examination of prenatal and childhood social adversity in a prospective cohort study. Psychoneuroendocrinology. Elsevier Ltd. 2015;51:403–13.
44. Entringer S, Kumsta R, Nelson EL, Hellhammer DH, Wadhwa PD, Wüst S. Influence of prenatal psychosocial stress on cytokine production in adult women. Dev Psychobiol. 2008;50:579–87.
45. Tyrka AR, Parade SH, Valentine TR, Eslinger NM, Seifer R. Adversity in preschool-aged children: effects on salivary interleukin-1beta. Dev Psychopathol. United States. 2015;27:567–76.
46. Copeland WE, Wolke D, Lereya ST, Shanahan L, Worthman C, Costello EJ. Childhood bullying involvement predicts low-grade systemic inflammation into adulthood. Proc Natl Acad Sci. 2014;111:7570–5.
47. Jonker I, Rosmalen JGM, Schoevers RA. Childhood life events, immune activation and the development of mood and anxiety disorders: the TRAILS study. Transl Psychiatry. Nature Publishing Group. 2017;7:1–9.
48. Ehrlich KB, Ross KM, Chen E, Miller GE. Testing the biological embedding hypothesis: is early life adversity associated with a later proinflammatory phenotype? Dev Psychopathol. 2016;28:1273–83.

49. Walsh K, Basu A, Werner E, Lee S, Feng T, Osborne LM, et al. Associations among child abuse, depression, and interleukin-6 in pregnant adolescents: paradoxical findings. Psychosom Med. 2016;78:920–30.
50. Bielas H, Jud A, Lips U, Reichenbach J, Landolt MA. Increased number of activated T cells in lymphocyte subsets of maltreated children: data from a pilot study. J Psychosom Res. Elsevier Inc. 2012;73:313–8.
51. Elwenspoek MMC, Hengesch X, Leenen FAD, Schritz A, Sias K, Schaan VK, et al. Proinflammatory T cell status associated with early life adversity. J Immunol. 2017;199:4046–55.
52. Hantsoo L, Jašarević E, Criniti S, McGeehan B, Tanes C, Sammel MD, et al. Childhood adversity impact on gut microbiota and inflammatory response to stress during pregnancy. Brain Behav Immun. 2019;75:240–50.
53. Hartwell KJ, Moran-Santa Maria MM, Twal WO, Shaftman S, DeSantis SM, McRae-Clark AL, et al. Association of elevated cytokines with childhood adversity in a sample of healthy adults. J Psychiatr Res. Elsevier Ltd. 2013;47:604–10.
54. Carpenter LL, Gawuga CE, Tyrka AR, Price LH. C-reactive protein, early life stress, and wellbeing in healthy adults. Acta Psychiatr Scand. 2012;126:402–10.
55. McDade TW, Hoke M, Borja JB, Adair LS, Kuzawa C. Do environments in infancy moderate the association between stress and inflammation in adulthood? Initial evidence from a birth cohort in the Philippines. Brain Behav Immun. Elsevier Inc. 2013;31:23–30.
56. Danese A, Moffitt TE, Harrington H, Milne BJ, Polanczyk G, Pariante CM, et al. Adverse childhood experiences and adult risk factors for age-related disease. Arch Pediatr Adolesc Med. 2009;163:1135–43.
57. Carpenter LL, Gawuga CE, Tyrka AR, Lee JK, Anderson GM, Price LH. Association between plasma IL-6 response to acute stress and early-life adversity in healthy adults. Neuropsychopharmacology. Nature Publishing Group. 2010;35:2617–23.
58. Janusek LW, Tell D, Gaylord-Harden N, Mathews HL. Relationship of childhood adversity and neighborhood violence to a proinflammatory phenotype in emerging adult African American men: an epigenetic link. Brain Behav Immun. Elsevier Inc. 2017;60:126–35.
59. Taylor SE, Lehman BJ, Kiefe CI, Seeman TE. Relationship of early life stress and psychological functioning to adult C-reactive protein in the coronary artery risk development in young adults study. Biol Psychiatry. 2006;60:819–24.
60. Bertone-Johnson ER, Whitcomb BW, Missmer SA, Karlson EW, Rich-Edwards JW. Inflammation and early-life abuse in women. Am J Prev Med. Elsevier Inc. 2012;43:611–20.
61. Lacey RE, Kumari M, McMunn A. Parental separation in childhood and adult inflammation: the importance of material and psychosocial pathways. Psychoneuroendocrinology. Elsevier Ltd. 2013;38:2476–84.
62. Rooks C, Veledar E, Goldberg J, Bremner JD, Vaccarino V. Early trauma and inflammation: role of familial factors in a study of twins. Psychosom Med. 2012;74:146–52.
63. Slopen N, Lewis TT, Gruenewald TL, Mujahid MS, Ryff CD, Albert MA, et al. Early life adversity and inflammation in African Americans and whites in the midlife in the United States survey. Psychosom Med. 2010;72:694–701.
64. Runsten S, Korkeila K, Koskenvuo M, Rautava P, Vainio O, Korkeila J. Can social support alleviate inflammation associated with childhood adversities? Nord J Psychiatry. 2014;68:137–44.
65. Schwaiger M, Grinberg M, Moser D, Zang JCS, Heinrichs M, Hengstler JG, et al. Altered stress-induced regulation of genes in monocytes in adults with a history of childhood adversity. Neuropsychopharmacology. 2016;41:2530–40.
66. Norton MC, Hatch DJ, Munger RG, Smith KR. Family member deaths in childhood predict systemic inflammation in late life. Biodemography Soc Biol. Routledge. 2017;63:104–15.
67. Lin JE, Neylan TC, Epel E, O'Donovan A. Associations of childhood adversity and adulthood trauma with C-reactive protein: a cross-sectional population-based study. Brain Behav Immun. Elsevier Inc. 2016;53:105–12.
68. Gouin JP, Glaser R, Malarkey WB, Beversdorf D, Kiecolt-Glaser JK. Childhood abuse and inflammatory responses to daily stressors. Ann Behav Med. 2012;44:287–92.

69. Kiecolt-Glaser JK, Gouin JP, Weng NP, Malarkey WB, Beversdorf DQ, Glaser R. Childhood adversity heightens the impact of later-life caregiving stress on telomere length and inflammation. Psychosom Med. 2011;73:16–22.
70. Shirtcliff EA, Coe CL, Pollak SD. Early childhood stress is associated with elevated antibody levels to herpes simplex virus type 1. Proc Natl Acad Sci. 2009;106:2963–7.
71. Elwenspoek MMC, Sias K, Hengesch X, Schaan VK, Leenen FAD, Adams P, et al. T cell immunosenescence after early life adversity: association with cytomegalovirus infection. Front Immunol. 2017;8:1–12.
72. Boeck C, Krause S, Karabatsiakis A, Schury K, Gündel H, Waller C, et al. History of child maltreatment and telomere length in immune cell subsets: associations with stress- and attachment-related hormones. Dev Psychopathol. 2018;30:539–51.
73. Holt PG, Jones CA. The development of the immune system during pregnancy and early life. Allergy. John Wiley & Sons, Ltd. 2000;55:688–97.
74. Perusini JN, Fanselow MS. Neurobehavioral perspectives on the distinction between fear and anxiety. Learn Mem. United States. 2015;22:417–25.
75. Clark SM, Sand J, Francis TC, Nagaraju A, Michael KC, Keegan AD, et al. Immune status influences fear and anxiety responses in mice after acute stress exposure. Brain Behav Immun. Elsevier Inc. 2014;38:192–201.
76. Baumeister D, Akhtar R, Ciufolini S, Pariante CM, Mondelli V. Childhood trauma and adulthood inflammation : a meta-analysis of peripheral C-reactive protein , interleukin-6 and tumour necrosis factor-α. Nature Publishing Group. 2015;21:642–9.
77. Singh T, Newman AB. Inflammatory markers in population studies of aging. Ageing Res Rev. Elsevier. 2011;10:319–29.
78. Baker DJ, Perez-Terzic C, Jin F, Pitel KS, Niederländer NJ, Jeganathan K, et al. Opposing roles for p16Ink4a and p19Arf in senescence and ageing caused by BubR1 insufficiency. Nat Cell Biol. Nature Publishing Group, A Division of Macmillan Publishers Limited. All Rights Reserved. 2012;14:649.
79. Xu W, Larbi A. Markers of T cell senescence in humans. Int J Mol Sci. 2017;18:1–13.
80. Verhoeven JE, Révész D, van Oppen P, Epel ES, Wolkowitz OM, Penninx BWJH. Anxiety disorders and accelerated cellular ageing. Br J Psychiatry. Cambridge University Press. 2015;206:371–8.
81. Ogrodnik M, Zhu Y, Langhi LGP, Tchkonia T, Krüger P, Fielder E, et al. Obesity-induced cellular senescence drives anxiety and impairs neurogenesis. Cell Metab. Cell Press. 2019;29:1061–1077.e8.

3 Immunity as a Common Risk Pathway for Psychiatric and Medical Comorbidity

Joshua D. Rosenblat and Roger S. McIntyre

3.1 The Association Between Psychiatric and Chronic Medical Conditions

"Comorbidity" is defined as the simultaneous presence of two chronic conditions in a single person [1]. Replicated epidemiological studies have demonstrated a clear association between psychiatric and medical conditions with high rates of comorbidity [2–4]. The US National Comorbidity Survey Replication (NCS-R), a rigorously designed national epidemiological study, revealed that comorbidity between chronic medical and psychiatric disorders is the rule rather than the exception; ~70% of adults with a psychiatric disorder had at least one general medical disorder, and ~30% of those with a medical disorder had a comorbid psychiatric condition [4, 5]. Indeed, almost all psychiatric disorders are associated with increased rates of medical comorbidity and vice versa. Given the high rates of comorbidity, an entire subspeciality within psychiatry has been created with this focus in mind. This subspeciality has a variety of different titles, including consultation–liaison psychiatry, psychosomatic medicine and medical psychiatry [5]. The establishment of this

J. D. Rosenblat (✉)
Mood Disorder Psychopharmacology Unit, University Health Network, Toronto, ON, Canada

University of Toronto, Toronto, ON, Canada

Canadian Rapid Treatment Center of Excellence, Mississauga, ON, Canada
e-mail: joshua.rosenblat@uhn.ca

R. S. McIntyre
Mood Disorder Psychopharmacology Unit, University Health Network, Toronto, ON, Canada

University of Toronto, Toronto, ON, Canada

Canadian Rapid Treatment Center of Excellence, Mississauga, ON, Canada

Brain and Cognition Discovery Foundation, Toronto, ON, Canada
e-mail: Roger.McIntyre@uhn.ca

M. Berk et al. (eds.), *Immuno-Psychiatry*, https://doi.org/10.1007/978-3-030-71229-7_3

subspecialty field further emphasizes the high prevalence and importance of medical comorbidity in psychiatry [6].

Severe and persistent mental illness (SPMI), such as schizophrenia, bipolar disorder (BD) and severe treatment-resistant major depressive disorder (MDD), have been most strongly associated with high rates of medical comorbidity [7]. As the association between schizophrenia, MDD, BD and medical comorbidity has been more clearly established, these disorders will be the focus of the current chapter, while acknowledging that other common disorders, such as anxiety and related disorders, are also associated with increased rates of medical comorbidity, albeit to a lesser degree [5].

Classic inflammatory conditions include autoimmune disorders, such as systemic lupus erythematosus (SLE), inflammatory bowel disease (IBD), psoriasis, rheumatoid arthritis (RA), multiple sclerosis (MS), thyroiditis, autoimmune hepatitis, myocarditis and asthma. However, inflammation has been strongly implicated in most major chronic medical conditions as a key pathogenic factor, including cardiovascular disease, diabetes mellitus, cerebral vascular disease and chronic pain conditions [8, 9]. As such, when considering the role of inflammation, a plethora of chronic medical conditions may be considered, not only autoimmune conditions.

Major depressive disorder (MDD), especially severe treatment-resistant depression (TRD), has been associated with inflammatory medical comorbidities [4]. Estimates of MDD in chronic medical illness have been consistently reported to be greater than twofold higher than the general population [10]. Further, the presence of multiple medical conditions (e.g. "multimorbidity") appears to be associated with even higher rates of depression and poorer medical and psychiatric outcomes [11, 12].

Autoimmune disorders, such as IBD, SLE, psoriasis and RA, have been strongly linked to MDD, with MDD prevalence rates of 10–30% [13–22]. Inflammatory neurological disorders are also strongly linked with increased rates of MDD, with an estimated lifetime prevalence of 20–40% across stroke, epilepsy, multiple sclerosis (MS), traumatic brain injury (TBI) and Parkinson's disease (PD) [23–26]. Significantly elevated rates of MDD are also observed with cancer (lifetime prevalence of MDD of 10–20%), diabetes (6–20%), cardiovascular diseases (15–25%), human immunodeficiency viruses (HIV; 25–40%) and chronic obstructive pulmonary disease (COPD; 20–30%), all of which have strong immunologic components to their pathophysiology.

Similarly, BD has been associated with increased rates of several medical comorbidities compared to healthy controls and vice versa (Kupfer, 2005). Notably, the increased prevalence of medical comorbidities, particularly cardiovascular disease, is primarily responsible for the 10- to 20-year decrease in life expectancy in BD compared to the rest of the population [27]. Increased rates of IBD, SLE, autoimmune thyroiditis, psoriasis, Guillain–Barré syndrome (GBS), autoimmune hepatitis, MS and RA have all been observed in patients with BD [17, 28–33]. BD has also been strongly associated with increased rates of cardiovascular disease, diabetes and obesity [33–35], which all have strong inflammatory components to their pathophysiology and also predict poorer clinical outcomes and decreased life expectancy.

Schizophrenia has been associated with increased rates of early mortality secondary to medical comorbidity with medical conditions often underrecognized and undertreated [36]. Life expectancy is 13 to 30 years earlier in patients with schizophrenia compared to the general population [36]. This premature mortality is secondary to increased rates of cardiovascular disease primarily, as well as increased rates of cancer and diabetes [2, 37]. Indeed, schizophrenia has been strongly associated with increased rates of cardiovascular disease, diabetes, inflammatory neurological conditions and cognitive disorders, suggesting a strong link between psychotic disorders and inflammatory conditions [2, 37].

Taken together, psychiatric disorders are clearly associated with increased rates of medical comorbidity. Further, in chronic medical illnesses, MDD, BD and schizophrenia are all also associated with poorer medical outcomes, increased health care utilization, decreased treatment adherence and poorer health-related quality of life [7, 23, 38–40]. Increased all-cause mortality and disease progression have been associated with comorbid psychiatric illness; however, a causal relationship has never been clearly established [38, 39]. With these high rates of comorbidity and significant implications for prognosis and treatment, understanding the mediating and moderating factors of comorbidity is of great importance. Herein, we discuss further the potential role of immune dysfunction for observed comorbidity trends.

3.2 Immune Dysfunction as a Common Risk Pathway for Psychiatric and Medical Comorbidity

The aforementioned studies provide strong evidence for an association between psychiatric and inflammatory medical conditions. However, causation has yet to be definitively established. In favour of a causal bidirectional association is the replicated observation that acute flares of inflammatory conditions (e.g. flare of MS or IBD, etc.) are associated with acute worsening of psychiatric symptoms [30, 37, 41]. Similarly, psychiatric deterioration is associated with flare-ups of medical comorbid conditions. As discussed in other chapters, immune-brain pathways present as biologically plausible mechanisms linking acute worsening of medical and psychiatric symptoms. Further, numerous shared genetic, epigenetic and psychosocial risk factors, such as adverse childhood experiences, may increase the risk of immune dysfunction which would in turn increase the risk of developing both medical and psychiatric disorders in a given individual [42, 43].

Autoimmune disorders are the prototypic inflammatory conditions with immune dysfunction as the key etiological factor driving the onset and progression of the disorder. In autoimmune diseases, the immune system falsely recognizes normal host tissue as pathogenic and launches an immune response to destroy this tissue. At the local site of inflammation, immune cells will attempt to induce cell death and clearance of the tissue [44]. This local response also increases inflammatory cytokine levels systemically leading to an increased level of inflammatory processes throughout the body, including in the brain, leading to psychological effects, such as "sickness behaviours" [45]. While distal tissues will not be destroyed to the same extent as the site of the local inflammatory response, the subtler effects of low-grade systemic inflammation on off-target areas (e.g. the brain) have been increasingly recognized as important [46].

Most chronic medical conditions and autoimmune disorders are associated with chronic low-grade inflammation with acute-on-chronic "flare-ups" (e.g. relapse and recurrence of signs and symptoms) associated with increased signs and symptoms of the illness [44]. For example, psoriasis flares are associated chronic mild increases in inflammatory marked with markedly elevated inflammatory markers during a flare. While the psoriatic plaques present on the skin due to a local inappropriate inflammatory response, the increased pro-inflammatory cytokines are circulated systemically through the lymphatic and circulatory system and may have significant off-target effects on the central nervous system, potentially leading to mood, anxiety, cognitive and even psychotic symptomatology [47]. These effects are observed through increased psychological symptoms, primarily anxiety, depression, fatigue and cognitive dysfunction during flare-ups of numerous disorders, such as psoriasis, MS, IBD and SLE [17, 18, 26, 48].

While autoimmune disorders are the prototypic inflammatory conditions, many other medical comorbidities have immune dysfunction as a key factor in their pathophysiology, such as cardiovascular disease. Specifically, SPMI have been strongly associated with increased rates of cardiovascular disease, diabetes and obesity, which have all have immune dysfunction as central to their pathophysiology [2, 7, 36, 40]. For example, in cardiovascular disease, inflammations play a key role in the propagation of atherosclerotic plaques [49]. Type II diabetes mellitus has also been recognized as an inflammatory condition associated with chronic low-grade inflammation that is predictive of the progression of disease [50]. Central obesity has also been shown to be inflammatory in nature as excess adipose tissue produces adipokines and cytokines which chronically increase systemic levels of inflammation [51]. The increased coprevalence of these specific disorders with schizophrenia, BD and MDD provides further support for immune mechanisms mediating and moderating the association between psychiatric and medical comorbidities.

As discussed in other chapters, increases in inflammatory cytokines can have profound effects on brain function and neuronal signalling [52]. Indeed, numerous pathways exist where immune overactivation can lead to significant psychiatric symptoms via changes in monoamine levels and microglial overactivation leading to neuronal apoptosis and destruction of key brain circuits controlling mood and cognition [53]. Of note, however, numerous other factors are likely at play, such as overlapping psychosocial factors, behavioural factors (e.g. smoking, alcohol, sedentary lifestyle) and iatrogenic factors (e.g. psychiatric and medical adverse effects of medications) [54, 55].

3.3 Treatment Implications

Given that inflammation is likely a key pathophysiological nexus between psychiatric and medical comorbidity, targeting inflammation may potentially provide disease-modifying effects for both disease processes simultaneously [1, 46]. Understanding the factors that mediate or moderate the bidirectional interaction between psychiatric and medical comorbidities may serve to improve both medical and psychiatric outcomes. Towards this end, numerous anti-inflammatory agents have been evaluated in the treatment and prevention of mood and psychotic disorders [56]. Additionally, the use of anti-inflammatory agents has also been considered with specific symptom clusters, such as fatigue, cognitive function and anhedonia [57–59]. As inflammation is a transdiagnostic target, it may be that transdiagnostic symptom domains, such as cognitive function and anhedonia, may be more appropriate targets compared to targeting specific disorders [58, 60, 61].

Meta-analytic level data have suggested that anti-inflammatories may have antidepressant effects, at least in a subset of patients with immune dysfunction, such as patients with inflammatory conditions. In a meta-analysis assessing the effects of anti-inflammatory agents in the acute treatment of MDD, significant antidepressant effects were observed [62]. Thirty randomized clinical trials (RCTs) with a total of 1610 participants were identified and included in this meta-analysis. The overall pooled analysis suggested that anti-inflammatory agents reduced depressive symptoms (moderate effect size of 0.55) compared with placebo. Higher response (risk ratio (RR) 1.52) and remission rates (RR 1.79) were seen in the group receiving anti-inflammatory agents compared to placebo. Subgroup analysis demonstrated efficacy in both the monotherapy and adjunctive treatment groups. Subgroup analysis of nonsteroidal anti-inflammatory drugs, omega-3 fatty acids, statins and minocycline, respectively, demonstrated significant antidepressant effects, however, with significant heterogeneity in results with both positive and negative studies identified. This meta-analysis replicated and expanded upon similar previous meta-analyses demonstrating antidepressant effects of immune modulating agents [56, 63].

Similarly, anti-inflammatory agents have been evaluated in BD samples. In a meta-analysis conducted by our group, we identified ten RCTs assessing the acute antidepressant effects of adjunctive anti-inflammatory agents in the treatment of bipolar depression [64]. Eight RCTs (n = 312) assessing adjunctive NSAIDs, omega-3s, *N*-acetylcysteine (NAC) and pioglitazone were included in the quantitative analysis. The overall pooled effect size of adjunctive anti-inflammatories on depressive symptoms was 0.40 (95% confidence interval − 0.14 to −0.65 (P = 0.002)), indicative of a moderate and statistically significant antidepressant effect compared to conventional therapy alone. Notably, manic/hypomanic induction was equivalent to the control group. This proof-of-concept for anti-inflammatory agents for BD has been established in other meta-analyses and RCTs as well, however, has yet to be demonstrated in phase III trials [63].

Significant interest in anti-inflammatory agents for psychotic disorders has also been assessed with promising results. A recent meta-analysis examined anti-inflammatory agents (aspirin, celecoxib, omega-3 fatty acids, oestrogen, selective oestrogen receptor modulator, pregnenolone, NAC, minocycline, davunetide and erythropoietin) as augmenting treatments for schizophrenia. Sixty-two RCTs including a total of 2914 participants were included [65]. Significant moderate overall effects were found for anti-inflammatory agents for reducing total, positive and negative symptom scores in the Positive and Negative Syndrome Scale. Cognitive improvements were significant with minocycline and pregnenolone augmentation therapy. General functioning was significantly enhanced by overall anti-inflammatory agents. A previous meta-analysis had similar conclusions, however, emphasized that some, but not all agents with anti-inflammatory properties showed efficacy [66]. Effective agents were aspirin, oestrogens, minocycline and NAC. Subanalysis also revealed greater beneficial results on symptom severity in first episode psychosis, suggesting the potential importance of targeting the immune system early on in the trajectory of illness [66].

An important limitation of all the aforementioned meta-analyses is the small sample sizes used for the individual RCTs; clinical trials have primarily been phase II proof-of-concept studies rather than more definitive phase III RCTs required to establish efficacy for a new indication (e.g. use of anti-inflammatory agents for a psychiatric indication). As such, despite the promising results, anti-inflammatory agents are not indicated for psychiatric disorders as further larger phase III RCTs are still required to confirm or refute efficacy.

While there is significant promise in the use of anti-inflammatories in psychiatry as discussed further in other chapters, no single anti-inflammatory agent has been robustly demonstrated to have beneficial effects. However, inflammatory subgroups are the one to presumably benefit most. Patients with inflammatory comorbidities are likely to fall in this category. As such, anti-inflammatory agents might be most helpful in reducing psychological symptoms for patients with inflammatory comorbidities. For example, anti-inflammatory agents have demonstrated benefits for depressive symptoms in patients with psoriasis [67], IBD [41] and MS [68].

Outside of the biological implications of psychiatric and medical comorbidity, system level changes are also important and may have a role in modifying treatment outcomes [1]. As high rates of comorbidity are known, routine screening with care pathways may be considered in patients with inflammatory conditions who are at greater risk of psychiatric conditions and vice versa [10]. Indeed, numerous disorder specific clinics have adopted routine screening practices [69–71]. However, screening is only of benefits when a clear pathway to further assessment and treatment is in place. Collaborative care models have been established to integrate medical and psychiatric care, given the substantial overlap observed and recognition of reciprocally poorer outcomes with comorbidity [72, 73].

3.4 Conclusions

Medical and psychiatric disorders have tremendously high rates of comorbidity with numerous factors mediating and moderating the co-occurrence of disorders. Immune dysfunction presents as one key biological nexus that may be both a cause and effect of medical and psychiatric disorders, likely contributing to the high rates of comorbidity observed. As such, the immune system presents as a promising novel treatment target that may serve to simultaneously improve medical and psychiatric outcomes. However, use of anti-inflammatory agents for psychiatric disorders has yielded mixed results, and it remains unclear which specific immune modulating agents are beneficial and which specific subgroup of patients (based on symptoms, disorders, biomarkers, etc.) may benefit from immune treatments. Future longitudinal research to establish more clearly the mechanisms at play and effective means to modify immune-mediated pathological changes are needed to improve outcomes for this difficult to treat population with comorbid psychiatric and medical conditions.

References

1. Rosenblat JD, Kurdyak P, Cosci F, Berk M, Maes M, Brunoni AR, et al. Depression in the medically ill. Aust N Z J Psychiatry. 2020;54(4):346–66.
2. Jeste DV, Gladsjo JA, Lindamer LA, Lacro JP. Medical comorbidity in schizophrenia. Schizophr Bull. 1996;22(3):413–30.
3. Bahorik AL, Satre DD, Kline-Simon AH, Weisner CM, Campbell CI. Serious mental illness and medical comorbidities: findings from an integrated health care system. J Psychosom Res. 2017;100:35–45.
4. Kessler RC, Berglund P, Demler O, Jin R, Koretz D, Merikangas KR, et al. The epidemiology of major depressive disorder: results from the National Comorbidity Survey Replication (NCS-R). JAMA. 2003;289:3095–105.
5. Iacovides A, Siamouli M. Comorbid mental and somatic disorders: an epidemiological perspective. Curr Opin Psychiatry. 2008;21(4):417–21.
6. Chen KY, Evans R, Larkins S. Why are hospital doctors not referring to Consultation-Liaison Psychiatry?—a systemic review. BMC Psychiatry. 2016;16(1):390.
7. De Hert M, Correll CU, Bobes J, Cetkovich-Bakmas M, Cohen D, Asai I, et al. Physical illness in patients with severe mental disorders. I. Prevalence, impact of medications and disparities in health care. World Psychiatry. 2011;10:52–77.
8. Abeywardena MY, Leifert WR, Warnes KE, Varghese JN, Head RJ. Cardiovascular biology of interleukin-6. Curr Pharm Des. 2009;15:1809–21.
9. Iadecola C, Anrather J. The immunology of stroke: from mechanisms to translation. Nat Med. 2011;17:796–808.
10. Li M, Rosenblat J, Rodin G. Chapter 7: Depression. In: Levenson JL, editor. The American Psychiatric Association publishing textbook of psychosomatic medicine and Consultation-Liaison Psychiatry. 3rd ed. Philadelphia, PA: American Psychiatric Association; 2019. p. 245–60.
11. Gallo JJ, Hwang S, Joo JH, Bogner HR, Morales KH, Bruce ML, et al. Multimorbidity, depression, and mortality in primary care: randomized clinical trial of an evidence-based depression care management program on mortality risk. J Gen Intern Med. 2016;31(4):380–6.

12. Read JR, Sharpe L, Modini M, Dear BF. Multimorbidity and depression: a systematic review and meta-analysis. J Affect Disord. 2017;221:36–46.
13. Ali S, Stone MA, Peters JL, Davies MJ, Khunti K. The prevalence of co-morbid depression in adults with Type 2 diabetes: a systematic review and meta-analysis. Diabetic Med. 2006;23:1165–73.
14. Ciechanowski PS, Katon WJ, Russo JE. Depression and diabetes: impact of depressive symptoms on adherence, function, and costs. Arch Intern Med. 2000;160(21):3278–85.
15. Eshun-Wilson I, Siegfried N, Akena DH, Stein DJ, Obuku EA, Joska JA. Antidepressants for depression in adults with HIV infection. Cochrane Database Syst Rev. 2018;1:CD008525.
16. Geng Q, Zhang Q-E, Wang F, Zheng W, Ng CH, Ungvari GS, et al. Comparison of comorbid depression between irritable bowel syndrome and inflammatory bowel disease: a meta-analysis of comparative studies. J Affect Disord. 2018;237:37–46.
17. Han C, Lofland JH, Zhao N, Schenkel B. Increased prevalence of psychiatric disorders and health care-associated costs among patients with moderate-to-severe psoriasis. J Drugs Dermatol. 2011;10:843–50.
18. Palagini L, Mosca M, Tani C, Gemignani A, Mauri M, Bombardieri S. Depression and systemic lupus erythematosus: a systematic review. Lupus. 2013;22:409–16.
19. Penninx BWJH. Depression and cardiovascular disease: epidemiological evidence on their linking mechanisms. Neurosci Biobehav Rev. 2017;74:277–86.
20. Pérez-Stable EJ, Miranda J, Muñoz RF, Ying Y-W. Depression in medical outpatients: underrecognition and misdiagnosis. Arch Intern Med. 1990;150(5):1083–8.
21. Thom R, Silbersweig DA, Boland RJ. Major depressive disorder in medical illness: a review of assessment, prevalence, and treatment options. Psychosom Med. 2019;81:246–55.
22. Wang Y, Tang S, Xu S, Weng S, Liu Z. Association between diabetes and risk of suicide death: a meta-analysis of 3 million participants. Compr Psychiatry. 2016;71:11–6.
23. Bhattarai N, Charlton J, Rudisill C, Gulliford MC. Prevalence of depression and utilization of health care in single and multiple morbidity: a population-based cohort study. Psychol Med. 2013;43(7):1423–31.
24. Diniz BS, Butters MA, Albert SM, Dew MA, Reynolds CF. Late-life depression and risk of vascular dementia and Alzheimer's disease: systematic review and meta-analysis of community-based cohort studies. Br J Psychiatry. 2013;202:329–35.
25. Elger CE, Johnston SA, Hoppe C. Diagnosing and treating depression in epilepsy. Seizure. 2017;44:184–93.
26. Rickards H. Depression in neurological disorders: Parkinson's disease, multiple sclerosis, and stroke. J Neurol Neurosurg Psychiatry. 2005;76(suppl 1):i48–52.
27. Kessing LV, Vradi E, McIntyre RS, Andersen PK. Causes of decreased life expectancy over the life span in bipolar disorder. J Affect Disord. 2015;180:142–7.
28. Bachen EA, Chesney MA, Criswell LA. Prevalence of mood and anxiety disorders in women with systemic lupus erythematosus. Arthritis Rheum. 2009;61:822–9.
29. Eaton WW, Pedersen MG, Nielsen PR, Mortensen PB. Autoimmune diseases, bipolar disorder, and non-affective psychosis. Bipolar Disord. 2010;12:638–46.
30. Edwards LJ, Constantinescu CS. A prospective study of conditions associated with multiple sclerosis in a cohort of 658 consecutive outpatients attending a multiple sclerosis clinic. Mult Scler. 2004;10:575–81.
31. Hsu CC, Chen SC, Liu CJ, Lu T, Shen CC, Hu YW, et al. Rheumatoid arthritis and the risk of bipolar disorder: a nationwide population-based study. PLoS One. 2014;9:e107512.
32. Kupka RW, Nolen WA, Post RM, McElroy SL, Altshuler LL, Denicoff KD, et al. High rate of autoimmune thyroiditis in bipolar disorder: lack of association with lithium exposure. Biol Psychiatry. 2002;51:305–11.
33. Perugi G, Quaranta G, Belletti S, Casalini F, Mosti N, Toni C, et al. General medical conditions in 347 bipolar disorder patients: clinical correlates of metabolic and autoimmune-allergic diseases. J Affect Disord. 2014;170C:95–103.

34. Calkin C, van de Velde C, Ruzickova M, Slaney C, Garnham J, Hajek T, et al. Can body mass index help predict outcome in patients with bipolar disorder? Bipolar disorders. Bipolar Disord. 2009;11:650–6.
35. Fagiolini A, Kupfer DJ, Houck PR, Novick DM, Frank E. Obesity as a correlate of outcome in patients with bipolar I disorder. Am J Psychiatry. 2003;160(1):112–7.
36. Laursen TM. Causes of premature mortality in schizophrenia: a review of literature published in 2018. Curr Opin Psychiatry. 2019;32(5):388–93.
37. Fond G, Lançon C, Korchia T, Auquier P, Boyer L. The role of inflammation in the treatment of schizophrenia. Front Psych. 2020;11:160.
38. Cuijpers P, Vogelzangs N, Twisk J, Kleiboer A, Li J, Penninx BW. Comprehensive meta-analysis of excess mortality in depression in the general community versus patients with specific illnesses. Am J Psychiatry. 2014;171(4):453–62.
39. Machado MO, Veronese N, Sanches M, Stubbs B, Koyanagi A, Thompson T, et al. The association of depression and all-cause and cause-specific mortality: an umbrella review of systematic reviews and meta-analyses. BMC Med. 2018;16(1):112.
40. McIntyre RS, Konarski JZ, Soczynska JK, Wilkins K, Panjwani G, Bouffard B, et al. Medical comorbidity in bipolar disorder: implications for functional outcomes and health service utilization. Psychiatric Serv. 2006;57:1140–4.
41. Graff LA, Walker JR, Bernstein CN. Depression and anxiety in inflammatory bowel disease: a review of comorbidity and management. Inflamm Bowel Dis. 2009;15:1105–18.
42. Edwards VJ, Holden GW, Felitti VJ, Anda RF. Relationship between multiple forms of childhood maltreatment and adult mental health in community respondents: results from the adverse childhood experiences study. Am J Psychiatry. 2003;160(8):1453–60.
43. Kerker BD, Zhang J, Nadeem E, Stein REK, Hurlburt MS, Heneghan A, et al. Adverse childhood experiences and mental health, chronic medical conditions, and development in young children. Acad Pediatr. 2015;15(5):510–7.
44. Abbas AK, Lichtman AH, Pillai S. Cellular and molecular immunology. Vol. 7th. Philadelphia, PA: Elsevier Saunders; 2012. 545 p.
45. Dantzer R, O'Connor JC, Freund GG, Johnson RW, Kelley KW. From inflammation to sickness and depression: when the immune system subjugates the brain. Nat Rev Neurosci. 2008 Jan;9:46–56.
46. Rosenblat JD, Cha DS, Mansur RB, McIntyre RS. Inflamed moods: a review of the interactions between inflammation and mood disorders. Prog Neuro-Psychopharmacol Biol Psychiatry. 2014;53:23–34.
47. Walker JR, Graff LA, Dutz JP, Bernstein CN. Psychiatric disorders in patients with immune-mediated inflammatory diseases: prevalence, association with disease activity, and overall patient well-being. J Rheumatol Suppl. 2011;88:31–5.
48. Walker EA, Roy-Byrne PP, Katon WJ, Li L, Amos D, Jiranek G. Psychiatric illness and irritable bowel syndrome: a comparison with inflammatory bowel disease. Am J Psychiatry. 1990;147:1656–61.
49. Libby P, Ridker PM, Hansson GK. Leducq transatlantic network on A. Inflammation in atherosclerosis: from pathophysiology to practice. J Am Coll Cardiol. 2009;54:2129–38.
50. Boutzios G, Kaltsas G. Immune system effects on the endocrine system. In: De Groot LJ, Beck-Peccoz P, Chrousos G, Dungan K, Grossman A, Hershman JM, et al., editors. Endotext. South Dartmouth, MA: MDText.com, Inc.; 2000.
51. Matsuzawa Y. The metabolic syndrome and adipocytokines. FEBS Lett. 2006;580:2917–21.
52. Brydon L, Walker C, Wawrzyniak A, Whitehead D, Okamura H, Yajima J, et al. Synergistic effects of psychological and immune stressors on inflammatory cytokine and sickness responses in humans. Brain Behav Immun. 2009;23:217–24.
53. Frick LR, Williams K, Pittenger C. Microglial dysregulation in psychiatric disease. Clin Dev Immunol. 2013;2013:608654.

54. Danaei G, Ding EL, Mozaffarian D, Taylor B, Rehm J, Murray CJ, et al. The preventable causes of death in the United States: comparative risk assessment of dietary, lifestyle, and metabolic risk factors. PLoS Med. 2009;6:e1000058.
55. Gans RO. The metabolic syndrome, depression, and cardiovascular disease: interrelated conditions that share pathophysiologic mechanisms. Med Clin North Am. 2006;90:573–91.
56. Kohler O, Benros ME, Nordentoft M, Farkouh ME, Iyengar RL, Mors O, et al. Effect of anti-inflammatory treatment on depression, depressive symptoms, and adverse effects: a systematic review and meta-analysis of randomized clinical trials. JAMA Psychiatry. 2014;71(12):1381–91.
57. Rosenblat JD, Brietzke E, Mansur RB, Maruschak NA, Lee Y, McIntyre RS. Inflammation as a neurobiological substrate of cognitive impairment in bipolar disorder: evidence, pathophysiology and treatment implications. J Affect Disord. 2015;188:149–59.
58. Bedwell JS, Gooding DC, Chan CC, Trachik BJ. Anhedonia in the age of RDoC. Schizophr Res. 2014;160:226–7.
59. Almeida OP, Alfonso H, Jamrozik K, Hankey GJ, Flicker L. Aspirin use, depression, and cognitive impairment in later life: the health in men study. J Am Geriatr Soc. 2010;58:990–2.
60. Insel TR. The NIMH research domain criteria (RDoC) project: precision medicine for psychiatry. AJP. 2014;171(4):395–7.
61. Swardfager W, Rosenblat JD, Benlamri M, McIntyre RS. Mapping inflammation onto mood: inflammatory mediators of anhedonia. Neurosci Biobehav Rev. 2016;64:148–66.
62. Bai S, Guo W, Feng Y, Deng H, Li G, Nie H, et al. Efficacy and safety of anti-inflammatory agents for the treatment of major depressive disorder: a systematic review and meta-analysis of randomised controlled trials. J Neurol Neurosurg Psychiatry. 2020;91(1):21–32.
63. Husain MI, Strawbridge R, Stokes PR, Young AH. Anti-inflammatory treatments for mood disorders: systematic review and meta-analysis. J Psychopharmacol. 2017;31:1137–48.
64. Rosenblat JD, Kakar R, Berk M, Kessing LV, Vinberg M, Baune BT, et al. Anti-inflammatory agents in the treatment of bipolar depression: a systematic review and meta-analysis. Bipolar Disord. 2016;18:89–101.
65. Cho M, Lee TY, Kwak YB, Yoon YB, Kim M, Kwon JS. Adjunctive use of anti-inflammatory drugs for schizophrenia: a meta-analytic investigation of randomized controlled trials. Aust N Z J Psychiatry. 2019;53(8):742–59.
66. Çakici N, van Beveren NJM, Judge-Hundal G, Koola MM, Sommer IEC. An update on the efficacy of anti-inflammatory agents for patients with schizophrenia: a meta-analysis. Psychol Med. 2019;49(14):2307–19.
67. Tyring S, Gottlieb A, Papp K, Gordon K, Leonardi C, Wang A, et al. Etanercept and clinical outcomes, fatigue, and depression in psoriasis: double-blind placebo-controlled randomised phase III trial. Lancet. 2006;367:29–35.
68. Fiest KM, Walker JR, Bernstein CN, Graff LA, Zarychanski R, Abou-Setta AM, et al. Systematic review and meta-analysis of interventions for depression and anxiety in persons with multiple sclerosis. Mult Scler Relat Disord. 2016;5:12–26.
69. Andersen BL, DeRubeis RJ, Berman BS, Gruman J, Champion VL, Massie MJ, et al. Screening, assessment, and care of anxiety and depressive symptoms in adults with cancer: an American Society of Clinical Oncology guideline adaptation. J Clin Oncol. 2014;32:1605–19.
70. Hermanns N, Caputo S, Dzida G, Khunti K, Meneghini LF, Snoek F. Screening, evaluation and management of depression in people with diabetes in primary care. Prim Care Diabetes. 2013;7:1–10.
71. Kroenke K. Enhancing the clinical utility of depression screening. CMAJ. 2012;184(3):281–2.
72. Gilbody S, Bower P, Fletcher J, Richards D, Sutton AJ. Collaborative care for depression: a cumulative meta-analysis and review of longer-term outcomes. Arch Intern Med. 2006;166(21):2314–21.
73. Katon WJ, Lin EHB, Von Korff M, Ciechanowski P, Ludman EJ, Young B, et al. Collaborative care for patients with depression and chronic illnesses. N Engl J Med. 2010;363(27):2611–20.

4 Magnetic Resonance Imaging Measures of Neuroinflammation in Psychiatry

Maria A. Di Biase, Jordan A. Chad, and Ofer Pasternak

4.1 Magnetic Resonance Imaging (MRI)

Magnetic Resonance Imaging (MRI) is a powerful noninvasive technique that can provide diverse measures of brain structure and function. Many detailed resources regarding MRI physics are available (e.g., see [1, 2]). In brief, MRI applies a strong magnetic field that causes hydrogen nuclei in the brain to align with the direction of the field and to precess at a certain frequency that depends on the magnetic field strength. The signal used to create MR images is generated by transmitting a radiofrequency (RF) pulse (electromagnetic energy) at the precession frequency, which

Maria A. Di Biase and Jordan A. Chad authors contributed equally to this work.

M. A. Di Biase
Department of Psychiatry, Brigham and Women's Hospital, Harvard Medical School, Boston, MA, USA

Melbourne Neuropsychiatry Centre, Department of Psychiatry, University of Melbourne and Melbourne Health, Carlton South, VIC, Australia
e-mail: mdibiase1@bwh.harvard.edu

J. A. Chad
Department of Medical Biophysics, University of Toronto, Toronto, ON, Canada

Rotman Research Institute, Baycrest Health Sciences, Toronto, ON, Canada
e-mail: jchad@research.baycrest.org

O. Pasternak (✉)
Department of Psychiatry, Brigham and Women's Hospital, Harvard Medical School, Boston, MA, USA

Department of Radiology, Brigham and Women's Hospital, Harvard Medical School, Boston, MA, USA
e-mail: ofer@bwh.harvard.edu

M. Berk et al. (eds.), *Immuno-Psychiatry*, https://doi.org/10.1007/978-3-030-71229-7_4

is absorbed by hydrogen nuclei. Subsequently, hydrogen nuclei release the energy, which is detected by receiver coils and transformed into images. The energy from nuclei is released through an exponential decay process at different rates, governed by relaxation times known as T_1 and T_2. The relaxation times depend on the environment and interaction between molecules, which varies across tissues.

A range of MRI contrasts can be obtained by modifying imaging sequences and their parameters, as well as by combining data from several acquisitions. The resulting contrasts and measures can identify different processes and pathologies in the brain. Here, we specifically discuss MRI measures that can probe aspects of neuroinflammation—a dynamic multicellular reaction to restore tissue homeostasis (as described in Chap. 1).

4.2 Anatomical MRI Measures of Neuroinflammation

Anatomical MRI provides contrast that is weighted by relaxation times (i.e., T_1 or T_2) of different tissues [1, 2]. T_1 values relate to the physicochemical properties of macromolecules (such as proteins and phospholipids) and to macromolecular volume in general. T_1-weighted images provide high contrast between gray matter, white matter, and cerebrospinal fluid (CSF) and are thus useful for segmenting these broad tissue types as well as measuring their respective volumes. T_2 values relate to molecular motion and interactions between neighboring molecules. Accordingly, T_2 values are similar for gray and white matter, but higher in CSF and pathologies associated with excess water within tissue, such as vasogenic edema.

4.2.1 T_2-Weighted MRI

T_2-weighted MRI (Fig. 4.1a) forms part of routine clinical practice for identifying and monitoring brain lesions that are accompanied by vasogenic edema such as in multiple sclerosis (MS), stroke, and brain injuries, where T_2 hyperintensities reflect accumulated water content (prolonged T_2 values) [3]. As it is difficult to readily discern hyperintense lesions from CSF, T_2-weighted MRIs typically use fluid attenuation inversion recovery (FLAIR) sequences, which mitigate the effect of CSF to enhance hyperintensities [4]. FLAIR methods are commonly used to highlight hyperintensities associated with MS pathology. By contrast, hyperintensities encountered in psychiatric populations are subtle, albeit have been detected in schizophrenia [5], bipolar disorder [6], and depression [7], as well as several childhood neuropsychiatric disorders [8].

In such cases where hyperintensities are visually imperceptible (spatially constrained and/or subtle), quantifying the T_2 relaxation times may increase sensitivity to mild variations compared to qualitative visual inspection of T_2-weighted images. To this end, multiple T_2-weighted images are acquired with different echo times and are fit to the T_2 exponential decay model. If neuroinflammation is present, higher T_2 values are expected, as vasogenic edema increases extracellular water content, and the T_2 of free water is greater than that of tissue. Several studies have

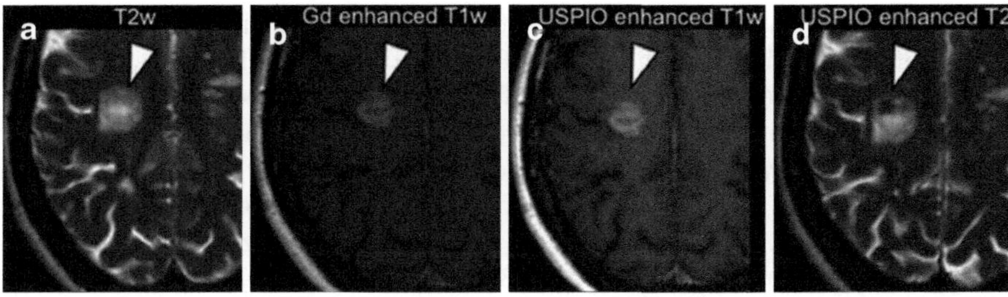

Fig. 4.1 Identifying neuroinflammation with anatomical MRI. Images from a relapsing–remitting MS patient. (**a**) T2-weighted (T2w), (**b**) Gd-enhanced T1-weighted (T1w), (**c**) ultrasmall superparamagnetic particles of iron oxide (USPIO)-enhanced T1w, and (**d**) USPIO-enhanced T2w maps from a relapsing–remitting multiple sclerosis patient demonstrate a large inflammatory lesion. The Gd enhancement reflects BBB breakdown, which is overlapping with USPIO enhancement (i.e., hyperintensity in T1w, and hypointensity in T2w) reflecting concomitant macrophage invasion. At the same time, the T2-hyperintensity suggests co-occurrence of vasogenic edema. Figure modified with permission from Tourdias and Dousset [29]

reported prolonged T_2 values in predominantly white matter of individuals with schizophrenia compared to healthy controls [9, 10].

While prolonged T_2 is often interpreted as neuroinflammation, it may reflect any change in water distribution (e.g., cerebral blood volume [11]) or in iron content [12, 13]. Therefore, caution is advised in extrapolating cellular or extracellular interpretations from T_2 findings. Interpretations of prolonged T_2 also vary within the context of psychiatry research. For example, studies in bipolar disorder have interpreted prolonged T_2 as reflecting vascular disruption [6], while studies in schizophrenia have construed prolonged T_2 as reflecting excessive interstitial water due to microstructural degeneration [9, 10]. To overcome challenges in specificity and elucidate potential sources underlying prolonged T_2 signals, studies have attempted to fit the T_2 decay curve to multiple compartments, such as free water and macromolecular-bound (myelin) water [14]. While this innovative approach can yield greater pathological specificity, it requires denser signal sampling (i.e., lengthier scan times) and elaborate mathematical fittings, which are not entirely stable.

Despite the aforementioned challenges of specificity, T_2 hyperintensities and quantitative T_2 values demonstrate high sensitivity to neuroinflammatory processes and may therefore rise in popularity for investigations in psychiatry.

4.2.2 Contrast-Enhanced MRI

T_1-weighted images are less sensitive to water content changes than T_2-weighted images. However, a contrast agent can be used to increase sensitivity of T_1-weighted images to other features of neuroinflammation. For example, gadolinium (Gd) is a nontoxic paramagnetic contrast-enhancement agent that can be injected during a T_1 scan. The interaction between Gd and hydrogen nuclei shortens the T_1 (and to a lesser extent, T_2) and, in turn, amplifies Gd signals in T_1-weighted images (Fig.

4.1b). As Gd molecules cannot pass an intact blood–brain barrier (BBB), increased signal outside blood vessels indicate BBB breakdown [15], which can result from neuroinflammation (e.g., accumulation of Aβ along brain blood vessels may cause vascular inflammation and BBB dysfunction) and/or induce neuroinflammatory processes (e.g., leaky BBB promotes macrophage infiltration) [16, 17]. Gd-enhanced T_1-weighted images have been used to characterize active lesions in MS (e.g., [18]) and brain tumors (e.g., [19]), but are less useful for characterizing neuroinflammatory processes in conditions where the BBB remains intact [20]. Gd-enhanced contrast is rarely applied to examine neuropathology in psychiatric disorders. The only schizophrenia study (to our knowledge) using Gd-enhanced contrast did not detect any discrete changes in BBB integrity in individuals with schizophrenia, although the sample size may have been too small ($n = 10$) to reveal significant differences [21].

Since this preliminary study, newer contrast agents and acquisitions have been developed, which may increase sensitivity to subtle BBB dysfunction (for a review, see [22]). For example, ultrasmall superparamagnetic particles of iron oxide (USPIO) have been developed as contrast agents for T_1- and T_2-weighted images (Fig. 4.1c, d), which may complement Gd signals [23]. Due to their physical properties and small size ($\approx$30 nm), USPIOs act as blood pool agents that are taken up by phagocytic cells (monocytes/macrophages), enabling direct information of immune cell infiltration. Studies in tumors (e.g., [24]) and MS (e.g., [25]) show that USPIO provides greater lesion enhancement than conventional Gd and therefore may detect subtle changes in vascular integrity. Another recent development provides noninvasive assessment of cerebral blood flow (i.e., without injecting contrast agents) via arterial spin labeling [26–28], although this approach may be less sensitive compared to contrast-based techniques.

Overall, added value may be gained by utilising contrast-enhanced MRI to capture immune dysregulation associated with BBB dysfunction.

4.3 Magnetization Transfer Imaging (MTI) Measures of Neuroinflammation

Magnetization Transfer Imaging (MTI) provides contrast based on the concentration of hydrogen nuclei bound to macromolecules relative to unbound hydrogen nuclei in free water. Under the assumption that inflammation increases extracellular water content, a decrease in the relative bound pool is considered a putative marker of inflammation.

MTI techniques exploit the fact that hydrogen nuclei bound to macromolecules experience off-resonance frequencies (due to variations in local magnetic fields) compared with unbound (free) hydrogen nuclei. The bound hydrogen nuclei interact with unbound hydrogen nuclei through chemical processes of diffusion and cross-relaxation [30]. MTI applies an initial preparation RF pulse at an off-resonance frequency such that it only excites the bound pool. Through chemical interactions, this magnetization is partially transferred from the bound pool to the unbound pool.

Thus, when the standard resonance RF pulse is subsequently applied, the unbound pool is already partially saturated, and the magnetization transfer can be measured by comparing the signal obtained in this acquisition with the signal obtained in another acquisition without the preparation pulse.

While the MTI contrast is qualitatively similar to a T1-weighted contrast, which is also sensitive to physiochemical environments, MTI provides a unique quantitative metric, namely the magnetization transfer ratio (MTR), which measures the ratio between the bound and unbound water pools [31]. Elevated water content by inflammatory processes leads to lower MTR values, as seen in MS patients with edema [32, 33]. MTI studies in psychiatry have reported lower MTR values in the cingulum bundle of individuals with schizophrenia relative to healthy controls [34]. Furthermore, lower MTR values have been observed in individuals with affective disorders, particularly in callosal and limbic brain regions [35–37]. More elaborate MTI models can provide measures of the cross-relaxation rate between bound and unbound water pools, as well as the volume fraction of each pool [38, 39]; however, these models have not been applied in psychiatry neuroimaging investigations.

The relative presence of bound and unbound protons probed by MTI can provide complementary information to anatomical MRI measures for detecting putative neuroinflammation. However, similar to T_2-weighted hyperintensities, MTI cannot yield direct or specific measures of inflammation. For instance, neuropathological [31] and translational animal studies [40, 41] have shown that MTI-derived metrics relate both to features of demyelination (i.e., less macromolecules) and to inflammation. Further experimental studies are needed to confirm the sources of MTI variation to enable more specific conclusions within disease-specific contexts.

4.4 Diffusion MRI Measures of Neuroinflammation

Whereas anatomical MRI and MTI index the relative presence of accumulated water, diffusion MRI measures the direction and amplitude of water motion. This is achieved by acquiring multiple images, each with a magnetic gradient applied along a given direction and by sensitizing the MRI signal to water molecule displacement along that direction [42]. Mathematical models can be applied to the diffusion MRI signal to extract quantitative metrics. The most common model employed in diffusion MRI is the diffusion tensor imaging (DTI) model [43]. DTI models diffusion as a 3D spherical ellipsoid (tensor), where the ellipsoid shape and orientation provide information about underlying white matter microstructure and the direction of white matter fibers. A variety of scalar measures can be derived from the diffusion tensor, such as the mean diffusivity (MD), which represents the average amplitude of diffusion within a voxel. DTI measures have shown high sensitivity and clinical utility across numerous neurological and psychiatric illnesses [44]. The MD measure was the first proposed diffusion MRI proxy for neuroinflammation, as higher diffusion coincides with higher water content in inflammatory injuries [45] and MS lesions [46, 47].

4.4.1 Free-Water Imaging

A fundamental limitation of DTI measures is that, like T_2 and MTI measures, they are inherently non-specific. Fluctuating MD signals can result from a variety of underlying processes, including inflammation or alterations in tissue microstructure [46, 47]. A more recent diffusion MRI method called free-water imaging attempts to address this issue by modeling diffusion with a two-compartment model: (a) the tissue compartment, modeled by a tensor, and (b) the free-water (FW) compartment, modeled as isotropic free diffusion [48], which captures extracellular water molecules that are free to diffuse, such as those found in CSF, blood and large enough pockets of interstitial fluid. FW is thus expected to provide a more specific diffusion MRI measure of vasogenic edema, characterized by extracellular fluid accumulation. Although direct validation studies are not yet available, initial support linking FW to inflammation derives from a recent animal study, which observed excess FW in the adult rat progeny of immune-challenged mothers (Fig. 4.2a). Importantly, the maternal immune activation model employed by this study is known to induce a robust neuroinflammatory response in the immune-challenged progeny reflected in increased levels of brain [50] and peripheral [51] proinflammatory cytokines as well as excessively activated microglia [52–56].

Free-water imaging has been applied to examine schizophrenia pathophysiology. A preliminary study observed widespread FW elevations in individuals with first episode psychosis (FEP) compared to controls [57] (Fig. 4.2b). These findings were since replicated in a larger sample of individuals presenting with FEP [58]. Interestingly, increased FW levels were not detected in individuals with prolonged illness duration, termed 'chronic schizophrenia' [59]. It was thus postulated that excess FW parallels acute psychosis onset or relapse. Consistent with this hypothesis, excess FW was observed in a subset of chronic schizophrenia patients presenting with (state-related) delusions compared to both chronic patients with remitted delusions and healthy controls [60]. The hypothesized time course of excess FW arising amid acute psychoses

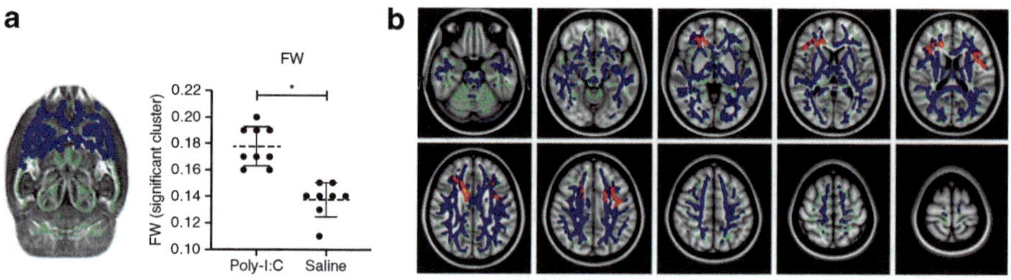

Fig. 4.2 Increased free water (FW). (**a**) Rats exposed to a prenatal immune challenge exhibit increased FW (blue) throughout callosal, external capsule, and striatal regions throughout the white matter skeleton (green) [49]. (**b**) Individuals with a first episode of psychosis showed a widespread increase in FW values (dark blue) throughout the white matter skeleton (green). Additionally, a focal reduction in free-water corrected (tissue-specific) fractional anisotropy (red) was found in frontal white matter. Figure (**a**) reproduced with permission from Di Biase and colleagues [49] and (**b**) from Pasternak and colleagues [57]

accords with the neuroinflammatory hypothesis that acute psychosis coincides with increased neuroinflammatory events [61]. Thus, while FW is not a direct measure of neuroinflammation, it may serve as a neuroinflammatory-linked biomarker for acute illness phases in schizophrenia. Applications of FW imaging in other psychiatric populations are underway; for example, widespread excess FW was recently reported in individuals with chronic bipolar disorder [62].

Aside from free-water imaging, FW can be extracted from diffusion MRI with models such as neurite orientation dispersion and density imaging (NODDI) [63]; diffusion basis spectrum imaging [64]; and multiple fascicle models [65]. The first of these—a variant of NODDI—has been applied to examine free-water levels in schizophrenia, which identified excess white matter FW in these individuals [66]. The tentative reproducibility of FW findings across studies, image acquisitions, and compartmental models lends support to its use in psychiatry for indexing putative neuroinflammatory processes linked to diffusional flow in blood, interstitial fluid, and CSF.

4.5 Magnetic Resonance Spectroscopy (MRS) Measures of Neuroinflammation

All of the aforementioned MRI modalities can examine whole-brain, voxelwise or regional inflammatory processes. Alternatively, magnetic resonance spectroscopy (MRS) probes molecular signatures of inflammation within specific regions or voxels. As mentioned above, nuclei in different chemical environments precess at different frequencies. As such, hydrogen nuclei that belong to different metabolites experience different frequency shifts (chemical shift). ^{1}H MRS quantifies metabolite concentrations based on the spectra of chemical shifts from the collection of hydrogen nuclei in a specified region [67]. The most prominent peak in ^{1}H MRS spectra is water, as the relative concentration of water to brain metabolites is about 10,000:1. Water can be suppressed from the spectra to enhance other peaks, and further spectral editing can reveal the presence of metabolites with relatively low concentrations, such as gamma-aminobutyric acid (GABA) (Fig. 4.3).

MRS studies have primarily targeted the following seven metabolites to examine neuroinflammatory processes in psychiatric disorders (refer to Table 4.1): (a) *N*-acetyl aspartate (NAA); (b) myo-inositol (MI); (c) choline (Cho); (d) creatine (Cr); (e) glutamate (Glu); (f) glutamine (Gln); and (g) glutathione (GSH).

NAA is the most dominant peak in the water suppressed ^{1}H MRS spectra and is located solely in neurons and not glial cells. As such, NAA is widely accepted as a neuronal marker. A large meta-analytic review of over 60 studies using ^{1}H MRS to measure NAA in schizophrenia concluded that NAA levels are reduced in broad-ranging regions of the brain in patients compared to controls [69]. Reduced NAA has further been reported in major depressive disorder [70] and bipolar disorder [71], suggesting that neuronal dysfunction may reflect a common pathophysiological feature across neuropsychiatric disorders. However, the precise function of NAA remains undetermined.

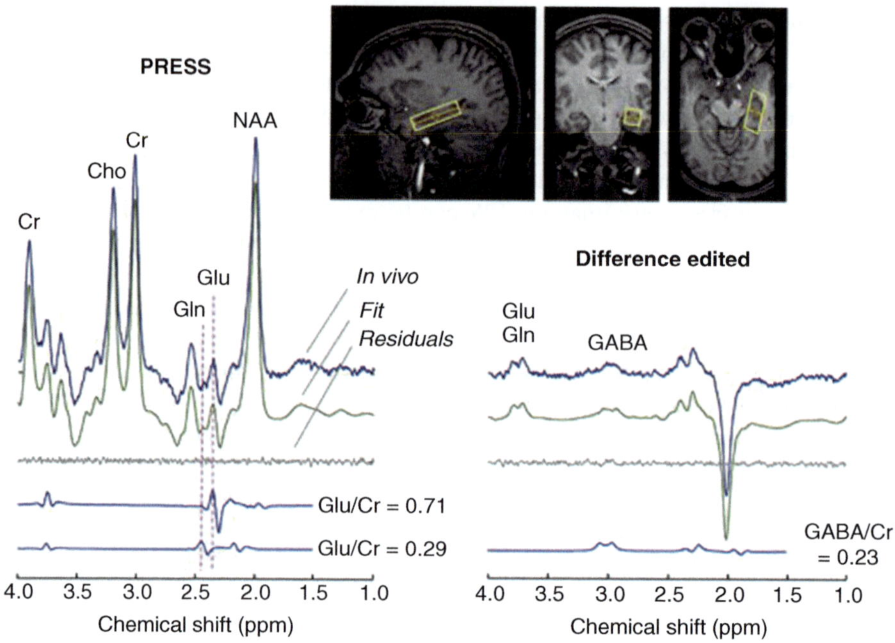

Fig. 4.3 Identifying molecular signatures of neuroinflammation with MRS. Representative MR spectra are displayed, as well as T1w images showing the brain voxel locations of spectra obtained from an individual with schizophrenia. Glutamate (Glu), glutamine (Gln), and gamma-aminobutyric acid (GABA) are shown with their concentration ratio to creatine. Point-Resolved Spectroscopy (PRESS) and difference-edited spectra are scaled equal. *NAA* = *N*-acetylaspartate. Reprinted with permission from Stan and colleagues [68]

Table 4.1 MRS-probed Metabolites Involved with neuroinflammatory processes

Proton MRS metabolite	Putative inflammatory marker	Neuroinflammatory phenomena
N-acetyl aspartate (NAA)	Neuronal viability and integrity	Neuronal degeneration, which may precede or follow neuroinflammatory events
Myo-inositol (MI)	Myeloid/glial cell activation, proliferation or signaling	Glial cell activation, which forms part of an immune response to infections or trauma in the brain
Choline (Cho)	Cell membranes turnover	Choline levels, where higher levels attenuate neuroinflammatory processes and suppress oxidative stress
Creatine (Cr)	Energy metabolism	Anti-inflammatory effects through inhibiting TNF-a
Glutamate (Glu)	Glutamate neurotransmitter release	Glutamate–glial–cytokine interactions. For example, glial cell activation could result in excess glutamate by decreasing the capacity of glial transporters to buffer and clear glutamate cell proliferation and apoptosis
Glutamine (Gln)	Glutamate synthesis	
Glutathione (GSH)	Antioxidant defense	

In addition to absolute NAA concentration, NAA is commonly reported relative to Cr or Cho, and decreases in the concentration ratios of these metabolites are also frequently reported across neuropsychiatric disorders. The biological interpretation of concentration ratios warrants caution, given the distinct functions and regional specificity of these metabolites. In particular, concentrations of Cho and Cr are two- to three-fold higher in glial cells compared to neurons [72]. The total creatine (tCr) peak includes both creatine and phosphocreatine, reflecting levels of cellular energy metabolites, while Cho is a marker of cell membrane metabolism and cellular turnover [73]. Given the complexity of these markers in isolation, concentration ratios (i.e., NAA/Cr and NAA/Cho) may be challenging to interpret, particularly in a psychiatric setting where disease mechanisms remain unclear.

In recent years, cumulative evidence has demonstrated glial alterations in neuropsychiatric disorders. MI is thought to be a marker of astrocytes and plays important roles in calcium-mediated glutamatergic signaling and maintenance of metabolism [74]. Whereas increases in MI concentration could reflect classic inflammatory responses, including glial cell activation, gliosis, or hyperosmolarity, decreases could reflect the converse—glial cell dysfunction due to reduced cell proliferation and signaling (e.g., reduced glutamate clearance from the synaptic cleft leading to glutamate excitotoxity) or hypoosmolarity. A recent meta-analysis reported a small but significant reduction in MI concentration in the medial prefrontal cortex of individuals with schizophrenia compared to controls [74]. In addition to schizophrenia, reduced MI is commonly reported as spatially distributed in childhood autism [75]. Conversely, MI is elevated in individuals with bipolar disorder; complementarily, reduced MI has been proposed as a measure of lithium treatment response [76].

Glial-mediated inflammation can disturb equilibrium in cortical excitation/inhibition, which is maintained by Glu and Gln—amino acid neurotransmitters concentrated in gray matter. Glu is the most abundant neurotransmitter and plays key roles in various neurodevelopmental processes including neural migration, differentiation, and metabolism. However, excessive glutamate action, induced, for example, by activated glia, could contribute to excitotoxicity and produce psychiatric phenotypes. Furthermore, activation of NMDA receptors by excessive Glu can trigger glial-mediated inflammation, which further perpetuates a neuroinflammatory cycle. The majority of Glu is synthesized by Gln, and hence, increased Gln may beget increased glutamatergic activity. At high MRI field strengths, ^{1}H-MRS can provide concentration estimates for Glu and Gln in isolation, but at lower field strengths, Glu and Gln signals are combined to yield Glx (i.e., Glx = Glu + Gln). Elevated levels of glutamatergic indices (Glu, Gln, Glx, Glu/Gln) have been reported in the medial prefrontal cortex and basal ganglia of medication-naïve schizophrenia individuals, and decreases have been reported following treatment and with increasing age/illness progression [77, 78]. Both higher and lower Glu concentrations have been reported in select brain regions in childhood autism [75] and affective disorders [79, 80]. Decreased Glu and Gln could indicate altered synaptic activity, altered glutamate receptor functioning, abnormal glutamine–glutamate cycling, or dysfunctional glutamate transport [78].

Glu is also used by the brain to synthesize glutathione (GSH), a major antioxidant involved in cell proliferation and apoptosis. GSH is highly concentrated in glia [81] and has thus become a popular putative index of neuroinflammation in psychiatry research [82]. A recent meta-analysis identified elevated GSH in bipolar disorder, but reduced GSH in schizophrenia in the anterior cingulate cortex, possibly suggesting divergent mechanisms in the cortical antioxidant system between psychotic and affective diagnoses [82]. These findings are notably consistent with elevated MI in bipolar disorder and reduced MI in schizophrenia, indicating that MI and GSH may provide complementary markers of glial function.

On one hand, MRS is limited by poor spatial resolution and minimal brain coverage, but on the other, it provides specific molecular signatures of neuroinflammation within such regions. One possibility to address poor spatial resolution (by virtue of large voxel size) is to increase scanning acquisition times; however, this may be unfeasible due to lengthy scan durations required by standard MRS acquisitions (up to ~10 min for 5 cm^3 voxel size depending on the acquisition technique). If scan time permits, applying additional magnetic gradients can achieve multivoxel MRS and, in turn, resolve the spectra in 2D or even 3D, capturing potential variation in the cellular dynamics of inflammation across distinct brain regions [83]. Moreover, MRS can be combined with MRI-based molecular imaging approaches, such as molecular labeling with contrast agents, to target specific facets of neuroinflammation [84].

4.6 Conclusions

MRI is paving the way for noninvasive, in-vivo measurement of putative neuroinflammatory processes. In recent years, psychiatry research has applied a range of inflammation-linked measures—T_2 hyperintensities and values, magnetization transfer ratios, diffusional free water, and putative markers of neuronal and glial dysregulation—to advance our knowledge regarding immune dysregulation in neuropsychiatric illness.

MRI-derived measures of neuroinflammation are increasingly applied to examine schizophrenia and affective disorders. These studies have shed light on regional variation of putative neuroinflammatory effects. For example, lower MTR values (elevated water content relative to macromolecules) are circumscribed to the cingulum in schizophrenia and spatially dispersed in affective disorders. In contrast, larger areas of T_2 hyperintensities are seen in individuals with schizophrenia relative to those with affective disorders. Furthermore, MRI studies have begun to elucidate the clinical relevance of putative inflammatory markers. For example, excess free-water movement is seen in early psychosis and in acute delusional states, which lends support to the neuroinflammatory hypothesis of acute psychosis. Lastly, the use of MRS has led to unprecedented insights regarding specific inflammatory processes, such as neuronal dysfunction (e.g., reduced N-acetyl aspartate, NAA) and glial dysfunction (e.g., reduced myo-inositol, MI), which were traditionally viewed as pathologies of classical neurodegenerative conditions.

The MRI measures reviewed in this chapter probe various aspects of neuroinflammation, such as accumulated water content (T_2-weighted MRI) and, more specifically, water content relative to macromolecules (MTI), increased water diffusion (diffusion MRI), and BBB dysfunction (Gd-enhanced T_1-weighted MRI). It is important to note, however, that these measures are not specific to inflammation but instead reflect a combination of molecular, cellular, geometric, and artefact-related factors that govern each signal. For instance, T_2-hyperintensities indicate accumulated water content, which may derive from a variety of inflammation-related (e.g., vasodilation, swollen glia, BBB dysfunction) and tissue-related (e.g., demyelination leading to increased extracellular water) sources. As such, future work will benefit from animal models to validate interpretations, as well as multimodal MRI approaches that can deconstruct potential pathologies. To this end, measures of water content can be combined with magnetic resonance spectroscopy to probe specific molecular signatures of inflammation (e.g., MI) and neuronal pathology (e.g., NAA) within brain regions exhibiting excess free water. Furthermore, water-linked measures in conjunction with perfusion measures, such as arterial-spin labeling and contrast-enhanced measures, could further distinguish whether excess water arises from blood vessel breakdown or enlarged interstitial space. Lastly, MRI data could be measured alongside positron emission tomography (PET) using specific radioligands for the translocator protein (TSPO) to concurrently index putative microglial activation. Collectively, these multimodal approaches may help to localize neuroinflammatory processes, pinpoint pharmacological targets, and differentiate patient subsets for clinical trials.

It will be crucial moving forward to assess whether neuroinflammation-linked MRI measures can predict symptom/functional outcomes and treatment response in psychiatry. Given the established sensitivity of these measures to psychiatric disorders, as well as their ease of access and use, it stands to reason that immune-related MRI measures hold enormous potential for enhancing diagnostic and prognostic efforts in psychiatry.

References

1. Mansfield P, Morris PG. NMR imaging in biomedicine. New York: Academic Press; 1982.
2. Haacke EM, Brown RW, Thompson MR, Venkatesan R. Magnetic resonance imaging: physical principles and sequence design. New York: Wiley; 1999.
3. Husstedt H, Sickert M, Köstler H, Haubitz B, Becker H. Diagnostic value of the fast-FLAIR sequence in MR imaging of intracranial tumors. Eur Radiol. 2000;10(5):745–52.
4. Castillo M, Mukherji SK. Clinical applications of FLAIR, HASTE, and magnetization transfer in neuroimaging. Semin Ultras CT MRI. 2000;21(6):417–27.
5. Persaud R, Russow H, Harvey I, Lewis SW, Ron M, Murray RM, du Boulay G. Focal signal hyperintensities in schizophrenia. Schizophr Res. 1997;27(1):55–64.
6. Beyer JL, Young R, Kuchibhatla M, Krishnan KRR, Hyperintense MRI. lesions in bipolar disorder: a meta-analysis and review. Int Rev Psychiatry. 2009;21(4):394–409.
7. Agid R, Levin T, Gomori JM, Lerer B, Bonne O. T2-weighted image hyperintensities in major depression: focus on the basal ganglia. Int J Neuropsychopharmacol. 2003;6:215–24.

8. Amat JA, Bronen RA, Saluja S, Sato N, Zhu H, Gorman DA, Royal J, Peterson BS. Increased number of subcortical hyperintensities on MRI in children and adolescents with Tourette's syndrome, obsessive-compulsive disorder, and attention deficit hyperactivity disorder. Am J Psychiatr. 2005;163(6):1106–8.
9. Pfefferbaum A, Sullivan EV, Hedehus M, Moseley M, Lim KO. Brain gray and white matter transverse relaxation time in schizophrenia. Psychiatry Res. 1999;91(2):93–100.
10. Du F, Cooper A, Cohen BM, Renshaw PF, Öngür D. Water and metabolite transverse T2 relaxation time abnormalities in the white matter in schizophrenia. Schizophr Res. 2012;137(1–3):241–5.
11. Anderson C, Kaufman M, Lowen S, Rohan M, Renshaw P, Teicher M. Brain T2 relaxation times correlate with regional cerebral blood volume. MAGMA. 2005;18(1):3–6.
12. Vymazal J, Hajek M, Patronas N, Giedd JN, Bulte JW, Baumgarner C, et al. The quantitative relation between T1-weighted and T2-weighted MRI of normal gray matter and iron concentration. J Magn Reson Imaging. 1995;5(5):554–60.
13. Vymazal J, Brooks RA, Baumgarner C, Tran V, Katz D, Bulte JW, et al. The relation between brain iron and NMR relaxation times: an in vitro study. Magn Reson Med. 1996;35(1):56–61.
14. Alonso-Ortiz E, Levesque IR, Pike GB. MRI-based myelin water imaging: a technical review. Magn Reson Med. 2015;73(1):70–81.
15. Brück W, Bitsch A, Kolenda H, Brück Y, Stiefel M, Lassmann H. Inflammatory central nervous system demyelination: correlation of magnetic resonance imaging findings with lesion pathology. Ann Neurol. 1997;42(5):783–93.
16. Kinnecom C, Lev M, Wendell L, Smith E, Rosand J, Frosch M, et al. Course of cerebral amyloid angiopathy–related inflammation. Neurology. 2007;68(17):1411–6.
17. Godbout JP, Johnson RW. Age and neuroinflammation: a lifetime of psychoneuroimmune consequences. Immunol Allergy Clin N Am. 2009;29(2):321–37.
18. Grossman RI, Gonzalez-Scarano F, Atlas SW, Galetta S, Silberberg D. Multiple sclerosis: gadolinium enhancement in MR imaging. Radiology. 1986;161(3):721–5.
19. Claussen C, Laniado M, Schörner W, Niendorf H-P, Weinmann H-J, Fiegler W, et al. Gadolinium-DTPA in MR imaging of glioblastomas and intracranial metastases. Am J Neuroradiol. 1985;6(5):669–74.
20. Rausch M, Hiestand P, Baumann D, Cannet C, Rudin M. MRI-based monitoring of inflammation and tissue damage in acute and chronic relapsing EAE. Magn Reson Med. 2003;50(2):309–14.
21. Szymanski S, Ashtari M, Zito J, Degreef G, Bogerts B, Lieberman J. Gadolinium-DTPA enhanced gradient echo magnetic resonance scans in first episode of psychosis and chronic schizophrenic patients. Psychiatry Res. 1991;40(3):203–7.
22. Heye AK, Culling RD, Valdés Hernández Mdel C, Thrippleton MJ, Wardlaw JM. Assessment of blood-brain barrier disruption using dynamic contrast-enhanced MRI. A systematic review. Neuroimage Clin. 2014;6:262–74.
23. Corot C, Robert P, Idée J-M, Port M. Recent advances in iron oxide nanocrystal technology for medical imaging. Adv Drug Deliv Rev. 2006;58(14):1471–504.
24. Taschner CA, Wetzel SG, Tolnay M, Froehlich J, Merlo A, Radue EW. Characteristics of ultrasmall superparamagnetic iron oxides in patients with brain tumors. Am J Roentgenol. 2005;185(6):1477–86.
25. Vellinga MM, Oude Engberink RD, Seewann A, Pouwels PJ, Wattjes MP, van der Pol SM, et al. Pluriformity of inflammation in multiple sclerosis shown by ultra-small iron oxide particle enhancement. Brain. 2008;131(3):800–7.
26. Hales PW, Clark CA. Combined arterial spin labeling and diffusion-weighted imaging for noninvasive estimation of capillary volume fraction and permeability-surface product in the human brain. J Cereb Blood Flow Metab. 2013;33(1):67–75.
27. Lin Z, Li Y, Su P, Mao D, Wei Z, Pillai JJ, et al. Non-contrast MR imaging of blood-brain barrier permeability to water. Magn Reson Med. 2018;80(4):1507–20.
28. Shao X, Sj MA, Casey M, D'Orazio L, Ringman JM, Wang DJJ. Mapping water exchange across the blood-brain barrier using 3D diffusion-prepared arterial spin labeled perfusion MRI. Magn Reson Med. 2019;81(5):3065–79.

29. Tourdias T, Dousset V. Neuroinflammatory imaging biomarkers: relevance to multiple sclerosis and its therapy. Neurotherapeutics. 2013;10(1):111–23.
30. Henkelman R, Stanisz G, Graham S. Magnetization transfer in MRI: a review. NMR Biomed. 2001;14(2):57–64.
31. Sled JG. Modelling and interpretation of magnetization transfer imaging in the brain. NeuroImage. 2018;182:128–35.
32. Laule C, Vavasour IM, Kolind SH, Li DK, Traboulsee TL, Moore GW, et al. Magnetic resonance imaging of myelin. Neurotherapeutics. 2007;4(3):460–84.
33. Vavasour IM, Laule C, Li DKB, Traboulsee AL, MacKay AL. Is the magnetization transfer ratio a marker for myelin in multiple sclerosis? J Magn Reson Imaging. 2011;33(3):710–8.
34. Palaniyappan L, Al-Radaideh A, Mougin O, Das T, Gowland P, Liddle PF. Aberrant myelination of the cingulum and Schneiderian delusions in schizophrenia: a 7T magnetization transfer study. Psychol Med. 2019;49:1890–6.
35. Kumar A, Gupta RC, Thomas MA, Alger J, Wyckoff N, Hwang S. Biophysical changes in normal-appearing white matter and subcortical nuclei in late-life major depression detected using magnetization transfer. Psychiatry Res. 2004;130(2):131–40.
36. Gunning-Dixon FM, Hoptman MJ, Lim KO, Murphy CF, Klimstra S, Latoussakis V, et al. Macromolecular white matter abnormalities in geriatric depression: a magnetization transfer imaging study. Am J Geriatr Psychiatry. 2008;16(4):255–62.
37. Bruno S, Barker G, Cercignani M, Symms M, Ron M. A study of bipolar disorder using magnetization transfer imaging and voxel-based morphometry. Brain. 2004;127(11):2433–40.
38. Yarnykh VL. Pulsed Z-spectroscopic imaging of cross-relaxation parameters in tissues for human MRI: theory and clinical applications. Magn Reson Med. 2002;47(5):929–39.
39. Yarnykh VL, Yuan C. Cross-relaxation imaging reveals detailed anatomy of white matter fiber tracts in the human brain. NeuroImage. 2004;23(1):409–24.
40. Stanisz GJ, Webb S, Munro CA, Pun T, Midha R. MR properties of excised neural tissue following experimentally induced inflammation. Magn Reson Med. 2004;51(3):473–9.
41. Odrobina EE, Lam TY, Pun T, Midha R, Stanisz GJ. MR properties of excised neural tissue following experimentally induced demyelination. NMR Biomed. 2005;18(5):277–84.
42. Le Bihan D, Turner R, Douek P, Patronas N. Diffusion MR imaging: clinical applications. Am J Roentgenol. 1992;159(3):591–9.
43. Basser PJ, Mattiello J, Le Bihan D. MR diffusion tensor spectroscopy and imaging. Biophys J. 1994;66(1):259–67.
44. Assaf Y, Pasternak O. Diffusion tensor imaging (DTI)-based white matter mapping in brain research: a review. J Mol Neurosci. 2008;34(1):51–61.
45. Lodygensky GA, West T, Stump M, Holtzman DM, Inder TE, Neil JJ, In vivo MRI. analysis of an inflammatory injury in the developing brain. Brain Behav Immun. 2010;24(5):759–67.
46. Tievsky AL, Ptak T, Farkas J. Investigation of apparent diffusion coefficient and diffusion tensor anisotropy in acute and chronic multiple sclerosis lesions. AJNR Am J Neuroradiol. 1999;20(8):1491–9.
47. Werring DJ, Clark CA, Barker GJ, Thompson AJ, Miller DH. Diffusion tensor imaging of lesions and normal-appearing white matter in multiple sclerosis. Neurology. 1999;52(8):1626–32.
48. Pasternak O, Sochen N, Gur Y, Intrator N, Assaf Y. Free water elimination and mapping from diffusion MRI. Magn Reson Med. 2009;62(3):717–30.
49. Di Biase MA, Katabi G, Piontkewitz Y, Cetin-Karayumak S, Weiner I, Pasternak O. Increased extracellular free-water in adult male rats following in utero exposure to maternal immune activation. Brain Behav Immun. 2019;83:283–7.
50. Garay PA, Hsiao EY, Patterson PH, McAllister AK. Maternal immune activation causes age- and region-specific changes in brain cytokines in offspring throughout development. Brain Behav Immun. 2013;31:54–68.
51. Romero E, Ali C, Molina-Holgado E, Castellano B, Guaza C, Borrell J. Neurobehavioral and immunological consequences of prenatal immune activation in rats. Influence of antipsychotics. Neuropsychopharmacology. 2007;32(8):1791.

52. Duchatel RJ, Meehan CL, Harms LR, Michie PT, Bigland MJ, Smith DW, et al. Late gestation immune activation increases IBA1-positive immunoreactivity levels in the corpus callosum of adult rat offspring. Psychiatry Res. 2018;266:175–85.
53. Hadar R, Dong L, del-Valle-Anton L, Guneykaya D, Voget M, Edemann-Callesen H, et al. Deep brain stimulation during early adolescence prevents microglial alterations in a model of maternal immune activation. Brain Behav Immun. 2017;63:71–80.
54. Murray KN, Edye ME, Manca M, Vernon AC, Oladipo JM, Fasolino V, et al. Evolution of a maternal immune activation (mIA) model in rats: early developmental effects. Brain Behav Immun. 2019;75:48–59.
55. Smolders S, Notter T, Smolders SMT, Rigo JM, Brone B. Controversies and prospects about microglia in maternal immune activation models for neurodevelopmental disorders. Brain Behav Immun. 2018;73:51–65.
56. Notter T, Coughlin JM, Sawa A, Meyer U. Reconceptualization of translocator protein as a biomarker of neuroinflammation in psychiatry. Mol Psychiatry. 2018;23(1):36–47.
57. Pasternak O, Westin CF, Bouix S, Seidman LJ, Goldstein JM, Woo TUW, et al. Excessive extracellular volume reveals a neurodegenerative pattern in schizophrenia onset. J Neurosci. 2012;32:17365–72.
58. Lyall AE, Pasternak O, Rbinson DG, Newell D, Trampush JW, Gallego JA, et al. Greater extracellular free water in first-episode psychosis predicts better neurocognitive functioning. Mol Psychiatry. 2018;23(3):701–7.
59. Pasternak O, Westin CF, Bahlben B, Bouix S, Kubicki M. The extent of diffusion MRI markers of neuroinflammation and white matter deterioration in chronic schizophrenia. Schizophr Res. 2015;161(1):113–8.
60. Oestreich LK, Lyall AE, Pasternak O, Kikinis Z, Newell DT, Savadjiev P, et al. Characterizing white matter changes in chronic schizophrenia: a free-water imaging multi-site study. Schizophr Res. 2017;189:153–61.
61. Monji A, Kato TA, Mizoguchi Y, Horikawa H, Seki Y, Kasai M, et al. Neuroinflammation in schizophrenia especially focused on the role of microglia. Prog Neuro-Psychopharmacol Biol Psychiatry. 2013;42:115–21.
62. Tuozzo C, Lyall AE, Pasternak O, James ACD, Crow TJ, Kubicki M. Patients with chronic bipolar disorder exhibit widespread increases in extracellular free water. Bipolar Disord. 2018;20(6):523–30.
63. Zhang H, Schneider T, Wheeler-Kingshott CA, Alexander DC. NODDI: practical in vivo neurite orientation dispersion and density imaging of the human brain. NeuroImage. 2012;61(4):1000–16.
64. Wang Y, Wang Q, Haldar JP, Yeh FC, Xie M, Sun P, et al. Quantification of increased cellularity during inflammatory demyelination. Brain. 2011;134(Pt 12):3590–601.
65. Scherrer B, Warfield SK. Parametric representation of multiple white matter fascicles from cube and sphere diffusion MRI. PLoS One. 2012;7(11):e48232.
66. Kraguljac NV, Anthony T, Monroe WS, Skidmore FM, Morgan CJ, White DM, et al. A longitudinal neurite and free water imaging study in patients with a schizophrenia spectrum disorder. Neuropsychopharmacology. 2019;44(11):1932–9.
67. Öz G, Alger JR, Barker PB, Bartha R, Bizzi A, Boesch C, et al. Clinical proton MR spectroscopy in central nervous system disorders. Radiology. 2014;270(3):658–79.
68. Stan AD, Ghose S, Zhao C, Hulsey K, Mihalakos P, Yanagi M, et al. Magnetic resonance spectroscopy and tissue protein concentrations together suggest lower glutamate signaling in dentate gyrus in schizophrenia. Mol Psychiatry. 2014;20:433.
69. Steen RG, Hamer RM, Lieberman JA. Measurement of brain metabolites by 1H magnetic resonance spectroscopy in patients with schizophrenia: a systematic review and meta-analysis. Neuropsychopharmacology. 2005;30:1949.
70. Chen C-S, Chiang I-C, Li C-W, Lin W-C, Lu C-Y, Hsieh T-J, et al. Proton magnetic resonance spectroscopy of late-life major depressive disorder. Psychiatry Res. 2009;172(3):210–4.

71. Kraguljac NV, Reid M, White D, Jones R, den Hollander J, Lowman D, et al. Neurometabolites in schizophrenia and bipolar disorder—a systematic review and meta-analysis. Psychiatry Res. 2012;203(2-3):111–25.
72. Brand A, Richter-Landsberg C, Leibfritz D. Multinuclear NMR studies on the energy metabolism of glial and neuronal cells. Dev Neurosci. 1993;15(3-5):289–98.
73. Chang L, Munsaka SM, Kraft-Terry S, Ernst T. Magnetic resonance spectroscopy to assess neuroinflammation and neuropathic pain. J NeuroImmune Pharmacol. 2013;8(3):576–93.
74. Das TK, Dey A, Sabesan P, Javadzadeh A, Théberge J, Radua J, et al. Putative astroglial dysfunction in schizophrenia: a meta-analysis of (1)H-MRS studies of medial prefrontal myo-inositol. Front Psychiatry. 2018;9:438.
75. Ford TC, Crewther DP. A comprehensive review of the 1H-MRS metabolite spectrum in autism spectrum disorder. Front Mol Neurosci. 2016;9:14.
76. Silverstone PH, McGrath BM, Kim H. Bipolar disorder and myo-inositol: a review of the magnetic resonance spectroscopy findings. Bipolar Disord. 2005;7(1):1–10.
77. Poels E, Kegeles L, Kantrowitz J, Slifstein M, Javitt D, Lieberman J, et al. Imaging glutamate in schizophrenia: review of findings and implications for drug discovery. Mol Psychiatry. 2014;19(1):20.
78. Marsman A, van den Heuvel MP, Klomp DWJ, Kahn RS, Luijten PR, Hulshoff Pol HE. Glutamate in schizophrenia: a focused review and meta-analysis of 1H-MRS studies. Schizophr Bull. 2011;39(1):120–9.
79. Taylor MJ. Could glutamate spectroscopy differentiate bipolar depression from unipolar? J Affect Disord. 2014;167:80–4.
80. Sanacora G, Gueorguieva R, Epperson CN, Wu Y-T, Appel M, Rothman DL, et al. Subtype-specific alterations of γ-aminobutyric acid and glutamate in patients with major depression. Arch Gen Psychiatry. 2004;61(7):705–13.
81. Janaky R, Cruz-Aguado R, Oja SS, Shaw CA. Glutathione in the nervous system: roles in neural function and health and implications for neurological disease. In: Lajtha A, Oja S, Schousboe A, Saransaari P, editors. Handbook of neurochemistry and molecular neurobiology: amino acids and peptides in the nervous system. New York: Springer; 2007.
82. Das TK, Javadzadeh A, Dev A, Sabesan P, Théberge J, Radua J. Palaniyappan L. Antioxidant defense in schizophrenia and bipolar disorder: a meta-analysis of MRS studies of anterior cingulate glutathione. Prog Neuro-Psychopharmacol Biol Psychiatry. 2019;91:94–102.
83. Tongarelli JM, Dawood M, Shariff MIF, Grover VPB, Crossey MME, Cox IJ, et al. Magnetic resonance spectroscopy: principles and techniques: lessons for clinicians. J Clin Exp Hepatol. 2015;5(4):320–8.
84. Hoehn M, Himmelreich U, Kruttwig K, Wiedermann D. Molecular and cellular MR imaging: potentials and challenges for neurological applications. J Magn Reson Imaging. 2008;27(5):941–54.

5 Cytokines as Biomarkers in Psychiatric Disorders: Methodological Issues

Olfa Khalfallah, Susana Barbosa, Emanuela Martinuzzi, Laetitia Davidovic, and Nicolas Glaichenhaus

5.1 Biomarkers in Psychiatry: Why Do We Need Them?

According to the National Institutes of Health (NIH), a biomarker is "a characteristic that is objectively measured as an indicator of normal biological processes, pathogenic processes, or pharmacologic responses to a therapeutic intervention" [1]. The NIH has identified five major types of biomarkers [2]: susceptibility biomarkers that measure the risk of developing a given disease in asymptomatic individuals; diagnostic biomarkers that enable detection or confirmation that symptomatic individuals are affected with a given disease; prognostic biomarkers that predict the likelihood of a clinical event such as disease recurrence or progression to occur in patients previously diagnosed with a given disease; predictive biomarkers that predict the likelihood of a beneficial or adverse effect to occur in response to a medical treatment; and monitoring biomarkers that reflect the nature and the severity of symptoms at a given time. Of note, in contrast to monitoring (or "state") biomarkers, susceptibility, diagnosis, prognosis, and predictive biomarkers are all independent on symptomatic changes and are therefore referred to as "trait" biomarkers [3].

In contrast to other fields of medicine, and despite extensive research to identify neuroimaging, electroencephalography, or blood-based biomarkers, neither trait nor state biomarkers are currently available in psychiatry. In schizophrenia (SCZ) for

O. Khalfallah · S. Barbosa · E. Martinuzzi · L. Davidovic
Université Côte d'Azur, Centre National de la Recherche Scientifique, Institut de Pharmacologie Moléculaire et Cellulaire, Valbonne, France
e-mail: khalfallah@ipmc.cnrs.fr; martinuzzi@ipmc.cnrs.fr; davidovic@ipmc.cnrs.fr

N. Glaichenhaus (✉)
Université Côte d'Azur, Centre National de la Recherche Scientifique, Institut de Pharmacologie Moléculaire et Cellulaire, Valbonne, France

Fondation FondaMental, Créteil, France
e-mail: nicolas.glaichenhaus@univ-cotedazur.fr

M. Berk et al. (eds.), *Immuno-Psychiatry*, https://doi.org/10.1007/978-3-030-71229-7_5

example, there is currently no biomarker to identify asymptomatic individuals who are at risk of presenting with SCZ later in life, to confirm that a symptomatic individual is affected with SCZ, or to predict response to treatment, relapse, or weight gain in a patient with SCZ treated with a given antipsychotic. Likewise, there is currently no biomarker that could be used to measure the severity of specific positive or negative symptoms in a patient with SCZ. Would such biomarkers be available, they could help clinicians to answer some of the simplest questions to which they are faced in their daily practice. For example:

- Will this recently diagnosed 23-year old patient with SCZ respond to olanzapine at the lowest possible dose, or should I prescribe a higher dose?
- The symptoms of this 30-year-old patient should be managed with olanzapine, but this antipsychotic often induces weight gain. I am afraid she would discontinue her treatment if this happens. Should I prescribe ziprasidone instead of olanzapine since weight gain is less common in patients treated with ziprasidone?
- This 40-year-old patient exhibits residual negative symptoms whatever antipsychotic he was given for the past 5 years. Could an add-on treatment with an anti-inflammatory drug help?

5.2 Cytokines as Biomarkers in Psychiatric Disorders: Why It Makes Sense?

Cytokines are a large group of small soluble proteins that are produced by various cells in the body including immune and nonimmune cell types [4]. All cytokines function by binding to specific cell surface receptors, which initiates a cascade of intracellular signals that result in an altered pattern of gene expression. While cytokines have been classified in superfamilies, families, and subfamilies, this classification may not always provide information on their biological function or mechanisms of action. For example, the name "interleukin" was initially given to cytokines that were produced by leukocytes and acted on leukocytes. However, it has since been found that many interleukins (IL) are produced by a wide variety of cells, which renders this term meaningless. The term "chemokine" has been applied to cytokines with chemotactic activity that exert their biological effects by interacting with G protein-linked transmembrane receptors. Cytokines of the Tumor Necrosis Factor (TNF) family are soluble proteins that are released by extracellular proteolytic cleavage of type II transmembrane proteins that contain a TNF homology domain. Other cytokines, such as interferons (IFN), have been classified based on the type of receptor through which they signal. Because most cell types express several cytokine receptors, cytokines are expected (and were actually demonstrated) to interact with each other in complex ways that may be additive, synergistic, or antagonistic or may involve the induction of one cytokine by another. Last but not least, most cytokines are pleiotropic which refers to their ability to address multiple targets and physiological effects. To summarize, while cytokines are well known for their role as regulatory and effector molecules of the immune system, they play a much broader role and regulate almost all physiological functions in the body.

There is ample evidence that immune dysfunction, and more specifically inflammation, is associated with severe psychiatric disorders such as SCZ, Bipolar Disorder (BD), Major Depressive Disorder (MDD), and autism spectrum disorder. Thus, the prevalence of autoimmune and allergic diseases in patients with mental disorders and/or their primary and secondary family members is higher compared with the general population [5]. Also, autoreactive antibodies directed to brain and central nervous system proteins are detected more frequently in patients with psychiatric disorders than healthy controls. Patients with severe psychiatric disorders often exhibit altered levels of cytokines in serum, plasma, and Cerebro Spinal Fluids (CSF) compared to sex- and age-matched healthy controls [6]. Last but not least, cancer patients treated with recombinant IFN-α often exhibit a mood/cognitive syndrome [7], and preclinical studies showed that administration of IL-1α or TNF-α induces depression-associated behavioral changes in mice [8]. Based on these latter results, many authors have proposed to use cytokines in biological fluids as diagnostic or prognostic biomarkers in psychiatric disorders.

5.3 Cytokines as Biomarkers in Psychiatric Disorders: What Has Been Done So Far?

Studies aimed at identifying cytokine biomarkers in psychiatric disorders have relied on clinical data and biological samples collected within the framework of naturalistic cohorts or Randomized Clinical Trials (RCT). Study samples varied between several dozens and several hundreds of volunteers. Clinical data such as sex, age, height, weight, past medical history, past and current treatments, tobacco smoking and alcohol drinking habits, as well as clinical scores relevant to the study objectives were recorded at baseline and at different time points. Biological samples and other clinical parameters such as heart rate and arterial pressure were collected at baseline and sometimes at later time points. Samples were eventually analyzed for the levels of various cytokines (see below) as well as other relevant analytes such as vitamin D [9], total and Low-Density Lipoprotein (LDL) cholesterol [10], C-reactive protein [11], and neurotransmitter metabolites. In a typical study, several dozens to several hundreds of categorical and continuous variables were collected at a given time point, with missing data occurring frequently. While most papers reported data on a single study sample, others used data from independent cohorts allowing for external validation. According to a widely cited research paper published in 2001 by Doug Laney, the 3Vs, i.e., volume, variety, and velocity, are three defining properties or dimensions of "big data" [12]. Volume refers to the amount of data, variety refers to the number of types of data, and velocity refers to the speed of data processing. Therefore, most studies aimed at identifying cytokines as biomarkers in psychiatric disorders DO NOT fall into the category of "big data"; i.e., datasets are measured in megabytes to a few gigabytes rather than in terabytes or petabytes.

Early studies aimed at identifying cytokines as biomarkers in psychiatric disorders have attempted to identify combinations of cytokines that could discriminate patients diagnosed with a given psychiatric disorder and healthy controls. These data have been summarized in several meta-analysis [13–20]. Other studies have focused on two groups of patients diagnosed with two different diseases, i.e., MDD and BD [21], or diagnosed with the same disease but exhibiting different symptoms [22, 23] or disease outcome [24, 25]. Unfortunately, and despite hundreds of papers in this field, no single cytokine, or combination of cytokines, has emerged as a biomarker that would be robust enough to be used in clinical settings. Here, we will argue that this failure may have been due at least in part to overlooked methodological issues not only for preparation, storage, and analysis of the biological samples but also for statistical analysis of the datasets. We will also propose some guidelines for future studies and advocate for the adoption of common Standard Operating Procedures (SOPs).

5.4 Biological Fluid and Matrix: Which One to Choose?

Cytokines can be detected in most biological fluids including the blood and the CSF. However, because venipuncture (to collect blood) is more acceptable in clinical practice than lumbar puncture (to collect CSF), most studies focusing on cytokines as biomarkers in psychiatric disorders have relied on blood-derived matrices such as plasma and serum. In most cases, an evacuated tube system (e.g., Becton-Dickinson Vacutainer®) is commonly used to collect blood in interchangeable glass or plastic tubes that contain either anticoagulants such as sodium citrate, heparin, EDTA or fluor for plasma preparation, or silica nanoparticles to activate coagulation for serum preparation. Tubes are then placed in a bench-top centrifuge and spun down to separate plasma or serum from insoluble materials. Plasma or serum are then transferred into cryogenic storage tubes and stored frozen at −80 °C until assessed for cytokine content using Ligand Binding Assays (LBA).

While serum and plasma samples are prepared daily in all clinical centers worldwide, differences in SOPs may have a significant impact on cytokine measurements as extensively reviewed elsewhere [26]. Serum is the liquid fraction of whole blood that is obtained after it has coagulated. It is prepared by leaving the blood undisturbed at room temperature for 30–60 min, by separating the clot from the liquid component (serum) by centrifugation in a refrigerated centrifuge and by immediately transferring the serum into a clean polypropylene tube using a Pasteur pipette. While most manufacturers of collections systems for serum samples recommend 30–60 min at room temperature for the clot to form, the longer the samples sit at room temperature, the more likely they are to experience cell lysis and the eventual release of intracellular cytokines that could contaminate the serum.

For plasma preparation, whole blood is collected into commercially available tubes that have been treated with different anticoagulants such as EDTA (lavender tops), citrate (light blue tops), or heparin (green tops). The cells are immediately removed by centrifugation, and the supernatant (plasma) is transferred into a polypropylene tube. While heparinized tubes are indicated for some applications, heparin is often contaminated with endotoxin which can stimulate white blood cells to release cytokines. More generally, each anticoagulant can impact the protein makeup in the plasma and more specifically the abundance of individual cytokines. As a result, plasma prepared from blood collected in the presence of EDTA, citrate, and heparin, may contain different levels of cytokines. Likewise, cytokine levels measured in serum and plasma could be very different [27, 28]. This is a particularly relevant issue for cytokines which are present in low pg/mL to subpg/mL levels in blood.

5.5 Serum and Plasma Samples: How to Handle Them?

Because serum and plasma samples are almost never assessed immediately for cytokine content, they should be stored for a certain period of time. As many other proteins, cytokine stability is expected to be both temperature-sensitive and temperature-dependent. A recent paper reviewed the results of 23 peer-reviewed articles which published data on the storage and freeze/thaw stability of 33 different cytokines and chemokines. Surprisingly, while the temperature at which serum and plasma samples are handled and stored and the number of freeze–thaw cycles a specimen undergoes have a major impact on the stability of some cytokines such as IL-4, IL-5, and IL-1RA; others such as IL-9, CCL11, and CXCL10 [29] appear to be remarkably stable. To stay on the safe side, investigators are therefore advised to process samples as quickly as possible, to use ice or cold packs for transport and handling steps, to initially partition serum and plasma specimens into small volumes to avoid multiple freeze–thaw cycles, to store samples at −80 °C or below and to use caution in interpreting cytokine concentration results after an extended period of storage.

5.6 Cytokine Measurements: Which Ligand Binding Assay to Choose?

Cytokine levels can be measured in serum and plasma using various LBAs which all rely on the binding of the cytokine of interest to a "capture" monoclonal Antibody (mAb) and on the detection of the bound cytokine by and enzyme-conjugated "detector" mAb. LBAs used to detect cytokines include the conventional Enzyme-Linked Immuno Sorbent Assay (ELISA) and other platforms with improved assay sensitivity such as Erenna® (Singulex), Imperacer® (Chimera Biotec GmbH), Ella™ (Protein Simple), Simoa HD-1 Analyzer™ (Quanterix), and ViBE® (Bioscale). Several multiplex immunoassay platforms which offer the possibility of simultaneously measuring the levels of several cytokines are also available including the bead-based immunoassays Luminex™ (Bio-Rad) and the BD™ Cytometric Bead

Array (BD Biosciences), the microtiter plate-based arrays V-plex™ (Mesoscale Discovery) and QPlex™ (Quansys BioSciences), and the slide-based array FastQuant™ (Vigene Tech).

Several papers aimed at comparing the performances of different immunoassays have been published [28, 30–32]. While inter-assay and intra-assay precision, analytical assay sensitivity, Frequency of Endogenous Analyte Detection (FEAD), and parallelism [33] differ from one platform to another for a given cytokine, they also differ from one cytokine to another on a given platform. For example, when serum samples from 10 MDD patients were analyzed for different cytokines, IL-4 levels measured using the Luminex™ and V-Plex™ platforms were above the Lower Limit Of Detection (LLOD) in 100% and 17.5% of the samples, respectively. In striking contrast, IL-15 was detected in all samples using the V-Plex™ platform but in none of them using the Luminex™ platform [28]. Furthermore, the absolute cytokine concentrations measured by the two platforms were often substantially different and exceeded tenfold for IL-6, IL-10, IL-17A, and TNF and 200-fold for IL-12p70 in plasma and/or sera [28]. Lastly, compared to the Luminex™ platform which provides three logs of linear dynamic range for most cytokines, it is up to five logs for the V-Plex™ platform, thereby reducing the need to run multiple dilutions. So, which LBA should be used to identify soluble biomarkers in psychiatric disorders? Compared to monoplex immunoassays, multiplex immunoassay platforms offer the possibility of simultaneously measuring the levels of several cytokines using a small volume of sample and at an affordable price. Multiplex immunoassays should therefore be preferred to monoplex immunoassays. Furthermore, because each platform detects at least some cytokines better than others, it may be worth analyzing the same samples on two different platforms in parallel. This would allow more cytokines to be detected in all samples which is a great advantage in discovery studies. On another but related topic, investigators should be aware that calibrators provided by different manufacturers are not always measured at the same concentration when tested on different platforms [34]. In other words—and in the absence of "gold standard calibrators"—the concentrations given by the different immunoassays should be regarded with caution.

5.7 Coefficients of Variation: Why They Should Be Measured?

Studies aimed at identifying cytokines as biomarkers in psychiatric disorders almost always require several immunoassays to be run sequentially. To ascertain the reliability of the results, serial dilutions of the calibrators (recombinant cytokines) should be prepared and run in duplicates within each immunoassay, so that the Coefficients of Variation (CVs) can be calculated. In general terms, the CV is a measure of the variability of the data and is defined as the Standard Deviation (SD) of a set of measurements divided by the mean of the set. Both intra-assay and inter-assay CVs can and should be calculated to reflect the performance of the assay in the hands of the user. For a given cytokine, CVs are calculated for each concentration of the calibrator that fall within the range of concentrations in the tested biological samples. The intra-assay and inter-assay CVs are the mean value of the CVs calculated for each concentration of the calibrator within each assay and between different assays, respectively. While there is no consensus on acceptable values for CVs, most authors consider that intra-assay and inter-assay CVs should be lower than 10% and 15%, respectively. While higher CVs may reflect various human and instrument errors (inaccurate pipetting technique, splashing of reagents between wells, inconsistent sample handling, uncalibrated pipettes, uncalibrated plate readers, etc.), cytokine concentrations measured in these assays should not be trusted and the assays should therefore be repeated.

5.8 Undetectable Cytokines: How to Handle Them?

Cytokines are typically present in low to subpg/mL levels in human blood, even when sensitive immunoassays are used. It is, therefore, common that cytokine measurements fall below either the Lower Limit Of Detection (LLOD) or the Lower Limit Of Quantification (LLOQ) in at least some samples. In general terms, the LLOD is the lowest quantity of an analyte that can be distinguished from the absence of that analyte (a blank value), but not necessarily quantified as an exact value, under the stated conditions of the assay. The LLOQ is the lowest concentration of an analyte in a sample which can be quantitatively determined with suitable precision and accuracy under the stated conditions of the assay. In practice, most authors define the LLOD as the lowest concentration of the analyte in the calibration curve whose readout is higher than 2.5 SD above that of the blank [35]. While several methods have been proposed to estimate the LLOQ, it is often defined as the lowest concentration of the calibrators for which the intra-assay CV is lower than 20%. While there is no consensus on the procedure to follow when cytokine measurements fall below the LLOD in some samples, some authors exclude cytokines from downstream analysis when they are below the LLOD in more than 10% of the samples. For the other cytokines, samples that fall below the LLOD should be given a substituted value (a process called imputation), but there is again no consensus on the method that should be used for this. Many authors impute to samples with measurements below the LLOD the value of half the LLOD threshold, but others have used different methods for imputation such as the Kaplan–Meier method (for censored data), generalized Wilcoxon test, and weighted quantile regression imputation [36]. Whatever methods authors use to deal with measurements that are below the LLOD should be clearly reported in the Material and Methods section of their manuscript. Unfortunately, this is not always the case.

5.9 Missing Data: How to Handle Them?

All studies aimed at identifying cytokines as biomarkers in psychiatric disorders require the collection and processing of demographic and clinical data such as sex, age, height, weight, smoking and drinking habits, diet, past medical history, current treatments, and clinical scores. Unfortunately, missing data are a common occurrence for most medical studies and should be processed before carrying out statistical analysis. Briefly, there are two ways to process missing data: listwise deletion and imputation [37]. In the listwise deletion method, a patient is excluded from the analysis if any single value is missing. The resulting dataset is referred to as "complete case." If values are missing at random, then listwise deletion does not introduce any bias, but it does decrease the power of the analysis by decreasing the effective sample size. In the imputation method, missing data are substituted with values based on other available information. Ideally, these replacements should not lead to significant changes in the distribution and composition of the dataset. Currently the best method for missing data imputation is through multiple imputation [38, 39]. In practice, several versions of the same dataset are created, analyzed, and then combined. When performed correctly, multiple imputation reduces bias, improves validity, increases precision, and results in robust statistics which are resistant to outliers (very high or very low data points). Some of the most commonly used software for creating multiple imputations in continuous, categorical, or mixture of continuous and categorical variables are the R packages "mice," "hmsic," "norm," "cat," and "mix."

5.10 Descriptive Statistics: What to Look at?

Descriptive statistics describe the basic features of a dataset. They are broken down into measures of central tendency, i.e., mean, median and mode, and measures of variability, i.e., range, quantiles, variance, and SD. Two other features are important to consider because they could have an impact on downstream statistical analysis: data distribution and outliers.

Data distribution is a function which shows all the possible values of the data and how often they occur. In some cases, the data fit a normal distribution which makes it easier to analyze in downstream analysis (of note, many methods are available to test the normality of observed data). If the data do not follow a normal distribution, it is possible to apply a range of transformations, such as the logarithmic function, to yield a normal distribution. Whatever the case, determining whether the data are normally distributed or not is critical as this determines which statistical test can be used in downstream analysis, for example, to determine if the means of two sets of data are significantly different from each other. Of note, cytokine levels in blood almost never follow a normal distribution. Log transformation helps for some cytokine datasets but not all.

Outliers are rare data points that differ significantly from other values in a dataset. They can be of two kinds: univariate and multivariate. Univariate outliers can be found when looking at a distribution of values in a single feature space, e.g., a blood concentration of LDL cholesterol of 250 mg/dL. Multivariate outliers can be found in a n-dimensional space, e.g., the levels of several cytokines in a given serum sample that all fall in the upper 1% percentile. Identifying and handling outliers is critical because they could interfere with downstream statistical analyses. While there is no general rule to define outliers, many statistical methods are available to identify extreme values such as Z-Score, Probabilistic and Statistical Modeling, Principal Component Analysis (PCA), Proximity-Based Models, and Information Theory Models. Outliers may be due to either human (data entry errors, data extraction or executing errors, experimental errors, data processing errors) or measurement (instrument error) errors. They may also correspond to a true value that reflects the natural interindividual variability in the measurement. Unfortunately, it is not always possible to tell apart the outliers that are due to an error from the others. Whatever the case, authors may decide to remove the outlier (and eventually use multiple imputation to replace the value), exclude the patient, or do nothing (and eventually use statistics that are robust to outliers).

Despite the impact of both data distribution and outliers on downstream analysis, these two issues are almost never discussed in papers that deal with medical datasets in general and cytokine datasets in particular. Furthermore, and although all authors report some descriptive statistics, these are often incomplete and therefore preclude the reader from capturing the complete characteristics of the dataset.

5.11 Univariate Analysis: Why We Should NOT Use Them?

The classical approach to identify biomarkers in psychiatric disorders is to perform statistical univariate tests, analyzing each cytokine separately. Various univariate methods are commonly used, including the Student's t test and ANalysis Of VAriance (ANOVA) both in its two-way or multiway (MANOVA) versions. However, those tests assume that the variance among the groups should be approximately equal (homogeneity of variance) that cytokines are independent of each other within each individual and that the data are normally distributed which may not always be the case even following transformation. While there are some non-parametric counterparts to these tests, like the Mann–Whitney U test and the Kruskal–Wallis H test with fewer assumptions to comply, the independence of variables is still a requirement and this is clearly not the case for cytokines. Additionally, univariate analysis does not allow for adjustment for variables that could impact the level of cytokines like sex, age, and smoking habits.

In a statistical hypothesis test, the significance probability or p-value denotes the probability that an extreme result will actually be observed if the null hypothesis is true [36]. It is common to use a threshold for statistical significance and set the type I error (the rejection of a true null hypothesis or a false positive) to $p = 0.05$, to decide if the result is likely to be random. However, along with publication bias, selective data analysis and selective reporting of outcomes focusing on the p-value in a statistical analysis seems to be at the core of the lack of reproducibility of a great number of published results [40]. The *p*-value is often used without realizing that the statistical power of a study is in most cases too low for p to assist the interpretation of the data and so that it is usually a poor test of the null hypothesis. A small sample that is not a satisfactory representation of the population under study will influence the *p*-values, and astonishingly, even when statistical power is close to 90%, the *p*-value is not stable and changes in subsequent replication studies. An alternative is to report the effect sizes estimates and their precision with confidence intervals [41–45].

Another issue is inherent to the parallel analysis of many cytokines. Multiple comparisons increase the probability that a spurious association is found and therefore the risk of type I errors. As an example, if twenty cytokines are measured in two groups of individuals, the null hypothesis is likely to be rejected just by chance for one cytokine if the significance threshold is set to $p < 0.05$ [46, 47]. With the aim of dealing with multiple comparisons, several authors including Bonferroni, Tukey, Scheffe, Dunnett, Newman-Keuls, and Ryan have developed Family-Wise Error Rate (FWER) procedures to adjust *p*-values or *p*-value thresholds to control for false positives while maintaining statistical power. For example, the False Discovery Rate (FDR) was introduced in the 90s as a less conservative approach that offers a balance between the number of true and false positives. It produces a *q* value, similar to the *p*-value, as a measure of statistical significance that is interpreted in terms of the FDR rather than the false positive rate [48].

To summarize, authors who aim at identifying biomarkers in psychiatric disorders should abandon univariate methods and exclusively use multivariate methods that can both take into consideration the correlation structure of the data and achieve the best compromise between the predictive ability (accomplished through the use of variable selection procedures) and exhaustivity [47].

5.12 Multivariable Analysis: Why Should We Use Them?

In recent years, there has been a surge in data-driven methodologies that can be used alone or in combination with previous knowledge to identify biomarkers in medicine in general and in psychiatry in particular [49]. The problem of selecting biomarkers from a pool of candidates can be seen as a variable selection problem in which variables are not independent of each other and do not always follow a normal distribution. A widely used method in variable selection is regression with stepwise selection [50], where the choice of predictive variables is carried out by going through a series of automated steps and is based on their statistical significance. At each step, candidate variables are evaluated one by one typically using univariate statistics. While regression with stepwise selection has been used in some papers in psychiatry [51], authors interested in cytokine biomarkers should step away from stepwise because of its many drawbacks: highly biased parameter estimates, incorrect standard errors, underestimated *p*-values due to multiple comparisons, and inconsistencies among model selection algorithms [52].

Several advanced multivariate methods have been used to analyze datasets in psychiatry in general and cytokine datasets in particular. These methods are categorized under the umbrella of supervised or unsupervised learning [49]. In contrast to supervised learning in which the algorithm builds a mathematical model from a set of data that contains both the input and the output variables, unsupervised learning is a type of self-organized learning that helps find previously unknown patterns in dataset without preexisting labels. With some noticeable exceptions [53, 54], most studies aimed at identifying biomarkers in psychiatric disorders have been based on supervised learning. There are two main types of supervised learning problems: classification that aims at predicting a class label, e.g., being responder or not to an atypical antipsychotic and regression that aim to predict a numerical value, e.g., a clinical score. Models are learned on training datasets with the algorithm using input variables (age, sex, smoking and drinking habits, blood cytokine levels) to predict the outcome class/value (output variable). The fitted model is subsequently used to predict the output in a test set based solely on the input variables. The performances of the model are evaluated by comparing the predicted output values with the known true values in the test set. Both classification and regression problems may have one or more independent variables of any data type, numerical, or categorical.

Two examples of supervised learning methods are Partial Least Squares regression (PLS) (when the outcome is numerical) and Partial Least Squares Discriminant Analysis (PLS-DA) (when the outcome is categorical). PLS first identifies a small set of input variables that are linear combinations of the original variables and then fits a linear model via least squares to the new variables. PLS makes use of the output variable in order to identify new features [55]. PLS is robust when the number of clinical and biological variables vastly exceeds the number of individuals (the $p >> n$ problem) and when some input variables are dependent on each other (which is the case with cytokines). However, one drawback of PLS-based approaches is that they often overfit and may not perform well on external datasets [55].

Other examples of supervised learning methods are penalized regression methods in which a penalty term is added to the log-likelihood function. While these methods were originally developed to handle high dimensional datasets, they can also be used with datasets that only contain several hundreds of patients and variables. Penalization results in the shrinkage of regression coefficients toward zero reducing model overfitting [56, 57]. Regression models that use L1 and L2 regularization techniques are called Least absolute shrinkage and selection operator (Lasso) and Regression Ridge (RR), respectively. Another model called Elastic Net (EN) uses both L1 and L2 regularization techniques allowing grouped selection of correlated variables [57]. In contrast, Lasso selects only one variable from the group of correlated variables seemingly at random, ignoring the relevance of other covariates. Of note, penalized regression methods are sensitive to outliers, but robust estimation methodologies are now available for EN [58]. Penalized regression methods have only begun to be used to identify blood biomarkers in psychiatry. For example, Bahn and her coworkers have used Lasso to identify 20 protein analytes (among 87) that discriminated patients with BD from healthy individuals with excellent predictive performances [Area Under the Curve (AUC) = 0.90] [59]. The same research group also used Lasso to analyze proteomic data (147 peptides from 77 proteins) from two independent collections of first-onset drug-naive SCZ patients and controls. The predictive performances of these models were good (AUC > 0.80) in both the discovery and the validation cohort [60].

Another supervised method is the bootstrap-enhanced EN [61] that combines nonparametric bootstrap with penalized regression to perform variable selection. The bootstrap-enhanced EN computes a Variable Inclusion Probability (VIP) which is the percentage of bootstrap resamplings in which a coefficient is estimated as different from zero. The VIP can be interpreted as the probability of including each variable in the model. After deciding on a threshold, the VIP can be used to select variables for further analysis [62]. Estimation of the prediction error is usually computed using resampling methods, such as leave-one-out, parametric, and nonparametric bootstrap, as well as repeated cross-validation methods and holdout [63]. Alternatively, postselection inference such as measuring *p*-values and confidence intervals could be performed in a different dataset [64]. We have recently applied the bootstrap-enhanced EN to identify a combination of cytokines that could discriminate BD and MDD patients in two independent study samples: a first cohort of 133 patients (among whom 40 with BD and 93 with MDD) and a second cohort of 204 patients (among whom 82 with BD and 122 with MDD) [65]. We measured the serum levels of 26 cytokines in all patients at baseline and applied the bootstrap-enhanced EN to these two datasets. Five and four cytokines with a VIP > 80% were identified in the first and the second datasets, respectively, with two being identified in both. The two models had a good predictive value (AUC = 0.8).

Lastly, supervised learning methods based on Artificial Neural Networks (ANNs) seem to have a promising future to identify biomarkers in psychiatric disorders [66]. Many different ANNs architectures have been developed, but they are basically an interconnected group of nodes in multiple layers in which the input and output nodes have clinical meaning [67]. While ANNs typically outperform other supervised learning methods when analyzing large datasets, they have also been successfully used to discriminate osteoarthritis and rheumatoid arthritis patients and healthy individuals using serum levels of 38 cytokines [68]. However, one problem with ANNs is that they learn a model too well when trained on relatively small datasets, a phenomenon called overfitting. Therefore, at the moment with the small datasets available, models generated using ANNs often fail to fit additional data or predict future observations reliably.

5.13 Unsupervised Methods: What for?

Unsupervised learning involves using methods to describe or extract relationships in data. Unsupervised learning uses only input data without output/outcome variables, and the performance cannot be compared to known labels/values. There are many types of unsupervised learning, but the most commonly used are clustering methods that allow to find groups in the data, projection methods that involves reducing the dimensionality of the data, and visualization that involves graphing or plotting data in different ways. Unsupervised clustering methods generally fall into two categories: hierarchical in which a dendrogram is derived with partitions of the data at all possible cluster levels and partitional where optimal clusters are found for a single k number of clusters. The most well-known hierarchical algorithms are single-link and complete-link, and the most popular and simplest partitional algorithm is "K-means" [69, 70]. Because unsupervised learning methods are designed to find previously unknown patterns in datasets [69], why would they be useful to identify biomarkers in psychiatric disorders? A good example is a very elegant study in which unsupervised learning methods were used to analyze functional Magnetic Resonance Imaging (fMRI) in a large multisite sample (n = 1188) of patients with depression [53, 54]. Data showed that patients with depression could be subdivided into four neurophysiological subtypes ("biotypes") defined by distinct patterns of dysfunctional connectivity in limbic and frontostriatal networks. Clustering patients on this basis enabled the development of diagnostic classifiers (biomarkers) with high (82–93%) sensitivity and specificity for depression subtypes in multisite validation (n = 711) and out-of-sample replication (n = 477) datasets. More recently, we have used unsupervised clustering methods to analyze cytokine data in 348 patients with first episode psychosis. This allowed for the identification of two subsets of patients that exhibited high and low levels of five pro-inflammatory cytokines, respectively. Further analysis showed that belonging to the "inflamed" subset was associated with increased odds of exhibiting severe negative symptoms after treatment with an atypical antipsychotic.

5.14 Model Performances: How to Measure Them?

Whatever the approach for biomarker identification, the performances of a model can be summarized using several metrics such as the Area Under the Receiver Operating Characteristics curve (AUROC), the specificity, the sensitivity, the accuracy, the Positive Predictive Value (PPV), the Negative Predictive Value (NPV), and the Brier score. Methods for evaluating a model's performance are divided into two categories: namely holdout and cross-validation. Both methods use a test set (i.e., data not seen by the model) to evaluate model performance. Cross-validation is a technique that involves partitioning the original observation dataset into a training set, used to train the model, and an independent set used to evaluate the analysis. In holdout evaluation, the dataset is randomly divided into three subsets: a training set, a validation set, and a test set. If a model fits to the training set much better than it fits the test set, overfitting is probably the cause. Holdout evaluation is considered to provide an unbiased estimate of learning performance.

Whatever method is used to evaluate the performance of a model on a given dataset, and because models tend to perform better on data on which they were constructed than on new data, it is of uttermost importance to assess how well the results of a predictive model generalize to an independent dataset, a process called external validation [71]. While this was done in a few studies aimed at identifying cytokines that discriminated patients with MDD [72, 73], BD [59], or SCZ [60, 74] from healthy individuals, these are more the exceptions than the rule.

5.15 Clinical Applications: Think Thoroughly

Apart from methodological issues, and as already pointed by Rothschild in his commentary entitled "A blood test for depression?" [75], both practitioners and researchers should think thoroughly about clinical applications before embarking in costly and time-consuming studies. For example, one may wonder what cytokine-based blood tests could add to the diagnosis and treatment of patients who already met criteria for SCZ, BD, or MDD? Would these diagnostic tests be more specific and sensitive than diagnosis by a board-certified psychiatrist or other health professional using DSM-5 criteria? Would they provide added value beyond what a trained clinician can do without the test? In contrast, if a cytokine-based blood test could influence health choices by clinicians for improved health care, e.g., predict whether the patient will respond to a given treatment before it is prescribed or predict risk in asymptomatic patients, it would definitively be worth it.

References

1. Biomarkers Definitions Working G. Biomarkers and surrogate endpoints: preferred definitions and conceptual framework. Clin Pharmacol Ther. 2001;69(3):89–95.
2. BEST (Biomarkers, EndpointS, and other Tools) Resource. Silver Spring (MD); 2016.
3. Lema YY, Gamo NJ, Yang K, Ishizuka K. Trait and state biomarkers for psychiatric disorders: importance of infrastructure to bridge the gap between basic and clinical research and industry. Psychiatry Clin Neurosci. 2018;72(7):482–9.
4. Dinarello CA. Historical insights into cytokines. Eur J Immunol. 2007;37(Suppl 1):S34–45.
5. Benros ME, Waltoft BL, Nordentoft M, et al. Autoimmune diseases and severe infections as risk factors for mood disorders: a nationwide study. JAMA Psychiatry. 2013;70(8):812–20.
6. Munkholm K, Vinberg M, Vedel Kessing L. Cytokines in bipolar disorder: a systematic review and meta-analysis. J Affect Disord. 2013;144(1–2):16–27.
7. Capuron L, Miller AH. Cytokines and psychopathology: lessons from interferon-alpha. Biol Psychiatry. 2004;56(11):819–24.
8. Dantzer R, O'Connor JC, Freund GG, Johnson RW, Kelley KW. From inflammation to sickness and depression: when the immune system subjugates the brain. Nat Rev Neurosci. 2008;9(1):46–56.
9. Akinlade KS, Olaniyan OA, Lasebikan VO, Rahamon SK. Vitamin D levels in different severity groups of schizophrenia. Front Psychiatry. 2017;8:105.
10. Pillinger T, Beck K, Stubbs B, Howes OD. Cholesterol and triglyceride levels in first-episode psychosis: systematic review and meta-analysis. Br J Psychiatry. 2017;211(6):339–49.
11. Johnsen E, Fathian F, Kroken RA, et al. The serum level of C-reactive protein (CRP) is associated with cognitive performance in acute phase psychosis. BMC Psychiatry. 2016;16:60.
12. Laney D. 3D Data Management: Controlling Data Volume, Velocity, and Variety. 2001. Accessed.
13. Miller BJ, Buckley P, Seabolt W, Mellor A, Kirkpatrick B. Meta-analysis of cytokine alterations in schizophrenia: clinical status and antipsychotic effects. Biol Psychiatry. 2011;70(7):663–71.

14. Modabbernia A, Taslimi S, Brietzke E, Ashrafi M. Cytokine alterations in bipolar disorder: a meta-analysis of 30 studies. Biol Psychiatry. 2013;74(1):15–25.
15. Dowlati Y, Herrmann N, Swardfager W, et al. A meta-analysis of cytokines in major depression. Biol Psychiatry. 2010;67(5):446–57.
16. Masi A, Quintana DS, Glozier N, Lloyd AR, Hickie IB, Guastella AJ. Cytokine aberrations in autism spectrum disorder: a systematic review and meta-analysis. Mol Psychiatry. 2015;20(4):440–6.
17. Upthegrove R, Manzanares-Teson N, Barnes NM. Cytokine function in medication-naive first episode psychosis: a systematic review and meta-analysis. Schizophr Res. 2014;155(1–3):101–8.
18. Ducasse D, Olie E, Guillaume S, Artero S, Courtet P. A meta-analysis of cytokines in suicidal behavior. Brain Behav Immun. 2015;46:203–11.
19. Black C, Miller BJ. Meta-analysis of cytokines and chemokines in suicidality: distinguishing suicidal versus nonsuicidal patients. Biol Psychiatry. 2015;78(1):28–37.
20. Goldsmith DR, Rapaport MH, Miller BJ. A meta-analysis of blood cytokine network alterations in psychiatric patients: comparisons between schizophrenia, bipolar disorder and depression. Mol Psychiatry. 2016;21(12):1696–709.
21. Wollenhaupt-Aguiar B, Librenza-Garcia D, Bristot G, et al. Differential biomarker signatures in unipolar and bipolar depression: a machine learning approach. Aust N Z J Psychiatry. 2019;2019:4867419888027.
22. Janelidze S, Mattei D, Westrin A, Traskman-Bendz L, Brundin L. Cytokine levels in the blood may distinguish suicide attempters from depressed patients. Brain Behav Immun. 2011;25(2):335–9.
23. Janelidze S, Ventorp F, Erhardt S, et al. Altered chemokine levels in the cerebrospinal fluid and plasma of suicide attempters. Psychoneuroendocrinology. 2013;38(6):853–62.
24. Mora C, Zonca V, Riva MA, Cattaneo A. Blood biomarkers and treatment response in major depression. Expert Rev Mol Diagn. 2018;18(6):513–29.
25. Carboni L, McCarthy DJ, Delafont B, et al. Biomarkers for response in major depression: comparing paroxetine and venlafaxine from two randomised placebo-controlled clinical studies. Transl Psychiatry. 2019;9(1):182.
26. Tuck MK, Chan DW, Chia D, et al. Standard operating procedures for serum and plasma collection: early detection research network consensus statement standard operating procedure integration working group. J Proteome Res. 2009;8(1):113–7.
27. Tvedt TH, Rye KP, Reikvam H, Brenner AK, Bruserud O. The importance of sample collection when using single cytokine levels and systemic cytokine profiles as biomarkers--a comparative study of serum versus plasma samples. J Immunol Methods. 2015;418:19–28.
28. Belzeaux R, Lefebvre MN, Lazzari A, et al. How to: measuring blood cytokines in biological psychiatry using commercially available multiplex immunoassays. Psychoneuroendocrinology. 2017;75:72–82.
29. Simpson S, Kaislasuo J, Guller S, Pal L. Thermal stability of cytokines: a review. Cytokine. 2020;125:154829.
30. Fu Q, Zhu J, Van Eyk JE. Comparison of multiplex immunoassay platforms. Clin Chem. 2010;56(2):314–8.
31. Soderstrom CI, Spriggs FP, Song W, Burrell S. Comparison of four distinct detection platforms using multiple ligand binding assay formats. J Immunol Methods. 2011;371(1–2):106–13.
32. Yeung D, Ciotti S, Purushothama S, et al. Evaluation of highly sensitive immunoassay technologies for quantitative measurements of sub-pg/mL levels of cytokines in human serum. J Immunol Methods. 2016;437:53–63.
33. Valentin MA, Ma S, Zhao A, Legay F, Avrameas A. Validation of immunoassay for protein biomarkers: bioanalytical study plan implementation to support pre-clinical and clinical studies. J Pharm Biomed Anal. 2011;55(5):869–77.

34. Nechansky A, Grunt S, Roitt IM, Kircheis R. Comparison of the calibration standards of three commercially available multiplex kits for human cytokine measurement to WHO standards reveals striking differences. Biomark Insights. 2008;3:227–35.
35. Chowdhury F, Williams A, Johnson P. Validation and comparison of two multiplex technologies, Luminex and Mesoscale Discovery, for human cytokine profiling. J Immunol Methods. 2009;340(1):55–64.
36. Lee M, Rahbar MH, Brown M, et al. A multiple imputation method based on weighted quantile regression models for longitudinal censored biomarker data with missing values at early visits. BMC Med Res Methodol. 2018;18(1):8.
37. Ibrahim JG, Chu H, Chen MH. Missing data in clinical studies: issues and methods. J Clin Oncol. 2012;30(26):3297–303.
38. Rubin DB. Multiple imputation for nonresponse in surveys. New York: John Wiley & Sons.; 1987.
39. Schafer JL. Analysis of incomplete multivariate data. UK: London; 1997.
40. Ioannidis JP. Why most published research findings are false. PLoS Med. 2005;2(8):e124.
41. Sterne JA, Davey Smith G. Sifting the evidence-what's wrong with significance tests? BMJ. 2001;322(7280):226–31.
42. Button KS, Ioannidis JP, Mokrysz C, et al. Power failure: why small sample size undermines the reliability of neuroscience. Nat Rev Neurosci. 2013;14(5):365–76.
43. Colquhoun D. An investigation of the false discovery rate and the misinterpretation of p-values. R Soc Open Sci. 2014;1(3):140216.
44. Halsey LG, Curran-Everett D, Vowler SL, Drummond GB. The fickle P value generates irreproducible results. Nat Methods. 2015;12(3):179–85.
45. Wasserstein RL, Schirm AL, Lazar NA. Moving to a world beyond "p < 0.05". Am Stat. 2019;73:1–19.
46. Genser B, Cooper PJ, Yazdanbakhsh M, Barreto ML, Rodrigues LC. A guide to modern statistical analysis of immunological data. BMC Immunol. 2007;8:27.
47. Robotti E, Manfredi M, Marengo M. Biomarkers discovery through multivariate statistical methods: a review of recently developed methods and applications in proteomics. J Proteomics Bioinform. 2014;S3:003.
48. Benjamini Y. Discovering the false discovery rate. J R Statist Soc B. 2010;72:405–16.
49. Iniesta R, Stahl D, McGuffin P. Machine learning, statistical learning and the future of biological research in psychiatry. Psychol Med. 2016;46(12):2455–65.
50. Efroymson MA. Multiple regression analysis. New York: Wiley; 1960.
51. Kopczynska M, Zelek W, Touchard S, et al. Complement system biomarkers in first episode psychosis. Schizophr Res. 2019;204:16–22.
52. Smith G. Step away from stepwise. J Big Data. 2018;5:32.
53. Drysdale AT, Grosenick L, Downar J, et al. Erratum: Resting-state connectivity biomarkers define neurophysiological subtypes of depression. Nat Med. 2017;23(2):264.
54. Drysdale AT, Grosenick L, Downar J, et al. Resting-state connectivity biomarkers define neurophysiological subtypes of depression. Nat Med. 2017;23(1):28–38.
55. Cramer RD. Partial least squares (PLS): its strengths and limitations. Perspect Drug Discov Design. 1993;1:269–78.
56. Tibshirani R. Regression shrinkage and selection via the lasso. J Roy Statist Soc. 1996;298(Series B (Methodological)):267–88.
57. Zou H, Hastie T. Regularization and variable selection via the elastic net. J R Statist Soc B. 2005;67(Part 2):301–20.
58. Kurnaz FS, Hoffmann I, Filzmoser P. Robust and sparse estimation methods for high-dimensional linear and logistic regression. Chemom Intell Lab Syst. 2018;172:221–2.
59. Haenisch F, Cooper JD, Reif A, et al. Towards a blood-based diagnostic panel for bipolar disorder. Brain Behav Immun. 2016;52:49–57.
60. Cooper JD, Han SYS, Tomasik J, et al. Multimodel inference for biomarker development: an application to schizophrenia. Transl Psychiatry. 2019;9(1):83.

61. Bunea F, She Y, Ombao H, Gongvatana A, Devlin K, Cohen R. Penalized least squares regression methods and applications to neuroimaging. NeuroImage. 2011;55(4):1519–27.
62. Abram SV, Helwig NE, Moodie CA, DeYoung CG, AW MD 3rd, Waller NG. Bootstrap enhanced penalized regression for variable selection with neuroimaging data. Front Neurosci. 2016;10:344.
63. Molinaro AM, Simon R, Pfeiffer RM. Prediction error estimation: a comparison of resampling methods. Bioinformatics. 2005;21(15):3301–7.
64. Terada Y, Shimodaira H. Selective inference after variable selection via multiscale bootstrap. 2019.
65. Glaichenhaus N, Belzeaux R, Courtet P, Martinuzzi E, Barbosa S, Ibrahim EC, inventors; CNRS, INSERM, Université Nice Sophia Antipolis, Assistance Publique Hôpitaux de Marseille, assignee. A method for diagnosing in vitro a bipolar disorder or a major depressive disorder. France. 2018.
66. Durstewitz D, Koppe G, Meyer-Lindenberg A. Deep neural networks in psychiatry. Mol Psychiatry. 2019;24:1583–98.
67. Shi H-Y, Lee K-T, Lee H-H, et al. Comparison of artificial neural network and logistic regression models for predicting in-hospital mortality after primary liver cancer surgery. PLoS One. 2012;7(4):e35781.
68. Heard BJ, Rosvold JM, Fritzler MJ, El-Gabalawy H, Wiley JP, Krawetz RJ. A computational method to differentiate normal individuals, osteoarthritis and rheumatoid arthritis patients using serum biomarkers. J R Soc Interface. 2014;11(97):20140428.
69. Jain AK. Data clustering: 50 years beyond K-means. Pattern Recogn Lett. 2010;31:651–66.
70. McDermott JE, Wang J, Mitchell H, et al. Challenges in biomarker discovery: combining expert insights with statistical analysis of complex omics data. Expert Opin Med Diagn. 2013;7(1):37–51.
71. Taylor JM, Ankerst DP, Andridge RR. Validation of biomarker-based risk prediction models. Clin Cancer Res. 2008;14(19):5977–83.
72. Papakostas GI, Shelton RC, Kinrys G, et al. Assessment of a multi-assay, serum-based biological diagnostic test for major depressive disorder: a pilot and replication study. Mol Psychiatry. 2013;18(3):332–9.
73. Bilello JA, Thurmond LM, Smith KM, et al. MDDScore: confirmation of a blood test to aid in the diagnosis of major depressive disorder. J Clin Psychiatry. 2015;76(2):e199–206.
74. de Witte L, Tomasik J, Schwarz E, et al. Cytokine alterations in first-episode schizophrenia patients before and after antipsychotic treatment. Schizophr Res. 2014;154(1–3):23–9.
75. Rothschild AJ. A blood test for depression? J Clin Psychiatry. 2015;76(2):e218–9.

Pro-inflammatory Cytokines and the Depressive Phenotype

6

Feyza Aricioglu, Ceren Sahin Ozkartal, and Brian E. Leonard

6.1 Introduction

6.1.1 The Concept of Psychoneuroimmunology

The idea that endogenous factors are responsible for the cognitive, affective, and behavioral dysfunction in major depression can be traced to antiquity. Hippocrates, about 400 BC, formulated the concept of Black Bile which he considered to be the cause of melancholia. This was associated with the autumn season in Europe and possibly a consequence of seasonal affective disorder.

Some 500 years later, the Roman physician Galen wrote that Black Bile (De Atrabile) described the depressive phenotype. This concept was further developed by the Oxford physician Robert Burton in his sixteenth-century monograph "The Anatomy of Melancholy" which also suggested that the symptoms of melancholia/depression are caused by an excess of Black Bile, an endogenous factor that affects the brain and causes "fear, sorrow, dullness, and heaviness that troubles the imagination." Burton considered melancholia/depression to be the disease of scholars due to their "sedentary life and excessive exertion of the brain."

The pathophysiological concept of depression changed radically in the late nineteenth century when specialized disciples came to dominate medicine, and the more holistic and integrated aspects were largely ignored. The immune system was largely considered to be confined to the peripheral areas while the brain was considered to be an immune-privileged organ.

F. Aricioglu · C. S. Ozkartal
Department of Pharmacology and Psychopharmacology Research Unit, University of Marmara, Istanbul, Turkey
e-mail: faricioglu@marmara.edu.tr

B. E. Leonard (✉)
Department of Pharmacology and Therapeutics, National University of Ireland, Galway, Ireland
e-mail: brian@psycholeonard.com

M. Berk et al. (eds.), *Immuno-Psychiatry*, https://doi.org/10.1007/978-3-030-71229-7_6

The current situation has changed in the past 25 years with evidence that inflammation involves changes in both peripheral organs and the brain. It is now apparent that small, but constant, rises in inflammatory mediators (termed chronic, low-grade inflammation) underlies the pathophysiology of major psychiatric disorders [1, 2] and also has important evolutionary significance [3]. The purpose of this contribution is to outline the possible mechanisms, whereby pro-inflammatory cytokines contribute to the depressive phenotype.

6.2 Neuroinflammation and Depression

The term "Neuroinflammation" is broadly used to describe immune-related processes within the central nervous system. Neuroinflammation occurs widely in both psychiatric and neurological diseases, brain injury, and severe psychological stress. In these situations, the innate immune cells in the brain, particularly the microglia which are the resident macrophages, are activated to produce cytokines, chemokines, and other inflammatory factors in response to the inflammatory stimulus. Whereas transient inflammatory stimuli are usually beneficial to the brain, chronic inflammation is maladaptive and profoundly affects neuronal plasticity and brain homeostasis [4].

There is ample clinical evidence that pro-inflammatory cytokines such as interleukin (IL-) 1, IL-6, and tumor necrosis factor-alpha (TNF-alpha) are raised in the serum of depressed patients [5, 6]. In addition, there is evidence that the inflammatory cytokine interferon-alpha, used therapeutically to treat hepatitis C and malignant melanoma, precipitates a depressive state in otherwise nondepressed patients [7]. These changes are ascribed to the endocrine and neurotransmitter changes as a consequence of the cytokine challenge [8].

In addition to the cytokine changes in depression, soluble cytokine receptors and plasma acute-phase proteins (such as alpha-1 acid glycoprotein and C-reactive protein) are also raised which results from the direct action of IL-6 on the liver. Effective antidepressant treatment generally (but not always!) attenuates these changes [9, 10].

The population of immune cells also changes in depression which reflects the increase in the inflammatory factors. Thus, there is an increase in the number of T-helper, T-memory cells, and activated T and B cells which act as a source of the plasma cytokines [11, 12]. The rise in the tissue concentrations of pro-inflammatory cytokines is associated with a decrease on the anti-inflammatory cytokines (such as IL-4 and IL-10). This implies that the pro-inflammatory Th-1 produced cytokines predominate over the anti-inflammatory Th-2 cytokines. Following effective antidepressant therapy, balance is usually established between the pro-and anti-inflammatory cytokines, a change which has been ascribed to the action of the Th-3 cytokine transforming growth factor-alpha (TGF-3) which is raised following effective antidepressant treatment [13].

The inflammatory changes found in depression occur in peripheral organs and the brain parenchyma. The pattern recognition receptor family, in particular the nod-like receptor-3 (NLRP-3) inflammasome, is of importance in initiating the pro-inflammatory cytokine response in the microglia. There is evidence that the density of the microglia is increased in depression and in schizophrenia [14], and the activated cells released not only pro-inflammatory cytokines but also inflammatory mediators such as prostaglandin E2 and nitric oxide as a consequence of the activation of cyclooxygenase 1 and 2 together with inducible nitric oxide synthase. Effective antidepressant treatment has been shown in some studies to reduce the concentration of PGE2 in the serum [15] which is raised in the serum and cerebrospinal fluid of untreated depressed patients [15]. As a result of the chronic exposure of the brain to inflammation, structural changes occur particularly in the frontal cortex and subcortical areas which have been implicated in depression [16]. This raises the question whether it is possible to prevent or even reverse these neurodegenerative changes by pharmacological interventions, thereby providing a novel target for the treatment of depression [17].

6.3 The Importance of Stress in the Link Between the Immune, Endocrine, and Neurotransmitter Systems

Clinical and experimental studies have demonstrated that acute stress and chronic stress are associated with neuroinflammation in depression [18, 19]. Chronic stress is commonly associated with depression and may trigger a depressive episode, exacerbate an existing episode, and significantly affect the course of the disorder [20]. Psychosocial stressors are known to initiate microglial activation in the hippocampus and many of the areas associated with the pathophysiology of depression, thereby providing a link between the stress axis and the disorder [21, 22]. Stress activates the macrophages and microglia by stimulating toll-like receptors (TLR's) on immune cells. This results in the activation of nuclear factor-kB (NF-kB) to liberate pro-IL-1 beta and TNF-alpha [23].

Stress activates both the HPA and the autonomic nervous system (ANS). Activation of the sympathetic branch of the ANS also occurs in the brain leading to an activation of the locus coeruleus and the release of noradrenaline. The increase in the activity of the SNS causes an imbalance in the ANS function and a reduction in the activity of the vagal nerve. As acetylcholine has an anti-inflammatory action in the brain [24], the reduction in the central cholinergic activity indirectly enhances the impact of inflammation. Chronic stress also precipitates resistance of the glucocorticoids receptors which are widely distributed throughout the body including the immune cells and the brain. This shifts the balance from glucocorticoid signaling to inflammation thereby leading to an increase in inflammatory factors despite the presence of elevated glucocorticoids [25].

In the periphery, stress activates visceral fat in addition to the macrophages. This provides an additional source of pro-inflammatory cytokines, chemokines, adipokines, leptin, resistin, and acute-phase proteins. Leptin occupies a central role in the regulation of food intake, a process linked to the activation of the dopaminergic system in the nucleus accumbens. In the nondepressed person, the dopaminergic system is implicated in maintaining the hedonic state and is assumed to be malfunction in anhedonia which is associated with chronic depression. Thus, the activation of leptin by pro-inflammatory cytokines provides a possible link between the changes in metabolism and central neurotransmitter function.

The metabolic effects of the glucocorticoids, which are an integral part of the stress response, initiate glucogenesis, mobilization of fatty acids, and, in the brain, a reduction in the synthesis of neurotrophic factors such as brain-derived neurotrophic factor (BDNF). This results in a decrease in neuronal repair [26] and contributes to the neurodegenerative changes in brain structure. In addition to the desensitization of the glucocorticoids receptors, chronic stress also results in insulin receptor hyposensitivity, an event which contributes to the cause of type 2 diabetes which frequently accompanies chronic depression [27]. Functional insulin insensitivity arises as a consequence of the glucocorticoids decreasing the insulin-mediated expression of the glucose transporter GLUT4 resulting in a reduction in the transport of glucose into the brain and peripheral cells [27]. Thus, chronic stress associated with depression is directly associated with insulin resistance, glucose intolerance, and type 2 diabetes [28].

6.4 The Role of the Inflammasome in the Link Between Inflammation and Depression

Recently, attention has been focused on some specialized inflammatory signaling pathways that initiates the resulting cytokine responses in neuroinflammation. In this context, NLRP3, a member of the pattern recognition receptor family and found in microglia, has shed new understanding of the role of pro-inflammatory cytokines in depression [29].

NLRP3 is a cytosolic receptor protein that recognizes danger signals that activate macrophages and microglia, thereby facilitating the release of IL-1 beta and IL-18 which are key cytokines involved in initiating inflammatory responses. When the NLRP3 is activated, the resulting complex is called the inflammasome. This structure activates caspase-1, which synthesizes and releases IL-1 and IL-18 from their inactive precursors. Despite the limitation of studies, there is now evidence that the inflammasome plays a role in depression [30]. Although studies in depression have so far been restricted to NLRP3, it is known that there are different types of inflammasome located in neurons and astroglial cells which may also be involved in the inflammatory responses in depression [31]. In order to better understand the role of the inflammasome in neuroinflammation, it is important to consider the pattern recognition receptors and their roles in the immune system [32–35].

6.4.1 Natural Immune System and Pattern Recognition Receptors

The recognition of various danger signals reaching the organism by the innate immune system takes place through various pattern recognition receptors.

Pattern recognition receptors are classified as; (a) Toll-like receptors (TLR), (b) NOD-like receptors (NLR), (c) C-type lectin receptors (CLR), (d) Retinoic acid-inducible gene (RIG)-like receptors (RIG), (e) Absent in melanoma-2 (AIM-2)—like receptors (ALR). Some of the pattern recognition receptors function in the recognition of signals reaching the extracellular environment by localization in the cell membrane (e.g., TLRs); some members are located at the intracellular level and are activated in the presence of danger stimuli reaching the cell (e.g., NLRs). Activation of pattern recognition receptors produces and releases pro-inflammatory mediators in order to eliminate the danger associated with pathogen/damage or restore tissue integrity. Although activation of the template recognition receptors is a defense mechanism that protects the organism against the danger stimulus in the first stage, chronic activation of these receptors is associated with the initiation of inflammatory diseases and associated pathophysiological processes [36]. TLRs are the human homologue of the TLRs, first described in Drosophila [37, 38]. Of the different types of pattern recognition receptors involved in initiating inflammation, the TLRs and NLRs have been implicated in depression. These will therefore be considered in more detail. Activation of TLRs leads to nuclear translocation of NF-κB to produce inflammatory mediators such as TNF-α, IL-6, and pro-IL-1β. TLRs play a role in the production of active IL-1β and IL-18 in coordination with NLRs, another pattern recognition receptor family located in the cell cytosol [36, 39].

6.4.2 NLR Family and Inflammasomes

NLR family can be activated by various pathogen and danger stimuli in the natural immune system. In this respect, it is an important family of pattern recognition receptors involved in initiating both pathogen-related and sterile inflammation responses [40]. NLRs located in the cell cytosol are composed of three basic structures. They carry a leucine rich repeat structure (LRR) at the carboxy-terminus, a nucleotide-binding oligomerization domain (NACHT) at the center, and a protein–protein interaction portion at the amino-terminus that can vary according to the subtype [40]. In the NLR family, five different subtypes have been identified (NLRA, NLRB, NLRC, NLRX, and NLRP). Among these five members, NLRPs, also known as pyrin structure, are the largest and most well-known NLR family that can create an inflammasome structure. NLRP members known to form inflammatory structure are NLRP1, NLRP2, NLRP3, NLRP6, and NLRP7; in addition, NLRC4 is also known to form inflammasome structure [39, 40].

The molecular structure of NLRPs is normally inactive in the cell. LRR at the C-terminal, NACHT at the central and N-terminal protein–protein interaction consists of three different parts of the pyrin structure [40]. Activation of NLRPs in the presence of a hazard stimulus results in the multiprotein complex structure (~700 kDa) by binding to ASC and pro-caspase-1 to the structure [36, 40]. The multiprotein complex of this oligomeric structure is called inflammasome. It is responsible for the initiation of the production and release of pro-inflammatory cytokines IL-1β and IL-18, leading to caspase-1 activation. İnflammasome-mediated caspase-1 activation may also initiate the process that activates the programmed cell death of pyroptosis [36–41].

6.4.3 CNS Inflammasomes

Although the role of inflammasomes in the organism's natural immune system responses is partially elucidated, only a few of them could be identified in the CNS [35]. The best-defined CNS inflammasomes are NLRP1, NLRP2, NLRP3, and AIM2 [39, 42–46].

NLRP1 is the first type of inflammasome to be expressed in the CNS neurons [42, 44] where it functions in the recognition of damage and pattern-related hazard signals. NLRP1 is demonstrated to be involved in spinal cord injury, traumatic brain injury, and stroke [47].

NLRP2 inflammasome which is widely distributed in the organism which is thought to play a role in astrocytes mediated neuroinflammation responses [46]. It has been shown that NLRP2 inflammasome is activated in ATP-induced astrocyte cells, accompanied by increased production of caspase-1 and IL-1β. The molecular organization of NLRP2 is similar to NLRP3. Inflammasome activation occurs as a result of binding of ASC and pro-caspase-1 to the structure [36, 48].

NLRP3 inflammasome is the most studied NLRP inflammasome which is characterized by its ability to recognize almost all types of distress signals [49]. It is known to most commonly expressed in microglia in the CNS [45, 50]. NLPP3, ASC and pro-caspase-1 binding occurs due to activation of the inflammasome. Caspase-1, on the other hand, initiates the conversion of active IL-1β and IL-18 from the biologically inert pro-IL-1β and pro-IL-18 [49].

AIM2 inflammasome is a different type of structure which is activated by the recognition of the bacterial, viral, and bilayer DNA molecules by the cytosolic AIM2 receptor [36, 47]. It is known that in the CNS it is expressed in neurons [43]. It has been shown to be activated by DNA released from dying cells in traumatic brain injury, followed by increased production of caspase-1 and IL-1β. AIM2 inflammation in cortical neurons occurs when pro-caspase-1 and ASC molecules are incorporated into the structure. AIM2 inflammasome is also known to induce programmed cell death pyroptosis in cortical neurons [36, 47].

6.4.4 Inflammasome Activation

As mentioned above, the immune responses are due to activation of the inflammasone. This begins when recognition receptors perceive danger stimuli within the organism. Hazard stimuli leading to activation of inflammasomes are divided into two as pathogens-related molecular patterns (PAMP) and damage-related molecular patterns (DAMP) [30, 31, 51]. Typical PAMPs known to cause activation of muramyl dipeptide, bacterial flagellin, bacterial LPS, lethal toxin, bacterial RNA, DNA, viral RNA, β-glucan, zymosan, and hemozoin due to bacterial, viral, fungal, or protozoal infections can be listed [51]. DAMPs, also known as sterile inflammatory activators, may be endogenous molecules released from dying or damaged cells in cases of cell damage, necrosis, or exogenous molecules that are ingested into the organism from outside and induce sterile inflammation. Endogenous DAMPs include ATP, uric acid crystals, cholesterol crystals, HMGB1, β-amyloid, hyaluronan, and glucose. The best-known exogenous DAMPs are UV radiation, asbestos, silica, and aluminum sulfate [39, 51].

Inflammasome is known to be activated by various DAMPs and PAMPs in structures other than CNS, while our knowledge of how this activation occurs within the CNS is still very limited [31]. The most potent inflammasome activator in the CNS has been shown to be increased extracellular ATP due to neuronal damage and stress [35, 47]. For example; hippocampal ATP levels were increased in rats exposed to immobilization stress; this was followed by activation of NLRP3 inflammasome and an increase in IL-1β production [52]. In another study, it has been shown that NLRP2 inflammasome is activated as a result of exogenous ATP application to human astrocyte cells [46]. It is known that high extracellular K + ion causes inflammasome activation in neurons and astrocytes due to opening of pannexin-1 channel. Amyloid-β plaques deposited in the brain have been reported to be microglial NLRP3 inflammasome activator, and based on these findings, NLRP3 inflammasome has become a possible therapeutic target for Alzheimer's disease [45, 53]. Another sterile activator in the CNS is saturated free fatty acid palmitate. It is known that palmitate leads to activation of NLRC4 inflammasome expressed in astrocytes [54]. In addition, reactive oxygen radicals are among the important inflammasome activators in CNS [55]. The ability to activate NLRP inflammasome in the presence of danger signals reaching the cell; two-stage signal transmission. The first stage involves the detection of the PAMP/DAMP ligands (e.g., LPS) by TLRs (particularly TLR-4) on the cell surface [29, 35]. This first step in which TLR-4 activation takes place is called the stimulation/firing phase [56]. As a result, transcription factor of NLRP, pro-IL-1β, and pro-IL-18 precursor cytokines is transcribed by activating NF-κB transcription factor. In the second stage, inactivated NLRP activates oligomerizes and binds with ASC and pro-caspase-1 to form the inflammasome complex. For this process, a second signal is required to reach the cell cytosol. During second signal, extracellular ATP is activated by purinergic 2X7 (P2X7) receptors located in the cell membrane. As a result, K + ion output occurs from the cell and low intracellular K + levels cause NLRP activation [49, 56]. In this stage, the activation of inflammasome activates the proteolytic caspase-1 and produces active and mature forms of IL-1β and IL-18 from pro-IL-1β and pro-IL-18 [39].

In addition to P2X7 receptors, P2X4 receptors and pannexin-1 channel activation are thought to play a critical role in the formation of inflammatory activation [57, 58] Following stress, trauma, or brain injury, ATP is released into the extracellular environment from dying cells to stimulate P2X4 receptors that are more susceptible than P2X7 activation by ATP [59]. Activation of P2X4 receptors results in the release of K + ions from the cell, and high extracellular K + levels lead to the opening of the pannexin-1 channel. Activation of the pannexin-1 channel contributes to further elevation of ATP levels in the extracellular environment. Further increases in extracellular ATP mediated by P2X4 receptors and pannexin-1 channel activation are stimulated by P2X7 receptors, resulting in increased K + output from the cell. A positive feedback in the form of "ATP-induced ATP release" with the ongoing cycle of pannexin-1 channel-P2X7 receptor activation occurs, and this cycle leads to further decrease of intracellular K + levels [31, 60]. It is still not known how low intracellular K + levels lead to activation of inflammasome [36]. In addition to inflammation-induced change, increased mitochondrial-induced reactive oxygen derivatives occur in cellular stress states, as well as various DAMPs in the phagocytosed crystal or particulate structures (such as silica uric acid crystals) cause lysosomal rupture leading to inflammasome activation [35, 39, 49, 61] (Fig. 6.1).

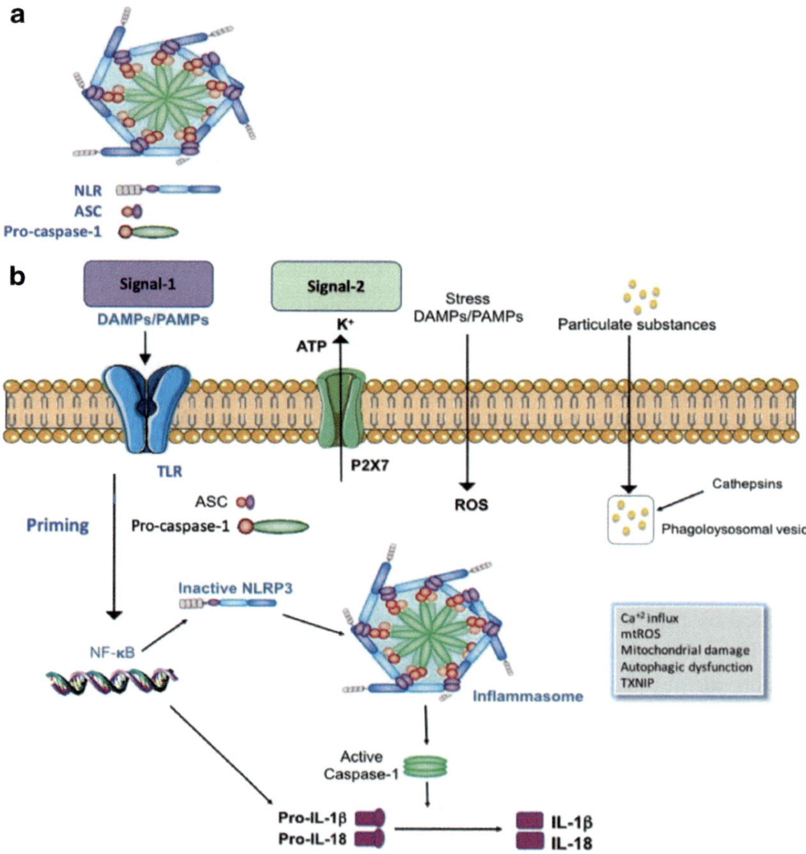

Fig. 6.1 Structure of NLRP3 inflammasome (**a**) and Illustration of the NLRP3 inflammasome pathway (**b**). Toll-like receptors (TLRs) can be phosphorylated by pathogen-associated molecular patterns (PAMPs) and/or danger-associated molecular patterns (DAMPs) which leads activation of NF-κB and transcription of NLRP3, proIL-1β, and proIL-18 (Signal-1). Extracellular ATP can induce potassium efflux through P2X7 receptors, which activates NLRP3 inflammasome (Signal-2). Environmental irritants form intracellular crystalline and/or particulate structures leading to lysosomal rupture also may lead NLRP3 inflammasome activation. (Modified from [62])

6.4.5 Pathologies Associated with Inflammasome Activation

The ability of NLRP inflammasomes to be activated by a wide variety of hazard signals whether exogenous or endogenous or pathogenic activations plays a role in the pathologies. In this context, metabolic and cardiovascular diseases such as obesity, type 2 diabetes, atherosclerosis, crystal-induced diseases such as gout, arthritis, exposure to environmental irritants, and various pathogen infections, especially autoimmune and autoinflammatory diseases, are among the main pathologies associated with activation of inflammasome [48, 63]. The importance of activation of inflammasome in host defense against pathogens in the organism has come to the fore as the first discovered inflammasome activators are PAMPs such as LPS, peptidoglycan, bacterial DNA, and bacterial and viral RNA. In mice whose NLRP3 gene was deleted, the susceptibility to Streptococcus pneumonia, Vibrio vulnificus, Candida albicans, and influenza A virus infections has been shown to increase [48]. The protective roles of NLRP3 inflammation activation are known to occur in chronic intestinal inflammatory diseases that are characterized by deterioration of the epithelial barrier in the intestinal tract and immune responses to beneficial bacteria [48, 64]. Protective models of NLRP3, NLRP6, NLRC4, ASC, and procaspase-1 have been demonstrated in colitis models where epithelial integrity is experimentally impaired [64]. In another study, it was reported that changes in intestinal microbiota composition that play a role in the development of inflammatory bowel diseases are reduced by the activity of the NLRP6 inflammasome [48]. In contrast to its protective roles in pathogen-induced inflammatory responses, activation of inflammasome is a disease factor involved in pathogenesis processes in various autoimmune and inflammatory component disorders accompanied by sterile inflammation [39, 65, 66].

6.4.6 The Link Between the Inflammasome Activation and the Metabolic Syndrome in Depression

High glucose levels associated with metabolic diseases such as obesity, type 2 diabetes, increased fatty acids such as increased palmitate due to high-fat diet, obesity, and islet amyloid polypeptide deposits in Alzheimer's disease are potent activators of NLRP3 inflammasome [56, 67, 68]. Based on this information, it is thought that inhibition of NLRP3 inflammasome may be a potential target in the treatment of diabetes. In support of this concept, some oral antidiabetic drugs, such as glyburide and glibenclamide, inhibit NLRP3 [29, 39, 56].

6.4.7 The Inflammasone in Neurological Disorders

Although research in this field is still limited, various studies have shown the role of different inflammasome structures in the pathologies associated with neurodegeneration such as traumatic brain injury and multiple sclerosis and particularly in

Alzheimer's disease [47]. Alzheimer's disease is a progressive and neurodegenerative disease characterized by accumulation of amyloid-β plaques and neurofibrillary tangles. Studies have shown that increased activation of microglia and triggered IL-1β-mediated neuroinflammation responses occur in Alzheimer's disease [69, 70]. In vitro cell culture studies show that amyloid plaques induce IL-1β release by activating NLRP3 inflammation in microglia cells [45, 53]. However, NLRP3 is not the only type of disease-related NLR in Alzheimer's disease [47]. For example, it has been suggested that NLRP1 gene expression is high in mice with genetic Alzheimer's model and some mutations in the gene may contribute to the etiology of the disease [71, 72]. In another study, NLRC4 and ASC expressions were reported to be high in postmortem brain tissues of sporadic Alzheimer's patients. In the same study, the activation of NLRC4 inflammasome caused by stimulation of isolated astrocyte cells with saturated fatty acid palmitate has been shown to increase IL-1β release and amyloid production in primary neurons [54]. In the light of these findings, it has been suggested that activation of astrocyte NLRC4 inflammasome may play a role in the pathogenesis of Alzheimer's disease [39].

6.4.8 Activation of Inflammasome by Stress and Depression

Recently, the involvement of the NLRP3 inflammasome pathway in depression has received attention. The potential relationship between stress and depression and activation of inflammasome was first noted by Iwata et al. [29]. Since 2014, experimental studies have been widely reported [29, 73–82], modified from Sahin Ozkartal [39], and a detailed summary is presented in Table 6.1.

In a study on mice, depressive-like behaviors in an acute inflammatory depression model induced by bacterial LPS were associated with activation of NLRP3 inflammasome [81]. It has been reported that brain NLRP3, ASC, caspase-1, and IL-1β gene expressions of mice considered to develop depression after acute LPS administration were increased compared to control group [81]. In addition, LPS administration has been shown to increase IL-1β protein expression. In the study, it was shown that irreversible caspase-1 inhibitor treatment reduced depressive-like behaviors in mice [81]. In another study of the same group, it was shown that serum IL-1β and IL-6 levels were increased by activating NLRP3 inflammasome in diencephalon in chronic burnout syndrome model where LPS and swimming stress were applied together. In the case of deletion of the NLRP3 gene, it was found that behavioral level improved and caspase-1 and IL-1β levels decreased in the diencephalon [83]. Thus, transgenic mice undergoing 30 days of chronic restraint stress did not show compulsory swimming, sucrose preference, social interaction, and nutrient consumption, which were accepted as the basic criteria of depression-like behavior. In addition, NLRP3 and IL-1β levels, which have been shown to increase in hippocampus and prefrontal cortex in healthy mice, and microglia activation have been shown to be unchanged in transgenic mice. In a subsequent study, deletion of the NLRP3 gene reported that depression did not occur and spontaneous anxiety-related depressive phenotype and the NLRP3 and IL-1 levels were unchanged [39, 74, 102].

Table 6.1 Stress and depression studies examining NLRP3 inflammasome activation (Given in chronological order)

Model/Disease	Organism	Tissue	Inflammasome component	Cytokine	Treatment	Method			Refs.
						PCR	Western blot	ELISA	
Acute restrain stress (1 h)	Rat	Hippocampus	NLRP3	IL-1β, TNF-α	P2X7 receptor antagonist (A-804598)	—	NLRP3	—	Iwata et al. [52]
Subchronic restrain stress (7 days)	Rat	Prefrontal Cortex Hippocampus	NLRP3, ASC Caspase-1 NF-κB	IL-1β, IL-18, IL-6, TNF-α, IL-2, IL-17, IFN-γ	Agmatine (acute)	NLRP3, ASC Caspase-1 NF-κB, IL-1β, IL-18, IL-6, TNF-α	—	IL-18	Sahin et al. [79]
Chronic restrain stress (30 days)	NLRP3$^{-/-}$ mice NLRP3$^{+/+}$ mice	Prefrontal Cortex Hippocampus	NLRP3	IL-1β	Minocycline	NLRP3, IL-1β	NLRP3, IL-1β	—	Alcocer-Gomez et al. [74]
LPS and swim stress	Wild-type mice NLRP3$^{-/-}$ mice	Diencephalon	NLRP3 Caspase-1 Procaspaz-1	IL-1β, Pro-IL-1β	—	NLRP3 Pro-IL-1β	NLRP3, Caspaz-1 Pro-caspase-1 IL-1β, Pro-IL-1β	—	Zhang et al. [83]
Early life LPS administration	Rat	Prefrontal Cortex Hippocampus	NLRP3, ASC Caspase-1	—	—	—	NLRP3, ASC Caspase-1	—	Lei et al. [84]
LPS (2 weeks)	Rat	Prefrontal Cortex Hippocampus	NLRP3 P2X7R	IL-1β, IL-6, TNF-α	Fish Oil	IL-1β IL-6	NLRP3, P2X7R	—	Dang et al. [85]

(continued)

Table 6.1 (continued)

Model/Disease	Organism	Tissue	Inflammasome component	Cytokine	Treatment	Method			Refs.
						PCR	Western blot	ELISA	
LPS administration	Mice	Hippocampus	NLRP3, ASC Caspase-1	IL-1β, IL-18, TNF-α IL-10	Caspaz-1 inhibitor (Ac-YVAD-CMK)	—	NLRP3, Caspaz-1 ASC	IL-1β, IL-18 TNF-α, IL-10	Zhu et al. [86]
CUMS (3 weeks)	Rat	Hippocampus	NLRP3, ASC Caspase-1	IL-1β	P2X7 receptor antagonists (BBG and A438079)	—	NLRP3, Caspase-1 ASC, IL-1β	—	Yue et al. [87]
CUMS (4 weeks)	Mice	Hippocampus	NLRP3, ASC Caspase-1	IL-1β	Caspaz-1 inhibitor (VX-765)	—	NLRP3, IL-1β, ASC	—	Zhang et al. [82]
CUMS (4 weeks)	NLRP3$^{-/-}$ mice NLRP3$^{+/+}$ mice	Hippocampus	NLRP3 NF-κB	IL-1β	—	—	NLRP3, NF-κB	IL-1β	Su et al. [88]
CUMS (5 weeks)	Rat	Hippocampus	NLRP3, ASC Caspase-1 NF-κB	IL-1β, TNF-α	Flavonoid extract (Icariin) Fluoxetine	IL-1β, TNF-α CD11b, iNOS	NLRP3, Caspase-1 ASC, NF-κB, iNOS	IL-1β, TNF-α	Liu et al. [89]
CUMS (6 weeks)	Mice	Hippocampus	NLRP3, ASC Caspase-1	IL-1β, IL-6, TNF-α	Thymol Fluoxetine	IL-1β, IL-6 TNF-α	NLRP3,Caspase-1 ASC	—	Deng et al. [90]
CUMS (6 weeks)	Mice	Prefrontal Cortex	NLRP3, ASC Caspase-1 NF-κB	IL-1β, IL-6, TNF-α	Geraniol, Fluoxetine	IL-1β, IL-6 TNF-α	NLRP3, Caspase-1 NF-κB, ASC	IL-1β	Deng et al. [91]

CUMS (6 weeks)	Mice	Hippocampus	NLRP3 Caspase-1	IL-1β, IL-6, TNF-α	L-Menthone, Fluoxetine	—	NLRP3, Caspase-1	IL-1β, IL-6 TNF-α	Xue et al. [80]
CUMS (6 weeks)	Rat	Prefrontal Cortex	NLRP3, ASC Caspase-1	IL-1β, IL-18	Apigenin (biflavonoid)	—	NLRP3, Caspase-1 ASC	IL-1β, IL-18	Li et al. [76]
CUMS (6 weeks)	Mice	Hippocampus	NLRP3, ASC Caspase-1	IL-1β, IL-18, TNF-α	Mangiferin (Mangifera indica) Fluoxetine	IL-1β, IL-18 TNF-α	NLRP3, ASC Caspase-1	—	Cao et al. [92]
CUMS (6 weeks)	Rat	Hippocampus	NLRP1,NLRP3, ASC, Caspase-1, P2X7	IL-1β, IL-18	Imipramine	IL-1β, IL-18	—	—	Sahin et al. [34]
CUMS (6 weeks)	Rat	Prefrontal Cortex	NLRP1,NLRP3, ASC, Caspase-1, P2X7	IL-1β, IL-6, NF-κB	P2X7 receptor antagonists (BBG)	IL-1β, IL-6, NF-κB	—	—	Aricioglu et al. [93]
CUMS (12 weeks)	Rat	Hippocampus Hypothalamus Prefrontal Cortex Liver	NLRP3, ASC Caspase-1	IL-1β	Banxia-houpu Fluoxetine	—	NLRP3, Caspase-1 ASC, IL-1β	IL-1β	Jia et al. [94]
CUMS (12 weeks)	Mice	Prefrontal Cortex	NLRP3 Caspase-1 NF-κB	IL-1β, IL-6, TNF-α	Ferulic acid Fluoxetine	IL-1β, IL-6 TNF-α	NLRP3 Caspase-1 NF-κB	IL-1β	Liu et al. [95]
Learned helplessness	Wild-type $TLR4^{-/-}$ mice	Hippocampus	NLRP3 Caspase-1 NF-κB	IL-1β	—	TLR4	NLRP3, Caspase-1 NF-κB	IL-1β	Cheng et al. [96]

(continued)

Table 6.1 (continued)

Model/Disease	Organism	Tissue	Inflammasome component	Cytokine	Treatment	Method			Refs.
						PCR	Western blot	ELISA	
Prenatal stress	Rat	Prefrontal Cortex Hippocampus	NLRP3, ASC Caspase-1	IL-1β, TNF-α, IL-6 IL-18, CCL2	Fractalkine CX3CL1	IL-1β, TNF-α, IL-6, IL-18, CCL2	NLRP3, Caspase-1 ASC	IL-1β, TNF-α, IL-6, IL-18, CCL2	Slusarczyk et al. [97]
Ovariectomy-induced depression-like syndrome	Mice	Hippocampus	NLRP3, ASC Caspase-1 P2X7, TLR-4	IL-1β, IL-18	—	NLRP3, IL-1β, IL-18	NLRP3, Caspase-1 ASC, P2X7, TLR-4 Pro-IL-1β, Pro-IL-18 IL-1β, IL-18	IL-1β, IL-18	Xu et al. [98]
Ovariectomy-induced depression-like syndrome	Mice	Hippocampus	NLRP3, ASC Caspase-1	IL-1β, IL-18	Exercise	NLRP3	NLRP3, Caspase-1 ASC Pro-IL-1β, Pro-IL-18	IL-1β, IL-18	Wang et al. [99]
MDD Patients	Human	PMN Cells	NLRP3 Caspaz-1	IL-1β, IL-18	Amitriptyline	NLRP3, Caspaz-1, IL-1β	NLRP3	IL-1β, IL-18	Alcocer-Gomez et al. [73]
MDD Patients	Human	PMN Cells	AIM2, ASC	—	—	AIM2, ASC	—	—	Momeni et al. [100]
MDD Patients	Human	PMN Cells	NLRP3	IL-1β, IL-18	Fluoxetine, paroxetine, mirtazapine, venlafaxine, desvenlafaxine, agomelatine, amitriptyline, imipramine	NLRP3	—	IL-1β, IL-18	Alcocer-Gomez et al. [101]

CUMS chronic unpredictable mild stress, *LPS* lipopolysaccharides, *NLRP* nod-like receptor protein, *TLR* toll-like receptor, *P2X7* purinergic 2X7 (Modified from [39])

In 2016, Iwata et al. demonstrated that stress induced increased extracellular ATP secretion in the brain led to activation of inflammasome via P2X7 receptor stimulation [52]. In this study, acute immobilization stress was applied to rats for 1 h resulting in an increase in and hippocampal ATP, glutamate, IL-1β, and TNF-α levels as monitored by microdialysis. Hippocampal NLRP3 levels were also examined. As ATP is activated, increased cytokine release by stress while the NLRP3 activity is suppressed. This is associated with improved stress-induced anhedonia and anxiety behaviors. Thus, it would appear that stress triggers innate immune responses, most likely through the ATP/P2X7 receptor/NLRP3 inflammasome cascade, which may be of potential therapeutic importance [39, 52].

NLRP3 activation has also been investigated using the learned helplessness model of depression in mice, where it has been shown that the activation of the inflammasome in hippocampal tissue is accompanied by various inflammatory mediators such as chemokine, cytokines, and increased glycogen synthase kinase (GSK)-3β activity [96]. After the deletion of the TLR4 gene and the application of a GSK-3β inhibitor, it was shown that activation of cytokine and activation of NLRP3 inflammasome caused by stress was not achieved. Therefore, it was thought that GSK-3β and TLR4 signaling pathways may play a role in stress-induced neuroinflammation [96]. In another study, the prenatal stress model was used and has been shown that depressive-like behaviors develop in adulthood; this is accompanied by activation of prefrontal cortex NLRP3 inflammasome and increased inflammatory mediators [97]. In the same study, the application of fractalkine (CX3CL1), an endogenous chemokine, has been shown to reduce anti-inflammatory effect and improve depressive behavior in adult rats exposed to prenatal stress by reducing activation of NLRP3 inflammasome and neuroinflammatory responses [97]. In another study in which NLRP3 inflammasome activation was examined in vivo and in vitro, the effects of fluoxetine were investigated [103] and shown to attenuate the inflammatory response [39].

In in vitro studies, the effects of fluoxetine following a LPS challenge and in vitro ATP have been investigated in macrophage and microglia cells. Following fluoxetine, NLRP3 inflammasome activation, reactive oxygen derivatives, the protein kinase pathway, and IL-1β release have been shown to decrease. In studies of the chronic unpredictable mild stress (CUMS) model following 5 or 6 weeks of fluoxetine treatment, activation of the NLRP3 inflammasome and cytokine responses occurs [80, 90, 91, 103], thereby demonstrating that fluoxetine can regulate both central and peripheral NLRP3 inflammasome activation [103]. Pan et al. [78] also studied NLRP3 inflammasome activation in the CUMS depression model developed and studied the effects of 12 weeks chronic stress on the inflammasome inflammatory mediators in the prefrontal cortex. NLRP3 and inflammasome activation occurred in the prefrontal cortex of rats exposed to chronic stress. NLRP3, ASC, caspase-1, and levels of IL-1β and NF-κB were increased due to inflammasome activation. NLRP3, caspase-1, and NF-κB protein expressions were increased in stressed rats, while there are no significant changes in ASC levels. IL-1β protein levels significantly increased by activation of NLRP3 inflammasome in prefrontal cortex in stressed rats, but there is no significant change in CSF and serum levels. In addition to protein expression, gene expression levels of NLRP3 and IL-1β were investigated and a significant increase was reported in the stress group. In addition, it has been shown that the activation of NLRP3 inflammasome caused by stress is accompanied by microglial activation. In this study, 6-week chronic administration of fluoxetine has been shown to significantly reduce elevated IL-1β levels and suppress NLRP3 activation in the prefrontal cortex and prevent microglia activation [78]. By using the same model, activation of NLRP3 inflammasome has been shown to occur in mice [77]. Increased levels of hippocampal NLRP3, caspase-1, and IL-1β in mice exposed to chronic stress for 7 weeks and developed depression were evaluated as an activation of inflammasome pathway [77]. Stress was also shown to increase IL-1β levels in serum. In addition to IL-1β, the changes in hippocampal gene expression of pro-inflammatory cytokines and anti-inflammatory cytokines such as TNF-α and IL-6 were also investigated. Stress has been shown to increase hippocampal IL-1β, TNF-α, and IL-6 gene levels, while IL-10 levels have been reported to decrease. In addition, CD11b immunoreactivity, which is one of the indicators of microglia activation, was examined and immunoreactivity findings indicating microglia activation were found in stress groups. ATP-sensitive potassium channel opener, iptakalim, and fluoxetine treatments have shown that antidepressant effects, reduced the activation of hippocampal NLRP3 inflammasome which was increased by stress and suppressed cytokine responses and microglia-mediated neuroinflammation thereby contributes to hippocampal neurogenesis [77]. In another study, it was reported that hippocampal NLRP3, caspase-1, ASC and IL-1β protein and serum IL-1β and corticosterone levels were increased by the CUMS model, and both behavior and molecular changes could be regulated in case of chronic caspase-1 inhibitor [82]. In 2016, subchronic restraint stress was created for 7 days and NLRP3 inflammasome activation was examined in hippocampus and prefrontal cortex [79]. NLRP3, ASC, caspase-1, and NF-κB inflammasome components were used to evaluate the activation of NLRP3 inflammasome, and various pro- and anti-inflammatory cytokine levels were examined. In this study, NLRP3 inflammasome activation occurred in the hippocampus and prefrontal cortex of stress-exposed rats and increased pro-inflammatory cytokine levels (TNF-α, IFN-γ, IL-6, IL-2, IL-17) have been shown. In addition, the levels of anti-inflammatory cytokines such as IL-4 and IL-10 were found decreased in stress group. The findings showed that stress triggers inflammatory responses in both CNS and peripheral circulation and leads to activation of NLRP3 inflammasome [79]. It has also been shown that CUMS-induced anhedonia in rats was coupled with upregulated mRNA levels of NLRP1, NLRP3, ASC, caspase-1, IL-1β, and IL-18 in hippocampus which were downregulated by chronic imipramine treatment and suggested that the activation of not only NLRP3 but also NLRP1 inflammasome together may be involved in chronic stress-induced depression [104]. Involvement of P2X7R in the pathogenesis of depression is investigated with administration of selective P2X7R antagonist Brilliant Blue G (BBG) in a rat model of CUMS for 6 weeks. While *NLRP3* gene expression levels were unchanged in rats exposed to the CUMS protocol, expression levels of other inflammasome pathway factors NLRP1, caspase-1, ASC, NF-κB, IL-1β, IL-6, and P2X7R were found to be increased. The results of this study has shown that suppression of inflammasome-related neuroinflammatory responses and involvement of NLRP1 in depression [93]. In addition to the abovementioned models of depression created by stress or LPS administration, it has been also observed that inflammasome activation is associated with different experimental models such as depression-like behaviors and estrogen deficiency due to ovariectomy [39, 98, 99, 105].

6.4.9 Clinical Studies That Demonstrate the Effects of Antidepressants on NLR Activity

Compared to experimental studies, clinical findings are very limited. Activation of NLRP3 inflammasome was first reported in patients with major depression in a clinical trial published in 2014 [73]. NLRP3 and caspase-1 expressions and associated IL-1β and IL-18 serum levels were found to be higher in peripheral blood mononuclear cells isolated from depressed patients compared to healthy individuals. In the same study, it was shown that NLRP3 activation and associated cytokine responses decreased in patients treated with amitriptyline for at least 10 months [73]. In another clinical study conducted in patients with depression, AIM2 levels did not change significantly in depressed patients, while ASC levels have been shown to increase [100]. Although the possible role of AIM2 inflammasome activation in depression was ruled out with these findings, the importance of the increase in ASC levels of other NLR members (NLRP1, NLRP3, NLRC4) constituting inflammation formation was emphasized [39, 100].

However, a recent study by Momeni et al. [100] of fluoxetine, paroxetine, mianserin, mirtazapine, venlafaxine, desvenlafaxine, amitriptyline, imipramine, and agomelatine on NLRP3-inflammasome complex was investigated. Antidepressant treatments induced inflammasome inhibition and reduced serum levels of IL-1β and IL-18 and lower NLRP3 and IL-1β protein expression. NLRP3 inflammasome is suggested as a biomarker for antidepressant treatment in MDD patients, in addition to the monitoring IL-1β/IL-18 release. It has also been suggested that NLRP3 expression levels and pro-inflammatory cytokines might have a clinical value in medication selection. In the same study, stress-induced depressive behavior and inflammasome activation in C57Bl/6 mice were investigated. Deletion of key autophagy mediator Atg5 in embryonic fibroblasts (MEF cells) showed an autophagy dependent-NLRP3-inflammasome inhibition by antidepressant treatment and shown that antidepressant-mediated autophagy may have a role in restoration of certain metabolic and immunological pathways in MDD patients [101]. Nevertheless, a large body of evidence suggests that depression is accompanied by the activation of the inflammasome pathway in the increase in the blood and CSF concentrations of IL-1, IL-6 and TNF-alpha [106]. While there is evidence that effective antidepressant therapy reduces IL-1, antidepressants do not consistently reduce TNF or IL-6 [107]. This implies that while IL-1 may play an important role in treatment response, it could be a potential functional biomarker of depression. However, there are significant changes in inflammatory mediators which are not reduced by conventional antidepressant treatments. This emphasizes the importance of investigating other methods for reducing neuroinflammation in depression [39].

6.5 Conclusion

The insidious effects of chronic low-grade inflammation on neuronal structure and function may only become apparent many years after the onset of depression. This raises the question regarding attempts that need to be made to target the inflammasome complex as a major source inflammatory components originating from activated microglia. There are many different types of drugs that target inflammation occurring in conditions such as chronic arthritis (e.g., celecoxib which reduces the synthesis of the inflammatory mediator PGE2), while drugs such as minocycline, the statins, metformin, and a new generation of monoclonal antibodies, such as infliximab and adalimumab, not only reduce inflammation in inflammatory diseases but also have putative antidepressant actions. The potential value of such drugs has been discussed in detail elsewhere [108, 109]. However, the anti-inflammatory action of such drugs is primarily directed at the actions of the cytokines on their receptors, apart from minocycline which reduces the release of cytokines from activated microglia and metformin which targets the glucose transporter and reactivates the desensitized insulin receptor [110].

However, a major target to attenuate the synthesis of pro-inflammatory cytokines is the inflammasome complex. This complex requires modulation in such a way that the pro-inflammatory cytokines are reduced to physiologically relevant levels [111]. The pro-inflammatory cytokines are pleiotrophic molecules, in that physiological concentrations play a crucial role in neuronal structure and differentiation, while the concentrations associated with neuroinflammation are generally neurotoxic. Thus, it is important to modulate the inflammasome complex so that it is not activated by inflammatory triggers and continues to release cytokines at physiologically relevant concentrations. In the meantime, attention can be directed to refining and developing anti-inflammatory drugs that target inflammation. Hopefully, this review will help to stimulate interest in novel ways to develop a new generation of psychotropic drugs that target neuroinflammation.

Acknowledgments Some parts of this review were prepared from Ceren Sahin Ozkartal's Ph.D. dissertation thesis. *(in Turkish).*

References

1. Leonard BE. Inflammation and depression: a causal or co-incidental link to the pathophysiology? Acta Neuropsychiatrica. 2018;30:1–16.
2. Maes M, Song C, Lin A, De Jongh R, Van Gastel A, Kenis G, Bosmans E, De Meester I, Benoy I, Neels H, Demedts P, Janca A, Scharpé S, Smith RS. The effects of psychological stress on humans: increased production of proinflammatory cytokines and Th1-like response in stress induced anxiety. Cytokine. 1998;10:313–8.
3. Raison CL, Miller AH. The evolutionary significance of depression in pathogen host defence (PATHOS-D). Mol Psychiatry. 2013;18(1):15–37.
4. Lyman M, Lloyd DG, Ji X, Vizcaychipi MP, Ma D. Neuroinflammation: the role and consequences. Neurosci Res. 2014;79:1–12.

5. Maes M, Meltzer HY, Bosmans E, Bergmans R, Vandoolaeghe E, Ranjan R, Desnyder R. Increased plasma concentrations of IL-6, soluble IL-6, soluble IL-2 and transferrin receptor in major depression. J Affect Disord. 1995;34:301–9.
6. Raison CL, Capuron L, Miller AH. Cytokines sing the blues: inflammation and the pathogenesis of depression. Trends Immunol. 2006;27:24–31.
7. Hosoda S, Takimura H, Shibayama M, Kanamura H, Ikeda K, Kumada H. Psychiatric symptoms related to interferon therapy for chronic hepatitis: clinical features and prognosis. Psychiatry Clin Neurosci. 2000;54:565–72.
8. Valentine AD, Meyers CA, Kling MA, Richelson E, Hauser P. Mood and cognitive side effects of interferon therapy. Semin Oncol. 1998;25(Suppl.1):39–47.
9. Maes M, Scharpé S, Van Grootel L, Uyttenbroeck W, Cooreman W, Cosyns P, Suy E. Higher alpha-1 and antitrypsin, haptoglobin, ceruloplasmin and lower retinol binding protein during depression: further evidence for the existence of an inflammatory response during that illness. J Affect Disord. 1992;24:183–92.
10. Sluzewska A, Rybakowski JK, Laciak M, Mackiewicz A, Sobieska M, Wiktorowicz K. IL-6 levels in depressed patients before and after treatment with fluoxetine. Ann N Y Acad Sci. 1995;762:474–6.
11. Birmaher B, Rabin RA, Garcia MR, Jain U, Whiteside TL, Williamson DE, al-Shabbout M, Nelson BC, Dahl RE, Ryan ND. Cellular immunity in depressed, conduct disorder and normal adolescents: role of adverse life events. J Child Adolesc Psychiatry. 1994;33:671–8.
12. Maes M, Lambrechts J, Suy E, Vandervorst C, Bosmans E. Absolute number and percentage of circulating natural killer cells, non MHC restricted T-cytotoxic and phagocytic cells in unipolar depression. Neuropsychobiology. 1994;29:157–63.
13. Myint AM, Leonard BE, Steinbusch HW, Kim YK. Th-1,Th-2 and Th-3 cytokine alterations in major depression. J Affect Disord. 2005;88:167–73.
14. Steiner J, Bielau H, Brisch R, Danos P, Ullrich O, Mawrin C, Bernstein HG, Bogerts B. Immunological aspects in the neurobiology of suicide: elevated microglial density in schizophrenia and depression in association with suicide. J Psychiatr Res. 2008;42:151–7.
15. Campuzano O, Castillo-Ruiz MM, Acarin L, Castellano B, Gonzalez B. Distinct patterns ofmicroglial response, cyclooxygenase-2 and inducible nitric oxide synthase expression in aged rat brain after excitotoxic damage. J Neurosci Res. 2008;86:3170–83.
16. Kim YK, Won E. The influence of stress on neuroinflammation and alteration in brain structure and function in major depression. Behav Brain Res. 2017;329:6–11.
17. Leonard BE, Wegener G. Inflammation, insulin resistance and neuroprogression in depression. Acta Neuropsychiatr. 2019;12:1–9.
18. Ader R, Cohen N, Felten D. Psychoneuroimmunology: interactions between the nervous system and the immune system. Lancet. 1995;345:99–103.
19. Gold PW, Machado-Vieira R, Pavlatou MG. Clinical and biochemical manifestations of depression: relation to the neurobiology of stress. Neural Plast. 2015;2015:581976.
20. Evans DL, Charney DS, Lewis L, Golden RN, Gorman JM, Krishnan KR, Nemeroff CB, Bremner JD, Carney RM, Coyne JC, Delong MR, Frasure-Smith N, Glassman AH, Gold PW, Grant I, Gwyther L, Ironson G, Johnson RL, Kanner AM, Katon WJ, Kaufmann PG, Keefe FJ, Ketter T, Laughren TP, Leserman J, Lyketsos CG, McDonald WM, McEwen BS, Miller AH, Musselman D, O'Connor C, Petitto JM, Pollock BG, Robinson RG, Roose SP, Rowland J, Sheline Y, Sheps DS, Simon G, Spiegel D, Stunkard A, Sunderland T, Tibbits P Jr, Valvo WJ. Mood disorders in the medically ill: Scientific review and recommendations. Biol Psychiat. 2005;58:175–89.
21. Raison C. When not enough is too much: the role of insufficient glucocorticoids signalling in the pathophysiology of stress related disorders. Am J Phys. 2003;160:1554–65.
22. Sorrells SF, Caso JR, Munhoz CD, Sapolsky RM. The stressed CNS: when glucocorticoids aggregate in inflammation. Neuron. 2009;64:33–9.
23. Smyth GP, Stapleton PP, Freeman TA, Concannon EM, Mestre JR, Duff M, Maddali S, Daly JM. Glucocorticoid pretreatment induces cytokine over expression and nuclear factor-B activation in macrophages. J Surg Res. 2004;261:253–61.

24. Tracey K. Physiology and immunology of the cholinergic anti-inflammatory pathway. J Clin Invest. 2007;117:289–96.
25. Yeager M, Pioli P, Guyre P. Cortisol exerts bi-phasic regulation on inflammation in humans. Dose-Response. 2011;1949:332–47.
26. Herbert J, Goodyer I, Grossman AB, Hastings MH, de Kloet ER, Lightman SL, Lupien SJ, Roozendaal B, Seckl JR. Do glucocorticoids damage the brain? J Neuroendocrinol. 2006;18:393–411.
27. Winokur A, Maislui G, Phillipps JL, Amsterdam JD. Insulin resistance after oral glucose tolerance testing in patients with major depression. Am J Psychiatry. 1988;145:325–30.
28. Weinstein SP, Paquin T, Pritsker A, Haber RS. Glucocorticoid induced insulin resistance: dexamethasone inhibits the activation of both insulin related and non-insulin related stimuli. Diabetes. 1995;44:441–5.
29. Iwata M, Ota KT, Duman RS. The inflammasome: pathways linking psychological stress, depression, and systemic illnesses. Brain Behav Immun. 2013;31:105–14.
30. Fleshner M, Frank M, Maier SF. Danger signals and inflammasomes: stress-evoked sterile inflammation in mood disorders. Neuropsychopharmacology. 2017;42(1):36–45.
31. de Rivero Vaccari JP, Dietrich WD, Keane RW. Activation and regulation of cellular inflammasomes: gaps in our knowledge for central nervous system injury. J Cereb Blood Flow Metab. 2014;34(3):369–75.
32. Miller AH, Raison CL. The role of inflammation in depression: from evolutionary imperative to modern treatment target. Nat Rev Immunol. 2016;16(1):22–34.
33. Sahin C, Aricioglu F. Future directions of cytokine hypothesis in depression: NLRP3 inflammasome. Bull Clin Psychopharmacol. 2013;23(3):280–8.
34. Sahin C, Dursun S, Cetin M, Aricioglu F. The neuroinflammation perspective of depression: reuniting the outstanding mechanisms of the pathophysiology. Bull Clin Psychopharmacol. 2016b;26(2):196–206.
35. Kaufmann FN, Costa AP, Ghisleni G, Diaz AP, Rodrigues AL, Peluffo H, Kaster MP. Nlrp3 inflammasome-driven pathways in depression: clinical and preclinical findings. Brain Behav Immun. 2017;64:367–83.
36. Kigerl KA, de Rivero Vaccari JP, Dietrich WD, Popovich PG, Keane RW. Pattern recognition receptors and central nervous system repair. Exp Neurol. 2014;258:5–16.
37. Lemaitre B, Nicolas E, Michaut L, Reichhart JM, Hoffmann JA. The dorsoventral regulatory gene cassette spatzle/Toll/cactus controls the potent antifungal response in Drosophila adults. Cell. 1996;86: 973–83.
38. Taguchi T, Mitcham JL, Dower SK, Sims JE, Testa JR. Chromosomal localization of TIL, a gene encoding a protein related to the Drosophila transmembrane receptor Toll, to human chromosome 4p14. Genomics. 1996;32:486–8.
39. Sahin Ozkartal C. Investigating the association between NOD like receptor protein 3 inflammasome mediated inflammatory pathways and nitridergic system in a rat model of depression (Doctoral dissertation thesis). Marmara University, Institute of Health Sciences, 2017 (Supervisor: Prof. Feyza Aricioglu) *(in Turkish)*.
40. Di Virgilio F. The therapeutic potential of modifying inflammasomes and NOD-like receptors. Pharmacol Rev. 2013;65(3):872–905.
41. Martinon F, Burns K, Tschopp J. The inflammasome: a molecular platform triggering activation of inflammatory caspases and processing of proIL-beta. Mol Cell. 2002;10(2): 417–26.
42. Abulafia DP, de Rivero Vaccari JP, Lozano JD, Lotocki G, Keane RW, Dietrich WD. Inhibition of the inflammasome complex reduces the inflammatory response after thromboembolic stroke in mice. J Cereb Blood Flow Metab. 2009;29(3):534–44.
43. Adamczak SE, de Rivero Vaccari JP, Dale G, Brand FJ 3rd, Nonner D, Bullock MR, Dahl GP, Dietrich WD, Keane RW. Pyroptotic neuronal cell death mediated by the AIM2 inflammasome. J Cereb Blood Flow Metab. 2014;34(4):621–9.
44. de Rivero Vaccari JP, Lotocki G, Marcillo AE, Dietrich WD, Keane RW. A molecular platform in neurons regulates inflammation after spinal cord injury. J Neurosci. 2008;28(13): 3404–14.

45. Halle A, Hornung V, Petzold GC, Stewart CR, Monks BG, Reinheckel T, Fitzgerald KA, Latz E, Moore KJ, Golenbock DT. The NALP3 inflammasome is involved in the innate immune response to amyloid-beta. Nat Immunol. 2008;9(8):857–65.
46. Minkiewicz J, de Rivero Vaccari JP, Keane RW. Human astrocytes express a novel NLRP2 inflammasome. Glia. 2013;61(7):1113–21.
47. Freeman LC, Ting JP. The pathogenic role of the inflammasome in neurodegenerative diseases. J Neurochem. 2016;136(Suppl 1):29–38.
48. Kersse K, Bertrand MJ, Lamkanfi M, Vandenabeele P. NOD-like receptors and the innate immune system: coping with danger, damage and death. Cytokine Growth Factor Rev. 2011;22(5-6):257–76.
49. Schroder K, Tschopp J. The inflammasomes. Cell. 2010;140(6):821–32.
50. Shi F, Yang Y, Kouadir M, Fu Y, Yang L, Zhou X, Yin X, Zhao D. Inhibition of phagocytosis and lysosomal acidification suppresses neurotoxic prion peptide-induced NALP3 inflammasome activation in BV2 microglia. J Neuroimmunol. 2013;260(1-2):121–5.
51. Davis BK, Wen H, Ting JP. The inflammasome NLRs in immunity, inflammation, and associated diseases. Annu Rev Immunol. 2011;29:707–35.
52. Iwata M, Ota KT, Li XY, Sakaue F, Li N, Dutheil S, Banasr M, Duric V, Yamanashi T, Kaneko K, Rasmussen K, Glasebrook A, Koester A, Song D, Jones KA, Zorn S, Smagin G, Duman RS. Psychological stress activates the inflammasome via release of adenosine triphosphate and stimulation of the purinergic type 2X7 receptor. Biol Psychiatry. 2016b;80(1):12–22.
53. Heneka MT, Kummer MP, Stutz A, Delekate A, Schwartz S, Vieira-Saecker A, Griep A, Axt D, Remus A, Tzeng TC, Gelpi E, Halle A, Korte M, Latz E, Golenbock DT. NLRP3 is activated in Alzheimer's disease and contributes to pathology in APP/PS1 mice. Nature. 2013;493(7434):674–8.
54. Liu L, Chan C. Activation of NLC4 inflammasome in primary rat astrocytes by palmitate enhances Alzheimer's disease-like changes in primary neurons. Alzheimer's and Dementia. 2012;8(4):302.
55. Lane T, Flam B, Lockey R, Kolliputi N. TXNIP shuttling: missing link between oxidative stress and inflammasome activation. Front Physiol. 2013;4:50.
56. Choi AJ, Ryter SW. Inflammasomes: molecular regulation and implications for metabolic and cognitive diseases. Mol Cell. 2014;37(6):441–8.
57. de Rivero Vaccari JP, Bastien D, Yurcisin G, Pineau I, Dietrich WD, De Koninck Y, Keane RW, Lacroix S. P2X4 receptors influence inflammasome activation after spinal cord injury. J Neurosci. 2012;32(9):3058–66.
58. Silverman WR, de Rivero Vaccari JP, Locovei S, Qiu F, Carlsson SK, Scemes E, Keane RW, Dahl G. The pannexin 1 channel activates the inflammasome in neurons and astrocytes. J Biol Chem. 2009;284(27):18143–51.
59. North RA, Surprenant A. Pharmacology of cloned P2X receptors. Annu Rev Pharmacol Toxicol. 2000;40:563–80.
60. Bodin P, Burnstock G. ATP-stimulated release of ATP by human endothelial cells. J Cardiovasc Pharmacol. 1996;27(6):872–5.
61. Zhou R, Tardivel A, Thorens B, Choi I, Tschopp J. Thioredoxin-interacting protein links oxidative stress to inflammasome activation. Nat Immunol. 2010;11(2):136–40.
62. Shao BZ, Xu ZQ, Han BZ, Su DF, Liu C. NLRP3 inflammasome and its inhibitors. Front Pharmacol. 2015;6:1–9.
63. Ratsimandresy RA, Dorfleutner A, Stehlik C. An update on pyrin domain-containing pattern recognition receptors: from immunity to pathology. Front Immunol. 2013;4:440.
64. Bauer C, Duewell P, Mayer C, Lehr HA, Fitzgerald KA, Dauer M, Tschopp J, Endres S, Latz E, Schnurr M. Colitis induced in mice with dextran sulfate sodium (DSS) is mediated by the NLRP3 inflammasome. Gut. 2010;59(9):1192–9.
65. Guarda G, So A. Regulation of inflammasome activity. Immunology. 2010;130(3):329–36.
66. Kubota T, Koike R. Cryopyrin-associated periodic syndromes: background and therapeutics. Mod Rheumatol. 2010;20(3):213–21.
67. Masters SL, Dunne A, Subramanian SL, Hull RL, Tannahill GM, Sharp FA, Becker C, Franchi L, Yoshihara E, Chen Z, Mullooly N, Mielke LA, Harris J, Coll RC, Mills KH, Mok KH,

Newsholme P, Nunez G, Yodoi J, Kahn SE, Lavelle EC, O'Neill LA. Activation of the NLRP3 inflammasome by islet amyloid polypeptide provides a mechanism for enhanced IL-1beta in type 2 diabetes. Nat Immunol. 2010;11(10):897–904.
68. Wen H, Gris D, Lei Y, Jha S, Zhang L, Huang MT, Brickey WJ, Ting JP. Fatty acid-induced NLRP3-ASC inflammasome activation interferes with insulin signaling. Nat Immunol. 2011;12(5):408–15.
69. Blum-Degen D, Muller T, Kuhn W, Gerlach M, Przuntek H, Riederer P. Interleukin-1 beta and interleukin-6 are elevated in the cerebrospinal fluid of Alzheimer's and de novo Parkinson's disease patients. Neurosci Lett. 1995;202(1-2):17–20.
70. Vehmas AK, Kawas CH, Stewart WF, Troncoso JC. Immune reactive cells in senile plaques and cognitive decline in Alzheimer's disease. Neurobiol Aging. 2003;24(2):321–31.
71. Pontillo A, Catamo E, Arosio B, Mari D, Crovella S. NALP1/NLRP1 genetic variants are associated with Alzheimer disease. Alzheimer Dis Assoc Disord. 2012;26(3):277–81.
72. Tan MS, Tan L, Jiang T, Zhu XC, Wang HF, Jia CD, Yu JT. Amyloid-beta induces NLRP1-dependent neuronal pyroptosis in models of Alzheimer's disease. Cell Death Dis. 2014;5:1382.
73. Alcocer-Gomez E, de Miguel M, Casas-Barquero N, Nunez-Vasco J, Sanchez-Alcazar JA, Fernandez-Rodriguez A, Cordero MD. NLRP3 inflammasome is activated in mononuclear blood cells from patients with major depressive disorder. Brain Behav Immun. 2014;36:111–7.
74. Alcocer-Gomez E, Ulecia-Moron C, Marin-Aguilar F, Rybkina T, Casas-Barquero N, Ruiz-Cabello J, Ryffel B, Apetoh L, Ghiringhelli F, Bullon P, Sanchez-Alcazar JA, Carrion AM, Cordero MD. Stress-induced depressive behaviors require a functional NLRP3 inflammasome. Mol Neurobiol. 2016;53(7):4874–82.
75. Baune BT. Inflammation and neurodegenerative disorders: is there still hope for therapeutic intervention? Curr Opin Psychiatry. 2015;28(2):148–54.
76. Li R, Wang X, Qin T, Qu R, Ma S. Apigenin ameliorates chronic mild stress-induced depressive behavior by inhibiting interleukin-1beta production and NLRP3 inflammasome activation in the rat brain. Behav Brain Res. 2016;296:318–25.
77. Lu M, Yang JZ, Geng F, Ding JH, Hu G. Iptakalim confers an antidepressant effect in a chronic mild stress model of depression through regulating neuro-inflammation and neurogenesis. Int J Neuropsychopharmacol. 2014;17(9):1501–10.
78. Pan Y, Chen XY, Zhang QY, Kong LD. Microglial NLRP3 inflammasome activation mediates IL-1beta-related inflammation in prefrontal cortex of depressive rats. Brain Behav Immun. 2014;41:90–100.
79. Sahin C, Albayrak O, Akdeniz TF, Akbulut Z, Yanikkaya Demirel G, Aricioglu F. Agmatine reverses sub-chronic stress-induced nod-like receptor protein 3 (NLRP3) activation and cytokine response in rats. Basic Clin Pharmacol Toxicol. 2016a;119(4):367–75.
80. Xue J, Li H, Deng X, Ma Z, Fu Q, Ma S. L-Menthone confers antidepressant-like effects in an unpredictable chronic mild stress mouse model via NLRP3 inflammasome-mediated inflammatory cytokines and central neurotransmitters. Pharmacol Biochem Behav. 2015; 134:42–8.
81. Zhang Y, Liu L, Peng YL, Liu YZ, Wu TY, Shen XL, Zhou JR, Sun DY, Huang AJ, Wang X, Wang YX, Jiang CL. Involvement of inflammasome activation in lipopolysaccharide-induced mice depressive-like behaviors. CNS Neurosci Ther. 2014;20(2):119–24.
82. Zhang Y, Liu L, Liu YZ, Shen XL, Wu TY, Zhang T, Wang W, Wang YX, Jiang CL. NLRP3 inflammasome mediates chronic mild stress-induced depression in mice via neuroinflammation. Int J Neuropsychopharmacol. 2015;18:8.
83. Zhang ZT, Du XM, Ma XJ, Zong Y, Chen JK, Yu CL, Liu YG, Chen YC, Zhao LJ, Lu GC. Activation of the NLRP3 inflammasome in lipopolysaccharide-induced mouse fatigue and its relevance to chronic fatigue syndrome. J Neuroinflammation. 2016;13(1):71.
84. Lei Y, Chen CJ, Yan XX, Li Z, Deng XH. Early-life lipopolysaccharide exposure potentiates forebrain expression of NLRP3 inflammasome proteins and anxiety-like behavior in adolescent rats. Brain Res. 2017;1671:43–54.

85. Dang R, Zhou X, Tang M, Xu P, Gong X, Liu Y. Fish oil supplementation attenuates neuroinflammation and alleviates depressive-like behavior in rats submitted to repeated lipopolysaccharide. Eur J Nutr. 2018;57(3):893–906.
86. Zhu W, Cao FS, Feng J, Chen HW, Wan JR, Lu Q. NLRP3 inflammasome activation contributes to long-term behavioral alterations in mice injected with lipopolysaccharide. Neuroscience. 2017;343:77–84.
87. Yue N, Huang H, Zhu X, Han Q, Wang Y, Li B. Activation of P2X7 receptor and NLRP3 inflammasome assembly in hippocampal glial cells mediates chronic stress-induced depressive-like behaviors. J Neuroinflammation. 2017;14(1):102.
88. Su WJ, Zhang Y, Chen Y, Gong H, Lian YJ, Peng W. NLRP3 gene knockout blocks NF-kappaB and MAPK signaling pathway in CUMS-induced depression mouse model. Behav Brain Res. 2017;322(Pt A):1–8.
89. Liu B, Xu C, Wu X, Liu F, Du Y, Sun J. Icariin exerts an antidepressant effect in an unpredictable chronic mild stress model of depression in rats and is associated with the regulation of hippocampal neuroinflammation. Neuroscience. 2015;294:193–205.
90. Deng XY, Li HY, Chen JJ, Li RP, Qu R, Fu Q, Ma SP. Thymol produces an antidepressant-like effect in a chronic unpredictable mild stress model of depression in mice. Behav Brain Res. 2015a;291:12–9.
91. Deng XY, Xue JS, Li HY, Ma ZQ, Fu Q, Qu R, Ma SP. Geraniol produces antidepressant-like effects in a chronic unpredictable mild stress mice model. Physiol Behav. 2015b;152(Pt A):264–71.
92. Cao C, Su M, Zhou F. Mangiferin inhibits hippocampal NLRP3 inflammasome and exerts antidepressant effects in a chronic mild stress mice model. Behav Pharmacol. 2017;28(5):356–64.
93. Aricioglu F, Ozkartal CS, Bastaskin T, Tüzün E, Kandemir C, Sirvanci S, Kucukali CI, Utkan T. Antidepressant-like effects induced by chronic blockade of the purinergic 2X7 receptor through inhibition of nod-like receptor protein 1 inflammasome in chronic unpredictable mild stress model of depression in rats. Clin Psychopharmacol Neurosci. 2019;17(2):261–72.
94. Jia KK, Zheng YJ, Zhang YX, Liu JH, Jiao RQ, Pan Y. Banxia-houpu decoction restores glucose intolerance in CUMS rats through improvement of insulin signaling and suppression of NLRP3 inflammasome activation in liver and brain. J Ethnopharmacol. 2017;209:219–29.
95. Liu YM, Shen JD, Xu LP, Li HB, Li YC, Yi LT. Ferulic acid inhibits neuro-inflammation in mice exposed to chronic unpredictable mild stress. Int Immunopharmacol. 2017;45:128–34.
96. Cheng Y, Pardo M, de Souza Armini R, Martinez A, Mouhsine H, Zagury JF, Jope RS, Beurel E. Stress-induced neuroinflammation is mediated by GSK3-dependent TLR4 signaling that promotes susceptibility to depression-like behavior. Brain Behav Immun. 2016;53:207–22.
97. Slusarczyk J, Trojan E, Wydra K, Glombik K, Chamera K, Kucharczyk M, Budziszewska B, Kubera M, Lason W, Filip M, Basta-Kaim A. Beneficial impact of intracerebroventricular fractalkine administration on behavioral and biochemical changes induced by prenatal stress in adult rats: possible role of NLRP3 inflammasome pathway. Biochem Pharmacol. 2016;113:45–56.
98. Xu Y, Sheng H, Bao Q, Wang Y, Lu J, Ni X. NLRP3 inflammasome activation mediates estrogen deficiency-induced depression- and anxiety-like behavior and hippocampal inflammation in mice. Brain Behav Immun. 2016;56:175–86.
99. Wang Y, Xu Y, Sheng H, Ni X, Lu J. Exercise amelioration of depression-like behavior in OVX mice is associated with suppression of NLRP3 inflammasome activation in hippocampus. Behav Brain Res. 2016;307:18–24.
100. Momeni M, Ghorban K, Dadmanesh M, Khodadadi H, Bidaki R, Kazemi Arababadi M, Kennedy D. ASC provides a potential link between depression and inflammatory disorders: a clinical study of depressed Iranian medical students. Nord J Psychiatry. 2016;70(4):280–4.
101. Alcocer-Gomez E, Casas-Barquero N, Williams MR, Romero-Guillena SL, Canadas-Lozano D, Bullon P, Sanchez-Alcazar JA, Navarro-Pando JM, Cordero MD. Antidepressants induce autophagy dependent-NLRP3-inflammasome inhibition in Major depressive disorder. Pharmacol Res. 2017;121:114–21.

102. Iwata M, Ishida H, Kaneko K, Shirayama Y. Learned helplessness activates hippocampal microglia in rats: a potential target for the antidepressant imipramine. Pharmacol Biochem Behav. 2016a;150–151:138–46.
103. Du RH, Tan J, Sun XY, Lu M, Ding JH, Hu G. Fluoxetine inhibits NLRP3 inflammasome activation: implication in depression. Int J Neuropsychopharmacol. 2016;19:9.
104. Sahin Ozkartal C, Aricioglu F, Tuzun E, Kucukali CI. Chronic mild stress-induced anhedonia in rats is coupled with the upregulation of inflammasome sensors: a possible involvement of NLRP1. Psychiat Clin Psyhopharm. 2018;28(3):236–44.
105. Hu W, Zhang Y, Wu W, Yin Y, Huang D, Wang Y, Li W, Li W. Chronic glucocorticoids exposure enhances neurodegeneration in the frontal cortex and hippocampus via NLRP-1 inflammasome activation in male mice. Brain Behav Immun. 2016;52:58–70.
106. Dolati Y, Herrmann N, Swardfager W, Liu H, Sham L, Reim EK, Lanctot KL. A meta analysis of cytokines in major depression. Biol Psychiatry. 2010;67:446–57.
107. Hannestadt J, Della Giola N, Block M. The effect of antidepressant medication treatment on serum levels of inflammatory cytokines: a meta-analysis. Neuropsychopharmacology. 2011;36:2452–9.
108. Halaris A, Leonard BE. Unravelling the complex interplay of immunometabolic systems that contribute to the neuroprogression of psychiatric disorders. Neurol Psychiatry Brain Res. 2019;32:111–21.
109. Tyring S, Gottlieb A, Papp K, Gordon K, Leonardi C, Wang A, Lalla D, Woolley M, Jahreis A, Zitnik R, Cella D, Krishnan R. Etanercept, and clinical outcome, fatigue syndrome and depression in psoriasis: a double blind placebo controlled randomised trial. Lancet. 2006;367:29–35.
110. Levine J, Cholestoy A, Zimmerman J. Possible antidepressant effects of monocycline. Am J Psychiatry. 1996;153:582–5.
111. Haapakoski R, Ebmeier KP, Alenius H, Kivimaki M. Innate and adaptive immunity in the development of depression: an update on current knowledge and technological advances. Prog Neuro-Psychopharmacol Biol Psychiatry. 2016;66:63–72.

Role of the T-Cell Network in Psychiatric Disorders

7

Monojit Debnath, Charles L. Raison, Michael Maes, and Michael Berk

7.1 Introduction

Immunological dysregulation has been conceived as a predominant pathogenetic mechanism in many psychiatric disorders. Indirect evidence indexing such a link includes epidemiological studies that catalog correlations between maternal infection and long-term risk of neuropsychiatric disorders and a higher prevalence of autoimmune disorders in people with such disorders. Direct evidence supporting a connection between immune function and neuropsychiatric disorders was experimentally shown in the beginning of the 1980s. Several HLA antigens were noted to have higher frequencies in patients with neuropsychiatric disorders. Subsequent to this, a number of autoantibodies against synaptic and neuronal cell membrane proteins, other cellular components as well as autoantibodies that were stimulating dopamine receptors provided support towards an autoimmune basis of psychiatric

M. Debnath (✉)
Department of Human Genetics, National Institute of Mental Health and Neurosciences, Bangalore, Karnataka, India

C. L. Raison
Department of Human Development and Family Studies, School of Human Ecology, University of Wisconsin-Madison, Madison, WI, USA
e-mail: raison@wisc.edu

M. Maes
Department of Psychiatry, Chulalongkorn University, Bangkok, Thailand

M. Berk
Deakin University, IMPACT - The Institute for Mental and Physical Health and Clinical Translation, School of Medicine, Barwon Health, Geelong, VIC, Australia

Orygen, The Centre of Excellence in Youth Mental Health, the Department of Psychiatry and the Florey Institute of Neuroscience and Mental Health, The University of Melbourne, Melbourne, VIC, Australia
e-mail: michael.berk@deakin.edu.au

M. Berk et al. (eds.), *Immuno-Psychiatry*, https://doi.org/10.1007/978-3-030-71229-7_7

disorders like schizophrenia. In addition, the Macrophage and Macrophage T-cell theory proposed in the early 1990s incorporated evidence of the involvement of immune cell abnormalities, and aberrant cytokine responses in patients with depression and schizophrenia [1, 2]. These findings led to paradigmatic changes in our understanding of the pathogenesis of major psychiatric disorders. Large scale genetic studies have also argued in favor of a role of immune components in psychiatric disorders. Studies validating immune hypotheses have demonstrated altered levels and activities of various inflammatory immune mediators and immune cells in the cerebrospinal fluid (CSF) as well as postmortem brains of individuals with psychiatric disorders.

Despite rapid advances in the field of immuno-psychiatry, there is no consensus on which immune components and/or cells play the predominant role in the neurobiological mechanisms of psychosis. The most consistent finding across all the neuropsychiatric disorders is that of altered levels of proinflammatory cytokines, raising the possibility that many psychiatric conditions are disorders of chronic low-grade inflammation. Notably, inflammatory mediators have been associated with a number of risk factors/mechanisms of psychosis; such as inflammatory cytokines, (a) impairing crucial phases of neurodevelopment, (b) mediating developmental neuroinflammation, (c) acting as footprints of childhood adverse effects and other environmental risks, (d) contributing to brain morphometric changes, and (e) resulting in cognitive deficits and potentially treatment resistance. Despite these advances, the question of how cytokine production is dysregulated in psychiatric disorders remains elusive.

There is a growing recognition that changes in circulating lymphocytes may contribute to the immune dysfunction in neuropsychiatric disorders, given that lymphocytes, especially T lymphocytes are prolific producers of proinflammatory cytokines. There are different classes of lymphocytes which include natural killer (NK) cells, T cells, whose role is in adaptive cell-mediated immunity and B cells, which serve adaptive, antibody-driven humoral immunity. It is not known whether the genomic architecture of T cells undergoes priming, particularly epigenetic priming, to drive inflammatory responses in the face of environmental challenges. The recent discovery of the existence of the lymphatic system in the brain and T lymphocytes trafficking from the periphery to the brain have led to a conclusion that T lymphocytes play an important role in brain immune surveillance and immune homeostasis [3]. T lymphocytes modulate physiological brain development, brain functions, and behavior-related attributes. Amongst these, some of the core processes and features like hippocampal neurogenesis, cognition, learning, and memory are regulated by T cells. Over the past few years, multiple studies have also demonstrated the encephalitogenic potential of T lymphocytes. These data suggest that alterations in the T-cell network might contribute to the pathogenetic pathway of psychiatric disorders. In this article, we highlight the implications of T lymphocytes in the etiopathology, course, and treatment of psychiatric disorders.

7.2 Genesis and Biology of T Lymphocytes

T lymphocytes originate from bone marrow progenitors and migrate to the thymus for maturation and selection. The T-cell repertoire after thymic selection gets exported to the periphery. T lymphocyte subtypes can be identified based on the expression of a surface cluster of differentiation (CD) molecule, named CD3 and are grouped into two major subpopulations: CD4 and CD8. Peripheral T cells comprise different subsets and they perform different functions. For example, naïve T cells are known to respond to new antigens; memory T cells, which are derived from previous antigen activation, can maintain long-term immunity and regulatory T (Treg) cells are known for their ability to regulate and check immune responses. Based on the interaction with an antigen, the nature of the signal and their helper activities on other populations of cells, naïve CD4 T cells are differentiated into various distinct lineages, including Th1, Th2, Th9, Th17, and induced regulatory T (iTreg) cells. Each of these lineages displays a characteristic profile of cytokine production and functional diversity. Th1 cells are critically involved in mediating immunity to intracellular microorganisms, Th2 to many extracellular pathogens, including helminths, while Th17 cells respond to extracellular bacteria and fungi, especially at mucosal surfaces of the lungs, skin and gut. Functionally, Th1 and Th17 cells are involved in the promotion of inflammation, Th2 cells help B lymphocytes, and Treg cells regulate immunosuppressive responses. CD8+ T lymphocytes act as cytotoxic T lymphocytes (CTL) and are involved in killing target cells. CD8+ T cells are crucially involved in immune protection against invading microbes, especially viruses. During infection, naïve T lymphocytes undergo activation in secondary lymphoid organs and also undergo expansion to large numbers. After clearing an infection, a subset of the activated T cells differentiates into memory T cells. Some memory T cells that circulate through the blood and the secondary lymphoid organs are termed as central memory T cells (T_{CM} cells), while memory T cells that move between blood and the spleen have the ability to enter nonlymphoid tissues under the circumstances of reinfection and are known as effector memory T cells (T_{EM} cells). Recent understanding reveals that tissues that are common sites of reinfection are distinctly populated by a lineage of tissue-resident memory T cells (T_{RM} cells).

T lymphocytes play crucial roles in the establishment and maintenance of immune responses and coordinate various aspects of adaptive immunity, including responses to pathogens, allergens, and tumors throughout life [4]. However, the number and role of T lymphocytes in immune responses seem to vary across the body at different stages of life. Infancy and early childhood are marked by the presence of a greater number of naïve T cells, along with a significant number of Treg cells. After childhood, memory T cells gain predominance throughout the body. It is now becoming increasingly apparent that T lymphocytes can populate virtually every organ and tissue. This includes not only the primary and secondary lymphoid organs but also a host of other sites such as mucosal surfaces, exocrine organs, and even the brain and central nervous system. It is being demonstrated that T cells exert specialized and tissue-specific responses and the kinetics of such responses depends on age and tissue microenvironment. A list of T lymphocytes and their biological attributes are summarized in Fig. 7.1.

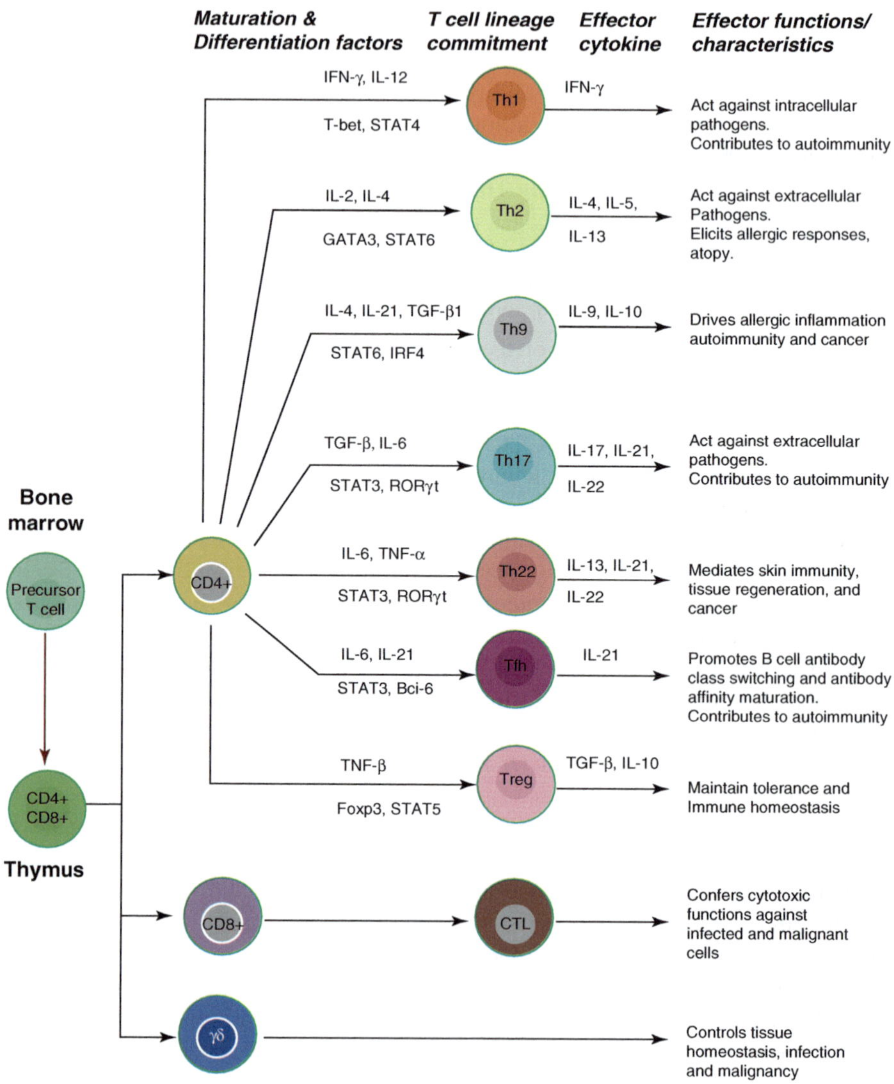

Fig. 7.1 Depiction of development, differentiation, and effector functions of T-cell subsets

7.3 Role of T Cells in CNS Homeostasis

It was long held that the central nervous system (CNS) is an immune-privileged organ that lacks a lymphatic system, fails to express major histocompatibility complex (MHC) molecules, and utilizes the blood-brain barrier (BBB) to limit the entry of peripheral immune cells into the brain. All these notions have recently been overturned. It is now established that brain cells express MHC molecules; and these molecules play important physiological roles in the brain, such as synaptic plasticity, learning, memory, etc. [5]. A recent landmark study demonstrated the presence of functional lymphatic vessels lining the dural sinuses in the CNS [3]. The role of T lymphocytes in CNS homeostasis is well established. The means by which T lymphocytes promote CNS homeostasis is highlighted below.

7.3.1 Neuroimmune Gateways: T Lymphocytes Homing into CNS

Various immune cells including T cells, B cells, NK cells, dendritic (DC) cells, monocytes, and macrophages are reported in the CNS under physiological conditions. These cells show differential distribution between meninges, choroid plexus, and parenchyma [6]. Besides this, in healthy individuals, 80% of the immune cells in CSF were found to be T cells [7] and 150,000 T lymphocytes are estimated to be in CSF [8]. The brain areas where T cells are found to be localized are also being elucidated. For example, under normal conditions CD4+ T cells are present in the meningeal space, meningeal lymphatic vessels, and choroid plex in the adult brain. This suggests that in steady state, the meningeal lymphatic system is involved in the trafficking of immune cells out of the CNS. Recent studies suggest that choroid plexus serves as an immunological niche within the CNS, which not only allows T lymphocytes to undergo proliferation and stimulation, but also to rapidly respond to peripheral inflammation [9].

Emerging research has helped in identifying the immune gateways as well as afferent and efferent immunological pathways that guide immune cells in mediating neuro-immune cross-talk. Converging evidence suggests that T lymphocytes serve as sentinel not only in carrying out immune surveillance in the brain but also in accomplishing neuro-immune cross-talk. However, the mechanism of immune surveillance in CNS, whether it is driven by resident immune cells or by peripheral immune cells that migrate to the brain, has been a subject of intense recent research. Several questions exist regarding migration of peripheral T cells into the brain. Do T lymphocytes require activation/priming to cross the BBB? Do all activated T lymphocytes have the ability to transmigrate?

Multiple studies have shown that naïve T cells are not able to migrate to the healthy brain parenchyma. T cells need to be primed or activated to cross the BBB. Two-photon laser scanning microscopy (TPLSM) studies have demonstrated that naïve T cells fail to migrate within the healthy, noninflamed brain parenchyma

[10]. It is also not very clear whether only antigen-specific T cells migrate to the brain. Recent understanding suggests that antigen specificity is not the central requirement for the migration of T cells into the brain. Rather, activation status is the key requirement for CD4+ T-cell migration into healthy CNS tissue. Besides this, emerging evidence suggests that the human brain is also surveyed by T_{RM} cells; and these cells are proposed to offer protection against neurotropic virus reactivation [11]. Contextually, such cells could act as an autonomous cytotoxic barrier in the brain against viral infection. Notably, most of the T cells in human CSF are central memory T cells, which not only patrol the CSF or perivascular space but also have the ability to return to the periphery through lymphatic vessels in the meningeal spaces [12].

7.3.2 Role of T Lymphocytes in Neurodevelopment and Neurogenesis

In addition to their role in regulating CNS immune surveillance, these immune cells play a critical role in brain development. During brain development, events like neurogenesis, gliogenesis, and synapse formation are carefully regulated by the immune system. T lymphocytes perform both immune and nonimmune functions in the brain. T lymphocytes are found in the brain from embryonic periods. In a study of mice, CD4+ T cells were present in the brain as early as embryonic day 16 and the proportion of T cells was shown to be stable throughout development [13]. Although the impact of various subsets of T lymphocytes on brain development and functions are largely unexplored, CD4+ T cells influence normal brain activity [14]. T cells and T cell-derived cytokines have been shown to regulate a number of neuronal- and plasticity-related processes during brain development.

Adult hippocampal neurogenesis is increasingly recognized as a key regulator of emotional regulation, cognition, learning and memory. Conversely, dysregulation of neurogenesis is increasingly considered to be one of the key factors in the pathogenesis and course of various neuropsychiatric disorders. Although the entire spectrum of factors involved in the regulation of adult neurogenesis is yet to be delineated, it is well-established that this process requires a neurogenic niche which supports and promotes neurogenesis through cell-cell contact as well as secretion of soluble factors/mediators. Immune players, not only those resident in the CNS but also peripheral immune cells, are involved in the regulation of hippocampal adult neurogenesis [14]. Among the immune components, an important role for T cells has been demonstrated by multiple studies. Studies on experimental animals have provided several important insights into the role of T cells in adult neurogenesis. T cell-deficient nude mice exhibit impaired adult neurogenesis [14]. In adult mice, T cells maintain normal baseline levels of neural precursor proliferation in the hippocampus [15]. Recent findings from experimental animal studies reveal that CD8+T lymphocytes are important mechanistic elements of an enriched environment that drives hippocampus-dependent behavior, hippocampal neurogenesis, and synaptic plasticity [16]. In mice, systemic depletion of CD4+ T lymphocytes, but not CD8+ cells, significantly reduces hippocampal neurogenesis [17]. However, the precise mechanism by which T cells contribute to variation in adult neurogenesis is not fully understood; however, recent understandings point to the possibility that adult neurogenesis may be driven by genetic background and the functional properties of T cells and/or proportions of CD8+ T versus CD4+ T lymphocytes. [18]. It is also necessary to understand the effects of activated T cells on adult neurogenesis. Activated T cells seemingly inhibit neurogenesis by impairing neuronal progenitor cell proliferation and differentiation by releasing Granzyme B [19]. Another chemokine induced by Th2 cells, namely eotaxin (CCL11), activates IL-2 stimulated T cells to adhesion and chemotaxis [20], and may rapidly pass the blood-brain barrier and accumulate in the brain [21]. The receptor for CCL11, namely CCR3 (C-C motif chemokine receptor 3) is expressed by microglia and neuronal cells and the CCR3-CCL11 complex may display neuroprotective properties and promote a Th2 phenotype [22]. Nevertheless, age-associated increases in CCL11 are associated with decreased neurogenesis [23] and with impaired cognitive functions including executive functions, episodic and semantic memory, and attention as well [24].

7.3.3 Role of T Lymphocytes in Learning, Memory, and Behavior

With a better understanding of the role of T lymphocytes in CNS homeostasis, it is now apparent that the essential components of the adaptive immune system like T lymphocytes have a substantial influence on cognitive performance, learning, and memory [25]. In a healthy senior population, better cognitive performance was shown to be associated with lower numbers of effector memory CD4+ T cells and higher numbers of naïve CD8+ T cells, implying an important role of immune system in healthy cognitive ageing [26]. In a study in patients with schizophrenia, peripheral immune cell populations were associated with cognitive deficits; more severe cognitive symptoms were associated with a decreased number of HLA-DR+ regulatory T-cells (Tregs) and CD4+ (CCR7+CD45RA-) central memory T cells and CD4+CD161+ naïve T cells [27]. Similar interesting results were obtained from experimental animal studies. Mice that were deficient in mature T cells were found to have cognitive deficits and behavioral abnormalities, and these changes could be reversed by T cell restoration [28]. Meninges are an important site for beneficial T-cell interaction with the CNS and facilitate cognitive task performance [29] and meningeal immunity plays an important role in learning and memory. T cells residing in meninges and IL-4 derived from these T cells play a crucial role in learning and memory. IL-4 deficient mice (*IL4 −/−* mice) exhibited cognitive deficits; however, adoptive transfer of T cells from wild type into *IL4 −/−* mice reversed this cognitive impairment [30]. Subsequent to this, T-cell derived cytokines, especially IFN-γ were shown to regulate neuronal connectivity as well as social behavior [31]. In addition, a restricted CD4+ T-cell receptor repertoire was shown to impair cognitive function by altering Th2 cytokine levels [32].

7.4 T Cells in the Brain: Protector or Destroyer?

The past several years have seen a debate within neuroimmunology regarding whether T cells can both provide neuroprotection and induce neurodegeneration [33]. Although evidence demonstrating neurotoxic effects of T cells is robust, data on their neuroprotective attributes are limited.

Peripheral T-cell abnormalities have been documented in a number of neurodegenerative diseases of immune origin or association. Though these findings reflect a link between T cells and underlying brain pathology, they do not shed any light on a precise mechanistic basis to account for these effects. Many animal as well as human postmortem brain studies have indicated T-cell infiltration into the brain in many neurodegenerative diseases including Parkinson's disease and Alzheimer's disease. The damaging effects of T cells after various pathological changes like stroke, etc. are shown in many studies. The traditional proposition was that the presence of activated immune cells, especially T lymphocytes in the CNS is a hallmark of ongoing pathology. This notion was specifically supported by studies which demonstrated the presence of activated T cells in injured CNS and their association with a poor prognosis and exacerbated neuronal loss.

In contrast to these findings, multiple studies have shown that T cells mediate a wide range brain processes and have a physiological role in normal brain functions. Amongst the T-cell subsets, Treg cells carry out specialized functions in tissue homeostasis and remodeling. However, the role of these cells in brain homeostasis and remodeling is inadequately known because a low number of Treg cells is reported in the brain in physiological conditions. Brain Treg cells exhibit some interesting features, in that they express some neural cell-specific genes like neuropeptide Y (npy) and the serotonin receptor type 7 (Htr7); this suggests their roles in brain-specific immune signaling. Brain Treg cells also respond to serotonin. The neuroprotective potential of T cells has been examined under various conditions. T cells are now thought to provide neuroprotective effects by down-regulating the synthesis of several components, including inflammatory mediators, reactive oxygen species, etc. and by up-regulating the expression of neurotrophic factors, such as brain-derived neurotrophic factor (BDNF) [34]. In *in vitro* co-culture experiments with T cells and astrocytes, glutamate secreted by T cells elicits release of neuroprotective thiols (cysteine, glutathione, and cysteinylglycine) and lactate from astrocytes, thus endowing astrocytes with a neuroprotective phenotype [35].

The longstanding view that T cells only mediate neuronal injury has been challenged by studies showing that T cells can also contribute to the repair and regeneration of the brain and thus play an important role in resolving damage after CNS injury. Robust support for this notion has come from several recent studies both in human and experimental animals. A massive accumulation of Treg cells was demonstrated in the mouse brain after ischemic stroke and this was associated with neural recovery during the chronic phase of ischemic brain injury by suppressing neurotoxic astrogliosis [36]. In an experimental mouse model of stroke, administration of serotonin or selective serotonin reuptake inhibitors was shown to increase the number of Treg cells in the brain and to reduce neurological dysfunction [36].

The above understanding undoubtedly suggests that T cell-mediated immunity has dual effects in the brain; they can either exacerbate neurotoxic response or provide neuroprotection.

7.5 Expanding Role of T Cells in Neuropsychiatric Disorders

There is an extensive body of data showing that major psychiatric disorders like schizophrenia, bipolar disorders, and major depressive disorders are associated with immune dysfunctions, driven at least in part by T-cell responses.

7.5.1 T Cells and Schizophrenia

Evidence linking T-cell abnormalities to schizophrenia dates back to early 1980s indicating that schizophrenia is accompanied by lowered T lymphocyte numbers as compared to controls [37]. Subsequent to this, the macrophage theory of schizophrenia was proposed in 1992 [38] and was further extended into the Macrophage-T lymphocyte theory of schizophrenia [2]. This theory was based on findings in the early 1990s showing increased levels of the soluble IL-2 receptor (sIL-2R) in schizophrenia, a marker of T-cell activation [39, 40]. Over the past 25 years, diverse lines of evidence have consistently highlighted the implications of T lymphocytes in schizophrenia pathobiology and this has been extensively reviewed in our previously published article [41].

Evidence linking T cell-mediated adaptive immunity with schizophrenia pathogenesis comes from studies showing altered percentages of various lineages of T lymphocytes and their ratio as well as an activation of the T-cell network. In one study, a lower level of CD4+ cells and a significantly higher percentage of CD4+45RA+ and CD8+ suppressor/cytotoxic T cell were reported in patients with schizophrenia [42]. In another study, a lower level of T-helper cells as well as a reduced CD4/CD8 ratio was reported during acute psychosis. However, after 6 weeks of medication, the counts of total T cell, T-helper cell, and T suppressor/cytotoxic cells increased significantly [43]. Similarly, another study examining the impact of antipsychotics demonstrated a significantly increased CD4/CD8 ratio in first episode patients; however, the ratio diminished following antipsychotic treatment, suggesting that this could be a state-related marker of psychosis in patients with schizophrenia [44].

Recently, Roomruangwong et al. [45] reviewed that different phenotypes of schizophrenia are accompanied by enhanced macrophage M1 and Th1, Th17, and Th2 activities as well as T regulatory (Treg) activities, indicating that different phenotypes are accompanied by an interrelated up-regulation of all immune functions. For example, in antipsychotic naïve first episode psychosis (FEP), there is an intertwined up-regulation of M1, Th1, Th17, Th2, and Treg cells, indicating a robust immune-inflammatory response [46]. In addition, increased levels of CCL11 in schizophrenia are significantly associated with formal thought disorders, deficits in sematic and episodic memory, and executive functions [24]. Another recent report indicates that those cognitive impairments in schizophrenia are strongly associated with peripheral aberrations in M1 (IL-1β and TNF-α) as well as Th2 (CCL11) functions [47].

Over the past few years, studies increasingly implicate other T-cell lineages, such as Th17 and Treg in schizophrenia [48, 49]. Further support for the involvement of Th17 cells comes from a study showing increased number of Th17 cells in patients with schizophrenia, with this increase positively correlating with plasma levels of IL-6, IL-17, and IFN-γ [50]. Consistent with this, elevated gene expression levels of the transcription factor (RORC), a master regulator of Th17 cells and plasma levels of cytokines like IL-6 and IL-22 were reported in drug naïve schizophrenia patients [51]. IL-6 drives Th17 cell differentiation, while IL-17 and IL-22 are hallmark effector cytokines of Th17 cells. These studies suggest that Th17 cells might play an important role in the immunopathogenesis of neuropsychiatric disorders. However, in contradiction to the above data, a recent study found no differences in the count of CD3+ and CD4+ T cells, although the proportion of Treg cells in schizophrenia patients was significantly greater than the healthy control subjects [52]. In addition to this, the strongest support of a dysregulated T-cell network comes from postmortem studies. Higher densities of T lymphocytes in the hippocampus and an increased frequency of activated lymphocytes in the CSF were reported in schizophrenia patients [53, 54].

The importance of T-cell immunity in schizophrenia is supported by genetic, epigenetic, and molecular studies. Genetic polymorphisms within genes such as CD28 and cytotoxic T lymphocyte antigen-4 (CTLA-4), which are known to regulate T-cell activity, were shown to be significantly associated with schizophrenia risk by candidate gene studies [55, 56]. In addition, pathway analyses performed on GWAS data indicated that certain genes involved in T-cell functions including antigen processing and cell adhesion, confer susceptibility to schizophrenia [57]. Data obtained from epigenetic studies provided further support by showing that certain genes involved in the activation of T cells were differentially methylated in schizophrenia [58]. An *in vitro* study on peripheral blood CD3+ pan T cells derived from schizophrenia patients, stimulated with anti-CD3 revealed significant physiological differences in T-cell responses. This included reduced proliferative responses of T cells to stimulation, alterations in T-cell subpopulations expressing CD45 isoforms, as well as changes in expression of genes regulating the cell cycle, cell signaling, oxidative stress, and metabolism [59].

7.5.2 T Cells and Mood Disorders

An important role of T lymphocytes in major depression was discovered in the 1990s as indicated by increased serum levels of sIL-2R [60] and activation markers on T lymphocytes including CD4+, CD4+CD45RA (T memory), HLA-DR, and CD25+ cells [61]. Moreover, using supervised machine learning, it was shown that major depression and melancholia constitute qualitatively distinct entities with regard to T-cell activation markers as compared with controls or minor depression

[62, 63]. T-cell activation was also reported in bipolar disorders as indicated by increased levels of sIL-2R [64]. Recent studies show increased proportions of activated T cells (CD4+CD25+), raised serum levels of sIL-2R, and increased p-ERK signaling in peripheral T-cell subsets [65–67]. In one study, the proliferation capacity of T lymphocytes was significantly reduced in bipolar disorder patients treated with lithium compared to healthy people. T lymphocytes from bipolar patients were more prone to apoptosis. When the impact of therapeutic doses of lithium or valproic acid was tested *in vitro* on T lymphocytes, these therapeutic agents protected T lymphocytes from apoptosis but did not enhance their proliferation capacity [68].

Treg cells (CD4+ CD25+ FOXP3+) play critical roles in suppressing excessive or inappropriate immune responses that are harmful to the host and/or immune responses against self-antigens in autoimmune diseases. Lower proportions of these cells are reported in patients with bipolar disorders in most studies [65, 67] that have examined the issue. On the other hand, a study reported increased percentages of CD4+ CD25+ FOXP3+ Treg cells and normal percentages of Th1, Th2, and Th17 cells in individuals with bipolar disorder [49].

Recent evidence also suggests that peripheral T cells may also influence structural and functional brain integrity in patients with bipolar disorder. For example, the percentage of circulating Th17 cells was positively correlated with higher fractional anisotropy in fiber tracts and circulating Treg cells were correlated positively with higher radial and mean diffusivity in patients with bipolar depression [69].

Defects in T-cell functioning have also been demonstrated in patients with major depressive disorder (MDD). Decreased percentages of Treg cells and an impaired ability of T-helper cells to differentiate into Th2 or Th17 cells were observed in MDD patients [70]. T-cell phenotype analysis suggests a shift in the CD4+ T cell compartment toward Treg cells, implying skewed T-cell differentiation in MDD [71], and significantly reduced surface expression of the chemokine receptors CXCR3 and CCR6 that are involved in T-cell differentiation and trafficking. In addition, a less diverse T-cell repertoire was found, based on the finding that the cell repertoire showed a trend for higher Gini-TCR indices in CD4+ cells. Based on this, it was concluded that the CD4+ TCR repertoire might be less evenly distributed in MDD [71]. Further evidence for the involvement of T cells in depression comes from animal studies. In mice during depression-like states, the number of Th17 cells increased in the brain, and inflammatory Th17 cells were found to promote depression-like behaviors [72]. Mice depleted of Treg cells were susceptible to chronic immobilization stress-induced depression-like behaviors [73].

The reasons behind the altered counts of T lymphocytes in various psychiatric disorders remain unknown. Some studies attempted to understand the effect of genetic and environmental risk factors on T-cell number variation in psychiatric disorders like schizophrenia and bipolar disorder. In twin studies, reductions in circulating T cells were associated with the liability to develop bipolar disorder; however, the authors emphasized that neither genetic nor environmental factors accounted for this association [74]. However, there are reports that environmental adversities like infection, nutritional deficiencies, stress, etc. known to be risks for psychiatric disorders can alter T-cell number and function. The notion that genetic factors may influence T cells function is supported by a recent study on 22q11.2 deletion syndrome patients, with or without psychosis. A high rate of schizophrenia has been reported in patients with 22q11.2 deletion syndrome, a condition that is predominantly marked by T-cell deficiency [75]. 22q11.2 deletion syndrome patients with psychotic symptoms displayed a partial T-cell deficiency, but had significantly higher percentages of inflammatory Th17 cells than deletion syndrome patients without psychosis [76].

Recently, a new immune theory of major depression and bipolar disorder was formulated, namely the IRS – CIRS immune theory [77]. This theory considers that both the IRS and CIRS (compensatory immune regulatory system) are involved in both affective disorders, whereby CIRS function attenuates a primary immune response thereby exerting protective functions including promoting spontaneous remission of the acute phase [77]. This theory also suggests that products of activated M1 (IL-1β, IL-6, TNF-α), Th1 (IL-2 and IFN-γ) as well as Th2 (CCL11, IL-4) cells may have neurotoxic activities thereby contributing to affective disorders.

7.6 The Mechanistic Relevance of T Cells to the Pathophysiology and Pathogenesis of Major Psychiatric Disorders

7.6.1 T Cells and Regulation of CNS Inflammatory State

Microglia are the macrophage-like resident immune cells in the central nervous system. Under physiological conditions, microglia survey the brain, provide a first line of defence, and participate in the maintenance and pruning of synapses. Given their scavenging potential, microglia are being considered as a sensor for pathological events including inflammation in the brain; they get rapidly activated in response to minor pathological changes in the brain. Activation of microglia marks a central event in neuroinflammation. Uncontrolled activation of microglia leads to exaggerated production of various substances like inflammatory cytokines, NO, PGE2, superoxide, etc., which, while having adaptive roles, can exert potentially toxic effects on neurons.

There is now evidence that microglia present antigens and stimulate CD4+ and CD8+ T cells. Like other antigen-presenting cells, microglia express major histocompatibility complex (MHC) class I and class II antigens. Microglia also express complement receptors, including CR1, CR2, and CR4, as well as Fc receptors. Microglia secrete pro- and anti-inflammatory cytokines, co-stimulatory molecules, intercellular adhesion molecule-1 (ICAM-1), B7-1, and B7-2. However, a pertinent question is how microglia derive their inflammatory potential? Do peripheral immune cells and mediators have any impact on inflammatory responses driven by microglia? A great deal of research suggests T cell-microglia cross-talk leading to inflammation and subsequently to deleterious consequences, such as impairing the BBB by increasing its permeability and thereby causing brain damage. Supporting the likelihood of this type of cross-talk are past studies demonstrating that there is a massive infiltration of T lymphocytes into the brain in various CNS pathologies/neurodegenerative disorders. Findings from animal studies also support the notion that T lymphocytes migrate into the brain from periphery across the blood and CSF barrier [78].

However, the question is, do all the T lymphocytes have the ability to home into the brain and mount an immune response, or is it the case that only a few selectively primed T cells can home into the brain? And under what circumstances might they do so? A study on experimental animals suggests that CD8+ T lymphocytes that are primed in the periphery provide time bound immune surveillance in the CNS [79]. Effector molecules released by various subsets of T cells like Th1 and Th17 have distinct effects on different glial cell subtypes and in amplifying inflammatory responses in the brain [80, 81]. These studies suggest that T lymphocyte subsets critically influence the outcome of microglial activation as well as neuroinflammation.

Neuroinflammation, elicited by activated microglia and infiltrating T cells is emerging as a prominent pathological feature in various neuropsychiatric conditions. Albeit limited, a few preliminary studies in postmortem brain samples suggest the presence of increased and/or activated immune cell populations in the brain of schizophrenia patients. Higher densities of CD3+ T lymphocytes as well as HLA-DR+ microglia were observed in the hippocampus of schizophrenia patients [53]. Cortical, thalamic, and mesiotemporal brain regions were found to have moderately or considerably increased numbers of CD3+ T lymphocytes. These and other recent findings on increased macrophage and altered endothelial gene expression in the frontal cortex of schizophrenia patients indicate immune cell transmigration into the brain of schizophrenia patients [82] as well as a possible role of neuroinflammation in the pathogenesis of schizophrenia.

7.6.2 T Cells as Mediators of Neuroprogression

Major psychiatric disorders like schizophrenia, bipolar disorder, and major depressive disorder can present a progressive course which is characterized by worsening of the clinical course, structural brain changes, and cognitive impairment as well as poorer response to pharmacotherapy as disease chronicity increases. There are renewed attempts to understand the neurobiological basis of clinical deterioration or neuroprogression in these neuropsychiatric disorders. Several mechanisms or factors such as neurotransmitter abnormalities, immunoinflammatory, oxidative, and nitrosative stress (IO&NS) pathway, mitochondrial dysfunction, tryptophan catabolite (TRYCAT) pathway, etc. have been proposed as interacting biological substrates of neuroprogression in major psychiatric disorders [83–85]. Among them, inflammatory and/or immune dysfunction has been proposed as a key mechanism. Despite these advances, the immune cell(s) or mediator that act as major toxic players in inducing neuroprogressive changes are yet to be precisely identified. Based on various lines of evidence, it is assumed that T cells may be crucially involved in this process. T cells have been implicated in neurodegenerative processes in several

CNS diseases in which they have been shown to actively contribute to neuronal damage. Encephalitogenic CD4+T cells such as Th1, Th17, GM-CSF producing CD4+ T cells and γδT-cells strongly induce chronic neuroinflammation. Neuroinflammation, which can be driven by an imbalance of inflammatory effector T cells and Tregs may lead to reduced neuroprotective effects and neuronal damage. The relevance of Th17 cells and the probable underlying mechanisms by which these cells may mediate neuroprogression in schizophrenia and major depressive disorders have been recently highlighted [86]. In a positron emission tomography (PET) scan study on recent onset schizophrenia patients, activated microglia were observed in the first few years of disease onset. It was proposed that during this period the disease process could be associated with immune-related neuronal damage [87].

7.6.3 T Cells as Mediators of Maternal Immune Activation-Induced Behavioral Changes

Maternal immune activation (MIA) due to prenatal infection has emerged as one of the predominant risk mechanisms of several neurodevelopmental disorders including schizophrenia. The identification of this and other prenatal risk factors and mechanisms interfering with crucial phases of neurodevelopment has led to the conceptualization of "fetal programming of neurodevelopmental disorders", and this process has been comprehensively reviewed in our previously published article [88]. In a recent study, the induction of MIA with staphylococcal enterotoxin A in C57BL/6 mice was shown to produce behavioral alterations akin to neurodevelopmental disorders. Notably, the induction of MIA was shown to be mediated prominently by T cells [89]. In addition to this, maternal immune stimulation was also found to shape the immunological phenotype of the offspring. This included lasting changes in inflammatory macrophages as well as components of adaptive immunity [90–92]. In experimental animal studies, prenatal infection-induced MIA resulted in hyperactivated immune responses in adult offspring through preferential development of Th17 cells as well as by inducing functional changes in CD4+ T cells [93, 94]. These studies suggest that T cells not only take part in maternal immune activation but also are crucially involved in mediating the lasting effect of MIA on brain and behavior.

7.6.4 T Cells and Neurotransmitters: Potential Interactions and Their Implications in Psychosis

The communication between the nervous system and immune system is bidirectional. The cells of the nervous system communicate with each other through neurotransmitters, while the cells of the immune system communicate with immune as well as nonimmune cells including cells of the nervous system by producing signaling molecules, predominantly cytokines. There is compelling evidence that lymphocytes express receptors for several neurotransmitters like dopamine, glutamate, serotonin, etc. [95]. These neurotransmitters activate T lymphocytes, and alter their function in ways that can also lead to autoimmunity or aberrant regulation of cell growth. For example, the dopaminergic system in peripheral blood lymphocytes plays a predominant role in neural-immune interactions in ways that have potential implications for neuropsychiatric disorders. The dopamine hypothesis of schizophrenia is the oldest and most enduring model and has parallels in bipolar disorder and depression [96, 97]. The immunomodulatory effects of dopamine are well-documented. It does so by directly interacting with the dopaminergic receptors expressed on the surface of T cells. Besides its role in migration, homing, and proliferation of T cells, dopamine can activate resting T cells by stimulating the release of cytokines and the expression of surface integrins. Conversely, it has also been shown that physiological concentrations of dopamine inhibited the proliferation and cytotoxicity of CD4+ and CD8+ T cells *in vitro* [98]. It is noteworthy that dopamine differentially favors CD4+ T-cell differentiation into Th1 or Th17 inflammatory cells; however, this is based on the activation of specific dopamine receptors on dendritic and T cells. For example, when the dopamine receptor D5 expressed on dendritic cells is stimulated, it potentiates Th17-mediated immunity [99].

Multiple studies demonstrated altered peripheral blood dopaminergic system in psychiatric disorders [100]. Significantly higher D3 and lower D4 receptor mRNA expression was reported in T cells of schizophrenia patients [101]. Importantly, studies have shown that mRNA levels of D2 and D3 receptor are correlated with the positive and negative symptom scale scores. Given these findings, it is not unreasonable to assume that dopamine plays an important role in the regulation of T cell-mediated immunity in schizophrenia and other disorders.

The balancing act of T cells and the possible mechanisms underlying T cell-mediated immunopathogenesis of neuropsychiatric disorders are depicted in Fig. 7.2.

7.7 T Cells and Antipsychotic Treatment Response

Antipsychotic drugs (APDs), which are commonly used to treat patients with major psychiatric disorders, have proven to have immunomodulatory functions. Importantly, some of the effects of APDs are manifested in peripheral blood lymphocytes. The effect of APDs on peripheral T cells number and functions have been examined in various neuropsychiatric disorders, with mixed findings.

In drug naïve schizophrenia patients, increased T suppressor lymphocytes were found, while in drug-treated patients there were increased numbers of T-helper lymphocytes [103]. In another study, higher CD3+ and CD4+ cells and a higher CD4/CD8 ratio were observed during the acute state, and became normalized during neuroleptic treatment [104]. These observations are supported by a meta-analysis reporting that the absolute levels of total lymphocytes, CD3 and CD4 cells as well as CD4/CD8 ratio are increased in drug-naïve first-episode psychosis, but the ratio of CD4/CD8 decreases following antipsychotic treatment [44]. In contradiction to this, one study reported that 6 weeks of medication normalized a lower level of

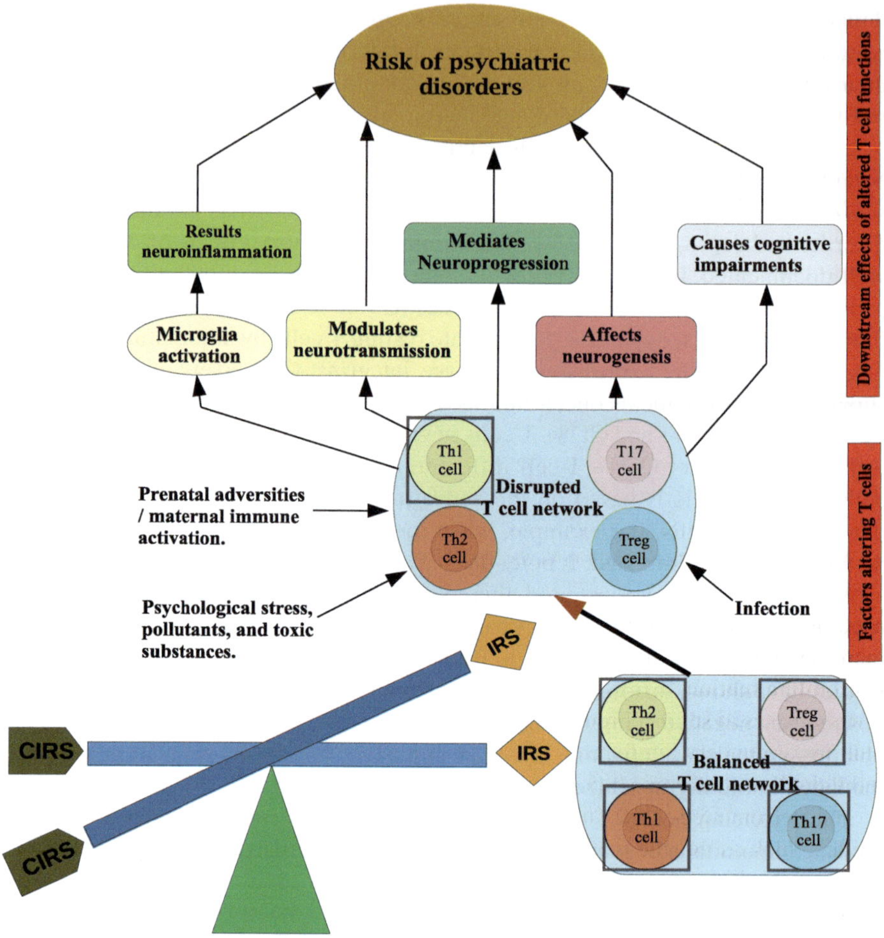

Fig. 7.2 Depicts disruption of T-cell balance in the face of various adversities and the summary of underlying mechanisms leading to neuropsychiatric disorders. The balance between immune-inflammatory response system (IRS) and compensatory immune regulatory system (CIRS) pathways determines which phenotypes prevail. There is some evidence that in MDD, BD, and SCZ, the IRS is activated and that the CIRS is insufficient to counteract the IRS response [45, 77]. Moreover, deficits in CIRS may predispose towards increased IRS responses as for example in deficit schizophrenia which is characterized by highly specific deficits in CIRS including lowered natural IgM responses to different oxidative-specific epitopes [102]

T-helper cells and a reduced CD4/CD8 ratio noted during acute psychosis [43]. The effects of APDs on Treg cells are evident in psychosis. Antipsychotic-medicated schizophrenia patients had significantly greater number of Treg cells compared to healthy control subjects and this correlated with fewer negative symptoms [52]. There is a growing discussion that these cells could emerge as crucial mediator of psycho-immune resilience and a potential player of immunotherapy in various neuropsychiatric disorders.

It is interesting to note that APDs can also influence the differentiation pattern of T lymphocytes. In an *in vitro* study, peripheral blood mononuclear cells (PBMCs) treated with clozapine or risperidone showed reduced differentiation of Th1 cells and T-bet expression, while, haloperidol reduced the expression of GATA3 and Th2 cell differentiation [105]. APDs like haloperidol and clozapine regulate expression of large number of genes in T lymphocytes. In another recent *in vitro* study, APD modulated mRNA-miRNA interactions and resulted in differential gene expression in genes related to cellular metabolism and oxidative stress in T lymphocytes [106]. In addition, several other studies have shown the immunomodulatory effects of APDs on Th1, Th2, Th17, and Treg pathway-related cytokines [107, 108].

Robust immunomodulatory effects of antidepressants have been documented in studies conducted both on experimental animals and human. This includes a variety of effects on cytokine levels, cytokine balance, immune cells count, and so on. In one of the earlier *in vitro* studies on human lymphocytes incubated with antidepressants, tricyclic antidepressants were found to induce apoptosis in T lymphocytes [109]. Another *in vitro* study examined the effect of antidepressants on cytokine synthesis by T lymphocytes and demonstrated that the tricyclic antidepressants inhibited the release of IFN-γ and IL-2 from activated T cells [110]. Besides this, several other studies have shown immuno-dampening effects of antidepressants, especially by down-regulating the expression of immuno-inflammatory cytokines. A recent study indicated IL-17, a hallmark cytokine of Th17 cells could serve as a novel T-cell biomarker for assessing differential treatment outcome with antidepressants [111]. Additionally, the impact of antidepressants on immuno-suppressive Treg cells has also been discussed in recent studies. Six weeks of treatment with antidepressants was shown to significantly increase the count of Treg cells and this was accompanied by decreased serum levels of IL-1β [112].

7.8 Conclusion

The understanding of neuro-immune cross-talk and the implications of such cross-talk in neuropsychiatric disorders has led to the conceptualization of a novel field, "Immunopsychiatry". This field has not only provided important insights into the neurobiological, trans-generational, gene-environmental bases of major psychiatric disorders, but has also pointed to a novel potential therapeutic avenue in treating patients with such disorders.

T cells have been implicated as a major driver of a large number of inflammatory and autoimmune diseases. The link between T cells and neurodegenerative and/or neurodevelopmental disorders has been the subject of intense research activity. With the discovery of a well-organized and functional lymphatic system and the identification of immune gateways in the brain, T lymphocytes have become a focus of researchers working on brain disorders having immunological underpinning. The ability of T cells to take part in brain tissue remodeling, their involvement in adult neurogenesis, and their determining role in learning, memory, and behavior, make them key immune cells in major psychiatric disorders. However, the factors that determine the dual- and often contradictory-behavior in the same tissue have remained a mystery. Though the mechanisms that ensure homing, molecular memory, stability, plasticity, and exhaustion of T lymphocytes are yet to be fully understood, genetic-epigenetic programming of T-cell responses are increasingly envisaged to be critical. Epigenetic regulation of T cell fate, function, and responses is shown to play a key role in health and in many immune-mediated diseases. Given ever-increasing implications of epigenetic processes in neuropsychiatric disorders, T cells could emerge as a potential missing link at the gene-environmental interface of psychiatric disorders. Animal modeling of neuropsychiatric disorders specifically targeting T lymphocytes under a controlled genetic/epigenetic environment could contribute to a greater understanding of immunopsychiatry.

References

1. Smith RS. The macrophage theory of depression. Med Hypotheses. 1991;35:298–306.
2. Smith RS, Maes M. The macrophage-T-lymphocyte theory of schizophrenia: additional evidence. Med Hypotheses. 1995;45:135–41.
3. Louveau A, Smirnov I, Keyes TJ, Eccles JD, Rouhani SJ, Peske JD, Derecki NC, Castle D, Mandell JW, Lee KS, Harris TH, Kipnis J. Structural and functional features of central nervous system lymphatic vessels. Nature. 2015;523:337–41.
4. Kumar BV, Connors TJ, Farber DL. Human T cell development, localization, and function throughout life. Immunity. 2018;48:202–13.
5. Elmer BM, Mcallister AK. Major histocompatibility complex class I proteins in brain development and plasticity. Trends Neurosci. 2012;35:660–70.
6. Korin B, Ben-Shaanan TL, Schiller M, Dubovik T, Azulay-Debby H, Boshnak NT, Koren T, Rolls A. High-dimensional, single-cell characterization of the brain's immune compartment. Nat Neurosci. 2017;20:1300–9.
7. Svenningsson A, Andersen O, Edsbagge M, Stemme S. Lymphocyte phenotype and subset distribution in normal cerebrospinal fluid. J Neuroimmunol. 1995;63:39–46.
8. Engelhardt B, Ransohoff RM. The ins and outs of T-lymphocyte trafficking to the Cns: anatomical sites and molecular mechanisms. Trends Immunol. 2005;26:485–95.
9. Strominger I, Elyahu Y, Berner O, Reckhow J, Mittal K, Nemirovsky A, Monsonego A. The choroid plexus functions as a niche for T-cell stimulation within the central nervous system. Front Immunol. 2018;9:1066.
10. Herz J, Paterka M, Niesner RA, Brandt AU, Siffrin V, Leuenberger T, Birkenstock J, Mossakowski A, Glumm R, Zipp F, Radbruch H. In vivo imaging of lymphocytes in the CNS reveals different behaviour of naive T cells in health and autoimmunity. J Neuroinflammation. 2011;8:131.
11. Smolders J, Heutinck KM, Fransen NL, Remmerswaal EBM, Hombrink P, TenBerge IJM, VanLier RAW, Huitinga I, Hamann J. Tissue-resident memory T cells populate the human brain. Nat Commun. 2018;9:4593.
12. Kivisakk P, Mahad DJ, Callahan MK, Trebst C, Tucky B, Wei T, Wu L, Baekkevold ES, Lassmann H, Staugaitis SM, Campbell JJ, Ransohoff RM. Human cerebrospinal fluid central memory CD4+ T cells: evidence for trafficking through choroid plexus and meninges via P-selectin. Proc Natl Acad Sci U S A. 2003;100:8389–94.
13. Tanabe S, Yamashita T. B-1a lymphocytes promote oligodendrogenesis during brain development. Nat Neurosci. 2018;21:506–16.
14. Ziv Y, Ron N, Butovsky O, Landa G, Sudai E, Greenberg N, Cohen H, Kipnis J, Schwartz M. Immune cells contribute to the maintenance of neurogenesis and spatial learning abilities in adulthood. Nat Neurosci. 2006;9:268–75.

15. Walker TL, Schallenberg S, Rund N, Gronnert L, Rust R, Kretschmer K, Kempermann G. T Lymphocytes contribute to the control of baseline neural precursor cell proliferation but not the exercise-induced up-regulation of adult hippocampal neurogenesis. Front Immunol. 2018;9:2856.
16. Zarif H, Nicolas S, Guyot M, Hosseiny S, Lazzari A, Canali MM, Cazareth J, Brau F, Golzne V, Dourneau E, Maillaut M, Luci C, Paquet A, Lebrigand K, Arguel MJ, Daoudlarian D, Heurteaux C, Glaichenhaus N, Chabry J, Guyon A, Petit-Paitel A. CD8(+) T cells are essential for the effects of enriched environment on hippocampus-dependent behavior, hippocampal neurogenesis and synaptic plasticity. Brain Behav Immun. 2018;69:235–54.
17. Wolf SA, Steiner B, Akpinarli A, Kammertoens T, Nassenstein C, Braun A, Blankenstein T, Kempermann G. CD4 positive T lymphocytes provide a neuroimmunological link in the control of adult hippocampal neurogenesis. J Immunol. 2009;182:3979–84.
18. Huang GJ, Smith AL, Gray DH, Cosgrove C, Singer BH, Edwards A, Sims S, Parent JM, Johnsen A, Mott R, Mathis D, Klenerman P, Benoist C, Flint J. A genetic and functional relationship between T cells and cellular proliferation in the adult hippocampus. PLoS Biol. 2010;8:e1000561.
19. Wang T, Lee MH, Johnson T, Allie R, Hu L, Calabresi PA, Nath A. Activated T-cells inhibit neurogenesis by releasing granzyme B: rescue by Kv1.3 blockers. J Neurosci. 2010;30:5020–7.
20. Jinquan T, Quan S, Feili G, Larsen CG, Thestrup-Pedersen K. Eotaxin activates T cells to chemotaxis and adhesion only if induced to express CCR3 by IL-2 together with IL-4. J Immunol. 1999;162:4285–92.
21. Erickson MA, Morofuji Y, Owen JB, Banks WA. Rapid transport of CCL11 across the blood-brain barrier: regional variation and importance of blood cells. J Pharmacol Exp Ther. 2014;349:497–507.
22. Wainwright DA, Xin J, Mesnard NA, Politis CM, Sanders VM, Jones KJ. Effects of facial nerve axotomy on Th2- and Th1-associated chemokine expression in the facial motor nucleus of wild-type and presymptomatic mSOD1 mice. J Neuroimmunol. 2009;216:66–75.
23. Villeda SA, Luo J, Mosher KI, Zou B, Britschgi M, Bieri G, Stan TM, Fainberg N, Ding Z, Eggel A, Lucin KM, Czirr E, Park JS, Couillard-Despres S, Aigner L, Li G, Peskind ER, Kaye JA, Quinn JF, Galasko DR, Xie XS, Rando TA, Wyss-Coray T. The ageing systemic milieu negatively regulates neurogenesis and cognitive function. Nature. 2011;477:90–4.
24. Sirivichayakul S, Kanchanatawan B, Thika S, Carvalho AF, Maes M. Eotaxin, an endogenous cognitive deteriorating chemokine (ECDC), is a major contributor to cognitive decline in normal people and to executive, memory, and sustained attention deficits, formal thought disorders, and psychopathology in schizophrenia patients. Neurotox Res. 2019;35:122–38.
25. Kipnis J, Gadani S, Derecki NC. Pro-cognitive properties of T cells. Nat Rev Immunol. 2012;12:663–9.
26. Serre-Miranda C, Roque S, Santos NC, Portugal-Nunes C, Costa P, Palha JA, Sousa N, Correia-Neves M. Effector memory CD4(+) T cells are associated with cognitive performance in a senior population. Neurol Neuroimmunol Neuroinflamm. 2015;2:e54.
27. Fernandez-Egea E, Vertes PE, Flint SM, Turner L, Mustafa S, Hatton A, Smith KG, Lyons PA, Bullmore ET. Peripheral immune cell populations associated with cognitive deficits and negative symptoms of treatment-resistant schizophrenia. PLoS One. 2016;11:e0155631.
28. Kipnis J, Cohen H, Cardon M, Ziv Y, Schwartz M. T cell deficiency leads to cognitive dysfunction: implications for therapeutic vaccination for schizophrenia and other psychiatric conditions. Proc Natl Acad Sci U S A. 2004;101:8180–5.
29. Radjavi A, Smirnov I, Derecki N, Kipnis J. Dynamics of the meningeal CD4(+) T-cell repertoire are defined by the cervical lymph nodes and facilitate cognitive task performance in mice. Mol Psychiatry. 2014;19:531–3.
30. Derecki NC, Cardani AN, Yang CH, Quinnies KM, Crihfield A, Lynch KR, Kipnis J. Regulation of learning and memory by meningeal immunity: a key role for IL-4. J Exp Med. 2010;207:1067–80.

31. Filiano AJ, Xu Y, Tustison NJ, Marsh RL, Baker W, Smirnov I, Overall CC, Gadani SP, Turner SD, Weng Z, Peerzade SN, Chen H, Lee KS, Scott MM, Beenhakker MP, Litvak V, Kipnis J. Unexpected role of interferon-gamma in regulating neuronal connectivity and social behaviour. Nature. 2016;535:425–9.
32. Song EJ, Jeon SG, Kim KA, Kim JI, Moon M. Restricted CD4+ T cell receptor repertoire impairs cognitive function via alteration of Th2 cytokine levels. Neurogenesis (Austin). 2017;4:e1256856.
33. Walsh JT, Watson N, Kipnis J. T cells in the central nervous system: messengers of destruction or purveyors of protection? Immunology. 2014;141:340–4.
34. Kerschensteiner M, Gallmeier E, Behrens L, Leal VV, Misgeld T, Klinkert WE, Kolbeck R, Hoppe E, Oropeza-Wekerle RL, Bartke I, Stadelmann C, Lassmann H, Wekerle H, Hohlfeld R. Activated human T cells, B cells, and monocytes produce brain-derived neurotrophic factor in vitro and in inflammatory brain lesions: a neuroprotective role of inflammation? J Exp Med. 1999;189:865–70.
35. Garg SK, Banerjee R, Kipnis J. Neuroprotective immunity: T cell-derived glutamate endows astrocytes with a neuroprotective phenotype. J Immunol. 2008;180:3866–73.
36. Ito M, Komai K, Mise-Omata S, Iizuka-Koga M, Noguchi Y, Kondo T, Sakai R, Matsuo K, Nakayama T, Yoshie O, Nakatsukasa H, Chikuma S, Shichita T, Yoshimura A. Brain regulatory T cells suppress astrogliosis and potentiate neurological recovery. Nature. 2019;565:246–50.
37. Nyland H, Naess A, Lunde H. Lymphocyte subpopulations in peripheral blood from schizophrenic patients. Acta Psychiatr Scand. 1980;61:313–8.
38. Smith RS. A comprehensive macrophage-T-lymphocyte theory of schizophrenia. Med Hypotheses. 1992;39:248–57.
39. Maes M, Meltzer HY, Bosmans E. Immune-inflammatory markers in schizophrenia: comparison to normal controls and effects of clozapine. Acta Psychiatr Scand. 1994;89:346–51.
40. Rapaport MH, Lohr JB. Serum-soluble interleukin-2 receptors in neuroleptic-naive schizophrenic subjects and in medicated schizophrenic subjects with and without tardive dyskinesia. Acta Psychiatr Scand. 1994;90:311–5.
41. Debnath M. Adaptive immunity in schizophrenia: functional implications of T cells in the etiology, course and treatment. J NeuroImmune Pharmacol. 2015;10:610–9.
42. Cazzullo CL, Saresella M, Roda K, Calvo MG, Bertrando P, Doria S, Clerici M, Salvaggio A, Ferrante P. Increased levels of CD8+ and CD4+ 45RA+ lymphocytes in schizophrenic patients. Schizophr Res. 1998;31:49–55.
43. Steiner J, Jacobs R, Panteli B, Brauner M, Schiltz K, Bahn S, Herberth M, Westphal S, Gos T, Walter M, Bernstein HG, Myint AM, Bogerts B. Acute schizophrenia is accompanied by reduced T cell and increased B cell immunity. Eur Arch Psychiatry Clin Neurosci. 2010;260:509–18.
44. Miller BJ, Gassama B, Sebastian D, Buckley P, Mellor A. Meta-analysis of lymphocytes in schizophrenia: clinical status and antipsychotic effects. Biol Psychiatry. 2013;73:993–9.
45. Roomruangwong C, Noto C, Kanchanatawan B, Anderson G, Kubera M, Carvalho AF, Maes M. The role of aberrations in the immune-inflammatory reflex system (IRS) and the compensatory immune-regulatory reflex system (CIRS) in different phenotypes of schizophrenia: the IRS-CIRS theory of schizophrenia. Preprints. 2018;2018:2018090289. https://doi.org/10.20944/preprints201809.0289.v1.
46. Noto MN, Maes M, Nunes SOV, Ota VK, Rossaneis AC, Verri WA Jr, Cordeiro Q, Belangero SI, Gadelha A, Bressan RA, Noto C. Activation of the immune-inflammatory response system and the compensatory immune-regulatory system in antipsychotic naive first episode psychosis. Eur Neuropsychopharmacol. 2019;29:416–31.
47. Al-Hakeim HK, Almulla AF, Maes M. The neuroimmune and neurotoxic fingerprint of major neurocognitive psychosis or deficit schizophrenia: a supervised machine learning study. Neurotox Res. 2020;37:753–71.
48. Debnath M, Berk M. Th17 pathway-mediated immunopathogenesis of schizophrenia: mechanisms and implications. Schizophr Bull. 2014;40:1412–21.

49. Drexhage RC, Hoogenboezem TH, Versnel MA, Berghout A, Nolen WA, Drexhage HA. The activation of monocyte and T cell networks in patients with bipolar disorder. Brain Behav Immun. 2011;25:1206–13.
50. Ding M, Song X, Zhao J, Gao J, Li X, Yang G, Wang X, Harrington A, Fan X, Lv L. Activation of Th17 cells in drug naive, first episode schizophrenia. Prog Neuro-Psychopharmacol Biol Psychiatry. 2014;51:78–82.
51. Subbanna M, Shivakumar V, Talukdar PM, Narayanaswamy JC, Venugopal D, Berk M, Varambally S, Venkatasubramanian G, Debnath M. Role of IL-6/RORC/IL-22 axis in driving Th17 pathway-mediated immunopathogenesis of schizophrenia. Cytokine. 2018;111:112–8.
52. Kelly DL, Li X, Kilday C, Feldman S, Clark S, Liu F, Buchanan RW, Tonelli LH. Increased circulating regulatory T cells in medicated people with schizophrenia. Psychiatry Res. 2018;269:517–23.
53. Busse S, Busse M, Schiltz K, Bielau H, Gos T, Brisch R, Mawrin C, Schmitt A, Jordan W, Muller UJ, Bernstein HG, Bogerts B, Steiner J. Different distribution patterns of lymphocytes and microglia in the hippocampus of patients with residual versus paranoid schizophrenia: further evidence for disease course-related immune alterations? Brain Behav Immun. 2012;26:1273–9.
54. Nikkila H, Muller K, Ahokas A, Miettinen K, Andersson LC, Rimon R. Abnormal distributions of T-lymphocyte subsets in the cerebrospinal fluid of patients with acute schizophrenia. Schizophr Res. 1995;14:215–21.
55. Frydecka D, Beszlej A, Karabon L, Pawlak-Adamska E, Tomkiewicz A, Partyka A, Jonkisz A, Monika SB, Kiejna A. The role of genetic variations of immune system regulatory molecules CD28 and CTLA-4 in schizophrenia. Psychiatry Res. 2013;208:197–8.
56. Liu J, Li J, Li T, Wang T, Li Y, Zeng Z, Li Z, Chen P, Hu Z, Zheng L, Ji J, Lin H, Feng G, Shi Y. CTLA-4 confers a risk of recurrent schizophrenia, major depressive disorder and bipolar disorder in the Chinese Han population. Brain Behav Immun. 2011;25:429–33.
57. Aberg KA, Liu Y, Bukszar J, Mcclay JL, Khachane AN, Andreassen OA, Blackwood D, Corvin A, Djurovic S, Gurling H, Ophoff R, Pato CN, Pato MT, Riley B, Webb T, Kendler K, O'Donovan M, Craddock N, Kirov G, Owen M, Rujescu D, St. Clair D, Werge T, Hultman CM, Delisi LE, Sullivan P, Van Den Oord EJ. A comprehensive family-based replication study of schizophrenia genes. JAMA Psychiatry. 2013;70:573–81.
58. Liu J, Chen J, Ehrlich S, Walton E, White T, Perrone-Bizzozero N, Bustillo J, Turner JA, Calhoun VD. Methylation patterns in whole blood correlate with symptoms in schizophrenia patients. Schizophr Bull. 2014;40:769–76.
59. Craddock RM, Lockstone HE, Rider DA, Wayland MT, Harris LJ, Mckenna PJ, Bahn S. Altered T-cell function in schizophrenia: a cellular model to investigate molecular disease mechanisms. PLoS One. 2007;2:e692.
60. Maes M, Bosmans E, Suy E, Vandervorst C, De Jonckheere C, Raus J. Immune disturbances during major depression: upregulated expression of interleukin-2 receptors. Neuropsychobiology. 1990;24:115–20.
61. Maes M, Lambrechts J, Bosmans E, Jacobs J, Suy E, Vandervorst C, De Jonckheere C, Minner B, Raus J. Evidence for a systemic immune activation during depression: results of leukocyte enumeration by flow cytometry in conjunction with monoclonal antibody staining. Psychol Med. 1992;22:45–53.
62. Maes M, Stevens WJ, Declerck LS, Bridts CH, Peeters D, Schotte C, Cosyns P. Significantly increased expression of T-cell activation markers (interleukin-2 and HLA-DR) in depression: further evidence for an inflammatory process during that illness. Prog Neuro-Psychopharmacol Biol Psychiatry. 1993;17:241–55.
63. Maes M, VanDerPlanken M, Stevens WJ, Peeters D, Declerck LS, Bridts CH, Schotte C, Cosyns P. Leukocytosis, monocytosis and neutrophilia: hallmarks of severe depression. J Psychiatr Res. 1992;26:125–34.
64. Maes M, Bosmans E, Calabrese J, Smith R, Meltzer HY. Interleukin-2 and interleukin-6 in schizophrenia and mania: effects of neuroleptics and mood stabilizers. J Psychiatr Res. 1995;29:141–52.

65. Barbosa IG, Rocha NP, Assis F, Vieira EL, Soares JC, Bauer ME, Teixeira AL. Monocyte and lymphocyte activation in bipolar disorder: a new piece in the puzzle of immune dysfunction in mood disorders. Int J Neuropsychopharmacol. 2014;2014:18.
66. Breunis MN, Kupka RW, Nolen WA, Suppes T, Denicoff KD, Leverich GS, Post RM, Drexhage HA. High numbers of circulating activated T cells and raised levels of serum IL-2 receptor in bipolar disorder. Biol Psychiatry. 2003;53:157–65.
67. Do Prado CH, Rizzo LB, Wieck A, Lopes RP, Teixeira AL, Grassi-Oliveira R, Bauer ME. Reduced regulatory T cells are associated with higher levels of Th1/TH17 cytokines and activated MAPK in type 1 bipolar disorder. Psychoneuroendocrinology. 2013;38:667–76.
68. Pietruczuk K, Lisowska KA, Grabowski K, Landowski J, Witkowski JM. Proliferation and apoptosis of T lymphocytes in patients with bipolar disorder. Sci Rep. 2018;8:3327.
69. Poletti S, DeWit H, Mazza E, Wijkhuijs AJM, Locatelli C, Aggio V, Colombo C, Benedetti F, Drexhage HA. Th17 cells correlate positively to the structural and functional integrity of the brain in bipolar depression and healthy controls. Brain Behav Immun. 2017;61:317–25.
70. Grosse L, Hoogenboezem T, Ambree O, Bellingrath S, Jorgens S, De Wit HJ, Wijkhuijs AM, Arolt V, Drexhage HA. Deficiencies of the T and natural killer cell system in major depressive disorder: T regulatory cell defects are associated with inflammatory monocyte activation. Brain Behav Immun. 2016;54:38–44.
71. Patas K, Willing A, Demiralay C, Engler JB, Lupu A, Ramien C, Schafer T, Gach C, Stumm L, Chan K, Vignali M, Arck PC, Friese MA, Pless O, Wiedemann K, Agorastos A, Gold SM. T cell phenotype and T cell receptor repertoire in patients with major depressive disorder. Front Immunol. 2018;9:291.
72. Beurel E, Harrington LE, Jope RS. Inflammatory T helper 17 cells promote depression-like behavior in mice. Biol Psychiatry. 2013;73:622–30.
73. Kim SJ, Lee H, Lee G, Oh SJ, Shin MK, Shim I, Bae H. CD4+CD25+ regulatory T cell depletion modulates anxiety and depression-like behaviors in mice. PLoS One. 2012;7:e42054.
74. Snijders G, Brouwer R, Kemner S, Bootsman F, Drexhage HA, Hillegers MHJ. Genetic and environmental influences on circulating NK and T cells and their relation to bipolar disorder. Int J Bipolar Disord. 2019;7:4.
75. Monks S, Niarchou M, Davies AR, Walters JT, Williams N, Owen MJ, VanDenBree MB, Murphy KC. Further evidence for high rates of schizophrenia in 22q11.2 deletion syndrome. Schizophr Res. 2014;153:231–6.
76. Vergaelen E, Schiweck C, VanSteeland K, Counotte J, Veling W, Swillen A, Drexhage H, Claes S. A pilot study on immuno-psychiatry in the 22q11.2 deletion syndrome: a role for Th17 cells in psychosis? Brain Behav Immun. 2018;70:88–95.
77. Maes M, Carvalho AF. The compensatory immune-regulatory reflex system (CIRS) in depression and bipolar disorder. Mol Neurobiol. 2018;55:8885–903.
78. Strazielle N, Creidy R, Malcus C, Boucraut J, Ghersi-Egea JF. T-Lymphocytes traffic into the brain across the blood-CSFbarrier: evidence using a reconstituted choroid plexus epithelium. PLoS One. 2016;11:e0150945.
79. Young KG, Maclean S, Dudani R, Krishnan L, Sad S. CD8+ T cells primed in the periphery provide time-bound immune-surveillance to the central nervous system. J Immunol. 2011;187:1192–200.
80. Prajeeth CK, Huehn J, Stangel M. Regulation of neuroinflammatory properties of glial cells by T cell effector molecules. Neural Regen Res. 2018;13:234–6.
81. Prajeeth CK, Lohr K, Floess S, Zimmermann J, Ulrich R, Gudi V, Beineke A, Baumgartner W, Muller M, Huehn J, Stangel M. Effector molecules released by Th1 but not Th17 cells drive an M1 response in microglia. Brain Behav Immun. 2014;37:248–59.
82. Cai HQ, Catts VS, Webster MJ, Galletly C, Liu D, O'Donnell M, Weickert TW, Weickert CS. Increased macrophages and changed brain endothelial cell gene expression in the frontal cortex of people with schizophrenia displaying inflammation. Mol Psychiatry. 2018;25(4):761–75.

83. Anderson G, Maes M. Schizophrenia: linking prenatal infection to cytokines, the tryptophan catabolite (TRYCAT) pathway, NMDA receptor hypofunction, neurodevelopment and neuroprogression. Prog Neuro-Psychopharmacol Biol Psychiatry. 2013;42:5–19.
84. Davis J, Moylan S, Harvey BH, Maes M, Berk M. Neuroprogression in schizophrenia: pathways underpinning clinical staging and therapeutic corollaries. Aust N Z J Psychiatry. 2014;48:512–29.
85. Meyer JH. Neuroprogression and immune activation in major depressive disorder. Mod Trends Pharmacopsychiatry. 2017;31:27–36.
86. Slyepchenko A, Maes M, Kohler CA, Anderson G, Quevedo J, Alves GS, Berk M, Fernandes BS, Carvalho AF. T helper 17 cells may drive neuroprogression in major depressive disorder: proposal of an integrative model. Neurosci Biobehav Rev. 2016;64:83–100.
87. VanBerckel BN, Bossong MG, Boellaard R, Kloet R, Schuitemaker A, Caspers E, Luurtsema G, Windhorst AD, Cahn W, Lammertsma AA, Kahn RS. Microglia activation in recent-onset schizophrenia: a quantitative (R)-[11C]PK11195 positron emission tomography study. Biol Psychiatry. 2008;64:820–2.
88. Debnath M, Venkatasubramanian G, Berk M. Fetal programming of schizophrenia: select mechanisms. Neurosci Biobehav Rev. 2015;49:90–104.
89. Glass R, Norton S, Fox N, Kusnecov AW. Maternal immune activation with staphylococcal enterotoxin A produces unique behavioral changes in C57BL/6 mouse offspring. Brain Behav Immun. 2019;75:12–25.
90. Mandal M, Donnelly R, Elkabes S, Zhang P, Davini D, David BT, Ponzio NM. Maternal immune stimulation during pregnancy shapes the immunological phenotype of offspring. Brain Behav Immun. 2013;33:33–45.
91. Mandal M, Marzouk AC, Donnelly R, Ponzio NM. Maternal immune stimulation during pregnancy affects adaptive immunity in offspring to promote development of TH17 cells. Brain Behav Immun. 2011;25:863–71.
92. Onore CE, Schwartzer JJ, Careaga M, Berman RF, Ashwood P. Maternal immune activation leads to activated inflammatory macrophages in offspring. Brain Behav Immun. 2014;38:220–6.
93. Luan R, Cheng H, Li L, Zhao Q, Liu H, Wu Z, Zhao L, Yang J, Hao J, Yin Z. Maternal lipopolysaccharide exposure promotes immunological functional changes in adult offspring CD4+ T cells. Am J Reprod Immunol. 2015;73:522–35.
94. Mandal M, Marzouk AC, Donnelly R, Ponzio NM. Preferential development of Th17 cells in offspring of immunostimulated pregnant mice. J Reprod Immunol. 2010;87:97–100.
95. Kerage D, Sloan EK, Mattarollo SR, Mccombe PA. Interaction of neurotransmitters and neurochemicals with lymphocytes. J Neuroimmunol. 2019;332:99–111.
96. Berk M, Dodd S, Kauer-Sant'anna M, Malhi GS, Bourin M, Kapczinski F, Norman T. Dopamine dysregulation syndrome: implications for a dopamine hypothesis of bipolar disorder. Acta Psychiatr Scand Suppl. 2007;434:41–9.
97. Malhi GS, Berk M. Does dopamine dysfunction drive depression? Acta Psychiatr Scand Suppl. 2007;2007:116–24.
98. Saha B, Mondal AC, Majumder J, Basu S, Dasgupta PS. Physiological concentrations of dopamine inhibit the proliferation and cytotoxicity of human CD4+ and CD8+ T cells in vitro: a receptor-mediated mechanism. Neuroimmunomodulation. 2001;9:23–33.
99. Prado C, Contreras F, Gonzalez H, Diaz P, Elgueta D, Barrientos M, Herrada AA, Lladser A, Bernales S, Pacheco R. Stimulation of dopamine receptor D5 expressed on dendritic cells potentiates Th17-mediated immunity. J Immunol. 2012;188:3062–70.
100. Berk M, Bodemer W, VanOudenhove T, Butkow N. Dopamine increases platelet intracellular calcium in bipolar affective disorder and controls. Int Clin Psychopharmacol. 1994;9:291–3.
101. Boneberg EM, VonSeydlitz E, Propster K, Watzl H, Rockstroh B, Illges H. D3 dopamine receptor mRNA is elevated in T cells of schizophrenic patients whereas D4 dopamine receptor mRNA is reduced in CD4+ -T cells. J Neuroimmunol. 2006;173:180–7.

102. Maes M, Kanchanatawan B, Sirivichayakul S, Carvalho AF. In schizophrenia, deficits in natural IgM isotype antibodies including those directed to malondialdehyde and azelaic acid strongly predict negative symptoms, neurocognitive impairments, and the deficit syndrome. Mol Neurobiol. 2019;56:5122–35.
103. Masserini C, Vita A, Basile R, Morselli R, Boato P, Peruzzi C, Pugnetti L, Ferrante P, Cazzullo CL. Lymphocyte subsets in schizophrenic disorders. Relationship with clinical, neuromorphological and treatment variables. Schizophr Res. 1990;3:269–75.
104. Sperner-Unterweger B, Whitworth A, Kemmler G, Hilbe W, Thaler J, Weiss G, Fleischhacker WW. T-cell subsets in schizophrenia: a comparison between drug-naive first episode patients and chronic schizophrenic patients. Schizophr Res. 1999;38:61–70.
105. Chen ML, Tsai TC, Lin YY, Tsai YM, Wang LK, Lee MC, Tsai FM. Antipsychotic drugs suppress the AKT/NF-kappaB pathway and regulate the differentiation of T-cell subsets. Immunol Lett. 2011;140:81–91.
106. Gardiner E, Carroll A, Tooney PA, Cairns MJ. Antipsychotic drug-associated gene-miRNA interaction in T-lymphocytes. Int J Neuropsychopharmacol. 2014;17:929–43.
107. Noto C, Ota VK, Gouvea ES, Rizzo LB, Spindola LM, Honda PH, Cordeiro Q, Belangero SI, Bressan RA, Gadelha A, Maes M, Brietzke E. Effects of risperidone on cytokine profile in drug-naive first-episode psychosis. Int J Neuropsychopharmacol. 2014;2014:18.
108. Romeo B, Brunet-Lecomte M, Martelli C, Benyamina A. Kinetics of cytokine levels during antipsychotic treatment in schizophrenia: a meta-analysis. Int J Neuropsychopharmacol. 2018;21:828–36.
109. Xia Z, Karlsson H, Depierre JW, Nassberger L. Tricyclic antidepressants induce apoptosis in human T lymphocytes. Int J Immunopharmacol. 1997;19:645–54.
110. Xia Z, Depierre JW, Nassberger L. Tricyclic antidepressants inhibit IL-6, IL-1 beta and Tnf-alpha release in human blood monocytes and IL-2 and interferon-gamma in T cells. Immunopharmacology. 1996;34:27–37.
111. Jha MK, Minhajuddin A, Gadad BS, Greer TL, Mayes TL, Trivedi MH. Interleukin 17 selectively predicts better outcomes with bupropion-SSRI combination: novel T cell biomarker for antidepressant medication selection. Brain Behav Immun. 2017;66:103–10.
112. Himmerich H, Milenovic S, Fulda S, Plumakers B, Sheldrick AJ, Michel TM, Kircher T, Rink L. Regulatory T cells increased while IL-1 beta decreased during antidepressant therapy. J Psychiatr Res. 2010;44:1052–7.

Microglia and Psychiatric Disorders

8

Amalie C. M. Couch and Anthony C. Vernon

8.1 Introduction to Microglia: Origins, Heterogenicity and Function

About 10–20% of all cells in the CNS are microglia, to which immunological, developmental and homeostatic CNS functions have been attributed [1]. Microglia are generally considered to derive from C-KIT$^+$/CD41$^+$ erythromyeloid progenitor (EMP) cells of the haematopoietic yolk sac (YS) in the mesoderm [2]. These EMP cells are characteristically dependent upon PU.1 and Irf8 for fate determination and survival, respectively and differ from haematopoietic monocyte and macrophage development by virtue of Myb independence [3, 4]. Data from rodents suggest that a subset of these EMPs begin to express the chemokine receptor for fractalkine (CX_3CR1^+ cells), which migrate to the brain at embryonic day 9.5 to 10.5 post-conception (E9.5–10.5) [5]. After the blood-brain barrier is formed between E13.5 and 14.5, microglia begin to self-renew and distribute throughout the CNS [6, 7]. In humans, the migration of microglia into the prenatal developing brain begins at gestation week (gw) 4.5, where microglia have been observed in the forebrain [8]. Hence, microglia are found in the hindbrain metencephalon at gw 6 after peak haematopoiesis [9]. This is followed by further microglia found in the spinal cord at gw 9, and finally by gw 19 microglia have been shown in the midbrain [10].

In the periphery, circulating macrophages derived from the haematopoietic lineage, demonstrate a clear polarisation when activated in response to tissue injury or infection. M1 polarisation, or classical activation, of macrophages is predominantly directed by Toll-like receptor (TLR) activation from cytokines including interferons

A. C. M. Couch · A. C. Vernon (✉)
Department of Basic and Clinical Neuroscience, Maurice Wohl Clinical Neuroscience Institute, King's College London, London, UK

MRC Centre for Neurodevelopmental Disorders, New Hunt's House, Guy's Campus, King's College London, London, UK
e-mail: amalie.couch@kcl.ac.uk; anthony.vernon@kcl.ac.uk

M. Berk et al. (eds.), *Immuno-Psychiatry*, https://doi.org/10.1007/978-3-030-71229-7_8

(IFN) such as Th1-derived interferon (IFN)-γ, lipopolysaccharide (LPS), granulocyte macrophage colony-stimulating factor (GM-CSF) and tumour necrosis factor (TNF), with the purpose of providing immunity against pathogenic infection [11]. In contrast, M2 polarisation is associated with a beneficial homeostatic or reparative state, which is activated by interleukins (IL) 10 (IL-10) and IL-4, derived from Th2 cells and macrophage colony-stimulating factor (M-CSF) [11]. For some time it was thought, brain-resident microglia also adhered to this bipolar framework. Transcriptional profiling studies have however revealed that a variety of different microglial states can co-exist in the same tissue, each with potentially distinct functions [12]. By integrating genomic and genetic-based alterations with microenvironment and systemic signals, microglia are thus able to shift between varied functional states to play key roles in several brain processes including brain development and synaptic plasticity, aside from their classical roles in mitigating tissue injury, infection or disease. Data from the murine brain suggest that microglia acquire these functions in a stepwise manner, by virtue of activation of distinct transcriptional programs and chromatin structure across the development of microglia from embryonic origins to adulthood [13]. Specifically, three distinct phases of microglial regulation are suggested to appear through development, each with potentially distinct functional effects: firstly early microglia (cell cycle), then pre-microglia (synaptic pruning and development) and finally adult microglia (immune surveillance and homeostasis). Transitions between these stages are coordinated by specific regulatory signals, driven by changes in histone modifications, chromatin accessibility and expression programs with distinct markers [13]. For example, early-microglia are associated with the expression of Dab2, Mcm5 and Lyz2, moving to expression of Crybb1, Csf1 and Cxcr2 at the pre-microglia stage and hence finally MafB, Cd14 and Mef2a in adult microglia [13]. Understandably, the reinforcement of regulatory changes to microglial development is a delicate area, and changes to this stepwise program have the clear potential to result in adverse effects in microglial function, thus compromising brain development, homeostasis and immune protection. Such early disruption to microglia function thus has the clear potential to render an individual more vulnerable to onset of neurodevelopmental disease and brain disorders in later life.

As already alluded to, given that microglia are highly plastic cells, with a variety of transformation states it is not surprising that they are reported to have a diverse functional repertoire [14]. Aside from their primary function of immune defence, microglia play key roles in both the developing and adult brain (summarised in Table 8.1) [15]. As an immune cell, microglia act as a line of self-defence against tissue damage and infection by pathogen recognition, phagocytosis and antigen presentation. It is clear however, that microglia also influence CNS development by several mechanisms including, regulation of axon formation/guidance and the refinement of neural circuits. Specifically, there is evidence to suggest that microglia are involved in setting an optimal number of synapses in the developing brain, by regulating both synapse formation and elimination, as well as modulating proliferation and differentiation of neural precursor cells (NPCs) [14, 16]. As a result, microglial function balances between protecting the brain from infection and

Table 8.1 The multitude of microglial functions

	Immunological	Developmental	Homeostatic
Neurotoxic	Phagocytosis	Synaptic elimination Neuron cell death	
Neuroprotective		Synaptogenesis Neurite formation Astrocyte growth and activation Myelinogenesis Axon fasciculation NPC/OPC growth & differentiation Dendritogenesis	Neuronal surveillance function

Microglia functions can broadly fall into three categories: immunological, developmental and homeostatic [14, 15]. These functions are also separated by the spectrum of microglial transformation states, which holding gain or loss of function effects on the CNS, respectively

shaping the neural networks of the developing brain. It is also worth recognising that astrocytes also play a similar role in the development of synapses and NPCs [17], but the specific focus of this chapter is on microglia.

In the adult brain, microglia primarily maintain homeostasis, with much less functional diversity as compared to with the developing brain [18]. When activated in response to tissue injury, the result on the CNS ranges between anti-inflammatory and pro-inflammatory, with neuroprotective and neurotoxic effects, respectively (Fig. 8.1). Of note, heterogenic microglial subpopulations are present throughout different regions of the developing and adult rodent and human brain [14, 19]. Regional variation is demonstrated by response to ATP, purinergic receptor expression (involved in learning and memory, locomotor and feeding behaviour and sleep), an ability to induce neurotoxicity, microglial density, cell protrusion branching, lysosomal content and membrane polarisation properties [14]. Single-cell sequencing presented these heterogenic populations by not only brain region but also time points, without distinct clustering of states [20]. Heterogenic diversity is reduced when the homeostasis of the brain is altered, for example upon aging or injury, with signatures moving towards an inflammatory signal [20]. In theory, a potential homeostatic signal imbalance could therefore lead to a gain or loss of microglial function dependent on the microglia's functional state, from which pathogenic results could link with brain disorders.

Supporting this view is evidence from microglial depletion studies, which are associated with the development of behavioural abnormalities in the rodent, some of which have dimensional relevance for psychiatric disorders such as autism spectrum disorder and schizophrenia. Specifically, in rodents, chronic exposure to Colony Stimulating Factor-1 (CSF-1) antagonists leads to rapid and sustained depletion of central microglia, for as long as the drug is present [21]. The consequence of such depletion appears to depend on the timing. For example, microglia depletion during juvenile or early adolescent periods leads to disruption of microglial homeostasis particularly in the cerebellum, increased dendrite branching but decreased dendrite length in the cerebellar cortex and adversely affects both motor learning and social interaction [21]. Furthermore, increased overconnectivity to

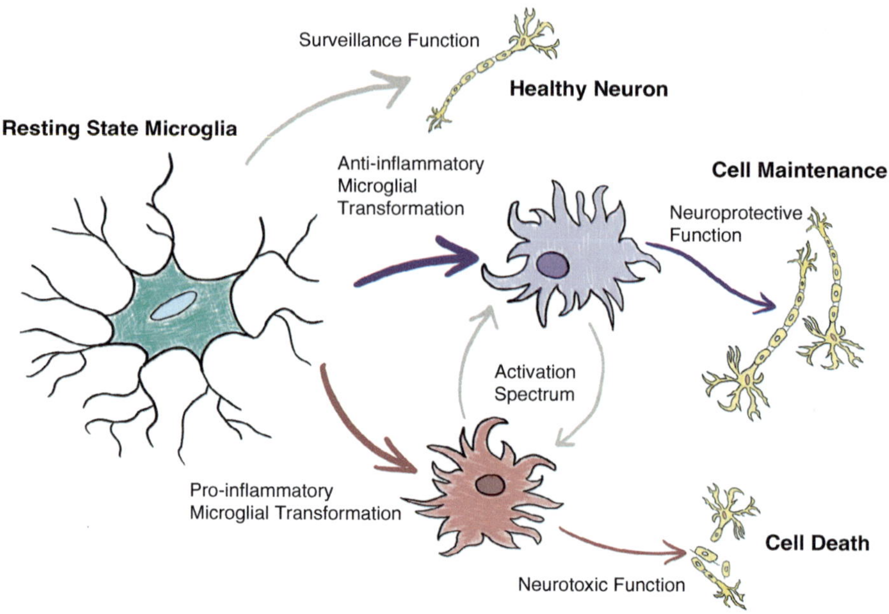

Fig. 8.1 The spectrum of microglial transformation states. Mature microglia have a surveillance function in the brain, maintaining homeostasis. Upon transformation by microenvironmental signals, microglia form a spectrum of functional states ranging from neurotoxic to neuroprotective, depicted by the red and green activation paths. These are deemed neurotoxic or neuroprotective by either a gain or loss of functions, to which the outcome could be toxic or protective to neurons. There is a spectrum of states between these polar ends, having similarly ranging effects on neurons

prefrontal neocortical regions from inflamed murine cerebellum has been demonstrated by MRI and associated with depressive and autism-like behaviours [22]. These behaviours were returned to normal by TNF-α inhibition [22]. Correspondingly, the depletion of macrophages including microglia prenatally in rodents also disrupts the density and function of fast-spiking parvalbumin (PV) inhibitory interneurons in a bi-phasic manner from the juvenile to the adult phase of life [23]. This finding is of particular interest given the long-standing evidence base for PV deficits in schizophrenia (SZ) [24], but also Autism Spectrum Disorder (ASD) [25]. Collectively, the growing evidence for the multi-faceted roles of microglia in brain development and the findings from depletion studies suggest a view that manipulating microglia form and function during critical periods of brain development can induce a behavioural state in the animal that has some potential relevance for psychiatric disorders. This raises the question of whether such microglia pathology is present in psychiatric disorders and if it is, can it be casual for such psychopathology in humans? To begin to address these questions, in this chapter we consider the evidence base for microglial involvement in human psychiatric disorders. We present converging lines of evidence from human genetics, post-mortem and in vivo neuroimaging studies, as well as rodent models where appropriate, that suggest microglia may be involved in the pathogenesis of psychiatric disorders with a putative neurodevelopmental origin, such as SZ and ASD. Furthermore, we briefly consider potential mechanistic pathways that may link microglial pathology and psychopathology and consider what unanswered questions remain in this context.

8.2 Evidence for Microglial Pathology in Psychiatric Disorders

The association of search terms 'Microglia' and 'Psychiatric disorders' has demonstrated an increase in research publications since the 2000s (Fig. 8.2). Notwithstanding the amounting publications, a clear decision of positive or detrimental effects that microglia have in the context of psychiatric disorders is still a topic of debate. Hence, we first consider the evidence base for microglial pathology in the context of SZ.

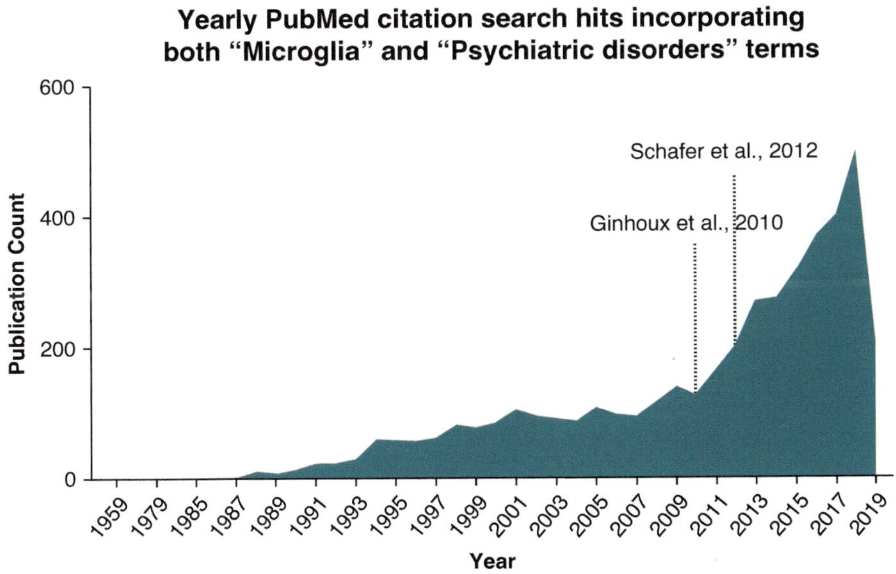

Fig. 8.2 PubMed publication hits retrieved from the search term 'Microglia' and 'Psychiatric disorders' by year. PubMed is a free publication database from the National Library of Medicine. Using Medical Subject Headings (MeSH) terms, the database is able to search publications for terms that link hierarchically with the term inputted into the database. Publications with matching journal names, author names, research investigator names, the title field, the author field, the publication date field and abstract field to the search term will be listed as hits. The number of hits associating with both 'Microglia' and 'Psychiatric disorders' per year were taken and presented here. Particularly prominent publications were: Florent Ginhoux et al., 'Fate mapping analysis reveals that adult microglia derive from primitive macrophages', Science (2010), cited 2667 times; Schafer et al., 'Microglia Sculpt Postnatal Neural Circuits in an Activity and Complement-Dependent Manner', Neuron (2012), cited 1223 times

8.2.1 Genetic Associations

Captivating evidence for immune activation in psychiatric disorders is the linkage of common genetic mutations in genes associated with inflammatory pathways and an increased risk for psychiatric disorders [26–28]. Genetic variants may increase susceptibility either through rare but highly penetrant variants. For example, 22q11.2 deletions are strongly associated with increased risk for both SZ and ASD [29]. The leukaemia inhibitory factor (*LIF*) gene locates to the 22q arm, to which polymorphic variants of the gene (rs929271, rs737812 and rs929273) associate particularly with hebephrenic SZ [30]. Interestingly, LIF plays a role in coordinating microglial function, suggesting dysregulation of microglial function as a possible mechanism (amongst many) to explain this association. Direct evidence for either microglial activation or gain/loss of function in 22q11.2 disorder patients is however currently lacking.

More typically, both SZ and ASD risk is associated with expression of many common risk variants of low penetrance; hence both are considered polygenic disorders. Genome-wide association studies (GWAS) have to date provided evidence for single nucleotide polymorphisms (SNPs) in >108 gene loci that are associated with increased risk for SZ, of which, the top 41 risk genes are highly expressed in neurons [26]. In particular, these top common risk variants appear to be enriched in expression in pyramidal cells, medium spiny neurons (MSNs) and certain interneurons based on recent mapping of GWAS data to a brain single-cell sequencing database [27]. Whilst it would seem that the majority of common genetic risk factors for SZ are thus associated with neurons, this does not rule out the possibility for involvement of other cell types, including microglia. Several genes included in these top 41 SNPs (including *ATP2A2, PSMA4, PBRM1, SERPING1* and *VRK2*) are also expressed in microglia, which may infer a role for microglia in SZ [26]. Studies on the impact of SNPs in the aforementioned genes on microglia form and function are however currently lacking, particularly in ether rodent or human model systems. In contrast to these is the very significant GWAS association for SZ with the human leukocyte antigen (HLA) locus, which encodes proteins to build the major histocompatibility complexes (MHCs) [31]. There is strong evidence for the linkage of SNPs within the MHC class-II gene locus, in the gene encoding complement factor 4 A/B (*C4A/B*) to an increased risk for SZ; moreover, knockout of *C4A/B* in rodents leads to aberrant synaptic pruning, a process in which glial cells, including microglia are strongly implicated [28]. It is worth noting then, that C4A expression is highest not only in microglia, but also in astrocytes and vascular leptomeningeal cells [27]. Hence, whilst not all cell types may be enriched in the expression of common risk variants for SZ, it is perhaps premature to conclude that other cell types, including microglia, may not play a role in the pathogenesis of SZ associated with distinct genotypes.

In support of this view is in vitro data garnered from human induced pluripotent stem cell (hiPSC) derived neurons and microglia, where microglial-mediated phagocytosis of synaptic material was found to be increased in such cells derived from individuals with a diagnosis of SZ, as compared to cells from otherwise healthy donors [32]. Of note, synaptic engulfment by these cells was also modulated to some degree by the *C4A/B* genotype of the patient-derived microglial cells [32]. These data are consistent with seminal observations in the rodent brain, whereby microglia are suggested to engulf synaptic material in a complement and activity-dependent manner [33]. Could such abnormalities in synaptic pruning however be causative for behavioural and brain phenotypes associated with either SZ or ASD? In support of this view, mice homozygous for the fractalkine receptor (*Cx3cr1−/−*), a critical mediator of neuron-microglia communication demonstrated delayed synaptic pruning, leading to excessive dendritic spine density and immature synapses in development [34]. This microglial-specific dysfunction resulted in both decreased brain functional connectivity between the prefrontal cortex and hippocampus (indexed by resting state functional magnetic resonance imaging [fMRI]) and abnormal social behaviour. Hence these data, provide the first evidence that a primary microglial dysfunction is causative for two key endophenotypes observed across psychiatric disorders and links this to defective synaptic pruning [35]. Translating these data to humans, it is notable that rare genetic variants in the CX_3CR1 G-protein coupled receptor (GPCR) solely expressed in the brain by microglia and disruption to its neuronally secreted ligand CX_3CL1 (also known as Fractalkine) are associated with increased risk for both ASD and SZ [36, 37]. Whilst debate continues in the literature with regard to the role of microglia in synaptic pruning per se, the aforementioned data suggest that risk variants in genes that encapsulate complement signalling (*Cx3cr1, C4A/B* and *CR3/C3)* are important leads for further research to understand how microglia may be involved in the pathology of psychiatric disorders. The identification of other key molecular signals aside from CX_3CR1 and the complement system that may mediate this process are however also important to elucidate the precise molecular code that defines which synapses are pruned and when, across both rodent and human model systems. Genotyping for genetic variation within complement C4A/B may also be a useful starting point to identify sub-groups of SZ or ASD patients whose illness may be related to dysfunction of the innate immune system, although this remains to be tested.

8.2.2 Post-mortem Studies

Supporting the evidence for microglial pathology in psychiatric disorders from genetics are observations made in human *post-mortem* brain tissue from SZ cases and controls regarding microglial pathology. Typically, such studies have focussed on identifying differences in the population of microglia by quantitative immunohistochemistry using a spectrum of surface marker proteins including CR3, ionised calcium-binding adapter molecule 1 (Iba-1), CD45, $CX_3CR1$and MHC class-II [15, 38]. A recent meta-analysis compared such data from *post-mortem* brain tissue in a total of 783 SZ patients and 762 healthy controls, across 41 studies [39]. In this study, the density of microglia was reported to be increased overall, specifically in the temporal cortex [39]. Other regions showing considerable heterogeneity, with no overall significant changes reported in the meta-analysis. Notably, there were no observed changes in astrogliosis in any brain region [39]. Consistent with these data, a second systematic review of 22 publications studying signs of microglial activation in SZ *post-mortem* brain tissue, again based on staining for microglial surface markers, found that 11/22 (50%) studies reported increased expression of microglial markers, 8/22 (36%) reported a decrease and 3/22 (14%) reported no change [40]. Collectively, these analyses suggest that there is evidence for microglial pathology in *post-mortem* brain tissue from SZ patients, although this is clearly not uniform across studies. Indeed, there is considerable variation between the included studies in both meta-analyses, with regard to both the microglial marker used and the method of quantification, which likely affected the overall pattern of the results. Moreover, to date there are no published transcriptomic studies of microglia isolated from human *post-mortem* brain tissue samples from either SZ, or ASD patients. This is relevant, since the aforementioned immunostaining data can only provide limited insights into the functional state of microglia in the brain in these disorders as morphology is often poorly correlated with function. Hence, we do not yet know if in the cases of SZ where increases in microglia density or surface maker expression are described, whether this represents a homeostatic, beneficial or a detrimental, pro-inflammatory response. In this context, a recent study suggests that microglia isolated from human *post-mortem* cortical tissue from bipolar disorder (BD) cases, were not activated towards a detrimental, pro-inflammatory state [41]. Such studies in SZ and ASD are thus eagerly awaited and now feasible given advances in isolation of microglia from *post-mortem* samples.

Were such studies available however, two other key limitations of the current human *post-mortem* data must be acknowledged. First, is the current lack of validated biomarkers with which to stratify patients into 'high' or 'low' inflammation populations for further study. One interesting advance in this context however, is the work of the Weickert group, who utilising a statistical clustering approach based on peripheral or central cytokine expression, has stratified SZ cases into such 'high' and 'low' inflammation categories. In doing so, they found evidence for increased MHC Class-II (*HLA-DR*), IL-1β, IL-8 and IL-6 inflammatory markers in the dorsolateral prefrontal cortex of SZ patients correlating with a decrease in BDNF mRNA [42]. These findings also extend to the ventral midbrain [43]. Hence, these studies provide evidence to suggest that focussing on defined subsets of patients will yield more informative data in due course, although the ideal means with which to stratify such patients remains debated.

The second important limitation in these studies is that the great majority of SZ cases will have been exposed to antipsychotic medication [44]. Here it is important to acknowledge that some findings in human *post-mortem* tissue from SZ cases with regard to microglial and cytokine gene expression have been replicated in a rodent model of maternal immune activation (MIA), which has pathological relevance for SZ (but also ASD) [43]. Hence, at least some of these mechanisms are likely intrinsic to the illness and not simply a medication effect. On the other hand, highly significant correlations between some (but not all) microglia and cytokine gene expression and the dose and duration of antipsychotic medication exposure have been reported in human studies [43]. Whilst it may be argued that this could simply reflect greater illness severity in these cases (thus requiring higher antipsychotic medication prescribing), it is also conceivable that antipsychotics themselves may influence microglia form and function. In support of this view, rodent studies using clinically comparable exposure to antipsychotics confirm that these drugs can influence both microglia density and morphology in a time-, dose- and region-dependent manner [45, 46]. The precise influence of antipsychotics on microglia function however, remains to be fully characterised and is an important gap in our knowledge.

8.2.3 In-Vivo Positron Emission Tomography (PET) Studies

Important to any disease research is the ability to study it in the living human body using non- or minimally-invasive measures, such as those based on neuroimaging methods. The application of neuroimaging (clinically comparable technology) may also facilitate translation from animal models to human clinical data and vice versa [47]. In this context, an in vivo neuroimaging marker for putative microgliosis is critical. To date, the only potential marker in use within clinical populations to index putative microgliosis is radioligands-specific for the 18 kDa Translocator protein (TSPO) combined with PET [48]. Both first and second generation TSPO radioligands with distinct strengths and weaknesses are in research use in SZ [49]. The TSPO protein is expressed on the outer mitochondrial membrane, particularly, but not exclusively, in microglia, where its functional role spans many contexts including respiration, inflammation, redox processes, cellular proliferation, apoptosis and steroidogenesis [50, 51]. Rodent microglia up-regulate expression of TSPO after transition to a pro-inflammatory state [52]. For example, rodents injected intracranially with the toll-like receptor 4 (TLR-4) agonist lipopolysaccharide (LPS) to induce pro-inflammatory polarisation showed an increased number of microglia, expressing TSPO, suggesting its role as a marker of pro-inflammatory state, although such changes were also seen in macrophages and astrocytes [53–55]. Supporting the rodent data, peripheral administration of LPS increases TSPO ligand binding in non-human primates [56]. Moreover, upon pharmacological depletion of microglia in non-human primates, TSPO ligand binding is significantly reduced and recovers 12 days after treatment [57]. Translating these data to humans, peripheral administration of LPS resulted in a measurable increase in TSPO ligand binding in a small sample of healthy volunteers [58], although such findings have yet to be more widely replicated in vivo. Collectively, these data confirm that TSPO is sensitive to microglial responses, but not specific to these cells [52]. What then is the evidence base for TSPO PET imaging changes in patients with SZ and other psychiatric disorders in which microgliosis is implicated?

Summarised in Table 8.2 are studies assessing changes in TSPO ligand binding in psychiatric disorders, which clearly shows a marked heterogeneity in findings with regard to TSPO binding between research groups for the main effects reported, the tracer used, the method of quantification, illness stage and medication status (Table 8.2). Attempting to summarise these data, a recent meta-analysis combined data from 12 published TSPO PET studies comprising 190 SZ patients and 200

Table 8.2 Summary of human PET studies using TSPO radiotracers in psychosis, SZ and ASD

References	Effect on TSPO ligand binding	Subjects and sample size	Tracer used	Tracer binding outcome measure	Comment
Bloomfield PS et al. Am J Psychiatry. 2016 [61]	Increase	Ultra-high psychosis ($n = 14$) and SZ patients ($n = 14$) with healthy matched controls ($n = 28$)	^{11}C-PBR28	V_T	Region of interest was total grey matter, then temporal and frontal lobe grey matter. TSPO binding was positively related to risk symptom severity
Ottoy J et al. J Nucl Med. 2018 [62]	Increase	SZ male patients ($n = 11$) and healthy controls ($n = 17$)	^{18}F-PBR111	V_T	Varied by age and genotype. Hippocampal and cortical grey matter showed increased binding
Suzuki, K et al. Archives of General Psychiatry. 2013 [63]	Increase	ASD Male Patients ($n = 20$) and matched controls ($n = 20$)	^{11}C-PK11195	BP_{ND}	Increased binding seen in cerebellum, midbrain, pons, fusiform gyri and the anterior cingulate and orbitofrontal cortices. No correlation between symptoms and TSPO binding signal
Van Der Doef TF et al. npj Schizophr. 2016 [64]	No difference	SZ patients ($n = 19$) and healthy controls ($n = 17$)	^{11}C-PK11195	V_T	Measurements assessed total grey matter, as well as grey matter from frontal cortex, temporal cortex, parietal cortex, striatum and thalamus

(continued)

Table 8.2 (continued)

References	Effect on TSPO ligand binding	Subjects and sample size	Tracer used	Tracer binding outcome measure	Comment
Doorduin J et al. J Nucl Med. 2009 [65]	Increase	SZ patients ($n = 7$) and healthy controls ($n = 8$)	^{11}C-PK11195	BP_{ND}	Significant increase in TSPO binding in the hippocampus, non-significant increase in total grey matter
Takano A et al. Int J Neuropsychopharmacol. 2010 [66]	No difference	SZ patients ($n = 14$) and matched healthy controls ($n = 14$)	^{11}C-DAA1106	BP_{ND}	Studied 11 regions of interest with no changes in TSPO binding between groups. Positive correlations between binding and positive symptom scores were noted in the medial frontal cortex, medial temporal cortex and occipital cortex
Kenk M et al. Schizophr Bull. 2015 [67]	No difference	SZ patients ($n = 18$) and matched controls ($n = 27$)	^{18}F-FE PPA	V_T	No changes seen in TSPO binding in any grey matter or white matter regions
Coughlin JM et al. Transl Psychiatry. 2016 [68]	No difference	SZ patients ($n = 12$) and healthy controls ($n = 14$)	^{11}C-DPA-713	V_T	Measured TSPO binding in insula, cingulate, parietal, frontal, temporal and occipital regions of the cortex, plus the hippocampus and amygdala. Trend towards decreases in frontal cortex but not statistically significant

(continued)

Table 8.2 (continued)

References	Effect on TSPO ligand binding	Subjects and sample size	Tracer used	Tracer binding outcome measure	Comment
Hafizi S et al. Am J Psychiatry. 2017 [69]	No difference	First episode psychosis (FEP) patients ($n = 19$) and controls ($n = 20$)	^{18}F-FEPPA	V_T	FEP with minimal medication exposure. Measured TSPO binding in cerebellum, grey matter or whole brain. No group differences
Holmes SE et al. Mol Psychiatry. 2016 [70]	Increase binding in medicated patients, no difference in antipsychotic-free patients	Medicated SZ patients ($n = 8$), antipsychotic-free SZ patients ($n = 8$) and healthy controls ($n = 16$)	^{11}C-PK11195	BP_{ND}	Elevated TSPO binding seen in prefrontal, anterior cingulate and parietal cortical brain regions of medicated patients only
Collste K et al., Mol Psychiatry. 2017 [71]	Decrease	Drug naïve first-episode psychosis patients ($n = 16$) and healthy controls ($n = 16$)	^{11}C-PBR28	V_T	Particularly measured in grey matter. No correlation between binding changes and cognitive or clinical symptoms

(continued)

Table 8.2 (continued)

References	Effect on TSPO ligand binding	Subjects and sample size	Tracer used	Tracer binding outcome measure	Comment
Di Biase MA et al., Transl Psychiatry. 2017 [72]	No difference	Ultra-high risk SZ patients ($n = 10$), recently diagnosed SZ patients ($n = 18$), chronic SZ patients ($n = 15$) and aged-matched healthy controls ($n = 27$)	^{11}C-PK11195	BP_{ND}	Measurements taken from dorsal frontal, orbital frontal, anterior cingulate, medial temporal, thalamus and insula. Correlation between binding potential and grey matter in the thalamus with age. No correlations between grey matter, peripheral cytokines or symptoms
De Picker L et al., Brain Behav Immun. 2019 [73]	Increase correlated with age	Male psychosis patients ($n = 14$) and age-matched healthy controls ($n = 17$)	^{18}F-PBR111	V_T	Change correlated with age, and positive symptoms correlated with cortical grey matter binding changes
Hafizi S et al., Neuropsycho Pharmacolo-gy. 2017 [74]	No difference	High-risk psychosis patients ($n = 24$, $n = 22$ antipsychotic naïve) and healthy controls ($n = 23$)	^{18}F-FEPPA	V_T	Measured changes in dorsolateral prefrontal cortex and hippocampus. In high-risk patients, ligand binding correlated with apathy and anxiety

(continued)

Table 8.2 (continued)

References	Effect on TSPO ligand binding	Subjects and sample size	Tracer used	Tracer binding outcome measure	Comment
van Berckel BN et al., Biol Psychiatry. 2008 [75]	Increase	Recently diagnosed SZ patients (n = 10) and age matched controls (n = 10)	^{11}C-PK11195	BP_P	Increase was noted in total grey matter. These patients were within 5 years of disease onset

Notes on the publication's conclusion and use of PET tracer are included. Method refers to method of TSPO binding quantification, either by volume of distribution (V_T), parameter binding potential (BP_P) or non-displaceable binding potential (BP_{ND}). Changes in TSPO ligand binding were compared with matched healthy controls, with sample size given in parentheses

controls, reporting no significant differences between SZ patients and controls when volume of distribution (V_T) was used to quantify TSPO ligand binding, with these studies predominantly using second generation TSPO tracers (e.g. PBR28) [60]. In contrast, increases in TSPO binding in grey matter were observed, particularly for studies using first generation TSPO tracers (e.g. PK11195) when binding potential (BP_{ND}) was used to quantify TSPO ligand binding [59], findings that have sparked an interesting debate with regards to how quantification methods may influence the outcome of TSPO PET studies. To address this point further, an individual patient data meta-analysis, including only studies using the second-generation TSPO-PET radioligands, in either first episode or SZ patients (n = 75) as compared to healthy controls (n = 77) has been conducted, which provides evidence for a *reduction* in TSPO binding in several brain regions, interpreted by the authors as reduced glial density or loss of function [60]. Taken together, these heterogenous data render it challenging to make a firm conclusion with regard to TSPO binding in the context of SZ and psychosis. A single study (see Table 8.2) has however found increased TSPO binding in ASD patients, although this needs to be replicated.

What may be driving this heterogeneity in the data? Aside from the debate around quantification methods, two other important limitations are hindering our interpretation of available TSPO PET imaging data in SZ. First, as already stated, TSPO is not specific to microglia and to what extent changes in other cell types may influence the results in SZ cases is not known [51]. Second, it is not straightforward to directly link in vivo imaging to biology in humans, hence we lack detailed information as to how a change in TSPO binding reflects microglia activation or functional state. For example, alterations in TSPO expression by microglia could reflect a multitude of microglial functions including increased steroidogenesis, respiration, redox processes, cellular proliferation and apoptosis [50, 51]. Although linked, these transformational microglial phenotypes do not necessarily equate to detrimental neuroinflammation. Human *post-mortem* studies of TSPO are also sparse. A single study to the best of our knowledge, has reported no increase in TSPO protein expression in *post-mortem* brain tissue from SZ patients, but also that TSPO protein levels were neither correlated with the expression of surface microglial activation markers, nor was TSPO protein expression restricted to microglia [41]. Of course, the same caveats apply here for interpretation of this data, including effects of age, medication exposure and non-stratification of cases, as already discussed in Sect. 8.2.2 for *post-mortem* studies of microglia in SZ. Hence, back-translating the human TSPO findings into relevant rodent or non-human primate models may be an alternative strategy to address the issues around TSPO in SZ, since invasive studies can be carried out to link neuroimaging signals to their cellular and molecular correlates. In this context, TSPO protein levels are reduced in the prefrontal cortex of mice exposed to maternal immune activation (MIA) early in gestation (GD9) [51], modelling a known environmental risk factor associated with increased risk for psychiatric disorders with a neurodevelopmental origin [51]. This decrease occurred in microglia, astrocytes and endothelial cells, confirming the non-specificity of TSPO for microglia. Of note, cytokine levels were increased in the frontal cortex of GD9-MIA offspring, but there were no overt changes in microglial density, morphology or expression of surface markers associated with microglial activation (e.g. CD68). Intra-hippocampal injection of kainic acid, however, triggered a marked increase in TSPO protein in all three-cell types, accompanied by robust microglial activation confirming that TSPO expression is also highly context dependent [51, 76]. In a rat MIA model with the exposure in mid-gestation (GD15), transcriptional analysis by RNAseq of microglia isolated from the hippocampus of MIA-exposed offspring confirmed an abnormal microglial phenotype, suggestive of a loss of function, as indexed by down-regulation of genes involved in the inflammatory response and phagocytosis [76]. TSPO binding and microglia density were however increased in the hippocampus, in a separate cohort of rats [76] in contrast to the work of Notter and colleagues (2018). Species differences (rats vs. mice) and the differential timing (GD9 vs. 15) of MIA could explain these discrepancies. Consistent with this view, TSPO levels have also been recently reported as increased in the cortex of rats exposed during the perinatal period to phencyclidine (PCP), modelling early glutamate dysfunction associated with psychosis [77]. These data confirm the non-specific nature of TSPO with regard to microglial expression and additionally highlight the context-dependent nature of changes in TSPO protein and/or ligand binding. As yet however, no studies have definitively linked a change in TSPO binding directly to microglial functional state (or that of astrocytes and endothelial cells) in the same animal.

In this context, potential species differences from rodent to human microglia also have to be considered [53, 78]. For example, whilst a nine-fold TSPO expression up-regulation was observed in rodent-derived microglia following pro-inflammatory challenge, TSPO was in fact reduced in primary human microglia [78]. Interestingly the direction of this finding is in agreement with the reduction in TSPO ligand binding reported in the meta-analysis of Plaven-Sigray and colleagues [60] and the data from the MIA model reported by Notter et al. [51]. Nonetheless, to what extent these in vitro studies accurately reflect in vivo human microglia responses, is however not clear. For instance, following isolation from the human brain microglia rapidly down-regulate microglia signature genes and adopt a more 'active' state [79]. Recent advances in differentiating microglia from human induced pluripotent stem cells (hiPSC), that replicate authentic microglia ontogeny and allow for co-culture with neurons to maintain a CNS-like phenotype, may be helpful to address this issue [80].

As already alluded to the potential influence of antipsychotic drugs on TSPO ligand binding also needs to be considered. A single TSPO PET study comparing SZ patients on long-acting injectable (LAI) antipsychotics to patients free of medication found elevated TSPO ligand binding (indexed using [^{11}C]-PK11195 BP_{ND}) in the frontal and parietal cortices of medicated patients, as compared to un-medicated patients who were not significantly different from controls on this measure [70]. This may suggest an influence of antipsychotics on TSPO ligand binding and whilst the patients in the medication group were older, including age as a co-variate did not change these results [70]. On the other hand, no effect of antipsychotic medication was reported in the meta-analysis by Plaven-Sigray and colleagues [60]. Back-translating these data to rodents, where the effects of antipsychotic medication can be studied free of any confounding illness effects, Bloomfield and colleagues [46] found no change in TSPO ligand binding (indexed using ^{3}H-PBR28 and quantitative receptor autoradiography) in the rat anterior cingulate cortex following a 2-week exposure to 0.05 mg/kg/day of haloperidol and no changes in either Iba1+ microglia density or morphology [46]. Since longer exposure to higher doses of antipsychotics does affect microglia density and morphology; however, it will be important to confirm these findings in future studies, including following exposure to other antipsychotics [45]. In support of this view, Danovich and colleagues found increased [^{3}H]-PK11195 binding in mitochondrial fractions isolated from the rat hippocampus following a 3-week exposure to clozapine (20 mg/kg/day) [81]. Interestingly, in the same region, 3-week exposure to sulpiride or risperidone actually decreased TSPO binding [81]. Moreover, in human *post-mortem* tissue from the ventral midbrain of SZ cases, TSPO mRNA expression was positively correlated with the mean daily dose of antipsychotics (in chlorpromazine equivalents) [43]. Hence, further work is still required to fully understand, what if any, is the effect of antipsychotic exposure on TSPO binding.

Collectively, these limitations likely explain the inconsistencies in TSPO binding studies in SZ cases, but also the decrease in the number of publications using TSPO PET scans in psychiatric disorders (Fig. 8.3). Data from animal or human model systems that directly link TSPO changes to microglial state and novel radioligands with greater sensitivity or selectivity for microglia are thus equally awaited. Such novel tracers are in development, for example, [^{11}C]-CPPC, which binds the CSF-1 receptor, the expression of which is essentially restricted to microglia within brain [82].

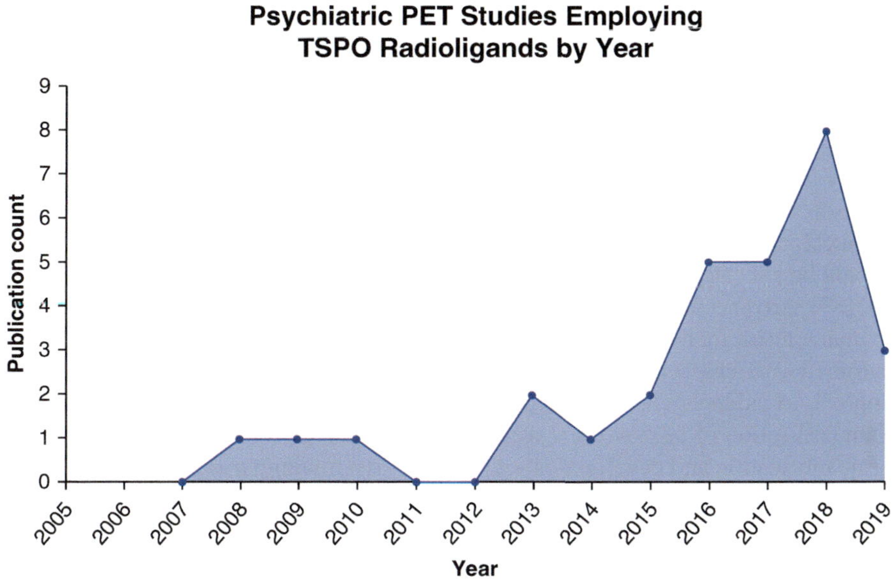

Fig. 8.3 Publications applying PET scanning methods to analyse microglial changes in vivo in psychiatric disorders, as described by Notter et al., 2018 [51]. Publication data were added from the years 2018 and 2019 to that already published by Notter et al. from 2007. The publication search used the same databases (PubMed and Web of Science™) with the same search terms: 'positron emission tomography', 'PET', 'translocator protein', 'TSPO', 'peripheral benzodiazepine receptor', 'PBR', 'neuroimaging', 'neuroinflammation', 'inflammation', 'microglial activation' and the addition of 'psychiatric disorder'. Thus, these publications uniquely addressed psychiatric disorders, disregarding neurological disorders such as neurodegenerative diseases

8.3 Outstanding Questions

Although often inconsistent, there is convergent evidence from genetics, *post-mortem* data and PET imaging to suggest that microglia pathology may be present, at least in a sub-set of SZ cases and potentially also in ASD [15]. However, a number of key questions remain to be addressed. Paramount amongst these is first, whether microglia pathology is causal for psychopathology, or merely an epiphenomenon of no consequence and second, what might be the potential mechanisms by which this could occur?

Before addressing the question of causality, it is worth considering how best to optimally characterise microglia and their distinct functions in both health and disease. The multitude of transformation phenotypes that microglia take is highly documented [83]. Yet in the context of disease, this inherent heterogenicity has been largely unstudied, particularly for psychiatric disorders. The term 'activation' when applied to microglia is also confounding due to their high plasticity (Table 8.1), particularly also when it alludes to the term 'neuroinflammation' which is often misused, as discussed elsewhere [51]. Given that there may be very heterogeneous populations of transformed microglia in the human brain, it becomes exceedingly hard to find a ground truth for comparison when studying disease states, since publications could be referring to inconstant transformed states of microglia, which themselves will hold different functions and transformation triggers. This is particularly apparent with the recent identification of 'dark' microglia, a phenotype associated with an increased synaptic pruning and pathological states as identified by electron microscopy [84]. Whether such 'dark' microglia are present in brain tissue from SZ cases, remains to be seen, but it is now being suggested that microglia should be subcategorised by their function in order to make studies more comparable [83]. Advances in isolation of microglia from the human brain [85] and methods to characterise their heterogeneity using single-cell RNA sequencing [19] or mass cytometry to characterise surface marker protein expression [86, 87] could be applied to address this issue in SZ or ASD cases as compared to controls. Standardisation of *post-mortem* tissue studies with regard to markers and methods of quantification and development of novel in vivo imaging tracers more specific to microglia will also be important advances to clarify the involvement of microglia in SZ and ASD. Combining these with new developments in stem cell-derived microglia [80], or induced microglia as embraced by Sellgren and colleagues also has the potential to provide mechanistic insights using a human model system [32]. We suggest that studies that cannot specify the distinct microglial function phenotype should conclude on microglial density and morphology rather than 'activation' state to not only from study to study, but globally in studies across species too.

With regard to causation, one key element to consider is where does the potential dysregulation of microglial developmental function originate? (Fig. 8.4) In both SZ and ASD, GWAS studies provide evidence for dysregulation of synapse transmission and neuron growth as evidenced by the enrichment of synaptic transmission-related genes in neurons, supporting the idea of synapse dysregulation [26]. As already discussed in this chapter, microglia play key roles in brain development related to synaptogenesis, neurite formation and axon fasciculation. The synaptic pruning model suggests that microglia phagocytose synaptic material during postnatal development, evidenced by studies in mice, linking the resting state microglial surveillance function to proper synaptic maturation [34]. As already discussed in Sect. 8.2.1, a gain or loss of this function caused by mutations in CX_3CR1/CX_3CL1, CR3/C3 and/or C4A/B could result in dysregulated synaptogenesis, for which there is some evidence in both SZ and ASD [28, 32–35]. Supporting this view, as already mentioned in Sect. 8.2.1 is the work of Sellgren et al. [32]. This study is the only to date which suggests, that human induced microglia from SZ patients are more likely to phagocytose synaptic material in either monoculture or co-culture with human neurons [32]. It may be anticipated that if such changes occur in vivo they would lead to circuit malformation and the emergence of abnormal behaviours. However, whether the dysregulation of synaptogenesis falls to a gain or loss of function by microglial regulation is still unexplained. Additionally, this model does not account for any potential epigenetic influences on microglia form or function. Evidence from rodents that gain or loss of microglia function, for example, by targeted depletion, or CX_3CR1 knock-out can induce behavioural changes in adult animals that

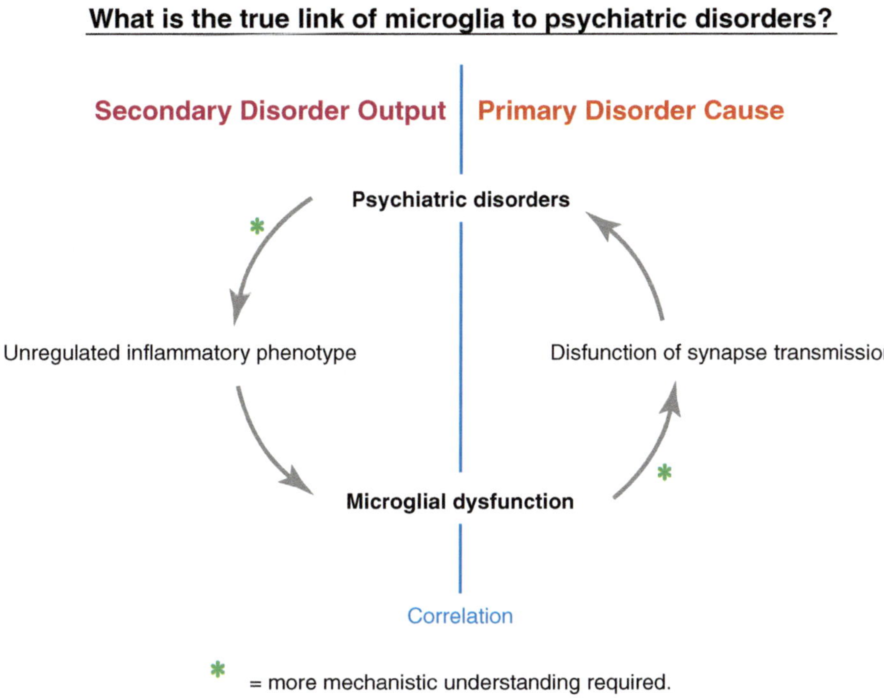

Fig. 8.4 Is microglial activation a primary cause of psychiatric disorders, or a secondary response to an origin elsewhere? Highlighted by the blue line, we have shown psychiatric disorders to correlate with changes in microglial activation and immune response. One side of the argument is that changes in microglial function are secondary to a psychiatric disorder origin which we are yet to uncover. On the other side, there is the argument that microglial dysfunction actually causes psychiatric disorder by dysfunction to synapse transmission. Green stared arrows denote areas of required research in order to elucidate whether this is a secondary symptom of the psychiatric disease, or a primary disorder causation

have dimensional relevance for psychiatric disorders is however, strongly suggestive that perturbing microglia function in critical periods could well be causative for serious mental illness in later life, in at least a subset of individuals.

Definitively demonstrating such causality in human patients has however yet to be achieved. Clinical trials with anti-inflammatory drugs provide mixed evidence for efficacy as adjunct treatments to standard antipsychotic drug therapy in SZ patients [88]. Anti-inflammatory treatment of ASD by Sulforaphane to regulate Nrf2- and NF-κB-related pathways associated with glial cell transformation has shown promising results in a clinical trial, given its ease in crossing the blood-brain barrier [89]. Other anti-inflammatories quoted to show promising results in reducing ASD symptoms are Oxytocin, Vitamin D and Resveratrol [90]. In the case of SZ, Celecoxib has shown a positive effect on symptoms particularly at early stages of disease presentation [91]. Acetylsalicylic acid (Aspirin) has also shown positive effects in both protecting against and symptom reduction in SZ [92]. However, there are some debate as to the reliability of these results [93]. Furthermore, the antibiotic minocycline has been shown to reduce negative SZ symptoms dramatically [94]. However, there have been contrasting results from randomised control trials of minocycline in SZ patients [95]. Importantly, most of these compounds are however, not specifically targeting microglia. Related to this context is a pressing need to better understand the influence of antipsychotic medications on microglia. It will therefore be important to support evidence from clinical trials of anti-inflammatory or microglia-targeting drugs with pre-clinical studies to dissect the influence of novel and existing medications on microglia form and function.

8.4 Conclusions

Microglia play key roles in the brain in both health and disease. Single-cell transcriptomics has uncovered a continuum of microglial signatures, rather than distinct clusters of activation states. Convergent lines of evidence from in vivo imaging, *post-mortem* tissue, genetics and epidemiological studies implicate microglia in the pathogenesis of psychiatric disorders including SZ and ASD. Whether microglia are causative for these disorders and the mechanisms driving any such effect remain however, unclear. The key role of microglia in brain development and maturation, particularly with regard to synapse formation and elimination is nonetheless, an active area of study in these contexts. Whether microglia pathology reflects gain or loss of function, is however also unknown. The precise effects of antipsychotic medication on microglia also remain incompletely characterised. Finally, it is evident the field of microglial research is heading towards a paradigm shift of microglial classification. Separate cell types with discrete functions require characterisation in order to compare more directly different microglial population signatures associated with disease environments.

To address these issues, we suggest future research in human tissues should therefore embrace advances in single-cell genomics and proteomics to more accurately classify and map microglia states and define microglia-neuron interactions using both human *post-mortem* tissue from disease cases as compared to controls, in combination with induced or hiPSC-derived microglia in co-culture with neurons or as organoids. The latter approach is particularly appealing since this could be done using somatic cell samples from either first-episode psychosis or clinical high-risk populations who are naïve with regard to antipsychotic medication exposure. Furthermore, such in vitro human models would also facilitate molecular studies of neuron-microglia interactions during development. Studying patient-derived and control microglia in a surrogate brain environment using chimeric models also offers potential in this regard, particularly to control for the potential impact of culturing human microglia-like cells in vitro [96]. Parallel studies in rodent models of clinically comparable antipsychotic dosing [97, 98] and in hiPSC microglia will also be useful to address potential medication confounds on microglia form and function. Overall however, progress in this field remains critically dependent on the identification of robust measures with which to accurately stratify psychiatric patients into potential sub-groups characterised by either putative central microgliosis (as indexed by PET imaging) or peripheral biomarkers suggestive of raised pro-inflammatory markers, to enable more specific comparisons with regard to microglia pathology and enrich a population who may benefit from anti-inflammatory or microglia-specific therapies.

References

1. Banati RB. Neuropathological imaging: in vivo detection of glial activation as a measure of disease and adaptive change in the brain. Br Med Bull. 2003;65:121–31. https://doi.org/10.1093/bmb/65.1.121.
2. Hoeffel G, et al. C-Myb+ erythro-myeloid progenitor-derived fetal monocytes give rise to adult tissue-resident macrophages. Immunity. 2015;42:665–78. https://doi.org/10.1016/j.immuni.2015.03.011.
3. Schulz C, et al. A lineage of myeloid cells independent of myb and hematopoietic stem cells. Science. 2012;335:86–90. https://doi.org/10.1126/science.1219179.
4. Kierdorf K, Prinz M. Factors regulating microglia activation. Front Cell Neurosci. 2013;7:44. https://doi.org/10.3389/fncel.2013.00044.
5. Kierdorf K, et al. Microglia emerge from erythromyeloid precursors via Pu.1-and Irf8-dependent pathways. Nat Neurosci. 2013;16:273–80. https://doi.org/10.1038/nn.3318.
6. Ginhoux F, et al. Fate mapping analysis reveals that adult microglia derive from primitive macrophages. Science. 2010;330:841–5. https://doi.org/10.1126/science.1194637.
7. Gomez Perdiguero E, et al. Tissue-resident macrophages originate from yolk-sac-derived erythro-myeloid progenitors. Nature. 2015;518:547–51. https://doi.org/10.1038/nature13989.
8. Bloom W, Bartelmez GW. Hematopoiesis in young human embryos. Am J Anat. 1940;67:21–53. https://doi.org/10.1002/aja.1000670103.
9. Migliaccio G, et al. Human embryonic hemopoiesis. Kinetics of progenitors and precursors underlying the yolk sac-liver transition. J Clin Invest. 1986;78:51–60. https://doi.org/10.1172/JCI112572.
10. Wierzba-Bobrowicz T, Gwiazda E, Poszwińska Z. Morphological study of microglia in human mesencephalon during the development and aging. Folia Neuropathol. 1995;33:77–83.
11. Martinez FO, Gordon S. The M1 and M2 paradigm of macrophage activation: time for reassessment. F1000Prime Reports. 2014;6. https://doi.org/10.12703/P6-13.
12. Ransohoff RM. How neuroinflammation contributes to neurodegeneration. Science. 2016;353:777–83.
13. Matcovitch-Natan O, et al. Microglia development follows a stepwise program to regulate brain homeostasis. Science. 2016;353. https://doi.org/10.1126/science.aad8670.
14. Wright-Jin EC, Gutmann DH. Microglia as dynamic cellular mediators of brain function. Trends Mol Med. 2019;25:967–79. https://doi.org/10.1016/j.molmed.2019.08.013.
15. Mondelli V, Vernon AC, Turkheimer F, Dazzan P, Pariante CM. Brain microglia in psychiatric disorders. Lancet Psychiatry. 2017;4:563–72. https://doi.org/10.1016/S2215-0366(17)30101-3.
16. Squarzoni P, et al. Microglia modulate wiring of the embryonic forebrain. Cell Rep. 2014;8:1271–9. https://doi.org/10.1016/j.celrep.2014.07.042.
17. Matias I, Morgado J, Gomes FCA. Astrocyte heterogeneity: impact to brain aging and disease. Front Aging Neurosci. 2019;11. https://doi.org/10.3389/fnagi.2019.00059.
18. Li Q, et al. Developmental heterogeneity of microglia and brain myeloid cells revealed by deep single-cell RNA sequencing. Neuron. 2019;101:207–223.e10. https://doi.org/10.1016/j.neuron.2018.12.006.
19. Masuda T, et al. Spatial and temporal heterogeneity of mouse and human microglia at single-cell resolution. Nature. 2019;566:388–92. https://doi.org/10.1038/s41586-019-0924-x.
20. Hammond TR, et al. Single-cell RNA sequencing of microglia throughout the mouse lifespan and in the injured brain reveals complex cell-state changes. Immunity. 2019;50:253–271.e6. https://doi.org/10.1016/j.immuni.2018.11.004.

21. Kana V, et al. CSF-1 controls cerebellar microglia and is required for motor function and social interaction. J Exp Med. 2019;216:2265–81. https://doi.org/10.1084/jem.20182037.
22. Yamamoto M, Kim M, Imai H, Itakura Y, Ohtsuki G. Microglia-triggered plasticity of intrinsic excitability modulates psychomotor behaviors in acute cerebellar inflammation. Cell Reports. 2019;28:2923–2938.e8. https://doi.org/10.1016/j.celrep.2019.07.078.
23. Thion MS, et al. Biphasic impact of prenatal inflammation and macrophage depletion on the wiring of neocortical inhibitory circuits. Cell Reports. 2019;28:1119–1126.e4. https://doi.org/10.1016/j.celrep.2019.06.086.
24. Bitanihirwe BKY, Lim MP, Kelley JF, Kaneko T, Woo TUW. Glutamatergic deficits and parvalbumin-containing inhibitory neurons in the prefrontal cortex in schizophrenia. BMC Psychiatry. 2009;9. https://doi.org/10.1186/1471-244X-9-71.
25. Lauber E, Filice F, Schwaller B. Parvalbumin neurons as a hub in autism spectrum disorders. J Neurosci Res. 2018;96:360–1. https://doi.org/10.1002/jnr.24204.
26. Ma C, Gu C, Huo Y, Li X, Luo XJ. The integrated landscape of causal genes and pathways in schizophrenia. Transl Psychiatry. 2018;8. https://doi.org/10.1038/s41398-018-0114-x.
27. Skene NG, et al. Genetic identification of brain cell types underlying schizophrenia. Nat Genet. 2018;50:825–33. https://doi.org/10.1038/s41588-018-0129-5.
28. Sekar A, et al. Schizophrenia risk from complex variation of complement component 4. Nature. 2016;530:177–83. https://doi.org/10.1038/nature16549.
29. Bassett AS, Chow EWC. Schizophrenia and 22q11.2 deletion syndrome. Curr Psychiatry Rep. 2008;10:148–57. https://doi.org/10.1007/s11920-008-0026-1.
30. Okahisa Y, et al. Leukemia inhibitory factor gene is associated with schizophrenia and working memory function. Prog Neuro-Psychopharmacol Biol Psychiatry. 2010;34:172–6. https://doi.org/10.1016/j.pnpbp.2009.10.020.
31. Mokhtari R, Lachman HM. The major histocompatibility complex (MHC) in schizophrenia: a review. J Clin Cell Immunol. 2016;7. https://doi.org/10.4172/2155-9899.1000479.
32. Sellgren CM, et al. Increased synapse elimination by microglia in schizophrenia patient-derived models of synaptic pruning. Nat Neurosci. 2019;22:374–85. https://doi.org/10.1038/s41593-018-0334-7.
33. Schafer DP, et al. Microglia sculpt postnatal neural circuits in an activity and complement-dependent manner. Neuron. 2012;74:691–705. https://doi.org/10.1016/j.neuron.2012.03.026.
34. Paolicelli RC, et al. Synaptic pruning by microglia is necessary for normal brain development. Science. 2011;333:1456–8.
35. Zhan Y, et al. Deficient neuron-microglia signaling results in impaired functional brain connectivity and social behavior. Nat Neurosci. 2014;17:400–6. https://doi.org/10.1038/nn.3641.
36. Ishizuka K, et al. Rare genetic variants in CX3CR1 and their contribution to the increased risk of schizophrenia and autism spectrum disorders. Transl Psychiatry. 2017;7. https://doi.org/10.1038/tp.2017.173.
37. Limatola C, Ransohoff RM. Modulating neurotoxicity through CX3CL1/CX3CR1 signaling. Front Cell Neurosci. 2014;8. https://doi.org/10.3389/fncel.2014.00229.
38. Frick LR, Williams K, Pittenger C. Microglial dysregulation in psychiatric disease. Clin Dev Immunol. 2013;2013. https://doi.org/10.1155/2013/608654.
39. Van Kesteren CFMG, et al. Immune involvement in the pathogenesis of schizophrenia: a meta-analysis on postmortem brain studies. Transl Psychiatry. 2017;7. https://doi.org/10.1038/tp.2017.4.
40. Trépanier MO, Hopperton KE, Mizrahi R, Mechawar N, Bazinet RP. Postmortem evidence of cerebral inflammation in schizophrenia: a systematic review. Mol Psychiatry. 2016;21:1009–26.
41. Sneeboer MAM, et al. Microglial activation in schizophrenia: is translocator 18 kDa protein (TSPO) the right marker? Schizophr Res. 2020;215:167–72. https://doi.org/10.1016/j.schres.2019.10.045.
42. Fillman SG, et al. Increased inflammatory markers identified in the dorsolateral prefrontal cortex of individuals with schizophrenia. Mol Psychiatry. 2013;18:206–14.
43. Purves-Tyson TD, et al. Increased levels of midbrain immune-related transcripts in schizophrenia and in murine offspring after maternal immune activation. Mol Psychiatry. 2021;26:849–63. https://doi.org/10.1038/s41380-019-0434-0.

44. Amato D, Vernon AC, Papaleo F. Dopamine, the antipsychotic molecule: a perspective on mechanisms underlying antipsychotic response variability. Neurosci Biobehav Rev. 2018;85:146–59. https://doi.org/10.1016/j.neubiorev.2017.09.027.
45. Cotel MC, et al. Microglial activation in the rat brain following chronic antipsychotic treatment at clinically relevant doses. Eur Neuropsychopharmacol. 2015;25:2098–107. https://doi.org/10.1016/j.euroneuro.2015.08.004.
46. Bloomfield PS, et al. The effects of haloperidol on microglial morphology and translocator protein levels: an in vivo study in rats using an automated cell evaluation pipeline. J Psychopharmacol. 2018;32:1264–72. https://doi.org/10.1177/0269881118788830.
47. Bracken MB. Why animal studies are often poor predictors of human reactions to exposure. J R Soc Med. 2009;102:120–2. https://doi.org/10.1258/jrsm.2008.08k033.
48. Bae K-R, Shim H-J, Balu D, Kim SR, Yu S-W. Translocator protein 18 kDa negatively regulates inflammation in microglia. J Neuroimmune Pharmacol. 2014;9:424–37.
49. Turkheimer FE, et al. The methodology of TSPO imaging with positron emission tomography. Biochem Soc Trans. 2015;43:586–92. https://doi.org/10.1042/BST20150058.
50. Owen DR, et al. TSPO mutations in rats and a human polymorphism impair the rate of steroid synthesis. Biochem J. 2017;474:3985–99.
51. Notter T, Coughlin JM, Sawa A, Meyer U. Reconceptualization of translocator protein as a biomarker of neuroinflammation in psychiatry. Mol Psychiatry. 2018;23:36–47. https://doi.org/10.1038/mp.2017.232.
52. Betlazar C, Harrison-Brown M, Middleton RJ, Banati R, Liu G-J. Cellular sources and regional variations in the expression of the neuroinflammatory marker translocator protein (TSPO) in the normal brain. Int J Mol Sci. 2018;19
53. Pannell M, et al. Imaging of translocator protein upregulation is selective for pro-inflammatory polarized astrocytes and microglia. Glia. 2020;68:280–97. https://doi.org/10.1002/glia.23716.
54. Saijo K, Crotti A, Glass CK. Regulation of microglia activation and deactivation by nuclear receptors. Glia. 2013;61:104–11. https://doi.org/10.1002/glia.22423.
55. Li X, et al. Microglia activation in the offspring of prenatal poly I: C exposed rats: a PET imaging and immunohistochemistry study. General Psychiatry. 2018;31
56. Hannestad J, et al. Endotoxin-induced systemic inflammation activates microglia: [11C]PBR28 positron emission tomography in nonhuman primates. NeuroImage. 2012;63:232–9. https://doi.org/10.1016/j.neuroimage.2012.06.055.
57. Hillmer AT, et al. Microglial depletion and activation: a [11C]PBR28 PET study in nonhuman primates. EJNMMI Res. 2017;7
58. Sandiego CM, et al. Imaging robust microglial activation after lipopolysaccharide administration in humans with PET. Proc Natl Acad Sci U S A. 2015;112:12468–73. https://doi.org/10.1073/pnas.1511003112.
59. Marques TR, et al. Neuroinflammation in schizophrenia: meta-analysis of in vivo microglial imaging studies. Psychol Med. 2019;49:2186–96. https://doi.org/10.1017/S0033291718003057.
60. Plavén-Sigray P, et al. Positron emission tomography studies of the glial cell marker translocator protein in patients with psychosis: a meta-analysis using individual participant data. Biol Psychiatry. 2018;84:433–42. https://doi.org/10.1016/j.biopsych.2018.02.1171.
61. Bloomfield PS, et al. Microglial activity in people at ultra high risk of psychosis and in schizophrenia: an [11C]PBR28 PET brain imaging study. Am J Psychiatr. 2016;173:44–52. https://doi.org/10.1176/appi.ajp.2015.14101358.
62. Ottoy J, et al. 18F-PBR111 PET imaging in healthy controls and schizophrenia: test-retest reproducibility and quantification of neuroinflammation. J Nucl Med. 2018;59:1267–74. https://doi.org/10.2967/jnumed.117.203315.
63. Suzuki K, et al. Microglial activation in young adults with autism spectrum disorder. Arch Gen Psychiatry. 2013;70:49–58. https://doi.org/10.1001/jamapsychiatry.2013.272.
64. Van Der Doef TF, et al. In vivo (R)-[11C]PK11195 PET imaging of 18kDa translocator protein in recent onset psychosis. NPJ Schizophrenia. 2016;2. https://doi.org/10.1038/npjschz.2016.31.

65. Doorduin J, et al. Neuroinflammation in schizophrenia-related psychosis: a PET study. J Nucl Med. 2009;50:1801–7. https://doi.org/10.2967/jnumed.109.066647.
66. Takano A, et al. Peripheral benzodiazepine receptors in patients with chronic schizophrenia: a PET study with [11C]DAA1106. Int J Neuropsychopharmacol. 2010;13:943–50. https://doi.org/10.1017/S1461145710000313.
67. Kenk M, et al. Imaging neuroinflammation in gray and white matter in schizophrenia: an in-vivo PET study with [18 F]-FEPPA. Schizophr Bull. 2015;41:85–93. https://doi.org/10.1093/schbul/sbu157.
68. Coughlin JM, et al. In vivo markers of inflammatory response in recent-onset schizophrenia: a combined study using [11C]DPA-713 PET and analysis of CSF and plasma. Transl Psychiatry. 2016;6:1–8. https://doi.org/10.1038/tp.2016.40.
69. Hafizi S, et al. Imaging microglial activation in untreated first-episode psychosis: a PET study with [18F]FEPPA. Am J Psychiatr. 2017;174:118–24. https://doi.org/10.1176/appi.ajp.2016.16020171.
70. Holmes SE, et al. In vivo imaging of brain microglial activity in antipsychotic-free and medicated schizophrenia: a [11C](R)-PK11195 positron emission tomography study. Mol Psychiatry. 2016;21:1672–9. https://doi.org/10.1038/mp.2016.180.
71. Collste K, et al. Lower levels of the glial cell marker TSPO in drug-naive first-episode psychosis patients as measured using PET and [11 C]PBR28. Mol Psychiatry. 2017;22:850–6. https://doi.org/10.1038/mp.2016.247.
72. Di Biase MA, et al. PET imaging of putative microglial activation in individuals at ultra-high risk for psychosis, recently diagnosed and chronically ill with schizophrenia. Transl Psychiatry. 2017;7. https://doi.org/10.1038/tp.2017.193.
73. De Picker L, et al. State-associated changes in longitudinal [18 F]-PBR111 TSPO PET imaging of psychosis patients: evidence for the accelerated ageing hypothesis? Brain Behav Immun. 2019;77:46–54. https://doi.org/10.1016/j.bbi.2018.11.318.
74. Hafizi S, et al. Imaging microglial activation in individuals at clinical high risk for psychosis: an in vivo PET study with [18F] FEPPA. Neuropsychopharmacology. 2017;42:2474–81. https://doi.org/10.1038/npp.2017.111.
75. van Berckel BN, et al. Microglia activation in recent-onset schizophrenia: a quantitative (R)-[11C]PK11195 positron emission tomography study. Biol Psychiatry. 2008;64:820–2. https://doi.org/10.1016/j.biopsych.2008.04.025.
76. Mattei D, et al. Maternal immune activation results in complex microglial transcriptome signature in the adult offspring that is reversed by minocycline treatment. Transl Psychiatry. 2017;7. https://doi.org/10.1038/tp.2017.80.
77. Lum JS, et al. Increased translocator protein (TSPO) binding throughout neurodevelopment in the perinatal phencyclidine rodent model of schizophrenia. Schizophr Res. 2019;212:243–5. https://doi.org/10.1016/j.schres.2019.07.041.
78. Owen DR, et al. Pro-inflammatory activation of primary microglia and macrophages increases 18 kDa translocator protein expression in rodents but not humans. J Cereb Blood Flow Metab. 2017;37:2679–90.
79. Gosselin D, et al. An environment-dependent transcriptional network specifies human microglia identity. Science. 2017;356:1248–59. https://doi.org/10.1126/science.aal3222.
80. Haenseler W, et al. A highly efficient human pluripotent stem cell microglia model displays a neuronal-co-culture-specific expression profile and inflammatory response. Stem Cell Reports. 2017;8:1727–42. https://doi.org/10.1016/j.stemcr.2017.05.017.
81. Danovich L, et al. The influence of clozapine treatment and other antipsychotics on the 18 kDa translocator protein, formerly named the peripheral-type benzodiazepine receptor, and steroid production. Eur Neuropsychopharmacol. 2008;18:24–33. https://doi.org/10.1016/j.euroneuro.2007.04.005.
82. Horti AG, et al. PET imaging of microglia by targeting macrophage colony-stimulating factor 1 receptor (CSF1R). Proc Natl Acad Sci U S A. 2019;116:1686–91. https://doi.org/10.1073/pnas.1812155116.

83. Stratoulias V, Venero JL, Tremblay M, Joseph B. Microglial subtypes: diversity within the microglial community. The EMBO J. 2019;38. https://doi.org/10.15252/embj.2019101997.
84. Bisht K, et al. Dark microglia: a new phenotype predominantly associated with pathological states. Glia. 2016;64:826–39. https://doi.org/10.1002/glia.22966.
85. Gerrits E, Heng Y, Boddeke EWGM, Eggen BJL. Transcriptional profiling of microglia; current state of the art and future perspectives. Glia. 2020;68:740–55. https://doi.org/10.1002/glia.23767.
86. Böttcher C, et al. Human microglia regional heterogeneity and phenotypes determined by multiplexed single-cell mass cytometry. Nat Neurosci. 2019;22:78–90. https://doi.org/10.1038/s41593-018-0290-2.
87. Sankowski R, et al. Mapping microglia states in the human brain through the integration of high-dimensional techniques. Nat Neurosci. 2019;22:2098–110. https://doi.org/10.1038/s41593-019-0532-y.
88. Sommer IE, et al. Efficacy of anti-inflammatory agents to improve symptoms in patients with schizophrenia: an update. Schizophr Bull. 2014;40:181–91. https://doi.org/10.1093/schbul/sbt139.
89. Singh K, et al. Sulforaphane treatment of autism spectrum disorder (ASD). Proc Natl Acad Sci U S A. 2014;111:15550–5. https://doi.org/10.1073/pnas.1416940111.
90. Li YJ, Zhang X, Li YM. Antineuroinflammatory therapy: potential treatment for autism spectrum disorder by inhibiting glial activation and restoring synaptic function. CNS Spectr. 2019; https://doi.org/10.1017/S1092852919001603.
91. Akhondzadeh S, et al. Celecoxib as adjunctive therapy in schizophrenia: a double-blind, randomized and placebo-controlled trial. Schizophr Res. 2007;90:179–85. https://doi.org/10.1016/j.schres.2006.11.016.
92. Laan W, et al. Adjuvant aspirin therapy reduces symptoms of schizophrenia spectrum disorders: results from a randomized, double-blind, placebo-controlled trial. J Clin Psychiatry. 2010;71:520–7. https://doi.org/10.4088/JCP.09m05117yel.
93. Müller N. COX-2 inhibitors, aspirin, and other potential anti-inflammatory treatments for psychiatric disorders. Front Psych. 2019;10 https://doi.org/10.3389/fpsyt.2019.00375.
94. Inta D, Lang UE, Borgwardt S, Meyer-Lindenberg A, Gass P. Microglia activation and schizophrenia: lessons from the effects of minocycline on postnatal neurogenesis, neuronal survival and synaptic pruning. Schizophr Bull. 2017;43:493–6. https://doi.org/10.1093/schbul/sbw088.
95. Solmi M, Correll CU. Adjunctive minocycline in schizophrenia: what one well-conducted study can tell us (and what it can't). Evid Based Ment Health. 2019;22:E3. https://doi.org/10.1136/ebmental-2018-300070.
96. Hasselmann J, et al. Development of a chimeric model to study and manipulate human microglia in vivo. Neuron. 2019;103:1016–1033.e10. https://doi.org/10.1016/j.neuron.2019.07.002.
97. Kapur S, Vanderspek SC, Brownlee BA, Nobrega JN. Antipsychotic dosing in preclinical models is often unrepresentative of the clinical condition: a suggested solution based on in vivo occupancy. J Pharmacol Exp Ther. 2003;305:625–31. https://doi.org/10.1124/jpet.102.046987.
98. Vernon AC, Natesan S, Modo M, Kapur S. Effect of chronic antipsychotic treatment on brain structure: a serial magnetic resonance imaging study with ex vivo and postmortem confirmation. Biol Psychiatry. 2011;69:936–44. https://doi.org/10.1016/j.biopsych.2010.11.010.

Human Endogenous Retrovirus as Missing Link in the Global Etiopathogenesis of Schizophrenia and Bipolar Disorder

9

Hervé Perron and Marion Leboyer

9.1 Introduction

Schizophrenia (SZ) and bipolar disorder (BD) are severe psychiatric disorders involving complex interactions between genetic and environmental factors [1–5].

Environmental factors, such as winter birth, urban environment, and maternal infection during pregnancy, in particular caused by Influenza virus, Herpesviruses or T. gondii, are associated with an increased risk for SZ and for BD [6–9]. Viruses or parasites have been associated with the pathogenesis of SZ or BD, but most studies were based on serology that essentially detects an immunological scar, i.e., specific immunoglobulin G antibody [10–12]. Nonetheless, though the period of infection can be debated, epidemiological data provide arguments for critical periods in life when they may have a significant impact, along with associated immune-mediated inflammation: (a) the perinatal period encompassing the embryonal development and the postnatal final steps of neurodevelopment and (b) the young adulthood period when infections with, e.g., Herpesviruses occur. These periods were further thought to correspond to the early acquisition of a

H. Perron (✉)
GeNeuro, Plan-Les Ouates, Geneva, Switzerland

GeNeuro-Innovation, Lyon, France

Université Claude Bernard Lyon-1, Lyon, France
e-mail: hperron@geneuro.com

M. Leboyer
University Paris Est Créteil (UPEC), Inserm, IMRB (Translational NeuroPsychiatry lab), AP-HP, DMU IMPACT, AP-HP, Fondation FondaMental, Créteil, France
e-mail: marion.leboyer@inserm.fr

M. Berk et al. (eds.), *Immuno-Psychiatry*, https://doi.org/10.1007/978-3-030-71229-7_9

"neurodevelopmental risk", followed by some triggering effects of new infections and/or particular stress factors in teenagers or young adults [12–17]. As illustrated in Fig. 9.1, such a lifelong scenario may integrate perinatal "priming" event(s) and "boosting" events later in life, which could be synergistic or substitutable, with a critical period for teenagers and young adults.

Genetic studies revealed a potential contribution of loci involved in the inflammatory/immune pathways, including the major histocompatibility complex region, in both SZ and BD [18–21], among other candidate genes [22, 23]. Structural genomic studies also highlighted significant modifications in psychotic patients, including copy number variations, deletions, or somatic modifications of the genomic DNA [24–26].

Nonetheless, the mechanisms possibly underlying interactions between genetic and environmental risk factors contributing to the clinical onset and/or to the progression of psychotic disorders remain to be understood. Moreover, the significant observations made in studies addressing different aspects from various disciplines should require a unifying, but missing, link to allow a global understanding.

Rather recently, the involvement of multicopy genetic elements of the human genome, such as Human Endogenous Retroviruses (HERVs), has been reported in SZ and BD [9, 13, 27].

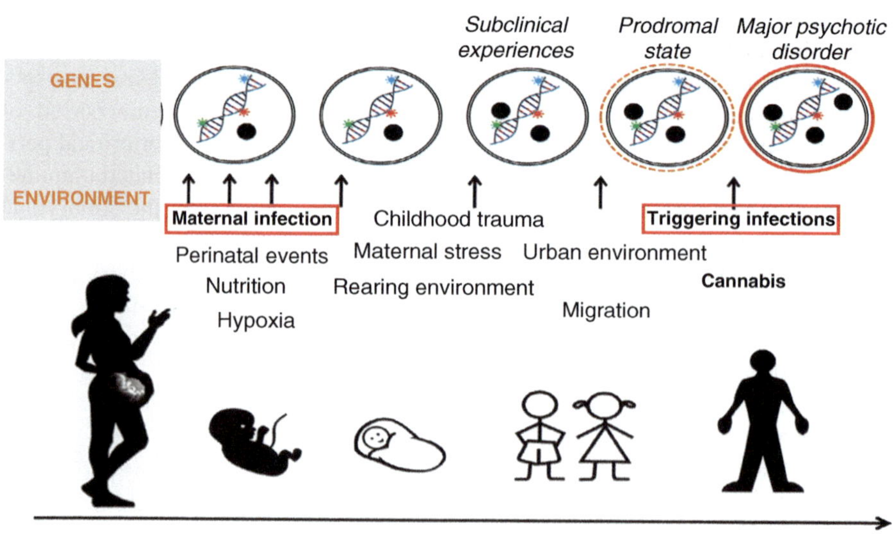

Fig. 9.1 Lifelong exposure to environmental factors impacting epigenetics and gene expression. Environmental triggers may influence gene expression but no direct link with disease was identified, nor directly targeted or involved genes. Epidemiological studies point to most critical periods of exposure to infectious factors, during the embryonal/postnatal period and during the teenage/young adult period. Black circles represent cumulated events having potentially impacted genomic regulation or structures. Colored stars on the drawing for DNA double helix represent potentially susceptible DNA sequences. Adapted from Rutten & Mills Sch. Bull. 2009

9.2 HERVs Represent a Disregarded but Important Part of the Human Genome with Original Genetic Features

HERVs are multicopy families of polygenic structures, represent 8% of the human genome and have retained characteristics of retroviruses. They entered the genome of species from ancient germ-line infections by exogenous retroviruses that have integrated their DNA genomic copy (cDNA) into the DNA of such host cells. Integration of retroviral genome cDNA reverse-transcribed from the virion RNA is a common characteristic of retroviruses, mediated by their encoded enzymes, reverse transcriptase, and integrase. Thus, nonlethal infection and integration of a retroviral genome within a chromosomal region that may not affect embryonal and adult development following gametes fusion, can lead to a hereditary transmission to the offspring. Multiple similar events, called "endogenization", with various retroviruses during evolution, led to multiple families of endogenous retroviruses (ERVs) within the genomes of species ending with numerous mutations, recombination events, and deletions within integrated sequences (provirus), as illustrated in Fig. 9.2.

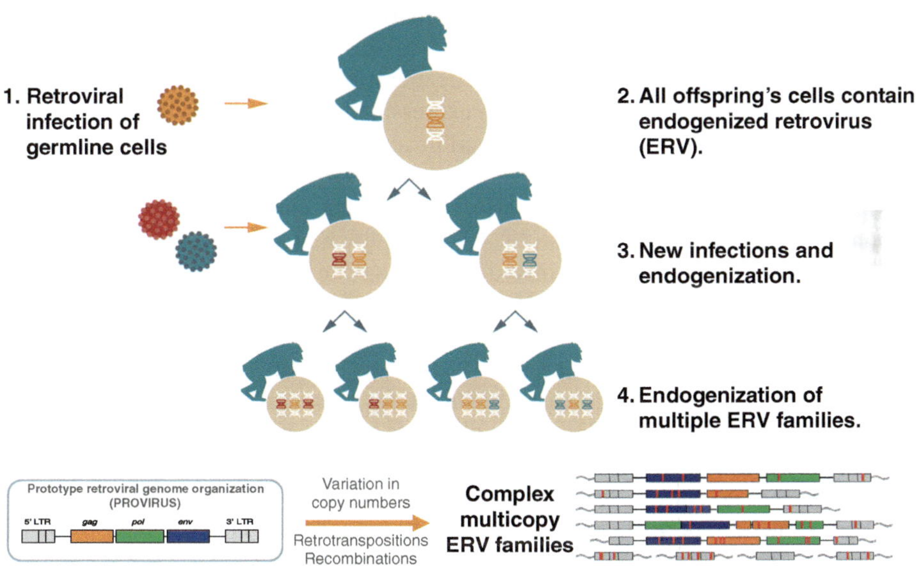

Fig. 9.2 Retroviral endogenizations and transmission to offspring. This illustration depicts the successive steps of retroviral endogenization in species, starting from infection of gametes, integration of a DNA retroviral copy (provirus) in a chromosome giving birth to a viable individual inheriting and retaining this copy in the DNA of all cells and transmitting it to its offspring. Throughout successive generations and species evolution, both endogenous retrotranspositions and re-infections of the germ line of certain individuals (as long as the exogenous strain is persisting in the environment) generate multiple and variable copy numbers in a final population. As shown in the lower panel, retroviral genomes integrated as proviruses are originally composed of two flanking long terminal regions of repeated sequences (LTR), with gag, pol, and env genes, respectively encoding viral capsid proteins, retroviral enzymes, and the envelope protein. They may undergo many somatic modifications during inheritance over generations and most elements are modified or inactivated. Nonetheless, few proviruses from various families may retain coding potential for proteins, if not for complete retroviral expression

HERVs, like other ERVs, belong to the superfamily of repeated and transposable elements (transposons, retrotransposons, and endogenous retroviruses) and altogether represent over 42% of the human genome. They were shown to have played a role in inter- and intra-species gene transmission between individuals. At the individual level, they are responsible of somatic modifications such as intracellular gene retro-transposition or recombination, and may undergo changes under selective environmental pressure or interactions with infectious pathogens.

HERVs are therefore components of the human genome that can be transmitted to subsequent generations through gametes, but have evolved differently from other host genes [28]. They have significant inter-individual copy number variations within the genome of healthy humans from different ethnic origins or simply between individuals [29–32], which would suggest inter-individual differences in potentially related genetic susceptibility.

9.3 HERVs in Schizophrenia and Bipolar Disorder

Interestingly, considering observed somatic rearrangements and copy number variation in psychotic patients' DNA, HERVs may generate such genetic rearrangements linked to their properties of mobile genetic elements [33]. This could even be triggered by microbial agents activating the expression of certain HERV copies or families [34–38]. Interestingly, structural modifications in the major histocompatibility complex (MHC) C4 gene were associated with characteristics of HERVs [29] and numerous HERV sequences were also found in the chromosomal region corresponding to MHC class II genes [39, 40]. In addition, the role of HERV inserts in the regulation of schizophrenia-linked genes has been described [41] and genomic differences between affected and nonaffected homozygous twins identified a differentially amplified HERV copy from the twin with SZ [42].

Thus, HERVs may link many observed genetic features in psychoses such as schizophrenia, while providing an explanation for an underlying mechanism driven by these remnants of "mobile genetic elements" in the human genome, since still functionally interacting with environmental pathogens.

However, a potentially unifying role should not be limited to the genomic level, as HERV-encoded proteins with well characterized and relevant pathogenic mode of action [43] were shown to be expressed in SZ or BD [44–49].

Although most of the contemporary copies of HERVs were inactivated by mutations or deletions or silenced by epigenetic modifications, as schematized in Fig. 9.2, their plasticity and potential responsiveness to environmental triggers are of particular relevance for gene–environment interactions [50]. Under certain conditions, undisrupted HERV sequences or copies may be expressed and display viral protein properties [51–53].

In schizophrenia, a sequence homologous to a human endogenous retrovirus originally identified in MS and previously named "Multiple Sclerosis-associated Retroviral element" (MSRV), was identified from differential DNA amplification in homozygote twins discordant for the disease [42]. MSRV sequences later permitted to unravel a previously unknown HERV family, now named HERV-W [54–56]. MSRV/HERV-W proteins or elevated RNA levels were further detected in patients with schizophrenia from different world areas and in independent studies [45, 47, 49]. Significantly elevated HERV-W transcriptional activity, though with different expression patterns, was also reported in patients with SZ or BD [44].

The HERV-W family and copies corresponding to its MSRV element, have now consistently been shown to be activated by infectious agents [35, 57–59]. In particular, HERV-W elements have been reported to be activated by T. gondii [60] as well as by Influenza virus in human cell lines [37], which is relevant for environmental infections incriminated in elevated risk, for e.g., schizophrenia. Such pathogenic activation of HERV-W elements [45, 61–63] may result in the production of its envelope protein (HERV-W Env) that strongly stimulates a pro-inflammatory cascade through the TLR4 receptor pathway [64] and displays neurotoxicity [43].

At the neuronal level, altered NMDA receptor (NMDAR) signaling plays a central role in psychosis [65] and this glutaminergic system has been extensively described to be part of several key physiological processes, such as synapse maturation [61, 62], spinogenesis [63, 66], and learning/memory [67]. Moreover, the regulation of NMDA receptor signaling is highly dependent on the surface diffusion of the receptor and its dynamic anchoring within postsynaptic densities [68]. A recent study showed that the effect of HERV-W-encoded envelope protein (HERV-W ENV) on glutamatergic NMDAR signaling was not mediated through direct action on channel physiology, but on its trafficking in the plasma membrane at the level of neuronal synapses [43]. This showed a potent link between exposure to HERV-W ENV and NMDAR surface dynamics with a pattern of response that was unique to HERV-W Env compared to all other tested compounds, including LPS, another TLR4 agonist. The effect also uniquely targeted gluN2B and not gluN2A receptors. The fact that these effects were not observed under glia-free conditions also suggested the implication of glia-dependent pathways in this process. The study showed the potential impact of HERV-W env expression, beyond its pro-inflammatory effects, on neuroreceptor dysregulation as observed in psychoses such as schizophrenia and bipolar disorder. Moreover, these specific effects were reproduced using HERV-W ENV serum from patient.

Most interestingly, this study also showed that consistent psychotic behavior was induced in an animal model consisting in rats expressing HERV-W ENV protein in hippocampal neurons transfected with *ENV* gene expressing plasmids in vivo. In addition, a specific monoclonal antibody targeting HERV-W ENV not only inhibited HERV-W ENV pathogenic effects in vitro but also significantly prevented abnormal behavioral signs in antibody-treated rats using intraperitoneal injections in this animal model, versus mock-transfected controls. This not only confirmed the specificity of the neuropathogenic effects of HERV-W ENV and of its behavioral correlates in vivo, but importantly paves the way toward a new therapeutic avenue with antibodies neutralizing this HERV protein.

Thus, HERVs should not only provide a link with previously described genomic features of SZ or BD but also with the abnormal expression of pathogenic endogenous proteins activated by environmental factors, in particular HERV-W envelope

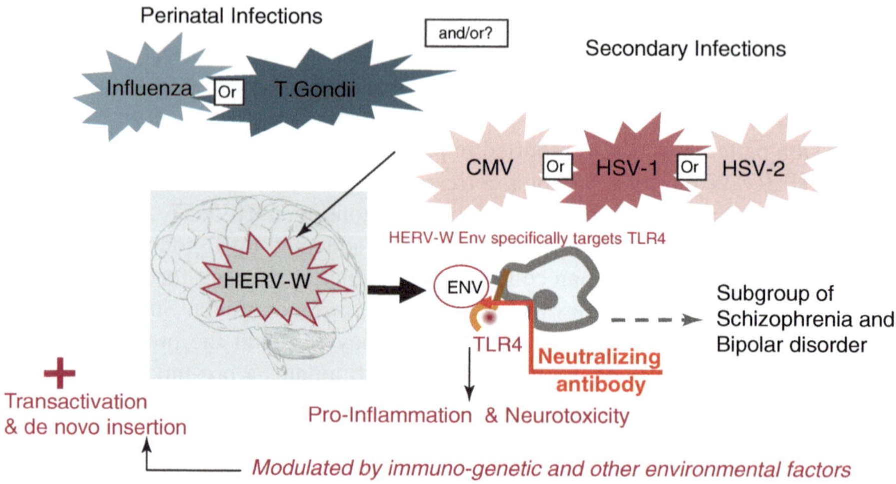

Fig. 9.3 Human Endogenous retroviruses (HERV-W): the missing link? As previously presented, infectious agents were associated with increased risk for schizophrenia or bipolar disorder but, according to their tropism and corresponding periods of infection, they can activate HERV-W elements as already shown in vitro. They would however have a relevant impact in two different periods of life. The early perinatal infections would mostly involve influenza virus or Toxoplasma gondii, while viruses from the Herpesvirus family (e.g., Cytomegalovirus-CMV; Herpes simplex virus type 1 and type 2 -HSV-1 or 2) are commonly acquired in teenagers and young adults

protein with a now evidenced mode of action on the distribution of neuronal receptors at the synapse level. Therefore, the involvement of certain HERV elements appears consistent with the previously evoked missing link between known features of these psychotic diseases and it may provide a global understanding of their pathogenesis, with gene-environment interactions and resulting endogenous neuropathogenic effector molecules. A global scenario summarizing the hypothesis resulting from the present data on the role of HERV-W envelope protein is proposed in Fig. 9.3.

9.4 Conclusion and Perspectives

In conclusion, a lifelong scenario of a detrimental interaction between infectious agents and HERV-W genes may decipher the actual development and course of schizophrenia or bipolar disorder. But, after the preclinical proof of concept provided with a monoclonal antibody neutralizing the pathogenic effects of HERV-W ENV in an animal model, further research and development followed by clinical studies are needed to find out if such a specific treatment strategy could neutralize the pathogenic effects of HERV-W ENV and/or reduce the expression of HERV-W, with appropriate endpoints in patients with schizophrenia or with bipolar disorder. Time may come when new therapeutic strategies targeting pathogenic and non-physiological agonists would allow treating, or possibly preventing, such psychiatric diseases without impairing physiological functions mediated by neuroreceptors and neurotransmitters.

References

1. Uher R. Gene-environment interactions in severe mental illness. Front Psychiatry. 2014;5:48.
2. Misiak B, Stramecki F, Gaweda L, Prochwicz K, Sasiadek MM, Moustafa AA, et al. Interactions between variation in candidate genes and environmental factors in the etiology of schizophrenia and bipolar disorder: a systematic review. Mol Neurobiol. 2018;55(6):5075–100.
3. Mas S, Boloc D, Rodriguez N, Mezquida G, Amoretti S, Cuesta MJ, et al. Examining gene-environment interactions using aggregate scores in a first-episode psychosis cohort. Schizophr Bull. 2020;46(4):1019–25.
4. Kano SI, Hodgkinson CA, Jones-Brando L, Eastwood S, Ishizuka K, Niwa M, et al. Host-parasite interaction associated with major mental illness. Mol Psychiatry. 2020;25(1):194–205.
5. Sahu G, Malavade K, Jacob T. Cognitive impairment in schizophrenia: interplay of BDNF and childhood trauma? A review of literature. Psychiatr Q. 2016;87(3):559–69.
6. Hamdani N, Daban-Huard C, Godin O, Laouamri H, Jamain S, Attiba D, et al. Effects of cumulative herpesviridae and toxoplasma gondii Infections on cognitive function in healthy, bipolar, and schizophrenia subjects. J Clin Psychiatry. 2017;78(1):e18–27.
7. Burgdorf KS, Trabjerg BB, Pedersen MG, Nissen J, Banasik K, Pedersen OB, et al. Large-scale study of toxoplasma and cytomegalovirus shows an association between infection and serious psychiatric disorders. Brain Behav Immun. 2019;79:152–8.
8. Parboosing R, Bao Y, Shen L, Schaefer CA, Brown AS. Gestational influenza and bipolar disorder in adult offspring. JAMA Psychiatry. 2013;70(7):677–85.
9. Arias I, Sorlozano A, Villegas E, de Dios Luna J, McKenney K, Cervilla J, et al. Infectious agents associated with schizophrenia: a meta-analysis. Schizophr Res. 2012;136(1–3):128–36.
10. de Witte LD, van Mierlo HC, Litjens M, Klein HC, Bahn S, Osterhaus AD, et al. The association between antibodies to neurotropic pathogens and schizophrenia: a case-control study. NPJ Schizophr. 2015;1:15041.
11. Tanaka T, Matsuda T, Hayes LN, Yang S, Rodriguez K, Severance EG, et al. Infection and inflammation in schizophrenia and bipolar disorder. Neurosci Res. 2017;115:59–63.
12. Dickerson F, Jones-Brando L, Ford G, Genovese G, Stallings C, Origoni A, et al. Schizophrenia is associated with an aberrant immune response to epstein-barr virus. Schizophr Bull. 2019;45(5):1112–9.
13. Leboyer M, Tamouza R, Charron D, Faucard R, Perron H. Human endogenous retrovirus type W (HERV-W) in schizophrenia: a new avenue of research at the gene-environment interface. World J Biol Psychiatry. 2013;14(2):80–90.
14. Allswede DM, Yolken RH, Buka SL, Cannon TD. Cytokine concentrations throughout pregnancy and risk for psychosis in adult offspring: a longitudinal case-control study. Lancet Psychiatry. 2020;7(3):254–61.
15. Thomas P, Bhatia T, Gauba D, Wood J, Long C, Prasad K, et al. Exposure to herpes simplex virus, type 1 and reduced cognitive function. J Psychiatr Res. 2013;47(11):1680–5.
16. Fruchter E, Goldberg S, Fenchel D, Grotto I, Ginat K, Weiser M. The impact of Herpes simplex virus type 1 on cognitive impairments in young, healthy individuals—a historical prospective study. Schizophr Res. 2015;168(1-2):292–6.
17. Hjorthoj C, Starzer MSK, Benros ME, Nordentoft M. Infections as a risk factor for and prognostic factor after substance-induced psychoses. Am J Psychiatry. 2020;177(4):335–41.
18. Nudel R, Benros ME, Krebs MD, Allesoe RL, Lemvigh CK, Bybjerg-Grauholm J, et al. Immunity and mental illness: findings from a Danish population-based immunogenetic study of seven psychiatric and neurodevelopmental disorders. Eur J Hum Genet. 2019;27(9):1445–55.
19. International Consortium on Lithium G, Amare AT, Schubert KO, Hou L, Clark SR, Papiol S, et al. Association of polygenic score for schizophrenia and HLA antigen and inflammation genes with response to lithium in bipolar affective disorder: a genome-wide association study. JAMA Psychiatry. 2018;75(1):65–74.
20. Calabro M, Drago A, Sidoti A, Serretti A, Crisafulli C. Genes involved in pruning and inflammation are enriched in a large mega-sample of patients affected by Schizophrenia and Bipolar Disorder and controls. Psychiatry Res. 2015;228(3):945–9.

21. Avramopoulos D, Pearce BD, McGrath J, Wolyniec P, Wang R, Eckart N, et al. Infection and inflammation in schizophrenia and bipolar disorder: a genome wide study for interactions with genetic variation. PLoS One. 2015;10(3):e0116696.
22. Forstner AJ, Fischer SB, Schenk LM, Strohmaier J, Maaser-Hecker A, Reinbold CS, et al. Whole-exome sequencing of 81 individuals from 27 multiply affected bipolar disorder families. Transl Psychiatry. 2020;10(1):57.
23. Nedic Erjavec G, Svob Strac D, Tudor L, Konjevod M, Sagud M, Pivac N. Genetic markers in psychiatry. Adv Exp Med Biol. 2019;1192:53–93.
24. Nishioka M, Bundo M, Iwamoto K, Kato T. Somatic mutations in the human brain: implications for psychiatric research. Mol Psychiatry. 2019;24(6):839–56.
25. Malhotra D, Sebat J. CNVs: harbingers of a rare variant revolution in psychiatric genetics. Cell. 2012;148(6):1223–41.
26. Green EK, Rees E, Walters JT, Smith KG, Forty L, Grozeva D, et al. Copy number variation in bipolar disorder. Mol Psychiatry. 2016;21(1):89–93.
27. Balestrieri E, Matteucci C, Cipriani C, Grelli S, Ricceri L, Calamandrei G, et al. Endogenous retroviruses activity as a molecular signature of neurodevelopmental disorders. Int J Mol Sci. 2019;20:23.
28. Feschotte C, Gilbert C. Endogenous viruses: insights into viral evolution and impact on host biology. Nat Rev Genet. 2012;13(4):283–96.
29. Pani MA, Wood JP, Bieda K, Toenjes RR, Usadel KH, Badenhoop K. The variable endogenous retroviral insertion in the human complement C4 gene: a transmission study in type I diabetes mellitus. Hum Immunol. 2002;63(6):481–4.
30. Wildschutte JH, Williams ZH, Montesion M, Subramanian RP, Kidd JM, Coffin JM. Discovery of unfixed endogenous retrovirus insertions in diverse human populations. Proc Natl Acad Sci U S A. 2016;113(16):E2326–34.
31. Thomas J, Perron H, Feschotte C. Variation in proviral content among human genomes mediated by LTR recombination. Mob DNA. 2018;9:36.
32. Shin W, Lee J, Son SY, Ahn K, Kim HS, Han K. Human-specific HERV-K insertion causes genomic variations in the human genome. PLoS One. 2013;8(4):e60605.
33. Weckselblatt B, Rudd MK. Human structural variation: mechanisms of chromosome rearrangements. Trends Genet. 2015;31(10):587–99.
34. Sutkowski N, Chen G, Calderon G, Huber BT. Epstein-Barr virus latent membrane protein LMP-2A is sufficient for transactivation of the human endogenous retrovirus HERV-K18 superantigen. J Virol. 2004;78(14):7852–60.
35. Ruprecht K, Obojes K, Wengel V, Gronen F, Kim KS, Perron H, et al. Regulation of human endogenous retrovirus W protein expression by herpes simplex virus type 1: implications for multiple sclerosis. J Neuro-Oncol. 2006;12(1):65–71.
36. Nellaker C, Yao Y, Jones-Brando L, Mallet F, Yolken RH, Karlsson H. Transactivation of elements in the human endogenous retrovirus W family by viral infection. Retrovirology. 2006;3:44.
37. Li F, Nellaker C, Sabunciyan S, Yolken RH, Jones-Brando L, Johansson AS, et al. Transcriptional derepression of the ERVWE1 locus following influenza A virus infection. J Virol. 2014;88(8):4328–37.
38. Charvet B, Reynaud JM, Gourru-Lesimple G, Perron H, Marche PN, Horvat B. Induction of proinflammatory multiple sclerosis-associated retrovirus envelope protein by human herpesvirus-6A and CD46 receptor engagement. Front Immunol. 2018;9:2803.
39. Kulski JK, Gaudieri S, Inoko H, Dawkins RL. Comparison between two human endogenous retrovirus (HERV)-rich regions within the major histocompatibility complex. J Mol Evol. 1999;48(6):675–83.
40. Andersson G, Svensson AC, Setterblad N, Rask L. Retroelements in the human MHC class II region. Trends Genet. 1998;14(3):109–14.
41. Suntsova M, Gogvadze EV, Salozhin S, Gaifullin N, Eroshkin F, Dmitriev SE, et al. Human-specific endogenous retroviral insert serves as an enhancer for the schizophrenia-linked gene PRODH. Proc Natl Acad Sci U S A. 2013;110(48):19472–7.

42. Deb-Rinker P, Klempan TA, O'Reilly RL, Torrey EF, Singh SM. Molecular characterization of a MSRV-like sequence identified by RDA from monozygotic twin pairs discordant for schizophrenia. Genomics. 1999;61(2):133–44.
43. Johansson EM, Bouchet D, Tamouza R, Ellul P, Morr A, Avignone E, et al. Human endogenous retroviral protein triggers deficit in glutamate synapse maturation and behaviors associated with psychosis. Sci Adv. 2020;6(29):eabc0708.
44. Perron H, Hamdani N, Faucard R, Lajnef M, Jamain S, Daban-Huard C, et al. Molecular characteristics of human endogenous retrovirus type-W in schizophrenia and bipolar disorder. Transl Psychiatry. 2012;2:e201.
45. Perron H, Mekaoui L, Bernard C, Veas F, Stefas I, Leboyer M. Endogenous retrovirus type W GAG and envelope protein antigenemia in serum of schizophrenic patients. Biol Psychiatry. 2008;64(12):1019–23.
46. Huang W, Li S, Hu Y, Yu H, Luo F, Zhang Q, et al. Implication of the env gene of the human endogenous retrovirus W family in the expression of BDNF and DRD3 and development of recent-onset schizophrenia. Schizophr Bull. 2010;37(5):988–1000.
47. Huang WJ, Liu ZC, Wei W, Wang GH, Wu JG, Zhu F. Human endogenous retroviral pol RNA and protein detected and identified in the blood of individuals with schizophrenia. Schizophr Res. 2006;83(2–3):193–9.
48. Karlsson H, Schroder J, Bachmann S, Bottmer C, Yolken RH. HERV-W-related RNA detected in plasma from individuals with recent-onset schizophrenia or schizoaffective disorder. Mol Psychiatry. 2004;9(1):12–3.
49. Karlsson H, Bachmann S, Schroder J, McArthur J, Torrey EF, Yolken RH. Retroviral RNA identified in the cerebrospinal fluids and brains of individuals with schizophrenia. Proc Natl Acad Sci U S A. 2001;98(8):4634–9.
50. Perron H, Lang A. The human endogenous retrovirus link between genes and environment in multiple sclerosis and in multifactorial diseases associating neuroinflammation. Clin Rev Allergy Immunol. 2010;39(1):51–61.
51. Duperray A, Barbe D, Raguenez G, Weksler BB, Romero IA, Couraud PO, et al. Inflammatory response of endothelial cells to a human endogenous retrovirus associated with multiple sclerosis is mediated by TLR4. Int Immunol. 2015;27(11):545–53.
52. Rolland A, Jouvin-Marche E, Saresella M, Ferrante P, Cavaretta R, Creange A, et al. Correlation between disease severity and in vitro cytokine production mediated by MSRV (multiple sclerosis associated retroviral element) envelope protein in patients with multiple sclerosis. J Neuroimmunol. 2005;160(1-2):195–203.
53. Perron H, Jouvin-Marche E, Michel M, Ounanian-Paraz A, Camelo S, Dumon A, et al. Multiple sclerosis retrovirus particles and recombinant envelope trigger an abnormal immune response in vitro, by inducing polyclonal Vbeta16 T-lymphocyte activation. Virology. 2001;287(2):321–32.
54. Perron H, Garson JA, Bedin F, Beseme F, Paranhos-Baccala G, Komurian-Pradel F, et al. Molecular identification of a novel retrovirus repeatedly isolated from patients with multiple sclerosis. The Collaborative Research Group on Multiple Sclerosis. Proc Natl Acad Sci U S A. 1997;94(14):7583–8.
55. Blond JL, Beseme F, Duret L, Bouton O, Bedin F, Perron H, et al. Molecular characterization and placental expression of HERV-W, a new human endogenous retrovirus family. J Virol. 1999;73(2):1175–85.
56. Perron H, Perin JP, Rieger F, Alliel PM. Particle-associated retroviral RNA and tandem RGH/HERV-W copies on human chromosome 7q: possible components of a 'chain-reaction' triggered by infectious agents in multiple sclerosis? J Neuro-Oncol. 2000;6(Suppl 2):S67–75.
57. Perron H, Bernard C, Bertrand JB, Lang AB, Popa I, Sanhadji K, et al. Endogenous retroviral genes, herpesviruses and gender in multiple sclerosis. J Neurol Sci. 2009;286(1–2):65–72.
58. Lafon M, Jouvin-Marche E, Marche PN, Perron H. Human viral superantigens: to be or not to be transactivated? Trends Immunol. 2002;23(5):238–9; author reply 9.
59. Perron H, Suh M, Lalande B, Gratacap B, Laurent A, Stoebner P, et al. Herpes simplex virus ICP0 and ICP4 immediate early proteins strongly enhance expression of a retrovirus harboured

by a leptomeningeal cell line from a patient with multiple sclerosis. J Gen Virol. 1993;74(Pt 1):65–72.
60. Frank O, Jones-Brando L, Leib-Mosch C, Yolken R, Seifarth W. Altered transcriptional activity of human endogenous retroviruses in neuroepithelial cells after infection with Toxoplasma gondii. J Infect Dis. 2006;194(10):1447–9.
61. Kelsch W, Li Z, Wieland S, Senkov O, Herb A, Gongrich C, et al. GluN2B-containing NMDA receptors promote glutamate synapse development in hippocampal interneurons. J Neurosci. 2014;34(48):16022–30.
62. Frank RA, Komiyama NH, Ryan TJ, Zhu F, O'Dell TJ, Grant SG. NMDA receptors are selectively partitioned into complexes and supercomplexes during synapse maturation. Nat Commun. 2016;7:11264.
63. Liu T, Kong D, Shah BP, Ye C, Koda S, Saunders A, et al. Fasting activation of AgRP neurons requires NMDA receptors and involves spinogenesis and increased excitatory tone. Neuron. 2012;73(3):511–22.
64. Rolland A, Jouvin-Marche E, Viret C, Faure M, Perron H, Marche PN. The envelope protein of a human endogenous retrovirus-W family activates innate immunity through CD14/TLR4 and promotes Th1-like responses. J Immunol. 2006;176(12):7636–44.
65. Tamminga CA, Zukin RS. Schizophrenia: evidence implicating hippocampal GluN2B protein and REST epigenetics in psychosis pathophysiology. Neuroscience. 2015;309:233–42.
66. Paoletti P, Bellone C, Zhou Q. NMDA receptor subunit diversity: impact on receptor properties, synaptic plasticity and disease. Nat Rev Neurosci. 2013;14(6):383–400.
67. Baez MV, Cercato MC, Jerusalinsky DA. NMDA receptor subunits change after synaptic plasticity induction and learning and memory acquisition. Neural Plast. 2018;2018:5093048.
68. Li B, Otsu Y, Murphy TH, Raymond LA. Developmental decrease in NMDA receptor desensitization associated with shift to synapse and interaction with postsynaptic density-95. J Neurosci. 2003;23(35):11244–54.

The Human Leukocyte Antigen System in Psychiatry: Where Do We Stand?

10

Ryad Tamouza, Rajagopal Krishnamoorthy, and Marion Leboyer

10.1 The HLA System

Since the first description of an association between HLA-B and Hodgkin lymphoma [1], genetic association between the highly polymorphic human leukocyte antigen (HLA) gene cluster and a large variety of immune/inflammatory disorders, ranging from infections to cancer, have consistently been observed [2]. Recently, a strong association between schizophrenia and the major histocompatibility complex (MHC) that hosts the HLA gene cluster was reported by the Psychiatry Genomic Consortium [3], extending the previous observation that dates back to 1975 [4]. Given the prominent role of HLA gene cluster in the regulation of immune-inflammatory processes, a genetically determined dysfunctional HLA system or

R. Tamouza (✉)
Laboratoire Neuro-Psychiatrie Translationnelle, INSERM U955, IMRB, Université Paris Est Créteil, Creteil, France

AP-HP, Département Medico-Universitaire de Psychiatrie et d'Addictologie (DMU IMPACT) and Fédération Hospitalo-Universitaire de Médecine de Précision en Psychiatrie (FHU ADAPT), Hôpitaux Henri Mondor, Créteil, France

Fondation FondaMental, Créteil, France

Service de Psychaitrie, Hopital Albert Chenevier, Créteil, France

R. Krishnamoorthy
Fondation FondaMental, Créteil, France

M. Leboyer
University Paris Est Créteil (UPEC), Inserm, IMRB (Translational NeuroPsychiatry lab), AP-HP, DMU IMPACT, AP-HP, Fondation FondaMental, Créteil, France
e-mail: marion.leboyer@inserm.fr

M. Berk et al. (eds.), *Immuno-Psychiatry*, https://doi.org/10.1007/978-3-030-71229-7_10

context-dependent inappropriate/aberrant response of the MHC complex very likely plays a major role in psychiatric settings. Indeed, a large subset of patients with autism, schizophrenia, or bipolar disorders have consistently been associated with immune dysfunction in a background of chronic low-grade inflammation and comorbid autoimmune diseases. The implication of HLA-related immune processes in psychiatric disorders could be related to its role in brain development as they regulate processes like microglia activation and synaptic pruning [5].

The MHC is a 4 Mb region located on the short arm of chromosome 6 (6p21.3-22.1) and is one of the most polymorphic and gene dense regions of the human genome [6]. This region hosts the HLA gene cluster, physically divided into three functionally distinct sub-regions:

1. The HLA-class I region that includes the classical HLA-A, HLA-B, and HLA-C genes as well as the non-classical HLA-E, HLA-F, and HLA-G loci; the former three are involved in antigen presentation to T CD8+ lymphocytes while the latter are mainly implicated in immunomodulatory functions.
2. The HLA class II region encompasses the HLA-DPA1, HLA-DPB1, HLA-DQA1, HLA-DRB1, HLA-DQB1, HLA-DQB2, HLA-DRA, HLA-DRB1, HLA-DRB2, HLA-DRB3, HLA-DRB4, and HLA-DRB5 genes which are involved in antigen presentation to T CD4+ lymphocytes.
3. The class III region consists of genes involved in inflammatory responses, leukocyte maturation, and some of the genetic components of the complement cascade.

While the encoded molecules of the HLA-A, -B, and -C genes play an essential role in the detection and elimination of virus-infected and tumoral cells through cellular-mediated cytotoxic processes, their HLA class II counterparts modulate humoral immune responses. Both gene sets are highly polymorphic with more than 26,000 alleles reported to date [7], the main function of which is to present self or foreign antigens to the T cell receptors (TCR) on the effector cells.

Since long, the HLA molecules are known to be involved in fine-tuning of the inflammatory processes, and any of their dysfunctions can cause a variety of immuno-pathological events including autoimmunity, a frequent comorbid condition in psychiatric disorders [8]. In recent years, evidences mount to show that the HLA molecules also play a role at a central level. Indeed, they modulate some of the core functions of the central nervous system (CNS) such as neurodevelopment, neuronal/synaptic plasticity, learning memory, and behavior [9]. In fact, neurons influence neuron-neuron interactions and neuro-signaling [10]. Their highest levels of expression were detected in post-synaptic hippocampal neurons [11]. Moreover, the HLA molecules are pivotal for the anatomical integrity of the CNS as exemplified by the enlarged ventricles observed in HLA-class I deficient murine models [12].

Despite evidences for the prominent immune dysfunctions in a significant subset of patients affected by major psychiatric disorders likely via the involvement of HLA molecules in neurodevelopment and neuronal function, further supported by HLA genetic association studies (that provide tags, but not direct proof), difficulties in deciphering the mechanistic link between the so-called classical HLA diversity (alleles corresponding to antigen-presenting molecules), and these disorders persist essentially due to the complex genetic architecture of the HLA system. Given the recent technological advances, it is now possible to perform a precise and deep characterization of the HLA gene cluster to understand the pathophysiological underpinnings of its diversity in conferring susceptibility to or protection against psychiatric disorders. In this review, we will discuss the current knowledge and prospects of HLA genetics in major psychiatric disorders.

10.2 The Genetic Complexity of the HLA Region

Since the discovery of the HLA system by Jean Dausset [13], the analysis of HLA polymorphism has undergone successive technological improvements over 20 years incorporating gradually DNA-based molecular approaches including the high throughput, and cost-effective next-generation sequencing (NGS) for reliable HLA genotyping, that could cover all the known HLA alleles. Nevertheless, such fine-tuned analysis and understanding of the potential of HLA diversity in genetic studies requires specially trained "histocompatibility expertise."

Despite such advances and available expertise, HLA and disease association studies are still hampered by several limitations including (i) the extreme rate of polymorphism, (ii) the ethno-geographical-dependent distribution of HLA alleles, (iii) disease-dependent variable pertinence of a given HLA allele. For example, the HLA-B27 association is prominently evident for Ankylosing Spondylitis while for other multi-genic and multifactorial disorders, evidence of disease association may not be that apparent because distinct alleles may have shared functions and (iv) further complexity of HLA polymorphism resides in the variability of allele expression [14–16]. Given these aspects, both the candidate gene approach which may ignore the degree of contribution of other interacting loci to the phenotype and the Genome-Wide Association Studies (GWAS) which covers imperfectly the extreme polymorphism of HLA loci (only 60% of the diversity accounted for) limit the power of HLA imputation-based methods.

To overcome these difficulties, one possible approach is to understand the evolution-based shaping of the present day HLA diversity stemming from a limited but manageable number of ancestral haplotypes (AH). Various genetic events, viz., crossing-overs, recombination and point mutations, have participated in that evolution [17, 18]. These AHs were selected under diverse geographic-specific environmental pressure, then conserved, and fully or partially transmitted to generations [18]. Hence, the study of the distribution of AHs in disease association studies has clarified issues raised by the scattered HLA allele association in a given disease and further allowed to predict, by features of commonality of these alleles, potential mechanisms in the disease process. One of the best examples is represented by the HLA-8.1AH, which is recognized as the most associated AH with immune disorders including infections, inflammation and autoimmunity, while being characterized by a steady-state pro-inflammatory background in healthy individuals [17, 19]. Consequently, such properties may explain why the 8.1AH was found to be protective against pathogens, a status likely due to positive (balancing) selection, however with a price to be paid by its inherent pro-inflammatory properties that could favor risk for chronic inflammation and autoimmunity [20].

Another way to apprehend the HLA functional diversity is to study allele-dependent expression status. Indeed, such diversity reflects the influence of HLA alleles per se. For example, single nucleotide polymorphisms (SNP) categorizing the HLA-DPB1 and HLA-C alleles into high and low expressed variants were shown to be strongly associated, respectively, with graft-versus host disease after hematopoietic stem cell transplantation and HIV infection [21–23].

Immersing further, it is relevant to note that the specific recognition of HLA-Peptide combination is mediated by the per se polymorphic T cell receptors (TCRs) on CD8+ T cells which bind class I molecules and on CD4+ T cells which bind class II molecules. The specificity of HLA-peptide-TCR tripartite interactions is fundamental in enabling the adaptive immune system to mount an efficient and appropriate response against infection while simultaneously being capable of preventing autoimmune processes [24–26].

Different mechanisms have been found in HLA-associated diseases such as atypical HLA-peptide-TCR binding orientation, low-affinity peptide binding that facilitates thymic escape, TCR-mediated stabilization of weak-peptide-HLA-interaction, or presentation of peptides in a different binding register [27], altogether adding a supplementary level of diversity.

Thus, while the GWAS allowed detection, among hundreds of genes, of the MHC/HLA genetic cluster as a pivotal region, specific HLA-dedicated expertise is needed to uncover meaningful functional haplotypes associated with disease subgroups of interest. It may even allow retro-stratification, based on their HLA type, into subgroups of the psychiatric patients who are essentially classified into clinical categories. Indeed, molecular retro-stratification may generate homogeneous subgroups, thus providing better insight into the pathophysiological underpinnings of these complex genetic disorders.

10.3 HLA Diversity in Major Psychiatric Disorders

In this section, we review the previously studied HLA gene candidate association in major psychiatric disorders, especially the risk/protection conferred by them not only on the disease category per se but also on specific sub phenotypes of a given disorder.

10.3.1 Schizophrenia (SZ)

Accumulated evidence from epidemiologic, immunological, genetic, imaging studies strongly argues in favor of the proposition that MHC confers risk to schizophrenia [28]. The first evidence supporting HLA as a schizophrenia susceptibility locus dates back to papers published in the 1970s [4, 29]. Since then, several associations have been reported in different ethnic populations, for example, the HLA-A9, HLA-A10, HLA-DRB1, HLA-DQB1 alleles [28]. In 2009, three GWAS and meta-analysis of these GWAS published in the same issue of *Nature* revealed strong association between the MHC region and schizophrenia [30–33]. These studies clearly established that the HLA hosting MHC is the strongest region of association with SZ, but without any precision on the location of a potential at risk loci albeit possible involvement of the HLA gene cluster.

Later, GWAS subjected to HLA imputation of classical HLA alleles strikingly revealed a dominant protective effect conferred by some HLA alleles namely, HLA-A*01, B*08, and DRB1*03 (Donnelly et al. 2012), all derived from the so-called 8.1 "autoimmune" ancestral haplotype (8.1AH) (A*01 ~ B*08 ~ DRB1*03 ~ DQB 1*02). This latter is the most associated HLA haplotype with inflammatory processes and autoimmune diseases including Type1 diabetes, celiac disease, Grave's disease, and myasthenia gravis [17].

Further dissection of the MHC/HLA region revealed a major contribution to SZ risk is represented by an elevated expression of the complement C4A molecules. Such raised gene expression is apparently due to increased C4A gene copy number. This fits very well with the plausible (experimentally demonstrated) contribution of C4A to exaggerated C4-dependant neuro-synaptic pruning [34]. The complement system is a set of immune proteins involved not only in first-line defense against pathogens but also as a major contributor of synaptic pruning during neurodevelopment [35]. Recent observations established a link between the C4 locus and classical HLA haplotype diversity in the modulation of risk to develop schizophrenia. Indeed, the protective status conferred by the above-mentioned 8.1 AH haplotype is likely related to the fact that this haplotype naturally lacks the C4 locus. We recently showed that one of the 8.1 AH-derived HLA haplotypes was significantly less frequent in SZ patients with early onset but gradually increased in frequency with the age at the onset of SZ (12.7% after 30 years, $Pc = 0.008$) [36]. This is probably explained by the fact that carrying the 8.1 AH decreased the C4 expression which leads to less cortical thinning (synaptic pruning), thus delaying the age at the onset of SZ while potentially favoring autoimmune processes due to its pro-inflammatory properties. By contrast, SZ patients not bearing 8.1 AH-derived HLA haplotypes have an active C4 complement and may suffer from a more severe form of the disorder, characterized by early age at onset, associated to increased synaptic pruning leading to cortical thinning. Simultaneously these SZ subjects will be expected to be less prone to develop autoimmune disorders. This is in line with previous observations that carriers of MHC-linked risk variants (*rs*2596532) have larger ventricles [37].

Altogether, these observations highlight the possibility that the HLA genetics will help identifying homogeneous sub-groups of patients with schizophrenia.

10.3.2 Autism Spectrum Disorder (ASD)

Several case-control-based analyses of potential associations between the HLA genetic diversity and autism spectrum disorders (ASD) provide only fragmented data without any functional clues albeit GWAS studies confirmed the ASD risk conferred by the MHC region [38, 39]. Recent HLA haplotype-based analysis brought further precisions by identifying both at risk for and protective HLA haplotypes against ASD [40]. More precisely: (i) the celiac disease-associated HLA-DRB*11 ~ DQB1*07 was found to be associated with the risk to develop ASD and in particular in those with higher scores for social and non-verbal functioning, the two proxies of disease severity, and also interestingly in agreement with the concept of gastro-intestinal involvement in ASD [41, 42], (ii) as in SZ, here again a protective status conferred by the HLA 8.1 AH. To remind, this haplotype lacks the synaptic pruning complement C4 component and confers raised degree of steady-state pro-inflammatory status, and (iii) in a subset of regressive autism, a subset of ASD characterized by immunological features, protection was shown to be conferred by a class II sub-haplotype, namely, HLA-DPA1*01-DPB1*04 [43].

10.3.3 Bipolar Disorder (BD)

Along the report of pharmacogenetic association of HLA antigen with response to lithium [44], ancestral haplotype derivation from observed HLA allelic combinations revealed an association between the 8.1 AH and bipolar disorder (BD), and in particular with BD subgroup having rapid cycling and/or history of suicidal behaviors [45]. Such association likely bears pathophysiological relevance since the pro-inflammatory 8.1 AH favors autoimmune processes. This is in line with the well-known association of BD with comorbid autoimmune conditions [46, 47]. This study also reported associations between disease onset by hypomanic episode or by psychotic symptoms, and HLA 57.1 AH and 7.1 AH, both previously associated with common inflammatory disorders. Consequently, it is likely that in BD, HLA-mediated pro-inflammatory processes are at work.

An interesting observation is the contrasting effect of the 8.1 AH; in SZ and ASD it is protective while in BD it confers increased risk to develop severe forms of BD. Similarly, Andreasen et al. [48] reported that the same HLA allele was shared between SZ and multiple sclerosis (MS), but not between MS and BD. Despite a large overlap of the genetic and some clinical features between BD and SZ, it is possible that their neurodevelopmental differences may be related to temporal differences in HLA-dependent immunogenetic influences [48, 49]. In summary given the relationship between the 8.1 AH and complement C4-mediated synaptic pruning on the one hand and the established shared genetic inheritance between SZ and BD, on the other, it is possible that the 8.1 AH-associated immunogenetic processes contribute to temporal neurodevelopmental specificities between these disorders.

10.4 Other Implications in Psychiatric Settings

10.4.1 HLA and "Auto-Immune Psychosis"

After the initial description by Dalmau in 2008 of "autoimmune limbic encephalitis" [50], the concept of "auto-immune psychosis" emerged [51]. Indeed, in typical psychiatric setting antibodies directed against the NMDAr disrupt the receptor function/signaling through a mechanism different from that occurs in NMDAr limbic encephalitis [52]. Only few studies have addressed the potential relationship between autoimmune psychosis/encephalitis with HLA polymorphism. While the HLA-B*07:02 was found associated with anti-NMDAR encephalitis in German population-groups [53], in Chinese patients such association involve the HLA class II DRB1*16:02 allele [54]. Potential implication of HLA in anti-NMDAR encephalitis was further suspected by the appearance of anti-NMDAr encephalitis a month after pulmonary infection in a 3-year-old boy with chromosomal deletion in HLA-DP cluster [55]. In this case, one could postulate that HLA-dependent altered immune response failed to resolve the infectious event compromising the tolerogenic process with consequent occurrence of autoimmunity.

Other autoantibodies for brain receptor targets have recently been described. In particular, a German study described a strong association between anti-leucine-rich glioma-inactivated1 (LGI1) encephalitis and the HLA-DRB1*07:01, DQA1*02:01 haplotype [53]. Whether and how the HLA system is involved in the autoimmune encephalitis/psychosis remains an open question.

10.4.2 HLA and Treatment Responses to Psychotropic Compounds

The HLA genetic diversity is also implicated in the modulation of treatment responses in psychiatric settings either in terms of adverse drug reaction (ADRs) or treatment efficacy. In the context of ADRs both candidate gene studies and GWAS demonstrated that clozapine-induced agranulocytosis is partly mediated by HLA alleles belonging to both HLA-class I and class II specificities [56]. In terms of efficacy of treatment response, we showed that a double amino-acid change in the HLA-A peptide-binding groove was associated with better response to psychotropic treatment in patients with SZ [57]. A recent large survey showed that treatment response to lithium in BD is strongly influenced by both SZ-linked polygenic score and the MHC/HLA genetic diversity [44]. The latter finding may be in line with the assumption that a major difference in the shared heritability between SZ and BD likely lie in the MHC cluster [48].

10.4.3 HLA and Human Endogenous Retrovirus Elements (HERV)

The human endogenous retroviruses (HERVs) are ancient retroviral-derived fragments integrated in human genome representing 8% of it. A majority of them are not expressed, but some of the undisrupted HERV sequences can be reactivated under certain triggering conditions, such as early infections, with consequent expression of proteins harboring viral properties. Such reactivation is known to be associated with various autoimmune/inflammatory disorders such as multiple sclerosis or rheumatoid arthritis implicating, respectively, two types of HERV family, namely, HERV-W and HERV-K [58].

Given the likely gene and environment framework of HERV reactivation leading possibly to the production of pro-inflammatory and neurotoxic proteins, HERV was the focus of studies in psychiatric disorders revealing associations especially between the HERV-W type and both SZ and BD at protein and/or at DNA/RNA levels further influenced by copy number variations [59, 60]. More recently, one of the HERV members, namely, HERV-K, as a potential risk component for SZ was envisaged. Indeed, Sekar et al. demonstrated that complement C4 long allele harboring the insertion of HERV-K expressed higher levels of C4A molecules with presumable exaggerated synaptic pruning, and cortical thinning [34]. It is thus amazing that different types of the HERV family members can be associated with the same disease and may represent different disease pathways. Finally, within the context of the present review, it is important to remind that the complement C4 is located in the HLA-class III region and that the HLA-8.1 ancestral haplotype is believed to exert a protective effect against SZ risk possibly because it is devoid of C4A gene.

10.4.4 Another Facet of the HLA Diversity: The Non-classical HLA-Class I Loci

Given the extreme diversity of environmental stressors, including infections, evolutionary forces have gradually shaped a highly multigenic and polymorphic biological system to handle these challenges: the immune system. Upon interaction with a trigger, the immune system mounts non-specific pro-inflammatory processes, if necessary, by adaptive cellular processes specific for the triggering event. Such sequence of events could at times be deleterious in case of uncontrolled inflammatory processes. Thus, in parallel, counteracting immune-modulatory genetic strategies have emerged and were positively selected by evolutionary constraints.

One of the best example of such “Dr Jekyll and Mr Hyde” biological system is represented by the HLA-class I classical and non-classical molecules. Within the same HLA-class I region lie (i) the classical HLA-class I-A, -B, and -C loci characterized by an extreme polymorphism essential for their antigen-presentation functions and maintained by balancing selection to cope up with a large variety of environmental pathogens and (ii) the non-classical HLA-E, G, and F genes remarkable by a very low rate of diversity that reflect more broad properties such as immunomodulation.

Among these latter, the non-classical HLA-G encodes cell surface molecules exerting powerful immunomodulatory functions, first demonstrated essential for the establishment and tolerance between the maternal immune system and the semi-allogeneic fetus at the fetal-placental interface [61]. These characteristics thus opened the way to study various immune-related disorders, especially those possibly starting in early life, in particular during pregnancy when neurodevelopmental windows are critical. In this context, we and others have demonstrated the likely implication of both HLA-G polymorphism and expression in psychiatric disorders including autism, SZ, and BD. In consecutive articles Guerini et al. demonstrated that genetically determined low expression of the tolerogenic HLA-G molecules at the fetal-mother interface, possibly leading to prenatal immune activation, is associated with ASD risk [62–65].

In addition, in SZ, another neuro-developmental psychiatric disorder, even if the potential influence of HLA-G polymorphism and expression was less investigated, it seems that low levels of HLA-G either genetically determined or at circulating level may influence disease onset and phenotype [66–69]. In bipolar disorders two studies performed on patient population of distant ethnicity, i.e., French and south Indian Tamils revealed that contrary to ASD and SZ, genetically determined HLA-G low expression confer protection against the BD which can suggest a possible difference mediated by HLA-G in the ontogeny of such disease [70, 71]. It is hence possible that in BD the protection conferred by low-grade immunomodulation may rather favor more efficient and intense pro-inflammatory anti-infectious response but outside the neurodevelopmental window.

10.5 Future

These findings and the fact that, predating human lineage, HLA-equivalent loci are found in non-vertebrates and still retained accumulating diversity are the indisputable proof of the pivotal role of HLA in human health and disease [72].

Accordingly, the potential involvement of the HLA system in psychiatric disorders makes them eligible to integrate the pool of immune disorders. However, the present knowledge concerning the intricacies between HLA and psychiatry is without any doubt the tip of the iceberg as, for example, the vast majority of the studies was focused on populations of European and Asian, ancestries leaving aside the African continent where the rate of the genetic diversity is the highest among humans. In this context, a recent study of SZ patients from south Africa, namely, the Xhosa population-group, revealed not only that the observed overall genetic diversity was more important than that of non-African populations but importantly uncover mutational events that could be hypothesized to be founder SZ causing variants, latter on submitted to further variations, and genetic dilution after migration out of Africa as we see in present day Europeans and Asians [73]. Studying further such ancient populations from where the human genome was shaped by various environmental pressures over time including a variety of social and microbial pressures will be pivotal for the understanding of psychiatric disorders.

Hence, we are at the beginning of the of HLA and PSYCHIATRY history.

References

1. Amiel JL. Study of the leukocyte phenotypes in Hodgkin's disease. In: Curtoni ES, Mattiuz PL, Tosi MR, editors. Histocompatibility testing. Copenhagen: Munksgaard; 1967. p. 79.
2. Dendrou CA, Petersen J, Rossjohn J, Fugger L. HLA variation and disease. Nat Rev Immunol. 2018;18:325–39.
3. Schizophrenia Working Group of the Psychiatric Genomics Consortium. Biological insights from 108 schizophrenia-associated genetic loci. Nature. 2014;511:421–7.
4. Eberhard G, Franzén G, Löw B. Schizophrenia susceptibility and HL-A antigen. Neuropsychobiology. 1975;1:211–7.
5. Mokhtari R, Lachman HM. The major histocompatibility complex (MHC) in schizophrenia: a review. J Clin Cell Immunol. 2016;7:479.
6. Trowsdale J, Knight JC. Major histocompatibility complex genomics and human disease. Annu Rev Genomics Hum Genet. 2013;14:301–23.
7. IMGT/HLA Database. https://www.ebi.ac.uk/ipd/imgt/hla/
8. Khandaker GM, Dantzer R, Jones PB. Immunopsychiatry: important facts. Psychol Med. 2017;47:2229–37.
9. Boulanger LM. Immune proteins in brain development and synaptic plasticity. Neuron. 2009;64:93–109.
10. Sterner KN, Weckle A, Chugani HT, et al. Dynamic gene expression in the human cerebral cortex distinguishes children from adults. PLoS One. 2012;7:e37714.
11. Goddard CA, Butts DA, Shatz CJ. Regulation of CNS synapses by neuronal MHC class I. Proc Natl Acad Sci U S A. 2007;104(16):6828–33.
12. Huh GS, Boulanger LM, Du H, Riquelme PA, Brotz TM, Shatz CJ. Functional requirement for class I MHC in CNS development and plasticity. Science. 2000;290(5499):2155–9.
13. Dausset J, Brecy H. Identical nature of the leucocyte antigens detectable in monozygotic twins by means of immune iso-leuco-agglutinins. Nature. 1957;180:1430.
14. Ramsuran V, Naranbhai V, Horowitz A, et al. Elevated HLA-A expression impairs HIV control through inhibition of NKG2A-expressing cells. Science. 2018;358:86–90.
15. D'Antonio M, Reyna J, Jakubosky D, et al. Systematic genetic analysis of the MHC region reveals mechanistic underpinnings of HLA type associations with disease. Elife. 2019;8:e48476.
16. Aguiar VRC, César J, Delaneau O, Dermitzakis ET, Meyer D. Expression estimation and eQTL mapping for HLA genes with a personalized pipeline. PLoS Genet. 2019;15:e1008091.
17. Price P, Witt C, Allcock R, et al. The genetic basis for the association of the 8.1 ancestral haplotype (A1, B8, DR3) with multiple immunopathological diseases. Immunol Rev. 1999;167:257–74.
18. Dawkins R, Leelayuwat C, Gaudieri S, et al. Genomics of the major histocompatibility complex: haplotypes, duplication, retroviruses and disease. Immunol Rev. 1999;167:275–304.
19. Gambino CM, Aiello A, Accardi G, Caruso C, Candore G. Autoimmune diseases and 8.1 ancestral haplotype: an update. HLA. 2018;92:137–43.
20. Crespi BJ, Go MC. Diametrical diseases reflect evolutionary-genetic tradeoffs: evidence from psychiatry, neurology, rheumatology, oncology and immunology. Evol Med Public Health. 2015;1:216–53.
21. Petersdorf EW, Malkki M, O'hUigin C, et al. High HLA-DP expression and graft-versus-host disease. N Engl J Med. 2015;373:599–609.

22. Thomas R, Apps R, Qi Y, et al. HLA-C cell surface expression and control of HIV/AIDS correlate with a variant upstream of HLA-C. Nat Genet. 2009;41:1290–4.
23. Apps R, Qi Y, Carlson JM, Chen H, et al. Influence of HLA-C expression level on HIV control. Science. 2013;340:87–91.
24. Woodsworth DJ, Castellarin M, Holt RA. Sequence analysis of T-cell repertoires in health and disease. Genome Med. 2013;5(10):98.
25. Morris GP. Allen PM How the TCR balances sensitivity and specificity for the recognition of self and pathogens. Nat Immunol. 2012;13:121–8.
26. Creusot RJ, Mitchison NA, Terazzini NM. The immunological synapse. Mol Immunol. 2002;38:997–1002.
27. Yin Y, Li Y, Mariuzza RA. Structural basis for self-recognition by autoimmune T-cell receptors. Immunol Rev. 2012;250:32–48.
28. Debnath M, Berk M, Leboyer M, Tamouza R. The MHC/HLA gene complex in major psychiatric disorders: emerging roles and implications. Curr Behav Neurosci Rep. 2018;5:179–88. https://doi.org/10.1007/s40473-018-0155-8.
29. Cazzullo CL, Smeraldi E. HLA system, psychiatry and psychopharmacology. Prog Neuropsychopharmacol. 1979;3:137–46.
30. International Schizophrenia Consortium, Purcell SM, Wray NR, et al. Common polygenic variation contributes to risk of schizophrenia and bipolar disorder. Nature. 2009;460:748–52.
31. Shi J, Levinson DF, Duan J, et al. Common variants on chromosome 6p22.1 are associated with schizophrenia. Nature. 2009;460:753–7.
32. Stefansson H, Ophoff RA, Steinberg S, et al. Common variants conferring risk of schizophrenia. Nature. 2009;460:744–7.
33. Irish Schizophrenia Genomics Consortium and the Wellcome Trust Case Control Consortium 2. Genome-wide association study implicates HLA-C*01:02 as a risk factor at the major histocompatibility complex locus in schizophrenia. Biol Psychiatry. 2012;72(8):620–8.
34. Sekar A, Bialas AR, de Rivera H, et al. Schizophrenia risk from complex variation of complement component 4. Nature. 2016;530:177–83.
35. Druart M, Le Magueresse C. Emerging roles of complement in psychiatric disorders. Front Psych. 2019;10:573.
36. Tamouza R, Krishnamoorthy R, Giegling I, Leboyer M, Rujescu D. The HLA 8.1 ancestral haplotype in schizophrenia: dual implication in neuro-synaptic pruning and autoimmunity? Acta Psychiatr Scand. 2020;141(2):169–71.
37. Agartz I, Brown AA, Rimol LM, et al. Common sequence variants in the major histocompatibility complex region associate with cerebral ventricular size in schizophrenia. Biol Psychiatry. 2011;70:696–8.
38. Cross-Disorder Group of the Psychiatric Genomics Consortium. Identification of risk loci with shared effects on five major psychiatric disorders: a genome-wide analysis. Lancet. 2013;381(9875):1371–9.
39. Wang HZ, Qin HD, Guo W, Samuels J, Shugart YY. New insights into the genetic mechanism of IQ in autism spectrum disorders. Front Genet. 2013;4:195.
40. Bennabi M, Gaman A, Delorme R, et al. HLA-class II haplotypes and autism spectrum disorders. Sci Rep. 2018;8:7639.
41. Vuong HE, Hsiao EY. Emerging roles for the gut microbiome in autism spectrum disorder. Biol Psychiatry. 2017;81:411–23.
42. Hughes HK, Rose D, Ashwood P. The gut microbiota and dysbiosis in autism spectrum disorders. Curr Neurol Neurosci Rep. 2018;18:81.
43. Tamouza R, Fernell E, Eriksson MA, et al. HLA polymorphism in regressive and non-regressive autism: a preliminary study. Autism Res. 2020;13:182–6.
44. Amare AT, Schubert KO, Hou L, et al. Association of polygenic score for schizophrenia and HLA antigen and inflammation genes with response to Lithium in bipolar affective disorder: a genome-wide association study. JAMA Psychiat. 2018;75:65–74.
45. Tamouza R, Oliveira J, Etain B, et al. HLA genetics in bipolar disorder. Acta Psychiatr Scand. 2018;138:464–71.

46. Padmos RC, Bekris L, Knijff EM, et al. A high prevalence of organ-specific autoimmunity in patients with bipolar disorder. Biol Psychiatry. 2004;56:476–82.
47. Jeppesen R, Benros ME. Autoimmune diseases and psychotic disorders. Front Psych. 2019;10:131.
48. Andreassen OA, Harbo HF, Wang Y, et al. Genetic pleiotropy between multiple sclerosis and schizophrenia but not bipolar disorder: differential involvement of immune-related gene loci. Mol Psychiatry. 2015;20:207–14.
49. Bergen SE, O'Dushlaine CT, Ripke S, et al. Genome-wide association study in a Swedish population yields support for greater CNV and MHC involvement in schizophrenia compared with bipolar disorder. Mol Psychiatry. 2012;17:880–6.
50. Dalmau J, Gleichman AJ, Hughes EG, et al. Anti-NMDA-receptor encephalitis: case series and analysis of the effects of antibodies. Lancet Neurol. 2008;7:1091–8.
51. Pollak TA, Lennox BR, Müller S, et al. Autoimmune psychosis: an international consensus on an approach to the diagnosis and management of psychosis of suspected autoimmune origin. Lancet Psychiatry. 2020;7:93–108.
52. Jézéquel J, Johansson EM, Dupuis JP, et al. Dynamic disorganization of synaptic NMDA receptors triggered by autoantibodies from psychotic patients. Nat Commun. 2017;8:1791.
53. Mueller SH, Färber A, Prüss H, et al. Genetic predisposition in anti-LGI1 and anti-NMDA receptor encephalitis. Ann Neurol. 2018;83:863–9.
54. Shu Y, Qiu W, Zheng J, et al. HLA class II allele *DRB1*16:02* is associated with anti-NMDAR encephalitis. J Neurol Neurosurg Psychiatry. 2019;90:652–8.
55. Verhelst H, Verloo P, Dhondt K, et al. Anti-NMDA-receptor encephalitis in a 3 year old patient with chromosome 6p21.32 microdeletion including the HLA cluster. Eur J Paediatr Neurol. 2011;15:163–6.
56. Numata S, Umehara H, Ohmori T, Hashimoto R. Clozapine pharmacogenetic studies in schizophrenia: efficacy and agranulocytosis. Front Pharmacol. 2018;9:1049.
57. Le Clerc S, Taing L, Fond G, et al. A double amino-acid change in the HLA-A peptide-binding groove is associated with response to psychotropic treatment in patients with schizophrenia. Transl Psychiatry. 2015;5:e608.
58. Greenig M. HERVs, immunity, and autoimmunity: understanding the connection. PeerJ. 2019;7:e6711.
59. Perron H, Hamdani N, Faucard R, et al. Molecular characteristics of human endogenous retrovirus type-W in schizophrenia and bipolar disorder. Transl Psychiatry. 2012;2:e201.
60. Leboyer M, Tamouza R, Charron D, Faucard R, Perron H. Human endogenous retrovirus type W (HERV-W) in schizophrenia: a new avenue of research at the gene-environment interface. World J Biol Psychiatry. 2013;14:80–90.
61. Ferreira LMR, Meissner TB, Tilburgs T, Strominger JL. HLA-G: at the interface of maternal-fetal tolerance. Trends Immunol. 2017;38:272–86.
62. Guerini FR, Bolognesi E, Chiappedi M, et al. An HLA-G(∗)14bp insertion/deletion polymorphism associates with the development of autistic spectrum disorders. Brain Behav Immun. 2015;44:207–12.
63. Guerini FR, Bolognesi E, Chiappedi M, et al. HLA-G coding region polymorphism is skewed in autistic spectrum disorders. Brain Behav Immun. 2018;67:308–13.
64. Guerini FR, Bolognesi E, Chiappedi M, et al. HLA-G∗14bp insertion and the KIR2DS1-HLAC2 complex impact on behavioral impairment in children with Autism spectrum disorders. Neuroscience. 2018;370:163–9.
65. Guerini FR, Bolognesi E, Sotgiu S, et al. HLA-G allelic distribution in Sardinian children with Autism spectrum disorders: A replication study. Brain Behav Immun. 2019;79:314–8.
66. Rajasekaran A, Shivakumar V, Kalmady SV, et al. Soluble human leukocyte antigen (sHLA)-G levels may predict early onset of schizophrenia in male patients. Tissue Antigens. 2015;86:36–7.
67. Rajasekaran A, Shivakumar V, Kalmady SV, et al. The impact of IL10 polymorphisms and sHLA-G levels on the risk of schizophrenia. Asian J Psychiatr. 2016;23:39–43.

68. Rajasekaran A, Shivakumar V, Kalmady SV, et al. The impact of HLA-G 3' UTR variants and sHLA-G on risk and clinical correlates of schizophrenia. Hum Immunol. 2016;77:1166–71.
69. Shivakumar V, Debnath M, Venugopal D, et al. Influence of correlation between HLA-G polymorphism and Interleukin-6 (IL6) gene expression on the risk of schizophrenia. Cytokine. 2018;107:59–64.
70. Debnath M, Busson M, Jamain S, et al. The HLA-G low expressor genotype is associated with protection against bipolar disorder. Hum Immunol. 2013;74(5):593–7.
71. Sundaresh A, Wu CL, Chinnadurai RK, et al. The HLA-G genetic contribution to bipolar disorder: a trans-ethnic replication. Immunol Investig. 2018;47:593–604.
72. De Tomaso AW, Nyholm SV, Palmeri KJ, et al. Isolation and characterization of a protochordate histocompatibility locus. Nature. 2005;438(7067):454–9.
73. Gulsuner S, Stein DJ, Susser ES, et al. Genetics of schizophrenia in the South African Xhosa. Science. 2020;367:569–73.

Testable Hypotheses Relating Complement Pathways to Elevated Risk for Schizophrenia

11

Lora McClain, Matthew Demers, Wenxiao Zheng, Maribeth Wesesky, Joel Wood, Leonardo D'Aiuto, Konsale Prasad, and Vishwajit Nimgaonkar

11.1 Introduction

Schizophrenia (SZ) is a life-long, potentially severe disorder characterized by impairment in cognition. The etiology of SZ is uncertain, though an inherited predisposition is undisputed, and a multi-factorial polygenic threshold model was proposed, based on family studies [1]. Family and twin studies suggest a substantial heritability for SZ (~0.70) [2]. Gene mapping studies were difficult to replicate, possibly because they were under-powered, but the use of larger samples and accurate next-generation molecular techniques has paved the way to a better

L. McClain
Department of Psychiatry, University of Pittsburgh, Pittsburgh, PA, USA

Veterans Affairs, Pittsburgh Health System, Pittsburgh, PA, USA
e-mail: mcclainll2@upmc.edu

M. Demers · W. Zheng · M. Wesesky · J. Wood · L. D'Aiuto
Department of Psychiatry, University of Pittsburgh, Pittsburgh, PA, USA
e-mail: demersm@upmc.edu; zhengw3@upmc.edu; weseskyma@upmc.edu; woodja@upmc.edu; daiutol@upmc.edu

K. Prasad
Department of Psychiatry, University of Pittsburgh, Pittsburgh, PA, USA

Veterans Affairs, Pittsburgh Health System, Pittsburgh, PA, USA

Department of Bioengineering, University of Pittsburgh, Pittsburgh, PA, USA
e-mail: prasadkm@upmc.edu

V. Nimgaonkar (✉)
Department of Psychiatry, University of Pittsburgh, Pittsburgh, PA, USA

Veterans Affairs, Pittsburgh Health System, Pittsburgh, PA, USA

Department of Human Genetics, University of Pittsburgh, Pittsburgh, PA, USA

Department of Psychiatry, Western Psychiatric Hospital, Pittsburgh, PA, USA
e-mail: VishwajitNL@upmc.edu

M. Berk et al. (eds.), *Immuno-Psychiatry*, https://doi.org/10.1007/978-3-030-71229-7_11

understanding of the molecular risks involved [3]. To enable larger samples, researchers pooled their resources and formed the Psychiatric Genomics Consortium (PGC) [4]. The first genome-wide association studies (GWAS) performed by the PGC for SZ amassed 28,799 cases and 356,986 controls, revealing 108 associated loci [3]. However, odds ratios (OR) were modest (most not exceeding 1.2); thus, the considerable fraction of genetic risk could not be explained. To further increase power to detect more associated loci, a meta-analysis was performed that combined the PGC data with the 'CLOZUK' study that identified 179 SZ risk variants mapping to 145 loci; the most significant locus mapped to the major histocompatibility (MHC) region, centered on the complement *C4* locus (OR = 1.28; $p = 2.12 \times 10^{-44}$) [5]. Efforts to increase sample sizes of case and control cohort to conduct new, updated GWAS by the PGC are ongoing. These studies estimate the single nucleotide polymorphism (SNP)-based heritability for SZ is approximately 0.45 [6].

As more risk variants are identified, a parallel challenge is an understanding of the mechanism/s by which these variants confer risk. One of the most daunting challenges rests in the MHC region. Pre-GWAS studies have consistently identified variants in the MHC region as risk factors for SZ (see Review by Farrell and colleagues [7]), and this region has emerged consistently as the most significantly associated region in GWAS [3, 5]. Yet, it has proven difficult to localize the variants primarily contributing to the risk, due to extensive linkage disequilibrium (LD) and repeat variation in the MHC region [8]. Elegant analyses based on genetic association and post-mortem gene expression analyses recently identified a copy number variation (CNV) as a plausible and substantial contributor to the MHC-associated risk [9]. Further, it was suggested that the risk was conferred primarily by *C4A*, an isotype of the complement component *C4* gene. The authors also proposed that the risk manifests through abnormal patterns of synaptic pruning during early development. Synaptic pruning is a part of healthy central nervous system (CNS) development; however, recent studies show evidence that aberrations in this process may be a risk factor for SZ [10]. In the following sections, we review the complement system, followed by a description of C4 structure, function, and its evolutionary conservation. We also discuss the synaptic pruning hypothesis alongside other plausible hypotheses. We close by providing an overview and a critique.

11.2 The Complement System

The role of the complement system and its factors in the development of mental disorders, including SZ, has been explored since the mid-1980s, albeit with conflicting interpretation [11]. As a part of the innate immune system, the complement system consists of an array of soluble inactive precursor proteins, cell surface receptors, and regulatory proteins that act in a sequential cascade following activation [12, 13]. The activation of this evolutionarily ancient system is triggered by three major, inter-connected pathways: classical, lectin, and alternative [14].

The classical pathway is activated by antigen-antibody complexes and is mediated by C1 activation [15]. The lectin pathway is activated via exposure to carbohydrate moieties and mediated by mannose-binding lectin or ficolins [15]. The alternative pathway is generally non-specific and is activated by foreign surfaces or exposure to C3 hydrolysis. All pathways lead to the downstream formation of the membrane attack complex (MAC) or the terminal complement complex (TCC), which are transmembrane channels composed of multiple proteins and located on the pathogen cell membrane [16]. The resultant transmembrane channels lead to pathogen cell lysis, enhanced phagocytosis, clearance of foreign debris, or enhanced functionality of cytokines [16].

The human immune response depends on the action of the complement system. C4 is a critical component of a robust immune response, yet the function/s of complement is not well understood within the central nervous system (CNS). Complement proteins are synthesized locally in the CNS [17]. Synthesis of most complement proteins of both classic and alternative complement pathways have been confirmed in microglia and astrocytes and are considered CNS "immune effector" cells [17]. In addition, complement proteins could have other functions in the CNS, like synaptic pruning, differentiation, and migration of neural progenitor cells during early embryonic brain development [18].

11.3 *C4* Gene Structure and Genetic Studies

The *C4* locus exists as two functionally distinct genes in humans, dubbed *C4A* and *C4B* [19]. Both *C4A* and *C4B* are 14.2 kilobases (kb), each containing 41 exons and 1744 amino acid residues. There is a difference in four amino acids that differentiate *C4A* from *C4B* (amino acids 1101–1106 encode for **PCP**V**LD** and **LS**PV**IH**, respectively) [20]. Though *C4A* and *C4B* have seemingly minor differences, they differ substantially in their hemolytic activities and antigen affinities [21]. C4A and C4B exist as either a long or a short transcript. The long transcript contains an additional 6.36 kb due to the retention of the ninth intron that includes a HERV-K retroviral sequence. Approximately 76% of *C4* gene copies encode this sequence; however, this sequence is spliced out of the final mRNA molecule and it is absent in the C4 protein [21].

C4 is encoded as part of a four-gene module that can occur in varying copy numbers in different individuals [22]. The three other genes in this module are serine/threonine kinase 19 *(RP1)*, steroid 21-hydroxylase (*CYP21*), and tenascin-X (*TNXB*; Fig. 11.1). The module, called "RCCX," can be duplicated in tandem [23]. An individual can have zero to eight copies of RCCX [9]. In addition to nucleotide polymorphisms, each RCCX can contain one, two, or three *C4* genes, and each *C4* locus may or may not contain the retained retroviral HERV-K sequence (Fig. 11.1a) [21]. Among European, East-Asian, and American persons, the distribution of the total number of *C4* genes among individuals is similar: ~25% have three copies, ~60% have four copies, and ~10% have five copies; the distribution of the *C4A* isotype copy number is similar, while *C4B* is skewed toward low copy number copies [24–26]. Some combinations of *C4* copy number, the HERV element, and flanking loci are described in Fig. 11.1a; however, complex configurations of *C4* copy numbers

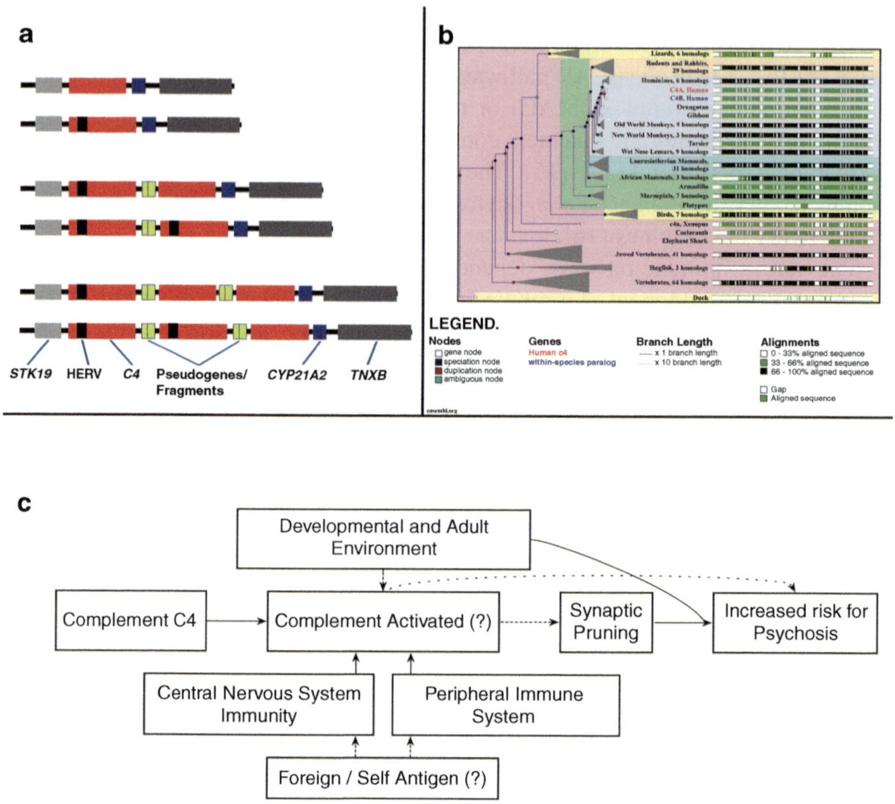

Fig. 11.1 Complement C4 variation and its putative role in schizophrenia pathogenesis. (**a**) Complement C4 Locus. Flanking C4 on chromosome 6 (shown with and without the retroviral element, "HERV") are the genes that produce the RCCX fragment. The RCCX fragment is composed of the following genes that lie sequentially along chromosome 6: *RP1(STK19)-C4-CYP21A2-TNXB*. Each individual has between 0–8 copies of RCCX. Pseudogenes and gene fragments composed of *CYP21A1P*, *RP1*, or *TNXB* may be present in some individuals. As an example, the configuration displayed at the top row in (**a**) show two chromosomes: one with the HERV sequence and the other without and two copies of *C4*; the middle configuration shows four copies of C4, where three contain HERV; the bottom configuration shows six copies of C4, where three contain HERV. (**b**) Gene Tree of complement *C4* across species. (**c**) Complement C4 genomic variation as a potential modulator in the multi-factorial polygenic threshold model of schizophrenia risk

arise when considering the absence or presence of the HERV sequence and the number of gene copies present on each chromosome.

The diversity in RCCX copy number could be an evolutionary advantage for an adaptive immune response. For example, the blood group antigens, Chido (Ch) and Rodgers (Rg), were identified on the C4 protein [27]. There are two Rg antigens, which are typically associated with C4A, and six Ch antigens associated with C4B, but in rare instances, Rg antigens may associate with C4B and vice versa [28].

Because of the highly variable nature of RCCX, Ch/Rg serotypes can be determined to be a complex mix of different C4A and C4B proteins with different antigenicities, which can be used to predict reactions to transfused blood or transplanted organs.

It is also of interest to study the evolution of the *C4* isotypes, in the context of the complement system as a highly conserved immune mechanism. The complement system is present in vertebrates and, given the absence of an antibody-based immune system, is an important defense mechanism for invertebrates, like insects or cnidaria. The complement system was likely present in a common ancestral species ~500 million years ago (mya) given its existence today in species like cnidaria [29]. At the protein level, the C4 protein structure is an α_2 macroglobulin molecule (α_2 macroglobulins are evolutionarily conserved to the worm) [30]. At the genetic level, *C4* is present in vertebrates (Fig. 11.1b), and *C4* duplication events likely occurred early in the evolutionary development of jawed vertebrates [31]. Jawed vertebrates, or gnathostomata, have been dated to 460 mya; other notable features of gnathostomata include an adaptive immune system and the presence of myelin on neurons [32, 33]. Other mammals do not encode both *C4A* and *C4B*: a single *C4* locus is present and highly conserved (Fig. 11.1b). This locus encodes proteins similar to *C4B*, suggesting that *C4A* evolved after a gene duplication event of *C4B* in a non-human primate ancestor [21, 34]. The HERV retroviral integration sequence is found in all Old World primates, before the hominoid-Old World monkey split [35]. Integration of the HERV sequence is estimated to have occurred 10–23 million years ago [36]. Figure 11.1b depicts a gene tree for *C4* across species. High homology is observed in many diverse organisms with the curious exception of the duck and platypus (Fig. 11.1b).

Given the recent developments linking *C4* with synaptic pruning and SZ in the CNS, the expression profile of C4 in the CNS was quantified by Sekar and colleagues using five post-mortem brain regions from 245 individual donors [9]. A proportional relationship in the expression of C4 mRNA and genomic copy number was observed in the CNS (similar to peripheral blood [37]), the expression of C4A was greater than C4B, and retroviral HERV element retention correlated with an increase of C4A:C4B ratio [9]. With regard to SZ, cases had increased expression of C4A than controls in five brain regions ($p < 0.0001$) [9], bolstering the evidence for *C4* variation in SZ etiology. These analyses indicate that increased transcription of *C4A* in the brain could be related to risk for SZ.

11.4 Hypothesis 1. C4, Synaptic Pruning and SZ Pathogenesis

Sekar et al. [9] first proposed that C4 mediates loss of synapses via increased synaptic pruning. Pruning of overproduced synapses during typical neurodevelopment is a physiological process that eventually leads to brain maturation. Pruning is particularly prominent during adolescence and young adulthood [38]. Overall, the number of synapses decreases in an age-related manner in humans [39] and these changes may underlie age-related gray matter reductions observed in neuroimaging studies of SZ [40]. Structural MRI studies that quantify gray matter alterations reported reductions in gray matter in children and adolescents [38], suggesting that synaptic pruning may be age-related.

Convergent animal [41], human developmental [42], neuroimaging [43], postmortem [44], and computational modeling [45] data suggest that increased neuropil loss predates [46] and continues after the onset of psychosis [47], and may also predict short-term outcome of SZ [48]. Such age-related abnormal pruning may occur before the onset of SZ clinical symptoms as shown in recent studies on clinical high-risk persons, who have up to 30 times higher risk for psychosis over 3 years, which consistently showed increased progressive reduction in gray matter as psychosis clinically manifested [49]. Similar longitudinal gray matter reduction was also observed among familial high-risk subjects [50] and during the early course of first-episode SZ [51] consistent with longitudinal gray matter loss reported by others [47]. However, it is unclear what proportion of variance of excessive synaptic pruning is associated with genetic variations, given that a significant portion of SZ risk is attributable to genetic factors [52].

Postmortem studies have consistently reported dendritic spine loss, one of the most consistently replicated findings in SZ research [44], as a proxy measure of synapse loss in SZ. Synaptic pruning has been demonstrated in the neuromuscular junction, prefrontal cortex, temporal cortex, visual cortex, dorsal lateral geniculate nuclei, cerebellum, and hippocampus; and the mechanisms likely differ by region [53]. Within the prefrontal and temporal cortex, lamina-specific dendritic spine loss has been observed rather than generalized spine loss in all layers [44]. Synaptic pruning is dependent on neural activity [54, 55]. Rodent models indicate that neural activity triggers the activation of complement protein C1q, leading to deposition of complement C3 on neural membranes, triggering microglial synaptophagy [56, 57], though the factors that spare neuronal process are still uncertain [58]. Others have also indicated a role for astrocytes [59], likely in conjunction with microglia [60]. From a neurodevelopmental perspective, the inappropriate activation of complement or the failure of complement to function correctly in the developing CNS could conceivably disrupt neuronal networks.

Based on functional links between C4 and C3 [57, 61], Sekar et al. [9] suggested that the *C4A*-SZ association is mediated through abnormal synapse elimination. This hypothesis is congruent with numerous neurodevelopmental abnormalities in SZ attributed to exaggerated synapse elimination [43]. The factors determining the type or timing of synaptic pruning are uncertain, though research suggests that immature synapses or those showing lower levels of activity are more likely to be eliminated [62].

11.5 Hypothesis 2. Signaling Cytokines and Complement in Schizophrenia Risk

Gestational viral infection could confer risk for SZ to offspring [63, 64]. The suspected viruses include herpes simplex, *T. gondii*, and rubella. Non-infectious environmental factors could also contribute to risk, including obstetric complications, perinatal hypoxia, environmental pollution, and even adverse childhood experiences [65, 66]. All these risk factors share a common thread, in that they are stressors that promote an inflammatory response. Inflammatory responses are accompanied by a release of signaling cytokines, and elevated levels of several cytokines, including IL-1B, IFN-g, TNF-a, and IL-6, have been consistently found in serum and cerebrospinal fluid of SZ patients [67].

Cytokines are important regulators of normal brain development, and disruption of cytokine-based signaling is believed to be detrimental [68]. Several cytokines are also known to regulate complement gene expression in a number of cell types [69, 70]. Most notably from the present perspective, C4 production and release is increased in cultured neurons in response to IFN-g and IL-6 [17, 71]. The complement system regulates CNS cell migration and differentiation [17], as well as synaptic pruning [9]. It is also possible that later in life, alterations in cytokine signaling activate complement pathways in the brain and lead to dysfunction in the central nervous system (CNS). Many complement proteins cannot cross the blood-brain barrier (BBB) [72], but inflammatory cytokines, which cross the BBB more readily, could still alter complement function in the CNS. Thus, we propose that gestational infections or other stressors in early life, and even stresses in adulthood, could initiate inflammatory responses that alter CNS function via the complement system.

11.6 Hypothesis 3. HERV Retroviral Sequence, C4 Expression, and SZ Risk

A third hypothesis of SZ pathogenesis states that increased *C4* expression, observed in persons with SZ, is mediated by the presence of the retroviral sequence HERV that exhibit enhancer-like activity. As noted above, HERV retroviral sequences can be present in the ninth intron of *C4A* and *C4B* sequences; if present, each allele is designated as "long" due to the increased number of nucleotides present. HERV likely originated from provirus HML-10, infecting a non-human primate 35 mya (see Review by Broecker and colleagues) [73]. HERV is likely integrated into the host genome by reverse transcription of an RNA intermediate [74] containing *gag*, *pol*, and *env* genes typically found in modern retroviruses [75].

Transcription of the *C4A*-containing HERV results in a mature RNA fragment that splices out HERV and is not contained in the resulting protein following translation [76]. However, there is evidence that the spliced retroviral fragments may function as an untranslated antisense RNA [73]. A different HTML10 retroviral element was found to regulate transcription for *DAP3* via antisense mechanisms [73]. This idea was explored for *C4*. The *C4A* locus was found to have increased enhancer activity at the HERV position; however, evidence supporting this claim for *C4B* was not supported [9]. Replication in relevant brain tissue would provide stronger support.

11.7 Critical Discussion and Conclusions

SZ is a complex disorder with an unknown etiology and only palliative treatment is available. Several clues to its etiology stem from genetics studies, particularly from recent GWAS. These population-based studies have consistently found association of the *C4* locus, in the MHC region of chromosome 6, with SZ. Further, the increased copy number of *C4A* is also a risk factor for SZ and also correlates with mRNA and protein level [9, 37]. Though the genetic associations have been related to SZ pathogenesis through altered synaptic pruning of neuronal cells within the CNS [57], we proposed that the genetic associations could also alter immune responses that could increase the risk for SZ pathogenesis through other routes.

Why do increased copies *of* C4 not elevate risk for SZ in all individuals bearing such alleles? The risk locus in *C4* only explains a small portion of the genetic risk but the risk allele is common in the population. Thus, it is conceivable that the mechanism/s underlying the onset of SZ involve a complex interaction between *C4*, other risk loci, and environmental factors. C4 may, in fact, operate as a modulator of other epigenetic processes, disrupting healthy brain development, including synaptic pruning. *C4* locus interactions, along with other critical factors, may occur only in a low proportion of the population, thus explaining the relatively low frequency of SZ prevalence (approximately 1%).

These complexities are evident when considering C4 copy number in relation to risk for autoimmunity and SZ. The prevalence of autoimmune diseases like systemic lupus erythematosus (SLE), Crohn's disease, and celiac disease can be elevated in not only patients with SZ but also their relatives; these data suggest a role for autoimmunity in SZ genesis [77–79]. Reduced C4 levels are observed in systemic lupus erythematosus (SLE) [80]. Homozygous genetic deficiency of C4 has also been associated with SLE [81]. The genetic association studies suggest that a deficit of serum C4 levels could be a *primary* event in the pathogenesis of these diseases, rather than an outcome of complement activation. The genetic studies have also been refined in relation to *C4A* and *C4B*. A recent carefully conducted case-control analysis of hospitalized Finnish patients indicated a significant genetic association with SLE (and celiac disease) was present among individuals with homozygous deficiency of *C4A*, but not in individuals with homozygous *C4B* deficiency (SLE: OR, 3.75, celiac disease: frequency 12.5% in *C4A* deficiency vs 0% in controls) [82]. These results are difficult to reconcile with the genetic association studies of SZ, in which *increased* C4 copy number and increased prevalence of autoimmune diseases are observed among patients with SZ.

We propose several hypotheses linking C4 with altered immune responses that could explain the pathogenesis of SZ. The biggest challenge in the generation of a unifying hypothesis of SZ would be to define the nature of the initial insult underlying its onset (see Fig. 11.1c).

References

1. Gottesman II, Shields J. A polygenic theory of schizophrenia. Proc Natl Acad Sci U S A. 1967;58(1):199–205.
2. Gottesman I. Schizophrenia genesis: the origins of madness. New York: WH Freeman; 1991.
3. Schizophrenia Working Group of the Psychiatric Genomics C. Biological insights from 108 schizophrenia-associated genetic loci. Nature. 2014;511(7510):421–7.
4. Sullivan PF. The psychiatric GWAS consortium: big science comes to psychiatry. Neuron. 2010;68(2):182–6.
5. Pardinas AF, Holmans P, Pocklington AJ, et al. Common schizophrenia alleles are enriched in mutation-intolerant genes and in regions under strong background selection. Nat Genet. 2018;50(3):381–9.
6. Zheng J, Erzurumluoglu AM, Elsworth BL, et al. LD Hub: a centralized database and web interface to perform LD score regression that maximizes the potential of summary level GWAS data for SNP heritability and genetic correlation analysis. Bioinformatics. 2017;33(2):272–9.
7. Farrell MS, Werge T, Sklar P, et al. Evaluating historical candidate genes for schizophrenia. Mol Psychiatry. 2015;20(5):555–62.
8. Miretti MM, Walsh EC, Ke X, et al. A high-resolution linkage-disequilibrium map of the human major histocompatibility complex and first generation of tag single-nucleotide polymorphisms. Am J Hum Genet. 2005;76(4):634–46.
9. Sekar A, Bialas AR, de Rivera H, et al. Schizophrenia risk from complex variation of complement component 4. Nature. 2016;530(7589):177–83.
10. Bearden CE, Forsyth JK. The many roads to psychosis: recent advances in understanding risk and mechanisms. F1000Res. 2018;7:1883.
11. Rudduck C, Beckman L, Franzén G, Jacobsson L, Lindström L. Complement factor C4 in schizophrenia. Hum Hered. 1985;35(4):223–6.
12. Walport MJ. Complement. First of two parts. N Engl J Med. 2001;344(14):1058–66.
13. Walport MJ. Complement. Second of two parts. N Engl J Med. 2001;344(15):1140–4.
14. Greco E, Domenica Guarino M, Ballanti E, Perricone R. The complement system. The novel factors of autoimmune diseases. London: Academic Press; 2019.
15. Gal P, Dobo J, Zavodszky P, Sim RB. Early complement proteases: C1r, C1s and MASPs. A structural insight into activation and functions. Mol Immunol. 2009;46(14):2745–52.
16. Hawlisch H, Kohl J. Complement and Toll-like receptors: key regulators of adaptive immune responses. Mol Immunol. 2006;43(1-2):13–21.
17. Veerhuis R, Nielsen HM, Tenner AJ. Complement in the brain. Mol Immunol. 2011;48(14):1592–603.
18. Tenner AJ, Stevens B, Woodruff TM. New tricks for an ancient system: physiological and pathological roles of complement in the CNS. Mol Immunol. 2018;102:3–13.
19. Carroll MC, Belt T, Palsdottir A, Porter RR. Structure and organization of the C4 genes. Philos Trans R Soc Lond Ser B Biol Sci. 1984;306(1129):379–88.
20. Kidmose RT, Laursen NS, Dobo J, et al. Structural basis for activation of the complement system by component C4 cleavage. Proc Natl Acad Sci U S A. 2012;109(38):15425–30.
21. Blanchong CA, Chung EK, Rupert KL, et al. Genetic, structural and functional diversities of human complement components C4A and C4B and their mouse homologues, Slp and C4. Int Immunopharmacol. 2001;1(3):365–92.
22. Wu YL, Savelli SL, Yang Y, et al. Sensitive and specific real-time polymerase chain reaction assays to accurately determine copy number variations (CNVs) of human complement C4A, C4B, C4-long, C4-short, and RCCX modules: elucidation of C4 CNVs in 50 consanguineous subjects with defined HLA genotypes. J Immunol. 2007;179(5):3012–25.
23. Yang Z, Mendoza AR, Welch TR, Zipf WB, Yu CY. Modular variations of the human major histocompatibility complex class III genes for serine/threonine kinase RP, complement component C4, steroid 21-hydroxylase CYP21, and tenascin TNX (the RCCX module). A mechanism for gene deletions and disease associations. J Biol Chem. 1999;274(17):12147–56.

24. Wu YL, Yang Y, Chung EK, et al. Phenotypes, genotypes and disease susceptibility associated with gene copy number variations: complement C4 CNVs in European American healthy subjects and those with systemic lupus erythematosus. Cytogenet Genome Res. 2008;123(1-4):131–41.
25. Yih Chen J, Ling Wu Y, Yin Mok M, et al. Effects of complement C4 gene copy number variations, size dichotomy, and C4A deficiency on genetic risk and clinical presentation of systemic lupus erythematosus in east Asian populations. Arthritis Rheumatol. 2016;68(6):1442–53.
26. Saxena K, Kitzmiller KJ, Wu YL, et al. Great genotypic and phenotypic diversities associated with copy-number variations of complement C4 and RP-C4-CYP21-TNX (RCCX) modules: a comparison of Asian-Indian and European American populations. Mol Immunol. 2009;46(7):1289–303.
27. Mougey R. A review of the Chido/Rodgers blood group. Immunohematology. 2010;26(1):30–8.
28. Giles CM. Antigenic determinants of human C4, Rodgers and Chido. Exp Clin Immunogenet. 1988;5(2–3):99–114.
29. Nonaka M. Evolution of the complement system. Subcell Biochem. 2014;80:31–43.
30. Sottrup-Jensen L, Stepanik TM, Kristensen T, et al. Common evolutionary origin of alpha 2-macroglobulin and complement components C3 and C4. Proc Natl Acad Sci U S A. 1985;82(1):9–13.
31. Nonaka MI, Terado T, Kimura H, Nonaka M. Evolutionary analysis of two complement C4 genes: ancient duplication and conservation during jawed vertebrate evolution. Dev Comp Immunol. 2017;68:1–11.
32. Cooper MD, Alder MN. The evolution of adaptive immune systems. Cell. 2006;124(4):815–22.
33. Nawaz S, Schweitzer J, Jahn O, Werner HB. Molecular evolution of myelin basic protein, an abundant structural myelin component. Glia. 2013;61(8):1364–77.
34. Dodds AW, Law SK. The phylogeny and evolution of the thioester bond-containing proteins C3, C4 and alpha 2-macroglobulin. Immunol Rev. 1998;166:15–26.
35. Reus K, Mayer J, Sauter M, Zischler H, Muller-Lantzsch N, Meese E. HERV-K(OLD): ancestor sequences of the human endogenous retrovirus family HERV-K(HML-2). J Virol. 2001;75(19):8917–26.
36. Dangel AW, Baker BJ, Mendoza AR, Yu CY. Complement component C4 gene intron 9 as a phylogenetic marker for primates: long terminal repeats of the endogenous retrovirus ERV-K(C4) are a molecular clock of evolution. Immunogenetics. 1995;42(1):41–52.
37. Yang Y, Chung EK, Zhou B, et al. Diversity in intrinsic strengths of the human complement system: serum C4 protein concentrations correlate with C4 gene size and polygenic variations, hemolytic activities, and body mass index. J Immunol. 2003;171(5):2734–45.
38. Gogtay N, Giedd JN, Lusk L, et al. Dynamic mapping of human cortical development during childhood through early adulthood. Proc Natl Acad Sci U S A. 2004;101(21):8174–9.
39. Huttenlocher PR, Dabholkar AS. Regional differences in synaptogenesis in human cerebral cortex. J Comp Neurol. 1997;387(2):167–78.
40. Giedd JN, Jeffries NO, Blumenthal J, et al. Childhood-onset schizophrenia: progressive brain changes during adolescence. Biol Psychiatry. 1999;46(7):892–8.
41. Mayilyan KR, Weinberger DR, Sim RB. The complement system in schizophrenia. Drug News Perspect. 2008;21(4):200–10.
42. Stanley JA, Kipp H, Greisenegger E, et al. Evidence of developmental alterations in cortical and subcortical regions of children with attention-deficit/hyperactivity disorder: a multivoxel in vivo phosphorus 31 spectroscopy study. Arch Gen Psychiatry. 2008;65(12):1419–28.
43. Prasad KM, Burgess AM, Keshavan MS, Nimgaonkar VL, Stanley JA. Neuropil pruning in early-course schizophrenia: immunological, clinical, and neurocognitive correlates. Biol Psychiatry Cogn Neurosci Neuroimaging. 2016;1(6):528–38.
44. Glausier JR, Lewis DA. Dendritic spine pathology in schizophrenia. Neuroscience. 2013;251:90–107.
45. Hoffman RE, McGlashan TH. Neural network models of schizophrenia. Neuroscientist. 2001;7(5):441–54.

46. Pantelis C, Velakoulis D, McGorry PD, et al. Neuroanatomical abnormalities before and after onset of psychosis: a cross-sectional and longitudinal MRI comparison. Lancet. 2003;361(9354):281–8.
47. Lieberman J, Chakos M, Wu H, et al. Longitudinal study of brain morphology in first episode schizophrenia. Biol Psychiatry. 2001;49(6):487–99.
48. Prasad K, Sahni SD, Rohm BR, Keshavan MS. Dorsolateral prefrontal cortex morphology and short-term outcome in first-episode schizophrenia. Psychiatr Res Neuroimaging. 2005;140(2):147–55.
49. Cannon TD, Chung Y, He G, et al. Progressive reduction in cortical thickness as psychosis develops: a multisite longitudinal neuroimaging study of youth at elevated clinical risk. Biol Psychiatry. 2015;77(2):147–57.
50. Bhojraj TS, Prasad KM, Eack SM, Francis AN, Montrose DM, Keshavan MS. Do inter-regional gray-matter volumetric correlations reflect altered functional connectivity in high-risk offspring of schizophrenia patients? Schizophr Res. 2010;118(1-3):62–68.
51. Bangalore SS, Goradia DD, Nutche J, Diwadkar VA, Prasad KM, Keshavan MS. Untreated illness duration correlates with gray matter loss in first-episode psychoses. Neuroreport. 2009;20(7):729–34.
52. Sullivan PF, Kendler KS, Neale MC. Schizophrenia as a complex trait: evidence from a meta-analysis of twin studies. Arch Gen Psychiatry. 2003;60(12):1187–92.
53. Riccomagno MM, Kolodkin AL. Sculpting neural circuits by axon and dendrite pruning. Annu Rev Cell Dev Biol. 2015;31:779–805.
54. Andjus PR, Zhu L, Cesa R, Carulli D, Strata P. A change in the pattern of activity affects the developmental regression of the Purkinje cell polyinnervation by climbing fibers in the rat cerebellum. Neuroscience. 2003;121(3):563–72.
55. Schafer DP, Lehrman EK, Kautzman AG, et al. Microglia sculpt postnatal neural circuits in an activity and complement-dependent manner. Neuron. 2012;74(4):691–705.
56. Paolicelli RC, Bolasco G, Pagani F, et al. Synaptic pruning by microglia is necessary for normal brain development. Science. 2011;333(6048):1456–8.
57. Stevens B, Allen NJ, Vazquez LE, et al. The classical complement cascade mediates CNS synapse elimination. Cell. 2007;131(6):1164–78.
58. Neniskyte U, Gross CT. Errant gardeners: glial-cell-dependent synaptic pruning and neurodevelopmental disorders. Nat Rev Neurosci. 2017;18(11):658–70.
59. Chung WS, Clarke LE, Wang GX, et al. Astrocytes mediate synapse elimination through MEGF10 and MERTK pathways. Nature. 2013;504(7480):394–400.
60. Bialas AR, Stevens B. TGF-beta signaling regulates neuronal C1q expression and developmental synaptic refinement. Nat Neurosci. 2013;16(12):1773–82.
61. Vasek MJ, Garber C, Dorsey D, et al. A complement-microglial axis drives synapse loss during virus-induced memory impairment. Nature. 2016;534(7608):538–43.
62. Jennings C. Developmental neurobiology. Death of a synapse. Nature. 1994;372(6506):498–9.
63. Manjunatha N, Math SB, Kulkarni GB, Chaturvedi SK. The neuropsychiatric aspects of influenza/swine flu: a selective review. Ind Psychiatry J. 2011;20(2):83–90.
64. Meyer U. Developmental neuroinflammation and schizophrenia. Prog Neuro-Psychopharmacol Biol Psychiatry. 2013;42:20–34.
65. Meyer U, Feldon J, Yee BK. A review of the fetal brain cytokine imbalance hypothesis of schizophrenia. Schizophr Bull. 2009;35(5):959–72.
66. Watanabe Y, Someya T, Nawa H. Cytokine hypothesis of schizophrenia pathogenesis: evidence from human studies and animal models. Psychiatry Clin Neurosci. 2010;64(3):217–30.
67. Miller BJ, Buckley P, Seabolt W, Mellor A, Kirkpatrick B. Meta-analysis of cytokine alterations in schizophrenia: clinical status and antipsychotic effects. Biol Psychiatry. 2011;70(7):663–71.
68. Stolp HB. Neuropoietic cytokines in normal brain development and neurodevelopmental disorders. Mol Cell Neurosci. 2013;53:63–8.
69. Volanakis JE. Transcriptional regulation of complement genes. Annu Rev Immunol. 1995;13:277–305.

70. Colten HR, Dowton SB. Regulation of complement gene expression. Biochem Soc Symp. 1986;51:37–46.
71. Veerhuis R, Janssen I, De Groot CJ, Van Muiswinkel FL, Hack CE, Eikelenboom P. Cytokines associated with amyloid plaques in Alzheimer's disease brain stimulate human glial and neuronal cell cultures to secrete early complement proteins, but not C1-inhibitor. Exp Neurol. 1999;160(1):289–99.
72. Yasojima K, Schwab C, McGeer EG, McGeer PL. Up-regulated production and activation of the complement system in Alzheimer's disease brain. Am J Pathol. 1999;154(3):927–36.
73. Broecker F, Horton R, Heinrich J, et al. The intron-enriched HERV-K(HML-10) family suppresses apoptosis, an indicator of malignant transformation. Mob DNA. 2016;7:25.
74. Gogvadze E, Buzdin A. Retroelements and their impact on genome evolution and functioning. Cell Mol Life Sci. 2009;66(23):3727–42.
75. Bannert N, Kurth R. The evolutionary dynamics of human endogenous retroviral families. Annu Rev Genomics Hum Genet. 2006;7:149–73.
76. Mack M, Bender K, Schneider PM. Detection of retroviral antisense transcripts and promoter activity of the HERV-K(C4) insertion in the MHC class III region. Immunogenetics. 2004;56(5):321–32. https://doi.org/10.1007/s00251-004-0705-y. Epub 2004 Aug 12.
77. Benros ME, Pedersen MG, Rasmussen H, Eaton WW, Nordentoft M, Mortensen PB. A nationwide study on the risk of autoimmune diseases in individuals with a personal or a family history of schizophrenia and related psychosis. Am J Psychiatry. 2014;171(2):218–26.
78. Benros ME, Eaton WW, Mortensen PB. The epidemiologic evidence linking autoimmune diseases and psychosis. Biol Psychiatry. 2014;75(4):300–6.
79. Kohler-Forsberg O, Petersen L, Gasse C, et al. A nationwide study in Denmark of the association between treated infections and the subsequent risk of treated mental disorders in children and adolescents. JAMA Psychiatry. 2019;76:271–9.
80. Yang Y, Chung EK, Zhou B, et al. The intricate role of complement component C4 in human systemic lupus erythematosus. Curr Dir Autoimmun. 2004;7:98–132.
81. Blanchong CA, Zhou B, Rupert KL, et al. Deficiencies of human complement component C4A and C4B and heterozygosity in length variants of RP-C4-CYP21-TNX (RCCX) modules in Caucasians. The load of RCCX genetic diversity on major histocompatibility complex-associated disease. J Exp Med. 2000;191(12):2183–96.
82. Liesmaa I, Paakkanen R, Järvinen A, Valtonen V, Lokki ML. Clinical features of patients with homozygous complement C4A or C4B deficiency. PLoS One. 2018;13(6):e0199305.

Gut Microbiome in Patients with Schizophrenia and Bipolar Disorder

12

Mohamed Genedi, Jenny Borkent, Magda Iouannou, Isabelle Janmaat, Benno Haarman, and Iris E. Sommer

12.1 Introduction

Approximately 23 million people worldwide suffer from schizophrenia-spectrum disorder (SSD), while for bipolar disorder, the estimated number of global patients is 60 million [1]. Although the introduction of antipsychotics in the 1950s has substantially improved clinical symptoms of SSD [2], patients still have considerable degrees of symptoms and increased mortality, with a mean life expectancy being 25–20 years shorter than that of healthy people [3]. In bipolar disorder, lithium is, for many years, the first-choice maintenance-treatment with anticonvulsants and antipsychotics as major alternatives. Yet, some 50% of bipolar disorder patients do not respond adequately and still suffer from affective episodes, often severely affecting daily functioning [4].

Patients with both disorders commonly report constipation/diarrhea and belly discomfort. Such complaints may be related to imbalances in the gut microbiome, which comprises the resident bacteria in the human intestine [5–7]. Dysbiosis (imbalance of the gut bacteria) can impair the tight junction of the gut, permitting bacterial fragments to reach the blood, causing an increased peripheral inflammatory status [8], and consequently alterations in the systemic immune system [9–11]. Increased intestinal permeability has been reported both for SSD and bipolar disorder, leading to translocation of bacterial and food-derived antigens from the intestinal lumen into the systemic circulation. Leaking bacteria trigger a strong immune

M. Genedi · J. Borkent · I. Janmaat · I. E. Sommer (✉)
Department of Biomedical Sciences, Cells & Systems, University Medical Centre Groningen, Groningen, The Netherlands
e-mail: Genedi@stud.uni-heidelberg.de; j.borkent@umcg.nl; i.e.janmaat@umcg.nl; i.e.c.sommer@umcg.nl

M. Iouannou · B. Haarman
Department of Psychiatry, University of Groningen, Groningen, The Netherlands
e-mail: m.ioannou@umcg.nl; b.c.m.haarman@umcg.nl

M. Berk et al. (eds.), *Immuno-Psychiatry*, https://doi.org/10.1007/978-3-030-71229-7_12

response, which can be measured as an increase in proinflammatory cytokines, such as IL-6 and IL-1b, through binding of the lipopolysaccharide (LPS) component of the bacterial cell walls to Toll-like receptors (TLRs; i.e. TLR-4), expressed at monocytes, macrophages, and in the brain at microglia. The increase in proinflammatory cytokines also affects the brain via the vagus nerve and more directly via the circumventricular organs (regions of the blood–brain barrier with relative permeability) [12, 13]. In addition to their role as macrophage-like cells, microglia are a main organizer in developing and shaping the central nervous system (CNS) neural circuitry [14]. Therefore, stimulation with proinflammatory cytokines, which triggers the immune response of microglia, can also affect patterning and wiring of the CNS [15–17].

Probiotics are living microorganisms that can have health benefits to the host when provided in adequate amounts [18]. The composition of probiotic formulae is variable. Bacterial species that are commonly used as a component in such formulae are the Lactobacillus and Bifidobacterium genera [18–21]. Probiotics are now available at drugstores, health food stores, webshops, and supermarkets in different forms such as tablets, capsules, sachets, wafers, but also as complete products such as fermented milks or drinks, yogurts, butter, cheese, and even in chocolates [22]. Not all forms are proven to be effective. Recent years have seen an interest in using probiotic products to improve symptoms and wellbeing in patients with mental disorders. Dinan et al. [23] even proposed the concept of "psychobiotics" to emphasize the potential of probiotics to improve brain status in psychiatric disorders. Hence, a better understanding of gut microbiome status and potential dysbalance in these disorders is needed. In this chapter, we summarize findings on dysbiosis and its involvement in the development of SSD and bipolar disorder. We will also summarize current clinical research using probiotic supplementation which has been performed to improve symptoms and/or cognition in patients with SSD and bipolar disorder.

12.2 The Gastro-Intestinal Tract

Data from both the MetaHit and the Human Microbiome Project isolated 2172 unique species from the human gastro-intestinal tract, classified into 12 different phyla, of which 93.5% belonged to the four large families (phyla): Proteobacteria, Firmicutes, Actinobacteria, and Bacteroidetes [24]. The Bacteroidetes and Firmicutes are conserved microbiotic species commonly present in almost all individuals, although the relative proportions of these phyla can vary [25]. When we look at the level of bacterial species within these families, variation in the composition of individual microbial communities is considerably greater than that observed at the phylum level [26].

So far, seven studies have assessed the gut microbiome composition in SSD and bipolar disorder, all published within the past 3 years. From these studies, 2 focused on SSD and 5 on bipolar disorder (Table 12.1).

Table 12.1 Clinical trials on gut microbiome dysbiosis in patients with schizophrenia and bipolar disorder

Publication	Sample size	Mean age (SD)	Gender (M/F)	Changes in taxonomic composition(in PT compared to NC)	Association with clinical features	Limitations
Nguyen et al. [18]	SCZ: 25NC: 25	SCZ: 52.9 (11.2)NC: 54.7 (10.7)	SCZ: 11/24NC: 10/15	Phylum level: ↓*Proteobacteria*Genus level: ↑*Anaerococcus* ↓ *Haemophilus*, *Sutterella*, and *Clostridium*	Greater severity of depressive symptoms was correlated with greater abundance of genus *Bacteroides* ($r = 0.70$; $p = 0.0002$) Increased negative symptoms were associated with decreased abundance of family *Ruminococcaceae* ($r = 0.74$; $p = 0.0002$). Overall self-reported mental well-being was positively correlated with phylum *Verrucomicrobia* ($r = 0.63$; $p = 0.002$).	– Cross-sectional – Small sample size – Co-morbid medical illnesses (e.g., diabetes, hypertension), which can cause microbial differences, were not taken into consideration
Shen et al. [19]	SCZ: 64NC: 53	SCZ: 42 ± 11NC: 39 ± 14	SCZ: 36/28NC: 35/18	Phylum level: ↑ *Proteobacteria, Fusobacteria* Genus level: ↑ *Succinivibrio, Megasphaera, Collinsella, Clostridium, Klebsiella*, and *Methanobrevibacter*↓ *Blautia, Coprococcus and Roseburia*	Several metabolic pathways differed significantly between NC and SCZ cohorts: Vitamin B6, fatty acid, starch and sucrose, tryptophan, cysteine, methionine, and linoleic acid metabolism, as well as the degradation of some xenobiotics	– Cross-sectional – Small sample size – Limited population (only Chinese Han nationality) – They did not, completely, eliminate the effect of antipsychotics on the gut microbiome

(continued)

Table 12.1 (continued)

Publication	Sample size	Mean age (SD)	Gender (M/F)	Changes in taxonomic composition(in PT compared to NC)	Association with clinical features	Limitations
Coello et al. [24]	BD: 113 UR: 39 NC: 77	BD: 31(26–39) UR: 28(22–34) NC: 29(24.5–40.5)	BD: 43/70 UR: 18/21 NC: 30/47	Phylum level: N/A Genus level: *Flavonifractor* was present in 61% of patients with BD, 42% of their unaffected relatives and 39% of healthy individuals. In BD PTs, which was associated with smoking and female sex	N/A	– Cross-sectional – Small UR sample size – Self-reported physical activity – No dietary information – No information on bowel movements or stool consistency
Painold et al. [26]	BD: 32 NC: 10	BD: 41.3 (14.7) NC: 31.4 (7.6)	BD: 18/14 NC: 4/6	Phylum level: ↑ *Actinobacteria* and *Coriobacteria* (class) Genus level: ↓*Ruminococcaceae* and *Faecalibacterium*	Negative correlation between microbial alpha-diversity and illness duration in BD ($R = -0.408$, $P = 0.021$). Identified bacterial clades associated with inflammatory status, serum lipids, TRP, depressive symptoms, oxidative stress, anthropometrics, and metabolic syndrome in individuals with BD. The phylum *Actinobacteria* (LDA = 4.82, $P = 0.007$) and the class *Coriobacteria* (LDA = 4.75, $P = 0.010$) significantly more abundant in BD PTs compared to NC. *Ruminococcaceae* (LDA = 4.59, $P = 0.018$) and *Faecalibacterium* (LDA = 4.09, $P = 0.039$) more abundant in NC compared with BD	– Cross-sectional – Small sample size – All BD in-patients in an acute episode of bipolar depression which may influence microbial diversity (stress associated by relapse, need of higher doses of medication and polypharmacy, lifestyle changes due to hospital admission; diet, physical activity, smoking habits, sleep quality) – No explicit assessment/ standardization of diet/ lifestyle parameters

Schwarz et al. [27]	FEP: 28 NC: 16	FEP: 25.9 (SD = 5.5) NC: 27.1 (SD = 6.0)	FEP: 16/12 NC: 8/8	Families: FEP ↑ *Lactobacillaceae, Halothiobacillaceae, Brucellaceae*, and *Micrococcineae*, ↓ *Veillonellaceae* Genera: FEP ↑ *Lactobacillus, Tropheryma, Halothiobacillus , Saccharophagus, Ochrobactrum, Deferribacter, and Halorubrum*↓ *Anabaena, Nitrosospira, and Gallionella*	*Lachnospiraceae, Bacteroides* spp., *Lactobacillus* correlated with increased psychotic symptoms. *Lachnospiraceae, Bacteroides* spp., and predominant bacteria [identified by the authors *Lachnospiraceae* (*Eubacterium rectale* group), *Ruminococcaceae* (*Clostridium leptum* group), *Bacteroides* spp., *Atopobium* group, *bifidobacteria, Lactobacillus*-group (genera *Lactobacillus, Leuconostoc, Pediococcus,* and *Weissella*)	– Small sample size – No community-level characteristics reported (alpha and beta-diversity) – A model predicting remission only used top five families rather than the entire population – More specific information about the/examination of the impact of AP medication use
Evans et al. [28]	BD: 115 NC: 64	BD: 50.2 (12.8) NC: 48.6 (16.6)	BD: 32/83 NC: 24/40	Phylum level: N/A Genus level: ↓*Faecalibacterium* ↓unclassified (Family level: *Ruminococcaceae*)	OTU00003 (*Faecalibacterium*) associated with improved physical health, depression, and sleep quality scores; OTU00024 (*Anaerostipes*) and OTU00025 (*Ruminococcaceae* family, unresolved at genus level) associated with improved physical health, while an unclassified genus from the family OTU00022 (*Enterobacteriaceae* family, unresolved at the genus level) associated with worse physical health scores	– Cross-sectional – Inability to control for medication use and compliance

(continued)

Table 12.1 (continued)

Publication	Sample size	Mean age (SD)	Gender (M/F)	Changes in taxonomic composition(in PT compared to NC)	Association with clinical features	Limitations
Flowers et al. [30]	BD on AP: 46 BD off AP: 69	BD on AP: 46.0 (12.0) BD off AP: 51.7 (13.5)	BD on AP: 12/34 BD off AP: 21/48	AP-treated PTs ↑ *Lachnospiraceae* Non-AP-treated PTs ↑ *Akkermansia and Sutterella*	*Akkermansia* ↓ in non-obese AP-treated PTs	– Illness' duration, disease's indicators, and symptom severity were not taken into consideration – Comorbid medical conditions/other metabolic biomarkers effect on microbiome needed further investigation – No dietary information

SCZ schizophrenia, *BD* bipolar disorder, *PT* patient, *NC* non-psychiatric comparison subject, *UR* unaffected first degree relative, *AP* antipsychotics, *FEP* first episode patients, *N/A* not available. ↑↓ arrows indicate an increase or decrease in relative abundance when referring to taxonomic differences
NB: All studies are arranged in a reversed chronological order (from the newest to oldest)

12.3 Schizophrenia-Spectrum Disorder

Regarding SSD, Nguyen et al. [27] was the first to provide evidence for an altered intestinal microbiome in 25 chronic patients in the United States in comparison to 25 nonpsychiatric controls. After controlling for demographic and clinical factors that may influence microbial composition, significant differences in the composition and levels of specific bacterial taxa in the intestinal microbiome emerged. These differences included decreased relative abundance of phylum Proteobacteria and genera Haemophilus, Sutterella, and Clostridium and increased abundance of genus Anaerococcus in SSD patients compared to controls. Importantly, they showed that the composition of the intestinal microbiome was associated with psychopathology; increased Ruminococcaceae was correlated with decreased negative symptoms while increased Bacteroides correlated with more severe depressive symptoms. These are interesting findings, even if causality cannot be assumed. Yet the study had a relatively small sample size. Another problem is that patients were using antipsychotic medication, while controls were not. Different types of medication can alter the intestinal flora and may have influenced results. Another important difference between the groups is that patients generally have less healthy lifestyles, including a high inflammatory diet, which will all be reflected in their intestinal microbiome.

A larger study, accessing 64 SSD patients and 53 controls [28] also observed significant differences in both phylum and genus levels, in intestinal microbiome. In this study, several metabolic pathways that are related to the intestinal flora (vitamin B6, fatty acid, starch and sucrose, tryptophan, cysteine, methionine, linoleic acid and the degradation of some xenobiotics) also differed significantly between the SSD patients and controls. This shows that dysbiosis also impacts nutrient and vitamin uptake. This study also introduced the idea of microbiome-based diagnosis for SSD; they could distinguish patients from controls, on the basis of 12 characteristic quantities of bacteria. A limitation of this study, similar to the study mentioned above, is that all patients were medicated, while controls were not.

Regarding the effect of antipsychotics on the gut microbiome, a large-scale in-vitro study investigated the effect of more than 1000 drugs on gut microbiome and found that nearly all antipsychotics exhibited anti-commensal activity. Moreover, similarity analysis indicated that all antipsychotics targeted a more similar pattern of species than would be expected from their chemical similarity. This means that direct bacterial inhibition may be relevant to the mechanism of action and/or side effects of antipsychotics [29]. The impact of atypical antipsychotics on the gut microbiota has been relatively well investigated. Olanzapine-induced weight gain was observed in both male and female rats, producing an altered microbiota profile with an increase in Firmicutes and a decrease in Bacteroidetes. This impact of olanzapine in rodents is not seen in germ-free animals, supporting the idea that antipsychotic-induced weight gain is mediated by the effect these drugs have on the gut microbiota. Other rodent studies showed that antipsychotic-induced weight gain is also attenuated when olanzapine is provided together with antibiotics or prebiotics [30, 31]. This is an intriguing finding, as it offers new leads to improve acceptability and tolerability of second-generation antipsychotics. The impact of chronic (>12 months) and short-term use of the atypical antipsychotic risperidone on the gut microbiome of underage psychiatric patients (most of them with autism-spectrum disorder) showed that a 10-month treatment with risperidone was associated with an increase in BMI and a significantly lower ratio of Bacteroidetes: Firmicutes as compared with antipsychotic-naıve psychiatric controls [32].

12.4 Bipolar Disorder

Five studies assessed intestinal microbiome dysbiosis in patients with bipolar disorder. Coello et al. [33] found that the microbial community of 113 bipolar disorder patients differed from that of 77 controls, but not from 39 unaffected first-degree relatives. This is very interesting, as it assumes a genetic factor to predispose for a specific microbiome. Most noticeable was the increase in Flavonifractor abundancy in the bipolar disorder group compared to controls and unaffected first-degree relatives. A possible bias could be caused by the higher prevalence of smoking in the bipolar group [34]. Painold et al. [35] confirmed the decreased abundance of Faecalibacterium and Ruminococcaceae in 32 bipolar patients in comparison to 10 controls. They also found that both the phylum Actinobacteria and the class Coriobacteria were more abundant in bipolar disorder compared to controls. Schwarz et al. [36] compared the microbiome of 28 first episode bipolar disorder patients to that of 16 controls. They found significant differences in multiple bacteria strains (detailed in Table 12.1) and concluded that the numbers of Lactobacillus were increased in the bipolar disorder patients, which correlated significantly to the severity of different symptoms domains. Stronger microbiome differences also indicated poorer response to 12 months of treatment.

Evans et al. [37] studied the gut-microbiome changes in bipolar disorder and controls and tested for associations with the burden of disease measurements. They reported that lower abundance of the strain of Faecalibacterium was associated with better physical health, lower depression scores, and better sleep quality. However, they did not take medication use into account while lithium, antidepressants, and mood stabilizers all have been shown to have an antibiotic effect [38]. An attempt to disentangle medication and disease factors on the intestinal microbiome was done by Flowers et al. [39]. They compared two groups of bipolar patients: 46 patients on atypical antipsychotics and 69 non-users. They showed differences in abundance in Lachnospiraceae (increased in the antipsychotic group), Akkermansia (decreased in the antipsychotic group), and Sutterella (decreased in the antipsychotic group). However, it is always difficult to differentiate between disease factors, medication effect, and effects due to illness-related behavior, especially in the field of microbiome, where these factors are heavily intertwingled. It can be concluded that there are clear differences between the microbiome of bipolar disorder patients and those of controls, but so far there is little overlap in observed differences in bacterial strains between the studies. Considering the effect of psychiatric medication (SSRI) on the gut microbiome, an in-vitro study showed fluoxetine and escitalopram to have differential antimicrobial effects. Remarkably, lithium, valproate, and aripiprazole significantly increased microbial species richness and diversity. At the genus level, several species belonging to Clostridium, Peptoclostridium, Intestinibacter, and Christenellaceae were increased following treatment with lithium, valproate, and aripiprazole when compared to baseline. Rats given escitalopram, venlafaxine, fluoxetine, and aripiprazole developed increased permeability in the ileum [31].

12.5 Oropharyngeal Microbiota

When the oropharynx microbiome of patients with SSD is investigated, substantial changes can be observed. A metagenomic study assessed the bacteriophage genomes in 41 SSD patients and 33 controls and found a significant difference in one bacteriophage genome, Lactobacillus phage phiadh, which correlated with the prevalence of immunological disorders as well as with the use of valproate [40]. Lactobacillus phage phiadh modulates the host bacteria level of Lactobacillus gasseri, which has been shown to modulate the immune system by alterations in the function of dendritic cells, enterocytes, and components of the innate immune system [41, 42]. Another metagenomic study including 16 SSD patients and 16 controls found high abundance of lactic acid bacteria in SSD patients, including species of Lactobacilli and Bifidobacterium, which have been shown to modulate chronic inflammation. A significant difference was observed in L. gasseri (about 400 times more abundant in SSD patients compared to with controls) [43].

Overall, in studies assessing the microbiome in both SSD and bipolar patients, a general trend can be observed in the commensal microorganisms of patients with these psychiatric disorders and controls. These differences have been found to correlate with symptoms severity. However, conclusions need to be taken with some consideration as all studies have major biases such as factors as medication use, metabolic syndrome, diet, and smoking, which have not been controlled.

12.6 Probiotics as a Therapeutic Option

To treat dysbiosis of the microbiome and to correct increased intestinal permeability, probiotic supplementation may be an option. Probiotics may elicit positive immunomodulatory effects by calibrating the responses of the host's immune system against pathogens and nonpathogenic organisms, as they stimulate pattern recognition receptors, which mediate bacterial antigen detection [44]. Animal studies assessing the effect of probiotics on hippocampal brain-derived neurotrophic factor (BDNF) in a model of low-grade colitis (AKR mice) showed that abnormal behavior could be reversed with probiotics. A possible route could be that in rats probiotics promote the expression of the neurotrophin under conditions of chronic stress, most likely by lowering microglia activation [45, 46]. Changes have also been observed in the expression of other neurotrophic factors such as glial-derived neurotrophic factor and nerve growth factor in mice who were treated with antibiotics

[47]. Another rodent study using obese-insulin resistant animals showed that hippocampal oxidative stress, apoptosis, and microglial activation were significantly decreased after probiotic supplementation, which promoted cognitive function [48].

Apart from potential beneficial effects on the brain, there is another reason to consider probiotic supplementation in patients with SSD and bipolar disorder. That is the high prevalence of gastrointestinal symptoms. In SSD patients, constipation is a prevalent symptom [49–51]. Probiotics have been shown to improve constipation in different populations but haven't yet been studied in SSD [52–54]. Bipolar disorder, in contrast, is associated with more common diarrhea and satiety, also gastrointestinal symptom for which probiotics are recognized to be efficacious [55]. Therefore, probiotics could form a potential add-on treatment in SSD and bipolar disorder, especially in those who have increased intestinal permeability.

12.7 Probiotic Studies in Patients with SSD or Bipolar Disorder

Currently, there are six clinical studies in which probiotics are administered in SSD or bipolar disorder patients (Table 12.2). Out of these six studies, there are four who included SSD patients and only two targeting bipolar disorder patients.

A recent study of Okubo et al. [56] provided Bifidobacterium breve strain A1 to 29 patients with SSD and found improvement in anxiety and depressive symptoms. Unfortunately, they found this potential effect in an open-label, single-arm study so a placebo effect cannot be excluded. In another study, the group of Yolken [57] found that the administration of probiotics for 22 male patients with SSD helped normalize *Candida albicans* antibody levels and *C. albicans*-associated gut discomfort. Tomasik et al. [58] measured 47 immune-related serum proteins in 57 chronic SSD patients after supplementation with probiotics. They found that probiotic add-on treatment significantly reduced the levels of von Willebrand factor and increased the levels of monocyte chemotactic protein-1 and BDNF, which suggests lower intestinal permeability. In addition, a borderline-significant difference in chemokine (C-C motif) ligand 5 and macrophage inflammatory protein-1 beta was found. A study including 55 SSD patients [59] did not find significant differences on the Positive and Negative Syndrome Scale (PANSS) score of probiotic supplementation compared to placebo. Patients diagnosed with SSD in the probiotic group did have lower severity of bowel difficulty over the course of the trial. Consistent in these studies is the finding that probiotics alleviate bowel discomfort, which is a common nuisance in SSD. However, the results of studies so far displayed limited consistency regarding the reduction of psychiatric symptoms.

Regarding clinical studies with probiotic supplementation in bipolar disorder, Dickerson et al. [60] found probiotics to be associated with a lower rate of rehospitalization in 66 patients who were recently discharged following hospitalization for mania. The probiotic's effect was increased in individuals with elevated levels of systemic inflammation at baseline. Another study by Reininghaus et al. [61] found a significant improvement in attention and psychomotor processing speed in 20

Table 12.2 Clinical trials on probiotic supplementation in patients with schizophrenia and/or bipolar disorder

Publication	Sample size (INT/PL)	Mean age	Sex (M/F)	Study compound (way of administration: orally)	Biomarker(s)/outcome measurements	Difference between INT and comparison groups	Association with clinical features	Limitations
Okubo et al. [56]	SCZ: 29	INT: 45 (16)	INT: 11/17	*Strain(s): Bifidobacterium breve* A-1 Daily amount: 10^{11} cfu Form: Sachet Frequency: Twice daily (w. food) Treatment time: 4 weeks	HADS, PANSS, blood test, faecal microbiome	HADS ($P = 0.037$), PANSS ($P = 0.004$)	Probiotic supplementation may reduce the severity of anxiety and depressive symptoms in SCZ by enhancement of gut epithelial barrier function	Short treatment duration (4 weeks) Open-label, single-arm study
Severance et al. [57]	SCZ: 56	INT: 44.7 (11.4) PL: 48.11 (9.6)	INT: 22/8 PL: 15/11	*Strain(s): Lactobacillus rhamnosus strain GG, Bifidobacterium animalis subs. Lactis strain Bb12* Daily amount: 10^9 cfu (per organism) Form: Tablet Frequency: Once daily (w. food) Treatment time: 14 weeks	Levels of antibodies to *C. albicans* and *S. cerevisiae*, PANSS, Query gastrointestinal functioning	*C. albicans IgG* level in males ($P < 0.001$), PANSS in seronegative *C. albicans* males ($P < 0.06$)	Probiotic supplementation may lead to improvement of bowel functions due to correction of yeast overgrowth	Interpretation of study results is limited by exploratory nature and small sample sizes

(continued)

Table 12.2 (continued)

Publication	Sample size (INT/PL)	Mean age	Sex (M/F)	Study compound (way of administration: orally)	Biomarker(s)/outcome measurements	Difference between INT and comparison groups	Association with clinical features	Limitations
Tomasik et al. [58]	SCZ: 57 (30/27)	INT: 44.8 (11.2) PL: 48.1 (9.2)	INT: 22/9 PL: 16/11	*Strain(s): Lactobacillus rhamnosus strain GG, Bifidobacterium animalis subs. Lactis strain Bb12* Daily amount: 10^9 cfu (per organism) Form: Tablet Frequency: Once daily (w. food) Treatment time: 14 weeks	47 immune-related serum proteins	Von Willebrand Factor ($P = 0.047$), Monocyte Chemotactic Protein 1 ($P = 0.054$), Brain-derived Neurotrophic Factor ($P = 0.063$), RANTES ($P = 0.069$), Macrophage Inflammatory Protein 1 beta ($P = 0.080$)	Probiotic supplementation may improve gastrointestinal leakage control in SCZ	Open-label, single-arm study Not able to detect all targeted cytokines in clinical samples Investigated SCZ patients on stable, long-term antipsychotics, but immune modularly effect still possible A small number of immune-related serum proteins identified as significantly or borderline different between two groups
Dickerson et al. [59]	SCZ: 65 (33/32)	INT: 44.4 (11.0) PL: 48.1 (9.4)	INT: 23/47 PL: 19/40	*Strain(s): Lactobacillus rhamnosus strain GG, Bifidobacterium animalis subs. Lactis strain Bb12* Daily amount: 10^9 cfu (per organism) Form: Tablet Frequency: Once daily (w. food) Treatment time: 14 weeks	PANSS, Query gastrointestinal functioning	PANSS ($P = 0.25$), Gastrointestinal functioning ($P = 0.003$)	Probiotic supplementation may make SCZ patients less likely to develop severe bowel difficulties	Not a detailed measurement of gastrointestinal functioning No complete history of participants' gastrointestinal symptoms and associated symptoms obtained

Dickerson et al. [60]	BD: 66 (33/33)	INT: 37.9 (11.7) PL: 33.3 (13.3)	INT: 9/24 PL: 15/18	*Strain(s): Lactobacillus rhamnosus strain GG, Bifidobacterium animalis subs. Lactis strain Bb12* Daily amount: >10^8 cfu Form: Tablet Frequency: Once daily (w. food) Treatment time: 24 weeks	Time to psychiatric inpatient rehospitalization, BPRS, Symptom assessment (YMRS), MADRAS	Time to psychiatric inpatient rehospitalization ($P = 0.017$). BPRS ($P < 0.0001$), YMRS ($P < 0.0001$)	Probiotic supplementation may alter clinical course following mania and lessen psychiatric symptom severity in BD	Treatment received after hospital discharge was not standardized The sample may not have fully representative of patients hospitalized for mania Effect of probiotics on gut microbiome/ inflammation in CNS is not directly measured
Reininghaus et al. [61]	BD: 20	INT: 51.5 (11.5)	INT: 11/9	*Strain(s): Lactobacillus casei W56, Lactobacillus acidophilus W22, Lactobacillus paracasei W20, Bifidobacterium lactis W51, Lactobacillus salivarius W24, Lactococcus lactis W19, Bifidobacterium lactis W52, Lactobacillus plantarum W62, Bifidobacterium bifidum W23* Daily amount: 2.25×10^{10} cfu Form: Sachet Frequency: Once daily (empty stomach) Treatment time: 12 weeks	TMT-A, digit symbol test, TMT-B. Digit-span-test, Mittenecker Pointing Test	Digit symbol test ($P < 0.001$), TMT-B ($P < 0.05$)	Probiotic supplementation may increase cognitive function in patients with BD	Open-label, single-arm study Small sample size Small cognitive test battery Medications/ Lifestyle changes were not taken into consideration

NB Publications are arranged in a reversed chronological order (from newest to oldest), *BD* bipolar disorder, *BPRS* Brief Psychiatric Rating Scale, *CNS* central nervous system, *HADS* Hospital Anxiety and Depression Scale, *INT* intervention, *MADRAS* Montgomery-Åsberg Depression Rating Scale, *PANSS* Positive and Negative Syndrome Scale, *PL* placebo, *SCZ* schizophrenia, *TMT-A* Trial Masking Test A, *TMT-B* Trial Masking Test B, *YMRS* Young mania rating scale patients and concluded that probiotic supplementation helps individuals with bipolar disorder to improve cognitive functioning. As a single arm study design was used, any influence of a placebo effect cannot be excluded.

As in SSD patients, these studies point to probiotic supplementation alleviating bowel discomfort, but effects on symptom severity are not noted. The available results seem to hint at improved cognition in at least bipolar disorder and possibly SSD. It would be valuable if future studies could take cognitive functioning into account, as well as subjective wellbeing and immunological/inflammatory biomarkers.

12.8 Intestinal Permeability

Several studies report that patients experiencing SSD or bipolar disorder have abnormal reactions to food-derived antigens, indicative for increased intestinal permeability. Patients with SSD had increased IgA for gliadin, b-lactoglobulin, and casein [62]. A cohort from the the clinical anti-psychotic trials for intervention effectiveness (CATIE) study demonstrated that 23.1% of patients with SSD had moderate-to-high levels of IgA to gliadin (IgAantigliadin antibodies) compared with only 3.1% in the control group [63]. Another study confirmed that patients with recent-onset of psychosis and patients with multi-episode SSD had increased levels of IgG and IgA antibodies to gliadin compared with controls. In this study, PANSS scores for negative symptoms correlated with casein a and b antibodies [64]. Dickerson et al. found that bipolar disorder patients also had elevated serum concentrations of IgG to gliadin and deamidated gliadin compared to controls [65]. In a follow-up study, patients with manic symptoms were found to have increased baseline IgG to gliadin, which normalized after 6 months of treatment [66]. In the same study, rehospitalized patients were more likely to have increased IgG to gliadin compared to baseline. Severance et al. compared serum samples of 141 individuals with SSD and 75 bipolar disorder to 78 controls and to 78 SSD patients who were antipsychotic-naïve. They assessed two markers of bacterial translocation, soluble CD14 (sCD14) and LPS-binding protein. sCD14 was significantly higher in both SSD and bipolar disorder. LPS-binding protein was higher in SSD than in bipolar disorder, but there was no significant difference between controls and cases. Both markers where significantly correlated with c-reactive protein [67].

12.9 Conclusion

Although the many interactions between the gut microbiota, the immune system, and the CNS have not been fully understood yet, current data indicate that there are differences in the microbiome in both patients with SSD and bipolar disorder patients as compared to controls. Part of these differences may be caused by medication use, smoking, and other lifestyle factors. Correlations between microbiome quantification and symptom severity have been observed in cross-sectional studies, but more replications are needed.

Probiotic supplementation was shown to alleviate gastrointestinal complaints in SSD and bipolar patients. Single studies showed reduction in rehospitalization rates, improvement on cognitive tasks, and improvement in symptom severity, but other studies could not find this.

Replication of findings as well as studies investigating the predictive role of biomarkers for intestinal permeability is needed. Although the term "probiotic" has gained substantial public attention and become part of the wider vocabulary, it is important to clarify that many commercially available strains marketed as probiotics have never been tested in clinical trials and therefore by definition may not meet the criteria of conferring a health benefit. For future studies, it would be important to tailor probiotic mixtures to deviations in the microbiota demonstrated in the patient group one is to focus on.

Acknowledgments The authors thank Anouk van Mourik, Bea Sloothaak, and Saskia van Hemert for their critical reading of the article. We would also like to thank Ahmed Eltokhi, Doaa Ali, Ahmed M. Disouky, Amr El-Araby, and Abdelrahman A. Fouad for their assistance and suggestions.

References

1. World Health Organization. Mental disorders. 2018. https://www.who.int/news-room/fact-sheets/detail/mental-disorders.
2. Tandon R, Nasrallah HA, Keshavan MS. Schizophrenia, 'just the facts' 5. Treatment and prevention. Past, present, and future. Schizophr Res. 2010;122:1–23.
3. Saha S, Chant D, McGrath J. A systematic review of mortality in schizophrenia: is the differential mortality gap worsening over time? Arch Gen Psychiatry. 2007;64:1123–31.
4. Perlis RH, Ostacher MJ, Patel JK, et al. Predictors of recurrence in bipolar disorder: primary outcomes from the systematic treatment enhancement program for bipolar disorder (STEP-BD). Am J Psychiatry. 2006;163:217–24.
5. Fond G, Boukouaci W, Chevalier G, et al. The 'psychomicrobiotic': targeting microbiota in major psychiatric disorders: a systematic review. Pathol Biol. 2015;63:35–42.
6. Nemani K, HosseiniGhomi R, McCormick B, FanX. Schizophrenia and the gut–brain axis. Prog Neuro-Psychopharmacol Biol Psychiatry. 2015;56:155–60.
7. Dickerson F, Severance E, Yolken R. The microbiome, immunity, and schizophrenia and bipolar disorder. Brain Behav Immun. 2017;62:46–52.
8. Ohland CL, Macnaughton WK. Probiotic bacteria and intestinal epithelial barrier function. Am J Physiol Gastrointest Liver Physiol. 2010;298:G807–19.
9. Anderson G, Maes M. Bipolar disorder: role of immune-inflammatory cytokines, oxidative and nitrosative stress and tryptophan catabolites. Curr Psychiatry Rep. 2015;17:8.
10. Rosenblat JD, Cha DS, Mansur RB, McIntyre RS. Inflamed moods: a review of the interactions between inflammation and mood disorders. Prog Neuro-Psychopharmacol Biol Psychiatry. 2014;53:23–34.
11. Leboyer M, Berk M, Yolken RH, et al. Immuno-psychiatry: an agenda for clinical practice and innovative research. BMC Med. 2016;14:173.

12. Daulatzai MA. Chronic functional bowel syndrome enhances gut–brain axis dysfunction, neuroinflammation, cognitive impairment, and vulnerability to dementia. Neurochem Res. 2014;39:624–44.
13. Kelly JR, Kennedy PJ, Cryan JF, et al. Breaking down the barriers: the gut microbiome, intestinal permeability and stress-related psychiatric disorders. Front Cell Neurosci. 2015;9:392.
14. Schafer DP, Lehrman EK, Kautzman AG, et al. Microglia sculpt postnatal neural circuits in an activity and complement-dependent manner. Neuron. 2012;74:691–705.
15. Maezawa I, Jin LW. Rett syndrome microglia damage dendrites and synapses by the elevated release of glutamate. J Neurosci. 2010;30:5346–56.
16. Lee AS, Azmitia EC, Whitaker-Azmitia PM. Developmental microglial priming in postmortem autism spectrum disorder temporal cortex. Brain Behav Immun. 2017;62:193–202.
17. Hui CW, St-Pierre A, El Hajj H, et al. Prenatal immune challenge in mice leads to partly sex-dependent behavioral, microglial, and molecular abnormalities associated with schizophrenia. Front Mol Neurosci. 2018;11:13.
18. Butel MJ. Probiotics, gut microbiota and health. Med Mal Infect. 2014;44:1–8.
19. Bercik P, Park AJ, Sinclair D, et al. The anxiolytic effect of Bifidobacterium longum NCC3001 involves vagal pathways for gut–brain communication. Neurogastroenterol Motil. 2011;23:1132–9.
20. Tillisch K, Labus J, Kilpatrick L, et al. Consumption of fermented milk product with probiotic modulates brain activity. Gastroenterology. 2013;144:1394–1401.e1–4.
21. Savignac HM, Kiely B, Dinan TG, Cryan JF. Bifidobacteria exert strain-specific effects on stress-related behavior and physiology in BALB/c mice. Neurogastroenterol Motil. 2014;26:1615–27.
22. McFarland LV. From yaks to yogurt: the history, development, and current use of probiotics. Clin Infect Dis. 2015;60(Suppl 2):S85–90.
23. Dinan TG, Stanton C, Cryan JF. Psychobiotics: a novel class of psychotropic. Biol Psychiatry. 2013;74:720–6.
24. Hugon P, Dufour JC, Colson P, et al. A comprehensive repertoire of prokaryotic species identified in human beings. Lancet Infect Dis. 2015;15:1211–9.
25. Lozupone CA, Stombaugh JI, Gordon JI, et al. Diversity, stability and resilience of the human gut microbiota. Nature. 2012;489:220–30.
26. Eckburg PB, Bik EM, Bernstein CN, et al. Diversity of the human intestinal microbial flora. Science. 2005;308:1635–8.
27. Nguyen TT, Kosciolek T, Maldonado Y, et al. Differences in gut microbiome composition between persons with chronic schizophrenia and healthy comparison subjects. Schizophr Res. 2019;204:23–9. [Epub ahead of print]
28. Shen Y, Xu J, Li Z, et al. Analysis of gut microbiota diversity and auxiliary diagnosis as a biomarker in patients with schizophrenia: a cross-sectional study. Schizophr Res. 2018. [Epub ahead of print]
29. Maier L, Pruteanu M, Kuhn M, et al. Extensive impact of nonantibiotic drugs on human gut bacteria. Nature. 2018;555:623–8.
30. Davey KJ, Cotter PD, O'Sullivan O, et al. Antipsychotics and the gut microbiome: olanzapine-induced metabolic dysfunction is attenuated by antibiotic administration in the rat. Transl Psychiatry. 2013;3:e309.
31. Cussotto S, Strain CR, Fouhy F, et al. Differential effects of psychotropic drugs on microbiome composition and gastrointestinal function. Psychopharmacology. 2018. [Epub ahead of print]
32. Bahr SM, Tyler BC, Wooldridge N, et al. Use of the second-generation antipsychotic, risperidone, and secondary weight gain are associated with an altered gut microbiota in children. Transl Psychiatry. 2015;5:e652.
33. Coello K, Hansen TH, Sorensen N, et al. Gut microbiota composition in patients with newly diagnosed bipolar disorder and their unaffected first degree relatives. Brain Behav Immun. 2019;75:112–8.

34. Biedermann L, Zeitz J, Mwinyi J, et al. Smoking cessation induces profound changes in the composition of the intestinal microbiota in humans. PLoS One. 2013;8:e59260.
35. Painold A, Morkl S, Kashofer K, et al. A step ahead: exploring the gut microbiota in inpatients with bipolar disorder during a depressive episode. Bipolar Disord. 2019;21:40–9. [Epub ahead of print]
36. Schwarz E, Maukonen J, Hyytiainen T, et al. Analysis of microbiota in first episode psychosis identifies preliminary associations with symptom severity and treatment response. Schizophr Res. 2018;192:398–403.
37. Evans SJ, Bassis CM, Hein R, et al. The gut microbiome composition associates with bipolar disorder and illness severity. J Psychiatr Res. 2017;87:23–9.
38. Lieb J. The immunostimulating and antimicrobial properties of lithium and antidepressants. J Infect. 2004;49:88–93.
39. Flowers SA, Evans SJ, Ward KM, et al. Interaction between atypical antipsychotics and the gut microbiome in a bipolar disease cohort. Pharmacotherapy. 2017;37:261–7.
40. Yolken RH, Severance EG, Sabunciyan S, et al. Metagenomic sequencing indicates that the oropharyngeal phageome of individuals with schizophrenia differs from that of controls. Schizophr Bull. 2015;41:1153–61.
41. Luongo D, Miyamoto J, Bergamo P, et al. Differential modulation of innate immunity in vitro by probiotic strains of Lactobacillus gasseri. BMC Microbiol. 2013;13:298.
42. Selle K, Klaenhammer TR. Genomic and phenotypic evidence for probiotic influences of Lactobacillus gasseri on human health. FEMS Microbiol Rev. 2013;37:915–35.
43. Castro-Nallar E, Bendall ML, Perez-Losada M, et al. Composition, taxonomy and functional diversity of the oropharynx microbiome in individuals with schizophrenia and controls. PeerJ. 2015;3:e1140.
44. Reid G, Younes JA, Van der Mei HC, et al. Microbiota restoration: natural and supplemented recovery of human microbial communities. Nat Rev Microbiol. 2011;9:27–38.
45. Bercik P, Verdu EF, Foster JA, et al. Chronic gastrointestinal inflammation induces anxiety-like behavior and alters central nervous system biochemistry in mice. Gastroenterology. 2010;139:2102–2112.e1.
46. Liang S, Wang T, Hu X, et al. Administration of Lactobacillus helveticus NS8 improves behavioral, cognitive, and biochemical aberrations caused by chronic restraint stress. Neuroscience. 2015;310:561–77.
47. Aguilera M, Cerda-Cuellar M, Martinez V. Antibiotic-induced dysbiosis alters host-bacterial interactions and leads to colonic sensory and motor changes in mice. Gut Microbes. 2015;6:10–23.
48. Chunchai T, Thunapong W, Yasom S, et al. Decreased microglial activation through gut–brain axis by prebiotics, probiotics, or synbiotics effectively restored cognitive function in obese-insulin resistant rats. J Neuroinflammation. 2018;15:11.
49. De Hert M, Dockx L, Bernagie C, et al. Prevalence and severity of antipsychotic related constipation in patients with schizophrenia: a retrospective descriptive study. BMC Gastroenterol. 2011;11:17.
50. De Hert M, Hudyana H, Dockx L, et al. Second-generation antipsychotics and constipation: a review of the literature. Eur Psychiatry. 2011;26:34–44.
51. Koizumi T, Uchida H, Suzuki T, et al. Oversight of constipation in inpatients with schizophrenia: a cross-sectional study. Gen Hosp Psychiatry. 2013;35:649–52.
52. Chmielewska A, Szajewska H. Systematic review of randomised controlled trials: probiotics for functional constipation. World J Gastroenterol. 2010;16:69–75.
53. Miller LE, Ouwehand AC. Probiotic supplementation decreases intestinal transit time: meta-analysis of randomized controlled trials. World J Gastroenterol. 2013;19:4718–25.
54. Dimidi E, Christodoulides S, Fragkos KC, et al. The effect of probiotics on functional constipation in adults: a systematic review and meta-analysis of randomized controlled trials. Am J Clin Nutr. 2014;100:1075–84.
55. Sherwin E, Sandhu KV, Dinan TG, Cryan JF. May the force be with you: the light and dark sides of the microbiota–gut–brain axis in neuropsychiatry. CNS Drugs. 2016;30:1019–41.

56. Okubo R, Koga M, Katsumata N, et al. Effect of Bifidobacterium breve A-1 on anxiety and depressive symptoms in schizophrenia: a proof-of-concept study. J Affect Disord. 2018;245:377–85.
57. Severance EG, Gressitt KL, Stallings CR, et al. Probiotic normalization of Candida albicans in schizophrenia: a randomized, placebo-controlled, longitudinal pilot study. Brain Behav Immun. 2017;62:41–5.
58. Tomasik J, Yolken RH, Bahn S, Dickerson FB. Immunomodulatory effects of probiotic supplementation in schizophrenia patients: a randomized, placebocontrolled trial. Biomark Insights. 2015;10:47–54.
59. Dickerson FB, Stallings C, Origoni A, et al. Effect of probiotic supplementation on schizophrenia symptoms and association with gastrointestinal functioning: a randomized, placebo-controlled trial. Prim Care Companion CNS Disord. 2014;16:219–222.
60. Dickerson F, Adamos M, Katsafanas E, et al. Adjunctive probiotic microorganisms to prevent rehospitalization in patients with acute mania: a randomized controlled trial. Bipolar Disord. 2018;20:614–21.
61. Reininghaus EZ, Wetzlmair LC, Fellendorf FT, et al. The impact of probiotic supplements on cognitive parameters in euthymic individuals with bipolar disorder: a pilot study. Neuropsychobiology. 2018;79:1–8. [Epub ahead of print]
62. Reichelt KL, Landmark J. Specific IgA antibody increases in schizophrenia. Biol Psychiatry. 1995;37:410–3.
63. Cascella NG, Kryszak D, Bhatti B, et al. Prevalence of celiac disease and gluten sensitivity in the United States clinical antipsychotic trials of intervention effectiveness study population. Schizophr Bull. 2011;37:94–100.
64. Dickerson F, Stallings C, Origoni A, et al. Markers of gluten sensitivity and celiac disease in recent-onset psychosis and multiepisode schizophrenia. Biol Psychiatry. 2010;68:100–4.
65. Dickerson F, Stallings C, Origoni A, et al. Markers of gluten sensitivity and celiac disease in bipolar disorder. Bipolar Disord. 2011;13:52–8.
66. Dickerson F, Stallings C, Origoni A, et al. Markers of gluten sensitivity in acute mania: a longitudinal study. Psychiatry Res. 2012;196:68–71.
67. Severance EG, Gressitt KL, Stallings CR, et al. Discordant patterns of bacterial translocation markers and implications for innate immune imbalances in schizophrenia. Schizophr Res. 2013;148:130–7.

Part II

Immune Dysfunctions and Psychiatric Disorders

13 Is Autism Spectrum Disorder Related to Immune Dysfunction(s)?

Florian Lejuste, Ryad Tamouza, and Marion Leboyer

13.1 Introduction

Autism spectrum disorder (ASD) is a heterogeneous neurodevelopmental disorder characterized by impairments in communication and social interactions as well as restricted patterns of interest or behavior. The most recent estimate indicates an increased prevalence with a rate of 1% worldwide. With a heritability estimate around 50%, autism is strongly influenced both by the human genetic diversity and by environmental factors. For example, while it has been known for more than 50 years, that congenital rubella infections increased the risk to develop autism from 0.05 to 13% [1], other pre-natal infections have been demonstrated to also increase this risk [2]. These data have stimulated research for possible abnormal immune functions. In order to review the potential role of immune dysfunctions in autism, we will summarize data along a developmental perspective: from specific

F. Lejuste (✉)
DMU IMPACT, Psychiatry and Addictology Department, Mondor University Hospital, University Paris-Est-Créteil, Créteil, France

INSERM U955, Translational Neuro-Psychiatry, Mondor Institute for Biomedical Research, Créteil, France

Service de psychiatrie, Hopital Albert Chenevier, Créteil, France

R. Tamouza
DMU IMPACT, Psychiatry and Addictology Department, Mondor University Hospital, University Paris-Est-Créteil, Créteil, France

INSERM U955, Translational Neuro-Psychiatry, Mondor Institute for Biomedical Research, Créteil, France

M. Leboyer
University Paris Est Créteil (UPEC), Inserm, IMRB (Translational NeuroPsychiatry lab), AP-HP, DMU IMPACT, AP-HP, Fondation FondaMental, Créteil, France
e-mail: marion.leboyer@inserm.fr

M. Berk et al. (eds.), *Immuno-Psychiatry*, https://doi.org/10.1007/978-3-030-71229-7_13

immuno-genetic backgrounds, to peri-natal factors such as auto-antibodies and early infections, to inflammation in childhood and adult dysimmune patterns.

13.2 Family History of Auto-Immune Diseases and Risk of ASD

Family history of auto-immune diseases has been linked to an increased risk of ASD in offsprings. In a recent meta-analysis, a family history of auto-immune disease increased the risk to 28%, while common non-psychiatric auto-immune diseases increased it even more, such as type 1 diabetes (49%), rheumatoid arthritis (51%), psoriasis (59%), or hypothyroidism (64%) [3].

Maternal auto-immune diseases have been associated with an increased risk of ASD in offsprings, with an overall odd ratio of 1.34 [4]. More specifically, mothers with auto-immune disease(s) with circulating antibodies able to cross placenta such as TPO-ab (anti-thyroid peroxidase, thyroid-related AD) or ß2GP1 (Anti-Beta-2-Glycoprotein I, antiphospholipid syndrome) are at an increased risk of having a child with ASD [5, 6]. In particular, a sub-group of mothers with auto-immune diseases were also found to have antibodies against fetal brain structures, while none were found in the group of mothers without AD [4]. Reasons for a history of auto-immune diseases in relatives being associated with ASD remain unknown. However, recent hypotheses incriminate the major histocompatibility complex (MHC) and its hosted human leukocytes antigen (HLA) cluster including loci encoding complement components [3].

13.3 Immunogenetic Background

Twin studies showed that heritability of ASD ranges approximately between 50% and 55% [7]. In approximately 10% of patients with ASD, especially those with intellectual disability, de novo copy number or single nucleotide variants affecting neurodevelopment were identified [8].

In transcriptomic analysis, two network modules have been identified, one related to down-regulation of genes involved in synaptic function and one related to over-expression of loci involved in immune processes and microglia activation [9]. This network comprises a highly expressed gene component which has a key role in immune system regulation, particularly in cytokine signaling pathways. Gandal et al. highlighted specific mutations in genes encoding microglial components in ASD, especially those linked to the complement pathways (C1QA and C1QB) and to the HLA system. These mutations were associated with an up-regulation of microglial activation [10].

Abnormalities in the MHC/HLA region in human have been linked to immune dysregulation and altered brain connectivity which are both observed in ASD. In this context, analysis of the genetic diversity of the classical HLA loci, known to be pivotal for both brain development and immune processes ranging from reduced anti-infectious responses to increased inflammation and auto-immunity, revealed associations between functionally important haplotypes called "ancestral haplotypes" and risk/protection status particularly in regressive autism [11, 12].

On the other side of the HLA system, HLA-G gene, known to encode molecules playing a key role in immune tolerance at the feto-maternal interface, was also implicated in increased ASD risk. The transmission of specific HLA-G variants from mother to children with ASD was demonstrated in several consecutive studies [13].

13.4 Infection, Inflammation, and Autoimmunity During Pregnancy

13.4.1 Maternal Infection During Pregnancy and ASD

In 1971, following a rubella epidemy, several studies reported an increased risk of ASD following congenital infection. Later, other infections have been implicated such as measles and mumps [14], CMV [15], influenza [16], bacteria [17], and viral and bacterial infections [18]. A recent meta-analysis by Jiang et al. found a significant association (OR: 1.14) regardless of infection site, trimester of pregnancy, or type of pathogen [19]. This result is consistent with a previous study, suggesting that infectious events may increase the risk of developing ASD regardless of the time of infection during pregnancy and the type of involved pathogen (virus, bacteria, parasite) [18]. Interestingly, the increase of ASD risk might not be correlated with maternal infection severity, as a study found similar odds ratio between urinary infection or respiratory/meningitis infections [2]. These results suggest a relatively non-specific role of pathogens, and a rather prominent role of maternal immune activation (MIA). Whatever the gestational exposure to a given infectious agent, MIA has repeatedly been found to induce neurodevelopmental abnormalities and was used to develop animal models of autism-like behavior [20]. Particularly, cytokines' role has been repeatedly linked to pathogenicity of this pro-inflammatory state. At a cellular level, pro-inflammatory cytokines produced during MIA might have a direct role on fetal neurons and glial cells homeostasis, thus affecting normal brain development [21].

13.4.2 Maternal Autoantibodies Against Fetal Brain Structures

The first study that identified autoantibodies against rat neuronal tissue was published in 2003 [22]. Later, Brauschweig et al. [23] identified auto-antibodies against fetal brain proteins in the serum of mothers of children with autism. This finding was replicated in several consecutive studies [24, 25]. In 2018, Jones and Van de Water reviewed the pathogenicity of mother-produced fetal brain autoantibodies. Such auto-antibodies have been found to be present in a subgroup of mothers whose children later develop ASD. These antibodies-positive mothers were more likely to have other autoimmune conditions, suggesting the involvement of a more global auto-immune process [26].

The mechanism of the induction of such autoimmunity in a subgroup of mothers (thus breaking immune tolerance during pregnancy) has not yet been elucidated.

However, some authors found an association between the presence of autoantibodies in the mother of children later developing ASD and a MET genetic variant: the "C" allele. MET is the tyrosine kinase promoter and has a tolerogenic role through IL-10 induction (a cytokine pivotal in down-regulation of inflammatory and immune reaction). The MET variant "C" allele was associated with decreased production of MET protein and decreased expression of IL-10 [27].

The presence of such autoantibodies was associated with various autistic traits later in life. Particularly, they were associated with delayed language acquisition and increased stereotyped behaviors [26]. In animal studies, injection of human autoantibodies in pregnant mice and monkeys resulted in restricted social behavior in offsprings and increased stereotyped behaviors [26].

These auto-antibodies are targeting various fetal brain proteins, now precisely identified: **LDH** *lactate dehydrogenase*, **STIP1** *stress-induced phosphoprotein 1*, **CRMP** *collapsin response mediator protein*, **YBX1** *Y-box-binding protein 1*, **GDA** *guanine deaminase.* All these proteins are directly implicated in neurodevelopmental processes [26].

Neuro-imaging studies using MRI have also found enlarged brain volume in male children prenatally exposed to autoantibodies [28]. Animal studies carried out on monkeys and mice exposed to autoantibodies during gestation produced similar results [26].

At a microscopic level, the brain tissue of embryonic mice injected with antibodies from the mother with ASD children was studied. Antibodies were found to strongly bind to radial glial cells in cortical parenchyma of embryonic mice. Their injection was also associated with a decrease in the number of dendritic spines in both prefrontal and occipital cortices in grown mice [26].

13.4.3 Post-natal Infections

There are contradictory results about an increased incidence of neonatal and childhood infections in children with ASD compared to the general population. However, several recent studies have found an association between early life infection and ASD diagnosis.

In a case-control study, Sabourin et al. found a significant increase in the incidence of infections in neonatal and childhood period with odds ratio of 1.8 and 1.7, respectively [29]. In a rat model exposed to lipopolysaccharide (LPS) which mimics bacterial infection in neonatal period with consequent immune activation, abnormalities were found in emotional response during adult life [30].

13.4.4 Maternal Inflammation, CRP, and Cytokines

13.4.4.1 CRP: Discrepant Data

The C-reactive protein (CRP) is an acute phase and non-specific inflammatory molecule. It is produced by liver cells under the control of pro-inflammatory interleukins, particularly interleukin 6 (IL6) and IL-1. An increased level of CRP in the first two trimesters of pregnancy was found to be associated with elevated ASD risk in offsprings [31]. In 2016, an increased level of CRP in pregnant mothers was found to be associated with a reduced risk [32], while a third prospective study did not find any association between the increase of CRP and the risk of autism [33]. Altogether, such apparently contradictory results between studies might be linked to a confounding factor: the mother's body mass index [33]. These discrepant results could also be related to the time-dependent variability of CRP circulating levels. Its evaluation at a single time point during pregnancy could not reflect the inflammatory state of the whole pregnancy.

13.4.4.2 Cytokines: Interleukins and Chemokines

Repeated studies of animal models show that disruption of cytokine levels during pregnancy is a risk factor for ASD [34]. In particular, a single injection of the pro-inflammatory IL-6 cytokine during pregnancy leads to abnormalities in the offspring, otherwise neutralized by the administration of anti-IL6 antibody. This effect was not seen with other pro-inflammatory cytokines [35].

In addition, IL-17alpha (IL-17a) seems to have a central role in fetal neurotoxicity linked to MIA. In mice, IL-17a expression in mother after exposure to infection or to an auto-immune disease has a pathological impact on the fetus' brain development. Strikingly, blocking IL-17a production prevents neuro-developmental abnormalities, suggesting an interesting therapeutic target [36]. Moreover, another study published in *Nature* in 2018 showed that IL-17a production in pregnant mice was strongly correlated with specific maternal gut bacteria. They demonstrated that some commensal bacteria were implicated in the production and the differentiation of T lymphocytes toward TH17 cells (which produce IL-17a). Segmented filamentous bacteria (SFB), which are strains of commensal bacteria, were particularly implicated. Indeed, the authors showed that mice treated with Vancomycin had reduced or no SFB in their gut. These treated pregnant mice were able to experience immune activation upon virus or poly(I:C) (mimicking virus) injections, but their offspring didn't develop the brain abnormalities expected after MIA. The authors concluded that specific commensal gut bacteria with the ability to induce TH17 cells in pregnant mother undergoing infection or auto-inflammation may increase the risk of abnormal neurodevelopment in offsprings [37].

Other cytokines during pregnancy have been associated with ASD, but with a less clear pathophysiological mechanism, and as for CRP with sometimes inconsistent results. High levels of IFN-γ, IL-4, IL-5 in pregnant mother have been associated with raised ASD risk in offspring. IL-2, IL-4 and IL-6 were found to be correlated with intellectual deficit without associated ASD [38]. Other authors couldn't find differences between the cytokine serum profiles of mothers of ASD and non-ASD children. However, when considering a subgroup of children with ASD and intellectual disability, they found mid-gestational elevated concentrations of inflammatory mediators, i.e., IFN-γ, IL-1α, and IL-6 [39].

Chemokines are involved in the attraction of leucocytes to the inflammatory sites. Monocyte chemoattractant protein-1 (MCP-1) is a chemokine with a known role in response to various viral and bacterial infection. MCP-1 was found in more elevated concentration in amniotic liquid of fetus developing ASD later in life. This could be a reflection of fetal inflammation, after maternal immune activation following infectious events [40, 41].

13.5 Abnormalities in Immune Function in Autism, from Children to Adults

Abnormalities in immune functions in children and adults with autism have also been reported, and linked to specific clinical dimensions, thus paving the way toward the identification of specific subgroups.

13.5.1 Brain Auto-Antibodies

In addition to maternal autoantibodies, circulating anti-brain immunoglobulins have been found in children and adults with autism compared to normal controls. In 2010 two different types of antibodies directed against cerebellar proteins in children were associated with ASD. Interestingly, their presence was associated with lower cognitive and adaptive function and with higher aberrant behavior. There was no correlation between children antibodies and mother anti-fetal brain antibodies [42]. Piras et al. confirmed that the presence of auto-antibodies was associated with greater severity (cognitive and behavioral) in children with ASD. However they couldn't confirm the association between their presence and an increased risk of ASD [43]. In fact, these auto-antibodies were found in neurotypical subject. Their pathological significance still needs to be explored. It might be linked to an alteration of the blood brain barrier in children with autism, due to another cause, allowing antibodies to cross the barrier and reach the central nervous system. The identification of auto-antibodies in autism needs thus to be validated and replicated in different samples. Also, the mechanism of action of auto-antibodies in brain targets the need to be explored at the synaptic level. For example, the presence of auto-antibodies against NMDA-R found in the serum of patient with autism does not imply that they have a pathogenic effect as shown by molecular brain imaging studies [44].

13.5.2 Immune Dysregulation

Natural killer cells have frequently been implicated in autism. High level of cell activation after in vitro stimulation was found in adults with autism without mental retardation suggesting, yet to be identified, viral infections [45].

13.5.3 Cytokine Profiles, Phenotype Characteristics, and Severity

Proteins of the peripheral immune system such as those encoded by cytokines complement proteins; and major histocompatibility complex loci have been found to have a key role in brain development such as neuronal differentiation and plasticity, axonal pathfinding, and synaptic pruning [46].

Various cytokines in neonatal serum of newborns have been associated with ASD. Abdallah et al. found decreased concentrations of IL-2 IL-4 IL-6, IL-10, and interferon gamma (IFNγ) in newborns later developing ASD [47]. Conversely, Krakowiak et al. found elevated concentrations of IL-4. Moreover higher concentration of IL-4 was associated with more severe ASD later in life [48].

Transforming growth factor beta (TGF-β) is a cytokine known for its modulatory role in both immune and central nervous systems [49, 50]. Its decreased concentration in children with ASD has been described and associated with more severe abnormal behaviors [51]. Similarly, another cytokine, the macrophage inhibitory factor (MIF), has been recently associated with ASD. Patients with the higher plasma concentrations of MIF had the more severe abnormal behavior [52, 53].

Mostafa et al. found that ASD children had an increased chemokine known as CXCL5 (or ENA-78). This chemokine is implicated in the attraction of neutrophils during inflammation, in multiple conditions. This increase in CXCL5 was positively correlated with increased auto-antibodies in children with ASD [54].

13.5.4 Gastro-Intestinal Inflammation

Gastro-intestinal tractus (GI-tract) dysfunctions (including diarrhea, constipation, and/or abdominal pain for example) are very frequent in children and adults with ASD compared to general population, with an odds ratio over 4 [55]. Histological studies have described an inflammatory infiltrate in the digestive mucosa of children with ASD and GI-tract symptoms. Inflammation implicated not only ileocolitis, but also oesophagitis, enteritis, and gastritis. Interestingly, GI-tract cytokine profiles showed specific patterns of inflammation, different when compared to those of inflammatory bowel diseases (IBD) (such as Crohn's disease and ulcerative colitis) [56]. Moreover, when considering mucosal gene expression, ASD patients with GI-tract symptoms showed overlaps with typical IBD having distinctive features. Pulled together, these results suggest a specific mucosal inflammatory condition in patients with ASD and GI-tract symptoms [57].

Recently, studies of the innate and adaptive immunity genetic diversity allowed to uncover the implication of (i) a variant encoded of the gene encoding the Dectin-1 molecule a pivotal player of intestinal antifungal immune responses and ASD severity [58] and (ii) specific HLA haplotype already described as a genetic risk factor for celiac disease [59].

13.5.5 Gut-Microbiota

In a review published in *Science* in 2019, Sherwin et al. highlighted the role of the gut microbiota in social behavior through neurodevelopment and inflammation. They emphasize that germ-free (GF) rodent models have abnormal social behaviors which can be partially corrected when the gut microbiota is reconstituted. One of the possible pathophysiological mechanisms is linked to microglia. Microglia derived from germ-free mice was immature and showed less activation to stimulation by bacterial LPS, and a reduced production of pro-inflammatory cytokines (IL-1β, IL-6 and TNF-α) [60]. Interestingly, abnormal microglia of GF mice could be normalized by postnatal supplementation of short-chain fatty acid (SCFA), normally produced by bacterial fermentation [61].

In a recent meta-analysis Xu et al. found that microbiota composition differed qualitatively between ASD subjects and controls: some bacterial strains being overrepresented (*Faecalibacterium* and *Lactobacillus)* while some others underrepresented (*Akkermansia, Bacteroides*, *Bi dobacterium*, *E. coli*, and *Enterococcus*) in participants with ASD. Such alterations could have an impact on brain development through inflammation and epithelial barrier integrity [62].

13.6 Conclusion

Here, we tentatively tried to draw a brief overview of the very complex and still misunderstood role of immune dysregulations in autism spectrum disorders. As it appears in our review, various immuno-inflammatory components or processes have been associated with ASD, at all developmental stages. An important and repeated discovery has been the presence of auto-antibodies in a sub-group of mothers of children with ASD, directed against fetal brain proteins, which might be linked to particular immune-genetic background. In this respect, genetic dissection of pivotal players of immune processes could allow not only to extend and refine the underlying pathophysiology of ASD, but also to identify possible markers of subgroups of ASD. Another field of research showing the role of the gut microbiota in ASD is also a very promising field of research, with diagnostic tools and therapeutic targets already considered. However, as we still lack a comprehensive natural and sequential view of the observed immune dysregulations, the need of pursuing research is strongly warranted.

References

1. Chess S. Autism in children with congenital rubella. J Autism Child Schizophr. 1971;1(1):33–47.
2. Al-Haddad BJS, Jacobsson B, Chabra S, Modzelewska D, Olson EM, Bernier R, et al. Long-term risk of neuropsychiatric disease after exposure to infection in utero. JAMA Psychiatry. 2019;76(6):594.
3. Wu S, Ding Y, Wu F, Li R, Xie G, Hou J, et al. Family history of autoimmune diseases is associated with an increased risk of autism in children: a systematic review and meta-analysis. Neurosci Biobehav Rev. 2015;55:322–32.

4. Chen S, Zhong X, Jiang L, Zheng X, Xiong Y, Ma S, et al. Maternal autoimmune diseases and the risk of autism spectrum disorders in offspring: a systematic review and meta-analysis. Behav Brain Res. 2016;296:61–9.
5. Abisror N, Mekinian A, Lachassinne E, Nicaise-Roland P, De Pontual L, Chollet-Martin S, et al. Autism spectrum disorders in babies born to mothers with antiphospholipid syndrome. Semin Arthritis Rheum. 2013;43:348–51. https://doi.org/10.1016/j.semarthrit.2013.07.001.
6. Brown AS, Surcel HM, Hinkka-Yli-Salomaki S, Cheslack-Postava K, Bao Y, Sourander A. Maternal thyroid autoantibody and elevated risk of autism in a national birth cohort. Prog Neuro-Psychopharmacol Biol Psychiatry. 2015;57:86–92. https://doi.org/10.1016/j.pnpbp.2014.10.010.
7. Colvert E, Tick B, McEwen F, Stewart C, Curran SR, Woodhouse E, et al. Heritability of autism spectrum disorder in a UK population-based twin sample. JAMA Psychiat. 2015;72(5):415–23.
8. Huguet G, Benabou M, Bourgeron T. The genetics of autism spectrum disorders. In: Sassone-Corsi P, Christen Y, editors. A time for metabolism and hormones. Cham (CH): Springer; 2016.
9. Voineagu I, Wang X, Johnston P, Lowe JK, Tian Y, Horvath S, et al. Transcriptomic analysis of autistic brain reveals convergent molecular pathology. Nature. 2011;474(7351):380–4.
10. Gandal MJ, Haney JR, Parikshak NN, Leppa V, Ramaswami G, Hartl C, et al. Shared molecular neuropathology across major psychiatric disorders parallels polygenic overlap. Science. 2018;359(6376):693–7.
11. Torres AR, Westover JB, Rosenspire AJ. HLA immune function genes in autism. Autism Res Treat. 2012;2012:959073. https://doi.org/10.1155/2012/959073.
12. Tamouza R, Fernell E, Eriksson MA, Anderlid B-M, Manier C, Mariaselvam CM, et al. HLA polymorphism in regressive and non-regressive autism: a preliminary study. Autism Res. 2020;13:182–6.
13. Guerini FR, Bolognesi E, Chiappedi M, Ghezzo A, Canevini MP, Mensi MM, et al. An HLA-G(∗)14bp insertion/deletion polymorphism associates with the development of autistic spectrum disorders. Brain Behav Immun. 2015;44:207–12.
14. Deykin EY, Macmahon B. Viral exposure and autism. Am J Epidemiol. 1979;109(6):628–38.
15. Maeyama K, Tomioka K, Nagase H, Yoshioka M, Takagi Y, Kato T, et al. Congenital cytomegalovirus infection in children with autism spectrum disorder: systematic review and meta-analysis. J Autism Dev Disord. 2018;48(5):1483–91.
16. Atladóttir HÓ, Henriksen TB, Schendel DE, Parner ET. Autism after infection, febrile episodes, and antibiotic use during pregnancy: an exploratory study. Pediatrics. 2012;130(6):e1447–54.
17. Zerbo O, Qian Y, Yoshida C, Grether JK, Van de Water J, Croen LA. Maternal infection during pregnancy and autism spectrum disorders. J Autism Dev Disord. 2015;45(12):4015–25.
18. Lee BK, Magnusson C, Gardner RM, Blomström Å, Newschaffer CJ, Burstyn I, et al. Maternal hospitalization with infection during pregnancy and risk of autism spectrum disorders. Brain Behav Immun. 2015;44:100–5.
19. Jiang H, Xu L, Shao L, Xia R, Yu Z, Ling Z, et al. Maternal infection during pregnancy and risk of autism spectrum disorders: a systematic review and meta-analysis. Brain Behav Immun. 2016;58:165–72.
20. Meyer U, Feldon J, Schedlowski M, Yee BK. Towards an immuno-precipitated neurodevelopmental animal model of schizophrenia. Neurosci Biobehav Rev. 2005;29(6):913–47.
21. Meyer U, Yee BK, Feldon J. The neurodevelopmental impact of prenatal infections at different times of pregnancy: the earlier the worse? The Neuroscientist. 2007;13(3):241–56.
22. Dalton P, Deacon R, Blamire A, Pike M, McKinlay I, Stein J, et al. Maternal neuronal antibodies associated with autism and a language disorder. Ann Neurol. 2003;53(4):533–7.
23. Braunschweig D, Ashwood P, Krakowiak P, Hertz-Picciotto I, Hansen R, Croen LA, et al. Autism: maternally derived antibodies specific for fetal brain proteins. Neurotoxicology. 2008;29(2):226–31.
24. Singer HS, Morris CM, Gause CD, Gillin PK, Crawford S, Zimmerman AW. Antibodies against fetal brain in sera of mothers with autistic children. J Neuroimmunol. 2008;194(1–2):165–72.

25. Brimberg L, Sadiq A, Gregersen PK, Diamond B. Brain-reactive IgG correlates with autoimmunity in mothers of a child with an autism spectrum disorder. Mol Psychiatry. 2013;18(11):1171–7.
26. Jones KL, Van de Water J. Maternal autoantibody related autism: mechanisms and pathways. Mol Psychiatry. 2019;24(2):252–65.
27. Heuer L, Braunschweig D, Ashwood P, Van de Water J, Campbell DB. Association of a MET genetic variant with autism-associated maternal autoantibodies to fetal brain proteins and cytokine expression. Transl Psychiatry. 2011;1:e48.
28. Nordahl CW, Braunschweig D, Iosif A-M, Lee A, Rogers S, Ashwood P, et al. Maternal autoantibodies are associated with abnormal brain enlargement in a subgroup of children with autism spectrum disorder. Brain Behav Immun. 2013;30:61–5.
29. Sabourin KR, Reynolds A, Schendel D, Rosenberg S, Croen LA, Pinto-Martin JA, et al. Infections in children with autism spectrum disorder: study to explore early development (SEED): autism spectrum disorder and infection. Autism Res. 2019;12(1):136–46.
30. Vojtechova I, Petrasek T, Maleninska K, Brozka H, Tejkalova H, Horacek J, et al. Neonatal immune activation by lipopolysaccharide causes inadequate emotional responses to novel situations but no changes in anxiety or cognitive behavior in Wistar rats. Behav Brain Res. 2018;349:42–53.
31. Brown AS, Sourander A, Hinkka-Yli-Salomäki S, McKeague IW, Sundvall J, Surcel H-M. Elevated maternal C-reactive protein and autism in a national birth cohort. Mol Psychiatry. 2014;19(2):259–64.
32. Zerbo O, Traglia M, Yoshida C, Heuer LS, Ashwood P, Delorenze GN, et al. Maternal mid-pregnancy C-reactive protein and risk of autism spectrum disorders: the early markers for autism study. Translational Psychiatry. 2016;6(4):e783.
33. Koks N, Ghassabian A, Greaves-Lord K, Hofman A, Jaddoe VWV, Verhulst FC, et al. Maternal C-reactive protein concentration in early pregnancy and child autistic traits in the general population: maternal CRP and child autistic traits. Paediatric Perinatal Epidemiol. 2016;30(2):181–9.
34. Hsiao EY. Immune dysregulation in autism spectrum disorder. Int Rev Neurobiol. 2013;113:269–302.
35. Smith SEP, Li J, Garbett K, Mirnics K, Patterson PH. Maternal immune activation alters fetal brain development through interleukin-6. J Neurosci. 2007;27(40):10695–702.
36. Choi GB, Yim YS, Wong H, Kim S, Kim H, Kim SV, et al. The maternal interleukin-17a pathway in mice promotes autism-like phenotypes in offspring. Science. 2016;351(6276):933–9.
37. Kim S, Kim H, Yim YS, Ha S, Atarashi K, Tan TG, et al. Maternal gut bacteria promote neurodevelopmental abnormalities in mouse offspring. Nature. 2017;549(7673):528–32.
38. Goines PE, Croen LA, Braunschweig D, Yoshida CK, Grether J, Hansen R, et al. Increased midgestational IFN-γ, IL-4 and IL-5 in women bearing a child with autism: a case-control study. Mol Autism. 2011;2(1):13.
39. Jones KL, Croen LA, Yoshida CK, Heuer L, Hansen R, Zerbo O, et al. Autism with intellectual disability is associated with increased levels of maternal cytokines and chemokines during gestation. Mol Psychiatry. 2017;22(2):273–9.
40. Patterson PH. Maternal infection and autism. Brain Behav Immun. 2012;26(3):393.
41. Abdallah MW, Larsen N, Grove J, Nørgaard-Pedersen B, Thorsen P, Mortensen EL, et al. Amniotic fluid chemokines and autism spectrum disorders: an exploratory study utilizing a Danish historic birth cohort. Brain Behav Immun. 2012;26(1):170–6.
42. Goines P, Haapanen L, Boyce R, Duncanson P, Braunschweig D, Delwiche L, et al. Autoantibodies to cerebellum in children with autism associate with behavior. Brain Behav Immun. 2011;25(3):514–23.
43. Piras IS, Haapanen L, Napolioni V, Sacco R, Van de Water J, Persico AM. Anti-brain antibodies are associated with more severe cognitive and behavioral profiles in Italian children with autism spectrum disorder. Brain Behav Immun. 2014;38:91–9.

44. Gréa H, Scheid I, Gaman A, Rogemond V, Gillet S, Honnorat J, et al. Clinical and autoimmune features of a patient with autism spectrum disorder seropositive for anti-NMDA-receptor autoantibody. Dialogues Clin Neurosci. 2017;19(1):65–70.
45. Bennabi M, Tarantino N, Gaman A, Scheid I, Krishnamoorthy R, Debré P, et al. Persistence of dysfunctional natural killer cells in adults with high-functioning autism spectrum disorders: stigma/consequence of unresolved early infectious events? Mol Autism. 2019;10:22.
46. Pramparo T, Pierce K, Lombardo MV, Carter Barnes C, Marinero S, Ahrens-Barbeau C, et al. Prediction of autism by translation and immune/inflammation coexpressed genes in toddlers from pediatric community practices. JAMA Psychiat. 2015;72(4):386.
47. Abdallah MW, Larsen N, Mortensen EL, Atladottir HO, Norgaard- Pedersen B, Bonefeld-Jorgensen EC, et al. Neonatal levels of cytokines and risk of autism spectrum disorders: an exploratory register-based historic birth cohort study utilizing the Danish Newborn Screening Biobank. J Neuroimmunol. 2012;252:75–82.
48. Krakowiak P, Goines PE, Tancredi DJ, et al. Neonatal cytokine profiles associated with autism spectrum disorder. Biol Psychiatry. 2017;81(5):442–51. https://doi.org/10.1016/j.biopsych.2015.08.007.
49. Letterio JJ, Roberts AB. Regulation of immune responses by TGF-beta. Annu Rev Immunol. 1998;16:137–61.
50. Gomes FC, Sousa Vde O, Romao L. Emerging roles for TGF-beta1 in nervous system development. Int J Dev Neurosci. 2005;23(5):413–24.
51. Ashwood P, Enstrom A, Krakowiak P, Hertz-Picciotto I, Hansen RL, Croen LA, et al. Decreased transforming growth factor beta1 in autism: a potential link between immune dysregulation and impairment in clinical behavioral outcomes. J Neuroimmunol. 2008;204:149–53.
52. Grigorenko EL, Han SS, Yrigollen CM, Leng L, Mizue Y, Anderson GM, et al. Macrophage migration inhibitory factor and autism spectrum disorders. Pediatrics. 2008;122(2):e438–45.
53. Goines P, Van de Water J. The immune system's role in the biology of autism. Curr Opin Neurol. 2010;23(2):111–7.
54. Mostafa GA, Al-Ayadhi LY. The possible link between elevated serum levels of epithelial cell-derived neutrophil-activating peptide-78 (ENA-78/CXCL5) and autoimmunity in autistic children. Behav Brain Funct. 2015;11:11.
55. McElhanon BO, McCracken C, Karpen S, Sharp WG. Gastrointestinal symptoms in autism spectrum disorder: a meta-analysis. Pediatrics. 2014;133(5):872–83.
56. Ashwood P, Anthony A, Torrente F, Wakefield AJ. Spontaneous mucosal lymphocyte cytokine profiles in children with autism and gastrointestinal symptoms: mucosal immune activation and reduced counter regulatory Interleukin-10. J Clin Immunol. 2004 Nov;24(6):664–73.
57. Walker SJ, Fortunato J, Gonzalez LG, Krigsman A. Identification of unique gene expression profile in children with regressive autism spectrum disorder (ASD) and ileocolitis. PLoS ONE. 2013;8(3):e58058.
58. Bennabi M, Delorme R, Oliveira J, Fortier C, Lajnef M, Boukouaci W, et al. Dectin-1 polymorphism: a genetic disease specifier in autism spectrum disorders? PLoS One. 2015;10(9):e0137339.
59. Bennabi M, Gaman A, Delorme R, Boukouaci W, Manier C, Scheid I, et al. HLA-class II haplotypes and autism spectrum disorders. Sci Rep. 2018;8(1):7639.
60. Sherwin E, Bordenstein SR, Quinn JL, Dinan TG, Cryan JF. Microbiota and the social brain. Science. 2019;366(6465):eaar2016.
61. Fung TC, Olson CA, Hsiao EY. Interactions between the microbiota, immune and nervous systems in health and disease. Nat Neurosci. 2017;20(2):145–55.
62. Xu M, Xu X, Li J, Li F. Association between gut microbiota and autism spectrum disorder: a systematic review and meta-analysis. Front Psych. 2019 Jul;17:10.

Inflammation and Immunity in Schizophrenia

14

Norbert Müller

14.1 Introduction

Well-regulated inflammation is an essential protective mechanism, for example, to eliminate bacterial and viral infections; however, excessive inflammatory processes can cause harm, as in autoinflammatory diseases such as multiple sclerosis. In the central nervous system (CNS), inflammation can also be either neuroprotective or neurotoxic [1]. The outcome of inflammation depends on interactions between environmental factors and the inflammatory response; genetics; and whether the inflammation is acute or chronic [2]. For example, acute inflammation in the CNS, such as encephalitis, can be fatal within a few hours or days, but a chronic, harmful inflammatory state can also continue over months or even years, such as in multiple sclerosis. In acute CNS inflammation, macrophages and B- and T-cells from the peripheral immune system are assumed to cross the blood-brain barrier. In contrast, chronic CNS inflammation is hypothesized to be related to the activity of the CNS-based immune system. In multiple sclerosis, for example, this local immune activity in the CNS is seen as disseminated activation of microglia [3]. Researchers have referred to these differences between THE involvement of the peripheral and central immune systems as "compartmentalization" [2, 4].

The pathogenetic mechanisms of multiple sclerosis and schizophrenia may show similarities because both affect the CNS, can be chronic, and are characterized by phases of active disease interspersed with phases of remission [5]. However, the inflammatory mechanisms in these two diseases differ. For example, a general neuroinflammatory state is typical for schizophrenia [6], whereas multiple sclerosis shows focal areas of neuroinflammation [3]. This chapter will review possible inflammatory mechanisms of schizophrenia and potential immune-based treatments.

N. Müller (✉)
Department of Psychiatry and Psychotherapy, Ludwig Maximilian University, Munich, Germany
e-mail: norbert.mueller@med.uni-muenchen.de

M. Berk et al. (eds.), *Immuno-Psychiatry*, https://doi.org/10.1007/978-3-030-71229-7_14

14.2 CNS Inflammation

Various components of the immune system are involved in inflammation in the CNS, including microglia, astrocytes, cytokines, and cells of the peripheral immune system, such as monocytes, macrophages, and T- and B-lymphocytes. These different parts of the immune system can be affected by a range of factors, including not only environmental toxins and pathogens but also genetics and secondary reactions to neuronal lesions resulting from trauma.

14.2.1 Microglia

Microglia make up 15% of cells in the CNS and are the most important component of the local immune defense system. They are activated in case of neuroinflammation, for example, resulting from injury or infection in the CNS [7]. Systemic infection also activates microglia, which contribute to the synthesis of proinflammatory cytokines in the CNS that cause so-called sickness behavior and other illness-related mental states [8, 9]. Although initially produced in response to an acute signal, proinflammatory cytokines may then continue to be released for up to 10 months; this finding led to the hypothesis that microglia may be involved in chronic inflammation [7]. In schizophrenia, in addition to activated microglia some studies found higher levels of pro-inflammatory cytokines and lower levels of anti-inflammatory cytokines (see below). As a caveat, one must note that the subdivision of cytokines into pro- and anti-inflammatory is an oversimplification because certain cytokines can show both properties; the respective activity of such cytokines depends on several factors, including the activating signal, timing, and type of target cell [10]. However, this topic is beyond the scope of this chapter.

14.2.2 Sensitization of the Immune System and the Effects of Stress

Microglia can also be "sensitized" or "primed" by various low-level stimuli [11], including ageing-related processes [12], neurodegeneration [13], and stress [14]. After sensitization, the response of microglia to a low-level stimulus such as minor infection is exaggerated and they show greater pro-inflammatory reactivity [15], perhaps leading to an exacerbation or re-exacerbation of a CNS immune response and affecting behavior. This process of sensitization is also seen in the peripheral immune system. As with microglia, an initial immune response to a stimulus, e.g., stress, strengthens the subsequent immune response or lowers the threshold for a response upon re-exposure to the same stimulus [16]. On the basis of earlier studies, researchers hypothesized that this process is related to a memory function in the acquired immune system [14, 17]. For example, later re-exposure to a stimulus that caused an early childhood infection can result in increased cytokine release and associated neurotransmitter disturbances [18]. Furthermore, in rats stress-related release of the cytokine interleukin-6 (IL-6) reactivated (prenatally) conditioned processes [19].

In addition to infections and trauma, stressful events can evoke a pro-inflammatory immune response [20]. Stress increases the levels of corticosterone, which activates the *N*-methyl-D-aspartate (NMDA) receptor, and this receptor activation causes microglia to proliferate [21]. The increased cytokine levels associated with this response can present as psychopathological symptoms and behavioral changes [22]. After an acute stressful event, the immune response is normally downregulated; however, studies have shown that chronic stress or repeated stressful events can lower the threshold for the physiological reactions to stress, including the immune system response or neurotransmitter changes [23]. Furthermore, the brains of aged animals were found to be in a proinflammatory state that sensitized them to peripheral infection and stress, so that they showed a greater cytokine response to these stimuli than younger animals [14]. In other animal studies, neurotransmitter responses to a cytokine, for example, tumor necrosis factor-alpha (TNF-α), were greater upon re-exposure [24, 25].

14.3 The Vulnerability-Stress-Inflammation Model of Schizophrenia

The vulnerability-stress model of schizophrenia was first proposed by Zubin and Spring over four decades ago [26]. The authors hypothesized that physical or mental stress can cause a psychotic episode. Because stress is known to be a cause of inflammation, and inflammation is known to be involved in schizophrenia, the model was further developed into the so-called vulnerability-stress-inflammation model. Evidence for the validity of this model is provided by animal studies, which show that offspring are more vulnerable to developing schizophrenia if an inflammatory response of the mother is stimulated in the second trimester or in the young offspring soon after birth [27]. Besides sensitization (see above), vulnerability to stress is also influenced by genetic factors, as proposed in the pathogen host defense hypothesis of depression [28]. Inflammatory markers and the effects of inflammation on neurotransmitter systems in schizophrenia are further elucidated.

14.3.1 Inflammatory Markers

An inflammatory process is hypothesized to be involved in the pathophysiology of at least a subgroup of patients with schizophrenia [29, 30], a theory that is supported by a range of findings. First, postmortem studies in schizophrenia have found degradation products of fibrin (a protein involved in coagulation and inflammation) in the brain [31] and cerebrospinal fluid (CSF) [32]. Furthermore, untreated patients with schizophrenia have a blunted type 1 cytokine response and an increased type 2 cytokine response [33]. Meta-analyses of studies in schizophrenia found higher levels of pro-inflammatory cytokines in the peripheral blood in patients with a first episode of the disease and those who had relapsed [34], including the inflammation-marker C-reactive protein [35]; in contrast, levels of some anti-inflammatory cytokines were lower than in healthy controls [34]. The results of a meta-analysis of studies on cytokines in the CSF were similar [36]. When examining these findings, however, one must consider the potential effects of confounding factors such as smoking, body mass index, sex, sleep, and medication. Moreover, blood levels of cytokines may not appropriately reflect their function because several cytokines have a primarily paracrine effect. Lastly, the brain is protected from peripheral inflammation by the blood-brain barrier, and an immune activation with increased pro-inflammatory cytokines in the blood does not necessarily reflect the situation in the brain [37].

14.3.2 Inflammation and Neurotransmitters

For a long time, research on the neurobiology of schizophrenia has focused mainly on disturbances in dopaminergic neurotransmission. Studies have clearly shown that the dopamine system is altered in schizophrenia [38], but the exact relationship remains unclear and results of studies on antidopaminergic drugs have been disappointing. At least two cytokines may be involved in the changes in neurotransmitter systems seen in schizophrenia: IL-1ß, which has been shown to cause rat mesencephalic progenitor cells to be converted into a dopaminergic phenotype [39–41], and IL-6, which shortens the survival of serotonergic neurons in the fetal brain [42].

The interaction between cytokines and neurotransmitters in certain brain regions and in particular during brain development has been shown to contribute to the pathophysiology of schizophrenia. In a mouse model, Winter et al. [43] found a significant increase in the dopamine levels in fetal brains after eliciting an immune response in the pregnant dams with a viral mimetic (poly I:C). The authors suggested that the poly I:C-induced immune response caused an excess of dopamine in the midbrain, a structure that is affected in patients with schizophrenia [43]. However, chronic administration of the cytokine interferon-alpha in animals was associated with a reduction in striatal dopamine release and with anhedonia [44]. Anhedonia is a characteristic negative symptom of schizophrenia, and negative symptoms are often found in chronic schizophrenia [45]. Other authors have proposed that latent persistent infections may result in imbalanced immune reactions [46]. Thus, inflammation may have diverse effects on dopaminergic neurotransmission and may be involved in the chronification of schizophrenia.

Another key neurotransmitter in the pathophysiology of schizophrenia is glutamate, the most abundant neurotransmitter in the CNS, which is involved in cytokine-directed tryptophan/kynurenine metabolism. Kynurenic acid, one of three or more intermediate neuroactive products in the kynurenine pathway, is the only known naturally occurring NMDA receptor antagonist in the human CNS [47]. In schizophrenia, a predominant type 2 immune response is proposed to inhibit indoleamine

2,3-dioxygenase (IDO), resulting in increased kynurenic acid production; kynurenic acid acts as an antagonist at NMDA receptors, which in turn decreases glutamate neurotransmission [48, 49]. Support for this hypothesis is provided by studies that found NMDA receptor antibodies in about 10% of untreated patients with acute schizophrenia [50, 51]. Some studies found higher kynurenic acid levels in the CSF [52, 53] and brains of patients with schizophrenia [54, 55] and in animal models of schizophrenia [56], and others found no changes in levels in the peripheral blood of patients with first-episode schizophrenia [57] or in other groups of schizophrenia patients [58]. Antipsychotic medication affects kynurenine metabolites and thus may be a confounder in studies [57–59].

14.4 Infection and Schizophrenia

Studies in animal models have shown that pre- and perinatal infections increase the likelihood of schizophrenia in offspring [60, 61]. For example, after prenatal exposure to viral agents animal offspring show symptoms typical of schizophrenia, including cognitive deficits and abnormalities in the startle reflex [62, 63]. The relationship between exposure to infections and a higher risk for schizophrenia appears to hold true in humans, too, and has been shown for prenatal or childhood viral exposure [64–67], respiratory infections [68], genital or reproductive tract infections [68, 69], *Toxoplasma gondii* infection [70], and other infections [71–74]. Findings on virus antibody titers in patients with schizophrenia are inconsistent [75], although this may be because the studies did not control for potential confounders, such as medication [76]. In an earlier study, we found higher titers of antibodies to various pathogens in patients with schizophrenia than in healthy controls, a phenomenon we named the "infectious index" [77]. Another study showed that the mothers of people with schizophrenia spectrum disorders had higher second-trimester levels of the pro-inflammatory cytokine IL-8 than controls [78].

Possible mechanisms of the association between early life infection and schizophrenia are of interest because schizophrenia is a disease of late adolescence/early adulthood. Many studies in animal models have shown that early infection or immune activation influences several neurodevelopmental processes, including dopaminergic and glutamatergic neurotransmission [40, 79]. In humans, studies on some infections [80] and a cohort study of bacterial infection are examples that support this explanation [68]. Furthermore, increased levels of cytokines or CRP in childhood predict an increased risk for schizophrenia [81].

Infection in adulthood also increases the risk of developing schizophrenia. A large epidemiological register study in Denmark found a higher risk for schizophrenia and schizophrenia spectrum disorders in people hospitalized for autoimmune disorders or severe infections, particularly in patients with both diseases [82]. However, the study found no evidence that early exposure to infections, including prenatal exposure, increased the risk for schizophrenia [82, 83].

14.5 Inflammation and CNS Volume Loss

Neuroimaging studies have not shown marked inflammation-related changes in schizophrenia, although they have found CNS volume reductions in first-episode schizophrenia and progressive volume loss in the further disease course [84–87]. People with schizophrenia showed decreased brain volume, i.e., lower volumes of the right posterior cingulum and left entorhinal cortex and higher volumes of the ventricles, after prenatal exposure to higher maternal IL-8 levels (measured in assays from archived prenatal sera) [88], and volume loss in schizophrenia was found to be associated with an increased genetic risk for greater production of the immune marker IL-1β [89].

The peripheral benzodiazepine receptor is expressed on microglia and is upregulated in inflammation [90]. Positron emission tomography (PET) studies therefore used radiolabeled PK11195, a ligand for the receptor, to estimate microglial activation in the CNS and found that binding of PK11195 is higher in schizophrenia, indicating neuroinflammation [91–93]. Another PET study used DAA1106, another marker of microglial activation, to investigate the brains of people with chronic schizophrenia and found a correlation between binding of the marker and positive symptoms, as well as the duration of the disease [94].

14.6 Anti-Inflammatory Treatment in Schizophrenia

Treatment with anti-inflammatory drugs, such as celecoxib (a cyclooxygenase-2 [COX-2] inhibitor) and acetyl salicylic acid, has positive effects in schizophrenia and schizophrenia spectrum disorders [95, 96], providing support for an involvement of inflammation in the disease. In a 6-week prospective, double-blind, randomized controlled trial in patients receiving risperidone for an acute schizophrenic episode, outcome was significantly better in the add-on celecoxib group ($n = 25$) than in the add-on placebo group ($n = 25$) [97]. Cognition also improved significantly more in the celecoxib group [98]. A pooled analysis ($n = 90$) of the data from this and another 6-week study of celecoxib add-on to risperidone found that the duration of illness influenced the effects of celecoxib; i.e., the drug was beneficial in patients with a duration of illness <2 years but not superior to placebo in case of a longer illness duration [99] (see Fig. 14.1).

Other studies also provided support for the hypothesis that duration of illness is an important factor in the efficacy of anti-inflammatory treatment in schizophrenia. In a 6-week study of celecoxib add-on treatment in patients with first-manifestation schizophrenia being treated with amisulpride, the Positive and Negative Syndrome Scale (PANSS) positive, negative, total, and general psychopathology scores improved more in the celecoxib add-on group than in the placebo add-on group [102]. However, an 8-week double-blind study comparing celecoxib and placebo augmentation in continuously ill outpatients with schizophrenia receiving stable antipsychotic treatment found no benefit of celecoxib [103]. In addition,

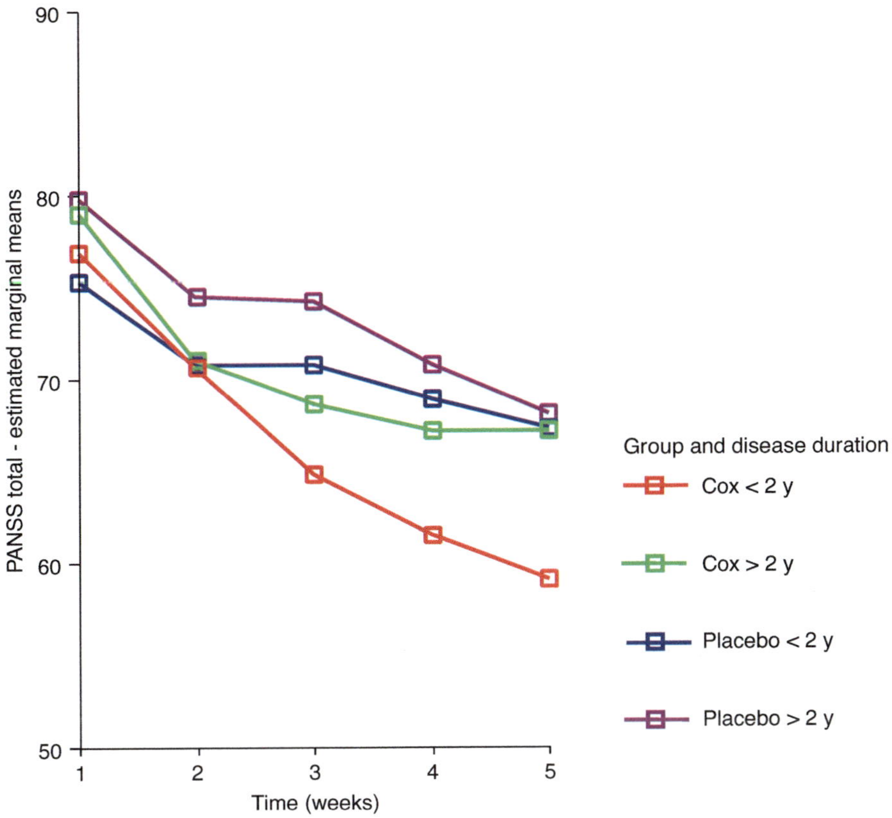

Fig. 14.1 Comparison of disease duration on the effects of celecoxib add-on therapy to risperidone. Patients with a disease duration <2 years and celecoxib treatment had a better outcome than patients with a disease duration >2 years and placebo and both groups of patients with a disease duration of more than 2 years (results not statistically significant). Reprinted from [100] by permission of Oxford University Press and [101] Copyright © 2017 Karger Publishers, Basel, Switzerland. *Cox* celecoxib, *PANSS* Positive and negative syndrome scale

a meta-analysis of eight studies (six of celecoxib and two of acetylsalicylic acid) found significant effects in first-episode but not chronic schizophrenia [104].

A possible explanation for the importance of the duration of illness for the efficacy of anti-inflammatory agents may be neuroprogression (Müller 2017). We know from studies of first- and second-generation antipsychotics that the efficacy of these treatments is worse in chronic schizophrenia than in acute schizophrenia. However, so far anti-inflammatory treatment in schizophrenia has been studied for a maximum of 8 weeks (see above). Furthermore, short-term anti-inflammatory treatment also has poor efficacy in chronic inflammatory diseases. Therefore, longer studies are needed to evaluate anti-inflammatory treatment in chronic schizophrenia [105].

Studies are also needed to investigate potential predictors of treatment response to anti-inflammatory treatment. Earlier studies found that a higher amount of inflammation is associated with worse response to antipsychotics [106–109]. The question remains open whether higher levels of inflammation predict a better outcome to anti-inflammatory treatment, as was shown for anti-TNF treatment and celecoxib in major depression [28, 110]. So far, no immune-related predictive markers for anti-inflammatory treatment have been identified.

14.7 Other Potential Inflammation-Related Treatments in Schizophrenia

As mentioned earlier, microglia play a role in CNS inflammation, and CNS inflammation is hypothesized to be involved in schizophrenia. Thus, studies have examined whether agents that can cross the blood-brain barrier and inhibit microglia activation may be useful in schizophrenia. One such drug is the antibiotic minocycline. Minocycline was studied in animal models of schizophrenia, where it was shown to have positive effects on cognition [111]. In a double-blind, placebo-controlled study, add-on minocycline improved negative symptoms of schizophrenia [112, 113]. In addition, case reports described positive effects on the overall symptom spectrum [114].

Studies have also found some positive effects of other anti-inflammatory substances, such as acetylcysteine and omega-3 fatty acids [115] and interferon-gamma, a cytokine that stimulates the monocytic type 1 immune response [116]. Interferon-gamma may not be a viable treatment option, though, because it can have adverse effects on the immune system and is thus probably a “double-edged sword” in psychiatric diseases, as it is in cancer [117].

Monoclonal antibodies to pro-inflammatory cytokines have also been proposed as a potential treatment for schizophrenia, and treatment appears to be feasible and potentially efficacious, warranting further research [118].

14.8 Conclusion

In the context of research on the immune system and inflammation, it is important to note that drug treatment, smoking, stress levels, sleep patterns, etc., can affect results. Nevertheless, research appears to support a role of immunological and inflammatory processes in the pathogenesis of schizophrenia. Data have been obtained from a range of approaches, including studies on the role of proinflammatory cytokines in the disease; the effects of cytokines on tryptophan/kynurenine metabolism and glutamatergic neurotransmission; the binding of markers of inflammation in imaging studies; genetics; and the effects of anti-inflammatory drugs. Further research is required, particularly into a potential association of inflammation with volume loss in the CNS and the importance of the duration of illness for treatment outcome. However, findings so far, in particular on the positive effects of anti-inflammatory treatment in schizophrenia, are encouraging.

Funding The work was supported by the foundation "Immunität und Seele."

Conflict of Interest None to declare.

References

1. Hohlfeld R, Kerschensteiner M, Meinl E. Dual role of inflammation in CNS disease. Neurology. 2007;68:S58–63; discussion S91–6
2. Kerschensteiner M, Meinl E, Hohlfeld R. Neuro-immune crosstalk in CNS diseases. Neuroscience. 2009;158:1122–32.
3. Elkjaer ML, Frisch T, Reynolds R, et al. Molecular signature of different lesion types in the brain white matter of patients with progressive multiple sclerosis. Acta Neuropathol Commun. 2019;7:205.
4. Meinl E, Krumbholz M, Derfuss T, et al. Compartmentalization of inflammation in the CNS: a major mechanism driving progressive multiple sclerosis. J Neurol Sci. 2008;274:42–4.
5. Hanson DR, Gottesman II. Theories of schizophrenia: a genetic-inflammatory-vascular synthesis. BMC Med Genet. 2005;6:7.
6. Anderson G, Berk M, Dodd S, et al. Immuno-inflammatory, oxidative and nitrosative stress, and neuroprogressive pathways in the etiology, course and treatment of schizophrenia. Prog Neuro-Psychopharmacol Biol Psychiatry. 2013;42:1–4.
7. Kreutzberg GW. Microglia: a sensor for pathological events in the CNS. Trends Neurosci. 1996;19:312–8.
8. van Dam AP. Diagnosis and pathogenesis of CNS lupus. Rheumatol Int. 1991;11:1–11.
9. Dantzer R. Cytokine-induced sickness behavior: where do we stand? Brain Behav Immun. 2001;15:7–24.
10. Cavaillon JM. Pro-versus anti-inflammatory cytokines: myth or reality. Cell Mol Biol (Noisy-le-Grand). 2001;47:695–702.
11. Perry VH. Stress primes microglia to the presence of systemic inflammation: implications for environmental influences on the brain. Brain Behav Immun. 2007;21:45–6.
12. Godbout JP, Johnson RW. Age and neuroinflammation: a lifetime of psychoneuroimmune consequences. Immunol Allergy Clin N Am. 2009;29:321–37.
13. Cunningham C, Wilcockson DC, Campion S, et al. Central and systemic endotoxin challenges exacerbate the local inflammatory response and increase neuronal death during chronic neurodegeneration. J Neurosci. 2005;25:9275–84.
14. Sparkman NL, Johnson RW. Neuroinflammation associated with aging sensitizes the brain to the effects of infection or stress. Neuroimmunomodulation. 2008;15:323–30.
15. Frank MG, Baratta MV, Sprunger DB, et al. Microglia serve as a neuroimmune substrate for stress-induced potentiation of CNS pro-inflammatory cytokine responses. Brain Behav Immun. 2007;21:47–59.
16. Schedlowski M, Pacheco-Lopez G. The learned immune response: Pavlov and beyond. Brain Behav Immun. 2010;24:176–85.
17. Furukawa H, del Rey A, Monge-Arditi G, et al. Interleukin-1, but not stress, stimulates glucocorticoid output during early postnatal life in mice. Ann NY Acad Sci. 1998;840:117–22.
18. Krusche J, Basse S, Schaub B. Role of early life immune regulation in asthma development. Semin Immunopathol. 2020;42:29–42.
19. Zhou D, Kusnecov AW, Shurin MR, et al. Exposure to physical and psychological stressors elevates plasma interleukin 6: relationship to the activation of hypothalamic-pituitary-adrenal axis. Endocrinology. 1993;133:2523–30.
20. Muller N, Krause D, Barth R, et al. Childhood adversity and current stress are related to pro- and anti-inflammatory cytokines in major depression. J Affect Disord. 2019;253:270–6.

21. Nair A, Bonneau RH. Stress-induced elevation of glucocorticoids increases microglia proliferation through NMDA receptor activation. J Neuroimmunol. 2006;171:72–85.
22. Lovelock DF, Deak T. Acute stress imposed during adolescence yields heightened anxiety in Sprague Dawley rats that persists into adulthood: sex differences and potential involvement of the medial amygdala. Brain Res. 2019;1723:146392.
23. Korte SM, Straub RH. Fatigue in inflammatory rheumatic disorders: pathophysiological mechanisms. Rheumatology (Oxford). 2019;58:v35–50.
24. Anisman H, Merali Z. Cytokines, stress and depressive illness: brain-immune interactions. Ann Med. 2003;35:2–11.
25. Hayley S, Wall P, Anisman H. Sensitization to the neuroendocrine, central monoamine and behavioural effects of murine tumor necrosis factor-alpha: peripheral and central mechanisms. Eur J Neurosci. 2002;15:1061–76.
26. Zubin J, Spring B. Vulnerability: a new view of schizophrenia. J Abnorm Psychol. 1977;86:103–26.
27. Khandaker GM, Zimbron J, Lewis G, et al. Prenatal maternal infection, neurodevelopment and adult schizophrenia: a systematic review of population-based studies. Psychol Med. 2013;43:239–57.
28. Raison CL, Rutherford RE, Woolwine BJ, et al. A randomized controlled trial of the tumor necrosis factor antagonist infliximab for treatment-resistant depression: the role of baseline inflammatory biomarkers. JAMA Psychiat. 2013;70:31–41.
29. Muller N, Schwarz MJ. Immune system and schizophrenia. Curr Immunol Rev. 2010;6:213–20.
30. Potvin S, Stip E, Sepehry AA, et al. Inflammatory cytokine alterations in schizophrenia: a systematic quantitative review. Biol Psychiatry. 2008;63:801–8.
31. Korschenhausen DA, Hampel HJ, Ackenheil M, et al. Fibrin degradation products in post mortem brain tissue of schizophrenics: a possible marker for underlying inflammatory processes. Schizophr Res. 1996;19:103–9.
32. Wildenauer DB, Korschenhausen D, Hoechtlen W, et al. Analysis of cerebrospinal fluid from patients with psychiatric and neurological disorders by two-dimensional electrophoresis: identification of disease-associated polypeptides as fibrin fragments. Electrophoresis. 1991;12:487–92.
33. Muller N, Schwarz MJ. Neuroimmune-endocrine crosstalk in schizophrenia and mood disorders. Expert Rev Neurother. 2006;6:1017–38.
34. Goldsmith DR, Rapaport MH, Miller BJ. A meta-analysis of blood cytokine network alterations in psychiatric patients: comparisons between schizophrenia, bipolar disorder and depression. Mol Psychiatry. 2016;21:1696–709.
35. Miller BJ, Culpepper N, Rapaport MH. C-reactive protein levels in schizophrenia: a review and meta-analysis. Clin Schizophr Relat Psychoses. 2014;7:223–30.
36. Wang AK, Miller BJ. Meta-analysis of cerebrospinal fluid cytokine and tryptophan catabolite alterations in psychiatric patients: comparisons between schizophrenia, bipolar disorder, and depression. Schizophr Bull. 2017.
37. Muller N, Bechter K. The mild encephalitis concept for psychiatric disorders revisited in the light of current psychoneuroimmunological findings. Neurol Psychiatry Brain Res. 2013;19:87–101.
38. Carlsson A. The current status of the dopamine hypothesis of schizophrenia. Neuropsychopharmacology. 1988;1:179–86.
39. Ling ZD, Potter ED, Lipton JW, et al. Differentiation of mesencephalic progenitor cells into dopaminergic neurons by cytokines. Exp Neurol. 1998;149:411–23.
40. Kabiersch A, Furukawa H, del Rey A, et al. Administration of interleukin-1 at birth affects dopaminergic neurons in adult mice. Ann N Y Acad Sci. 1998;840:123–7.
41. Potter ED, Ling ZD, Carvey PM. Cytokine-induced conversion of mesencephalic-derived progenitor cells into dopamine neurons. Cell Tissue Res. 1999;296:235–46.
42. Jarskog LF, Xiao H, Wilkie MB, et al. Cytokine regulation of embryonic rat dopamine and serotonin neuronal survival in vitro. Int J Dev Neurosci. 1997;15:711–6.

43. Winter C, Djodari-Irani A, Sohr R, et al. Prenatal immune activation leads to multiple changes in basal neurotransmitter levels in the adult brain: implications for brain disorders of neurodevelopmental origin such as schizophrenia. Int J Neuropsychopharmacol. 2009;12:513–24.
44. Felger JC, Mun J, Kimmel HL, et al. Chronic interferon-alpha decreases dopamine 2 receptor binding and striatal dopamine release in association with anhedonia-like behavior in nonhuman primates. Neuropsychopharmacology. 2013;38:2179–87.
45. Muller N, Ackenheil M. Immunoglobulin and albumin content of cerebrospinal fluid in schizophrenic patients: relationship to negative symptomatology. Schizophr Res. 1995;14:223–8.
46. Nikolich-Zugich J. Ageing and life-long maintenance of T cell subsets in the face of latent persistent infections. Nat Rev Immunol. 2008;8:512–22.
47. Stone TW. Neuropharmacology of quinolinic and kynurenic acids. Pharmacol Rev. 1993;45:309–79.
48. Muller N, Schwarz MJ. The immunological basis of glutamatergic disturbance in schizophrenia: towards an integrated view. J Neural Transm Suppl. 2007:269–80.
49. Muller N, Myint AM, Schwarz MJ. Kynurenine pathway in schizophrenia: pathophysiological and therapeutic aspects. Curr Pharm Des. 2011;17:130–6.
50. Steiner J, Walter M, Glanz W, et al. Increased prevalence of diverse N-methyl-D-aspartate glutamate receptor antibodies in patients with an initial diagnosis of schizophrenia: specific relevance of IgG NR1a antibodies for distinction from N-methyl-D-aspartate glutamate receptor encephalitis. JAMA Psychiat. 2013;70:271–8.
51. Vincent A, Bien CG. Anti-NMDA-receptor encephalitis: a cause of psychiatric, seizure, and movement disorders in young adults. Lancet Neurol. 2008;7:1074–5.
52. Erhardt S, Blennow K, Nordin C, et al. Kynurenic acid levels are elevated in the cerebrospinal fluid of patients with schizophrenia. Neurosci Lett. 2001;313:96–8.
53. Linderholm KR, Skogh E, Olsson SK, et al. Increased levels of kynurenine and kynurenic acid in the CSF of patients with schizophrenia. Schizophr Bull. 2012;38:426–32.
54. Schwarcz R, Rassoulpour A, Wu HQ, et al. Increased cortical kynurenate content in schizophrenia. Biol Psychiatry. 2001;50:521–30.
55. Sathyasaikumar KV, Stachowski EK, Wonodi I, et al. Impaired kynurenine pathway metabolism in the prefrontal cortex of individuals with schizophrenia. Schizophr Bull. 2011;37:1147–56.
56. Olsson SK, Andersson AS, Linderholm KR, et al. Elevated levels of kynurenic acid change the dopaminergic response to amphetamine: implications for schizophrenia. Int J Neuropsychopharmacol. 2009;12:501–12.
57. Condray R, Dougherty GG Jr, Keshavan MS, et al. 3-Hydroxykynurenine and clinical symptoms in first-episode neuroleptic-naive patients with schizophrenia. Int J Neuropsychopharmacol. 2011;14:756–67.
58. Myint AM, Schwarz MJ, Verkerk R, et al. Reversal of imbalance between kynurenic acid and 3-hydroxykynurenine by antipsychotics in medication-naive and medication-free schizophrenic patients. Brain Behav Immun. 2011;25:1576–81.
59. Ceresoli-Borroni G, Rassoulpour A, Wu HQ, et al. Chronic neuroleptic treatment reduces endogenous kynurenic acid levels in rat brain. J Neural Transm (Vienna). 2006;113:1355–65.
60. Buka SL, Tsuang MT, Torrey EF, et al. Maternal infections and subsequent psychosis among offspring. Arch Gen Psychiatry. 2001;58:1032–7.
61. Westergaard T, Mortensen PB, Pedersen CB, et al. Exposure to prenatal and childhood infections and the risk of schizophrenia: suggestions from a study of sibship characteristics and influenza prevalence. Arch Gen Psychiatry. 1999;56:993–8.
62. Meyer U, Feldon J. Prenatal exposure to infection: a primary mechanism for abnormal dopaminergic development in schizophrenia. Psychopharmacology. 2009;206:587–602.
63. Meyer U, Schwarz MJ, Muller N. Inflammatory processes in schizophrenia: a promising neuroimmunological target for the treatment of negative/cognitive symptoms and beyond. Pharmacol Ther. 2011;132:96–110.

64. Pearce BD. Schizophrenia and viral infection during neurodevelopment: a focus on mechanisms. Mol Psychiatry. 2001;6:634–46.
65. Buka SL, Cannon TD, Torrey EF, et al. Maternal exposure to herpes simplex virus and risk of psychosis among adult offspring. Biol Psychiatry. 2008;63:809–15.
66. Brown AS, Begg MD, Gravenstein S, et al. Serologic evidence of prenatal influenza in the etiology of schizophrenia. Arch Gen Psychiatry. 2004;61:774–80.
67. Brown AS, Cohen P, Greenwald S, et al. Nonaffective psychosis after prenatal exposure to rubella. Am J Psychiatry. 2000;157:438–43.
68. Sorensen HJ, Mortensen EL, Reinisch JM, et al. Association between prenatal exposure to bacterial infection and risk of schizophrenia. Schizophr Bull. 2009;35:631–7.
69. Babulas V, Factor-Litvak P, Goetz R, et al. Prenatal exposure to maternal genital and reproductive infections and adult schizophrenia. Am J Psychiatry. 2006;163:927–9.
70. Brown AS, Schaefer CA, Quesenberry CP Jr, et al. Maternal exposure to toxoplasmosis and risk of schizophrenia in adult offspring. Am J Psychiatry. 2005;162:767–73.
71. Boksa P. Maternal infection during pregnancy and schizophrenia. J Psychiatry Neurosci. 2008;33:183–5.
72. Gattaz WF, Abrahao AL, Foccacia R. Childhood meningitis, brain maturation and the risk of psychosis. Eur Arch Psychiatry Clin Neurosci. 2004;254:23–6.
73. Brown AS. The risk for schizophrenia from childhood and adult infections. Am J Psychiatry. 2008;165:7–10.
74. Dalman C, Allebeck P, Gunnell D, et al. Infections in the CNS during childhood and the risk of subsequent psychotic illness: a cohort study of more than one million Swedish subjects. Am J Psychiatry. 2008;165:59–65.
75. Yolken RH, Torrey EF. Viruses, schizophrenia, and bipolar disorder. Clin Microbiol Rev. 1995;8:131–45.
76. Leweke FM, Gerth CW, Koethe D, et al. Antibodies to infectious agents in individuals with recent onset schizophrenia. Eur Arch Psychiatry Clin Neurosci. 2004;254:4–8.
77. Krause D, Matz J, Weidinger E, et al. The association of infectious agents and schizophrenia. World J Biol Psychiatry. 2010;11:739–43.
78. Brown AS, Hooton J, Schaefer CA, et al. Elevated maternal interleukin-8 levels and risk of schizophrenia in adult offspring. Am J Psychiatry. 2004;161:889–95.
79. Meehan C, Harms L, Frost JD, et al. Effects of immune activation during early or late gestation on schizophrenia-related behaviour in adult rat offspring. Brain Behav Immun. 2017;63:8–20.
80. Brown AS, Schaefer CA, Wyatt RJ, et al. Maternal exposure to respiratory infections and adult schizophrenia spectrum disorders: a prospective birth cohort study. Schizophr Bull. 2000;26:287–95.
81. Metcalf SA, Jones PB, Nordstrom T, et al. Serum C-reactive protein in adolescence and risk of schizophrenia in adulthood: a prospective birth cohort study. Brain Behav Immun. 2017;59:253–9.
82. Benros ME, Nielsen PR, Nordentoft M, et al. Autoimmune diseases and severe infections as risk factors for schizophrenia: a 30-year population-based register study. Am J Psychiatry. 2011;168:1303–10.
83. Benros ME, Mortensen PB, Eaton WW. Autoimmune diseases and infections as risk factors for schizophrenia. Ann N Y Acad Sci. 2012;1262:56–66.
84. Gogtay N, Lu A, Leow AD, et al. Three-dimensional brain growth abnormalities in childhood-onset schizophrenia visualized by using tensor-based morphometry. Proc Natl Acad Sci U S A. 2008;105:15979–84.
85. Steen RG, Mull C, McClure R, et al. Brain volume in first-episode schizophrenia: systematic review and meta-analysis of magnetic resonance imaging studies. Br J Psychiatry. 2006;188:510–8.
86. Job DE, Whalley HC, McIntosh AM, et al. Grey matter changes can improve the prediction of schizophrenia in subjects at high risk. BMC Med. 2006;4:29.

87. Chakos MH, Schobel SA, Gu H, et al. Duration of illness and treatment effects on hippocampal volume in male patients with schizophrenia. Br J Psychiatry. 2005;186:26–31.
88. Ellman LM, Deicken RF, Vinogradov S, et al. Structural brain alterations in schizophrenia following fetal exposure to the inflammatory cytokine interleukin-8. Schizophr Res. 2010;121:46–54.
89. Meisenzahl EM, Rujescu D, Kirner A, et al. Association of an interleukin-1beta genetic polymorphism with altered brain structure in patients with schizophrenia. Am J Psychiatry. 2001;158:1316–9.
90. Filiou MD, Banati RB, Graeber MB. The 18-kDa translocator protein as a CNS drug target: finding our way through the neuroinflammation fog. CNS Neurol Disord Drug Targets. 2017;16:990–9.
91. Versijpt JJ, Dumont F, Van Laere KJ, et al. Assessment of neuroinflammation and microglial activation in Alzheimer's disease with radiolabelled PK11195 and single photon emission computed tomography. A pilot study. Eur Neurol. 2003;50:39–47.
92. van Berckel BN, Bossong MG, Boellaard R, et al. Microglia activation in recent-onset schizophrenia: a quantitative (R)-[11C]PK11195 positron emission tomography study. Biol Psychiatry. 2008;64:820–2.
93. Doorduin J, de Vries EF, Willemsen AT, et al. Neuroinflammation in schizophrenia-related psychosis: a PET study. J Nucl Med. 2009;50:1801–7.
94. Takano A, Arakawa R, Ito H, et al. Peripheral benzodiazepine receptors in patients with chronic schizophrenia: a PET study with [11C]DAA1106. Int J Neuropsychopharmacol. 2010;13:943–50.
95. Sommer IE, de Witte L, Begemann M, et al. Nonsteroidal anti-inflammatory drugs in schizophrenia: ready for practice or a good start? A meta-analysis. J Clin Psychiatry. 2012;73:414–9.
96. Laan W, Grobbee DE, Selten JP, et al. Adjuvant aspirin therapy reduces symptoms of schizophrenia spectrum disorders: results from a randomized, double-blind, placebo-controlled trial. J Clin Psychiatry. 2010;71:520–7.
97. Muller N, Riedel M, Scheppach C, et al. Beneficial antipsychotic effects of celecoxib add-on therapy compared to risperidone alone in schizophrenia. Am J Psychiatry. 2002;159:1029–34.
98. Muller N, Riedel M, Schwarz MJ, et al. Clinical effects of COX-2 inhibitors on cognition in schizophrenia. Eur Arch Psychiatry Clin Neurosci. 2005;255:149–51.
99. Müller N, Riedel M, Dehning S, et al. Is the therapeutic effect of celecoxib in schizophrenia depending from duration of disease? Neuropsychopharmacology. 2004;29:S176.
100. Muller N. Inflammation in schizophrenia: Pathogenetic aspects and therapeutic considerations. Schizophr Bull. 2018;44:973–82.
101. Müller N. Neuroprogression in schizophrenia and psychotic disorder: the possible role of inflammation. In: Halaris A, Leonard BE, editors. Neuroprogression in psychiatric disorders, Modern Trends Pharmacopsychiatry. Basel: Karger; 2017.
102. Muller N. COX-2 inhibitors as antidepressants and antipsychotics: clinical evidence. Curr Opin Investig Drugs. 2010;11:31–42.
103. Rapaport MH, Delrahim KK, Bresee CJ, et al. Celecoxib augmentation of continuously ill patients with schizophrenia. Biol Psychiatry. 2005;57:1594–6.
104. Nitta M, Kishimoto T, Muller N, et al. Adjunctive use of nonsteroidal anti-inflammatory drugs for schizophrenia: a meta-analytic investigation of randomized controlled trials. Schizophr Bull. 2013;39:1230–41.
105. Akhondzadeh S, Tabatabaee M, Amini H, et al. Celecoxib as adjunctive therapy in schizophrenia: a double-blind, randomized and placebo-controlled trial. Schizophr Res. 2007;90:179–85.
106. Lin A, Kenis G, Bignotti S, et al. The inflammatory response system in treatment-resistant schizophrenia: increased serum interleukin-6. Schizophr Res. 1998;32:9–15.
107. McAllister CG, van Kammen DP, Rehn TJ, et al. Increases in CSF levels of interleukin-2 in schizophrenia: effects of recurrence of psychosis and medication status. Am J Psychiatry. 1995;152:1291–7.

108. Mondelli V, Ciufolini S, Belvederi Murri M, et al. Cortisol and inflammatory biomarkers predict poor treatment response in first episode psychosis. Schizophr Bull. 2015;41:1162–70.
109. Zhang XY, Zhou DF, Cao LY, et al. Cortisol and cytokines in chronic and treatment-resistant patients with schizophrenia: association with psychopathology and response to antipsychotics. Neuropsychopharmacology. 2005;30:1532–8.
110. Abbasi SH, Hosseini F, Modabbernia A, et al. Effect of celecoxib add-on treatment on symptoms and serum IL-6 concentrations in patients with major depressive disorder: randomized double-blind placebo-controlled study. J Affect Disord. 2012;141:308–14.
111. Mizoguchi H, Takuma K, Fukakusa A, et al. Improvement by minocycline of methamphetamine-induced impairment of recognition memory in mice. Psychopharmacology (Berl). 2008;196:233–41.
112. Levkovitz Y, Mendlovich S, Riwkes S, et al. A double-blind, randomized study of minocycline for the treatment of negative and cognitive symptoms in early-phase schizophrenia. J Clin Psychiatry. 2010;71:138–49.
113. Chaudhry IB, Hallak J, Husain N, et al. Minocycline benefits negative symptoms in early schizophrenia: a randomised double-blind placebo-controlled clinical trial in patients on standard treatment. J Psychopharmacol. 2012;26:1185–93.
114. Ahuja N, Carroll BT. Possible anti-catatonic effects of minocycline in patients with schizophrenia. Prog Neuro-Psychopharmacol Biol Psychiatry. 2007;31:968–9.
115. Sommer IE, van Westrhenen R, Begemann MJ, et al. Efficacy of anti-inflammatory agents to improve symptoms in patients with schizophrenia: an update. Schizophr Bull. 2014;40:181–91.
116. Gruber L, Bunse T, Weidinger E, et al. Adjunctive recombinant human interferon gamma-1b for treatment-resistant schizophrenia in 2 patients. J Clin Psychiatry. 2014;75:1266–7.
117. Zaidi MR, Merlino G. The two faces of interferon-gamma in cancer. Clin Cancer Res. 2011;17:6118–24.
118. Miller BJ, Buckley PF. The case for adjunctive monoclonal antibody immunotherapy in schizophrenia. Psychiatr Clin North Am. 2016;39:187–98.

The Aberrant Immune System in Bipolar Disorder

15

Bartholomeus C. M. Haarman, Elissa L. Stam, Jenny Borkent, Magdalini Ioannou, and Hemmo A. Drexhage

15.1 Introduction

Bipolar disorder (BD) [1] is a mood disorder characterized by episodic pathologic disturbances in mood: (hypo)manic episodes and depressive episodes which alternate with euthymic periods, i.e., with normal mood. BD has to be distinguished from (unipolar) major depressive disorder (MDD), which is characterized by depressive episodes only.

According to DSM-5, the core criterion of a (hypo)manic episode is the occurrence of pathologic elated (euphoria), expansive or irritable mood and increased energy or activity lasting at least 1 week. In addition to these core criteria, there are other symptoms, of which three or more need to be present to a significant degree – namely, inflated self-esteem or grandiosity, decreased need for sleep, being more talkative than usual, flight of ideas, distractibility, increase in goal-directed activity

B. C. M. Haarman
Department of Psychiatry, University Medical Center Groningen, University of Groningen, Groningen, The Netherlands

Rob Giel Onderzoekscentrum, University of Groningen, Groningen, The Netherlands

Research School of Behavioural and Cognitive Neurosciences, University of Groningen, Groningen, The Netherlands
e-mail: b.c.m.haarman@umcg.nl

E. L. Stam · J. Borkent · M. Ioannou
Department of Psychiatry, University Medical Center Groningen, University of Groningen, Groningen, The Netherlands

Research School of Behavioural and Cognitive Neurosciences, University of Groningen, Groningen, The Netherlands
e-mail: e.l.stam@umcg.nl; j.borkent@umcg.nl; m.ioannou@umcg.nl

H. A. Drexhage (✉)
Department of Immunology, Erasmus MC, Rotterdam, The Netherlands
e-mail: h.drexhage@erasmusmc.nl

M. Berk et al. (eds.), *Immuno-Psychiatry*, https://doi.org/10.1007/978-3-030-71229-7_15

or psychomotor agitation, and excessive involvement in pleasurable activities that have a high potential for painful consequences. A depressive episode consists of at least one of the core symptoms: depressed mood and loss of interest or pleasure, completed with symptoms such as sleep problems, psychomotor changes, fatigue or loss of energy, feelings of worthlessness or excessive feelings of guilt, difficulty concentrating or making decisions, and recurrent thoughts of death [1].

Two types of BD are recognized: bipolar I disorder (BD-I) and bipolar II disorder (BD-II). Both types are characterized by the occurrence of extreme high and low mood episodes. Their main difference is the severity of manic episodes. Patients with BD-I experience full-blown manic episode(s), while BD-II patients experience only hypomanic episode(s). Manic, depressive, and mixed episodes can also be complicated by the presence of concurrent psychotic symptoms. Besides the mood symptoms, many patients with BD also show cognitive dysfunctions which may persist during euthymic periods, and which involve disturbances in various domains such as attention, verbal memory, and executive functioning [2, 3].

Worldwide, BD affects about 45 million people [4]. The lifetime prevalence of BD is about 2% across different countries, women being affected as frequently as men [5, 6]. Across the world, the disorder ranks sixth among all health conditions in terms of causing disability [7] with poor clinical and functional outcome [8], increased risk for suicidality [9], and significant societal costs [10].

Historically, treatment options for MDD, schizophrenia and partly BD, have focused on medications that modify the activity of monoamine neurotransmitter systems (i.e., dopamine, serotonin, and noradrenalin systems). Monoamines do play a role in the pathophysiology of these disorders, but the monoaminergic theory of illness has failed to deliver novel agents beyond the limited treatment options currently available.

The aim of this chapter is to provide an overview of various perspectives of the aberrant immune system in BD in light of the search of new therapy options. Nationwide epidemiologic analyses established a link between autoimmune liability, lifetime infections, psychosocial factors, and the presences of psychiatric disorders [11]. The "macrophage theory of mood disorders" postulates an aberrant pro-inflammatory state of monocytes/macrophages in patients with mood disorder and considers this aberrant state of the cells as a driving force behind the illness [12]. The theory was founded on the discovery in the 1980s and 1990s of increased serum or plasma levels of pro-inflammatory macrophage and T cell cytokines in patients. Also raised frequencies of auto-immune diseases and various T cell abnormalities were found in patients with BD [13], together with an aberrant expression of pro-inflammatory genes in circulating monocytes [11]. Moreover, although genome studies have linked BD to hundreds of variations, the stronger associations were found in the MHC immune region, such as the rs3130297 SNP, located in the NOTCH4 gene29.

The aberrant immune system is thought to have its effect on BD illness progression, via the tryptophan catabolic pathway and via glial cells, such as microglia and oligodendrocytes [14]. Therapeutic interventions targeting the immune system directly have thus far been mainly focused on non-steroid anti-inflammatory drugs

(NSAID), omega-3-fatty acids, and N-acetylcysteine (NAC) [15]. More recently, scientific attention has been given to the gut-brain-axis in BD, with emphasis on increased intestinal permeability and microbiome disturbances driving immune system dysregulation [16]. Based on the research that is becoming more extensive and global, this field seems promising for potential treatment options.

15.2 The Aberrant Immune System

15.2.1 Pro-Inflammatory Cytokines

The discovery of the various signal compounds (cytokines and growth factors) between the cells of the immune system in the 1980s and 1990s of the last century and the development of easy detection ELISA methods for their determination in serum and plasma made it possible to carry out extensive investigations to, e.g., interleukin (IL)-1β, IL-6, tumor necrosis factor (TNF)-α, their receptors, and BDNF in mood disorders. Increased levels were found in BD patients when compared to controls, although not in all studies [17, 18]. Initially, these seemingly contradicting results were not well understood. In 2018 Rowland et al. performed an extensive meta-analysis of cytokines, neurotrophins, and oxidative stress mediators in BD, including 53 studies comprising more than two thousand cases and controls. In this meta-analysis, a combination of high-sensitivity C-reactive protein (hsCRP)/IL-6, brain-derived neurotrophic factor (BDNF)/TNF-α, and soluble TNF-α receptor 1 (sTNFR1) alterations was found to be associated with specific mood phases in BD [19]. During depression BDNF and TNF-α were found to be decreased, while sTNFR1 and hsCRP/IL-6 were found to be normal. In euthymia hsCRP/IL6 were increased, while sTNFR1, TNF-α, and BDNF were found to be normal. During mania hsCRP/IL-6 remained high as in euthymia, but sTNFR1 and TNF-α were also increased; BDNF was decreased in mania. Apparently, the activity and phase of the disease is a determinant for alterations in the cytokine and growth factor serum levels.

It is also important to consider that aberrations in cytokine concentrations are a cross-diagnostic feature of severe mental illnesses, demonstrated by a recent meta-analysis [20]. In this analysis, comparing cytokine profiles in patients with schizophrenia, BD and MDD, manifest alterations in blood cytokine levels were demonstrated, which are consistent with an inflammatory and T-cell activation profile shared between the mental illnesses.

15.2.2 Autoimmune Thyroiditis

Considering the cytokine profile consistent with an inflammatory profile, it is not surprising that patients with BD have a raised prevalence of autoimmune diseases. We here focus as an example on Hashimoto's autoimmune thyroiditis [21–23], also because this is a frequent autoimmune complication of BD. Autoimmune thyroiditis is a chronic disease in which the body interprets components of the thyroid gland such as thyroid peroxidase (TPO) and thyroglobulin (Tg) as foreign (non-self). The body therefore mounts a specific destructive immune reaction toward its own thyroid cells. Although the attack is primarily orchestrated by inflammatory and cytotoxic T cells, the body also produces antibodies to TPO and Tg, which are used as easy-to-determine serum markers of the disease [24]. Autoimmune thyroiditis is considered an endophenotype of BD [13]. Not only BD patients but also their offspring (affected as well as non-affected) and their monozygotic (affected and non-affected) and dizygotic (affected, but not as much unaffected) co-twins have a raised prevalence of autoimmune thyroiditis [13, 25]. The intrinsic disturbances of monocytes and T cells in BD patients and their first degree family members are thought to be instrumental in the higher prevalence of autoimmune thyroiditis.

15.2.3 Monocyte Inflammatory Gene Expression

Stemming from the increased prevalence of autoimmune thyroiditis, it was hypothesized that an activated inflammatory response system in monocytes constitutes the shared susceptibility factor for both BD and thyroid autoimmunity. To investigate the pro-inflammatory state of monocytes in a more precise and robust manner, a quantitative polymerase chain reaction (q-PCR) analysis of purified monocytes was performed in which a signature of 22 discriminative mRNAs for inflammatory, chemokinesis/motility, cell survival/apoptosis, and mitogen-activated protein kinases (MAPKs) pathway molecules was detected and found to be increased in expression in monocytes in BD patients compared to that in controls [26]. In a subsequent study, this increased gene expression was found to be only present during mood episodes and not or hardly during euthymia [27]. The inflammation-related signature was also found to be associated with increased psychomotor symptoms [28]. In a follow-up study on well-controlled and euthymic relatively old bipolar patients, the inflammatory signature was even found to be decreased in expression in the patient monocytes, while a vascular repair factor (HGF) was found increased. This profile of gene expression is reminiscent of that of the vascular repair monocytes (so-called circulating angiogenic cells) seen in atherosclerotic disease and fitted well with the high prevalence of the metabolic syndrome seen in this relatively older patient group. Atherosclerotic diseases are nowadays also considered as partly belonging to the group of auto-inflammatory conditions.

15.2.4 T Lymphocytes

Important regulators of the inflammatory response are not only the cells belonging to the myeloid lineage (e.g., the monocytes, macrophages, and dendritic cells), but also the cells of the lymphoid lineage of the immune system (e.g., the different sets of T cells). T cells are generated in the thymus and all T cell are positive for an antigen-specific CD3+ T cell receptor. The CD3+ T cell population differentiates in the thymus into either the CD8+ T cytotoxic cells (with the capacity to kill, e.g., virus-infected cells and cancer cells) or CD4+ T helper cells (with the capacity to help other immune cells functioning). In the last decades, it was discovered that the latter CD4+ T helper population contains cells with the capacity to develop into 4 main types of T helper cells: the Th1 cells with the capacity to produce pro-inflammatory IFN-γ, the Th2 cells with the capacity to produce the anti-inflammatory, but B cell stimulating cytokine IL-4, the Th17 cells which produce IL-17, and the T regulatory cells which dampen all sorts of inflammatory responses by virtue of their production of IL-10 and TGF-β.

In BD, the different sets of T cells and T helper cells have not been examined as extensively as in MDD. However, many of the studies carried out by us on different cohorts have found slightly reduced levels of the total population of CD3+ T cells in euthymic BD patients [29], their children at risk for BD, and in affected and non-affected co-twins of BD patients [30]. In the latter group, the slight reduction in the total population of circulating CD3+ T cells was found to be associated with the familial liability to develop BD.

Despite these reduced levels of total T cells, a higher activation state (as measured by strong CD25 positivity) of the T cells has been demonstrated in both euthymic and symptomatic BD patients, compared to healthy controls [31]. We consider this activation as a compensatory reaction to counteract the slight T cell deficiency state of BD patients. Also circulating levels of T helper cells were found to be higher in euthymic BD as compared to healthy controls, but in particular to patients with active MDD [32]. Other investigators examining subpopulations of T cells also found reduced levels of T cells (particularly of T cytotoxic cells), but again in the presence of higher percentage of activated ($CD25^+$) T helper cells. In older euthymic BD patients, we found higher levels of IL-4-producing Th2 and IL-17-producing Th17 cells [29], and we again interpreted these findings of a higher production reactivity of the cells as a compensation for the reduced number of total T cells. With regard to children of a bipolar parent who are at risk for BD, we found next to the earlier mentioned slight reduction in T cells in general, an age-dependent change in the levels of the Th1, Th2, Th17, and T regulator populations [30]: In the bipolar offspring Th1, Th2, Th17, and the T regulatory cells followed a dynamic course over time with significantly reduced levels of Tregs in adolescence and reduced numbers of Th1 and Th17 cells in young adulthood. In post hoc analysis, the T regulatory cells were inversely associated with the pro-inflammatory monocyte state, which also occurred in adolescence in bipolar offspring irrespective of current psychopathology [33].

With regard to the T regulatory cell population, reduced percentages have in general been described in BD: Barbosa et al. described a lower percentage of IL-10 expressing T regulatory cells [34] and del Prado et al. also found lower levels of T regulatory cells in BD patients as compared to healthy controls [35]. We found the T regulatory cells to be dependent on age and significantly higher T regulatory cells were only found in BD patients under 40 years of age as compared to healthy controls; this was not the case in BD patients of over 40 years of age [36].

15.2.5 Conclusion on the Aberrant Immune System

Taken together, the immune system findings suggest a basic slight numerical T cell deficiency in BD patients irrespective of the phase of the disease and associated with the familial liability to develop BD in twins and offspring. Despite this numerical deficiency (or better probably due to the numerical deficiency), there are signs of a higher functional activation of the T system (high CD25 expression) and the capacity of T helper cells to produce higher levels of particularly IL-17 and IL-4. T regulatory cells are in general found to be reduced in BD patients, opening the gateway to a higher inflammatory state. We indeed found an inverse relationship of the level of T regulatory cells and the monocyte inflammatory state. However, it must be noted that age dependency, particularly also at teenage time, plays an important role in fluctuations of the populations of functional T helper cells and chronic monocyte inflammation patterns. The latter occurred particularly during active phases of the disease, something that has also been noted for the pro-inflammatory cytokine levels in serum and in plasma (Fig. 15.1).

15.3 Tryptophan Metabolism as an Intermediary Mechanism

Abnormal interactions between the immune system and the HPA-axis, as well as abnormal interactions between the immune system and the neuronal system acting via tryptophan catabolites and interacting with glial cells, have been suggested to result in mood disorder symptomatology.

In the tryptophan breakdown, several enzymes are of importance. Tryptophan hydroxylase is the enzyme that metabolizes the amino acid tryptophan down the pathway to the neurotransmitters serotonin and melatonin; both monoamines play an important role in emotion regulation and cognition. In addition, tryptophan is also metabolized down the kynurenine pathway via an alternative route. Two enzymes play a role in the first and rate-limiting step in this oxidative degradation of tryptophan to kynurenine: indoleamine-pyrrole 2,3-dioxygenase (IDO) and tryptophan 2,3-dioxygenase (TDO). IDO is particularly expressed in monocytes/macrophages and the IDO activity is enhanced by pro-inflammatory cytokines, e.g., by IFN-α, during viral infections. TDO is expressed in the liver and TDO activity is enhanced when there is physical or mental stress [37]. Under mentioned circumstances, tryptophan breakdown along the kynurenine branch is increased, while the availability of tryptophan for serotonin synthesis is decreased. Along the kynurenine pathway, tryptophan is first metabolized into kynurenine [38]. Subsequently, kynurenine is broken down via (1) a neuroprotective, kynurenic acid, NMDA receptor antagonist pathway, or (2) a neurotoxic, 3-hydroxy kynurenine, and quinolinic acid, NMDA receptor agonist pathway [39]. In the brain, the catabolism occurs in the astrocytes and microglia, where astrocytes produce mainly neuroprotective kynurenic acid while macrophages produce mainly neurotoxic metabolites, like quinolinic acid. Normally, formation of quinolinic acid is faster, while kynurenic acid has a counteractive protective role against quinolinic acid [40]. Based on the above, it

A MODEL OF THE DYNAMIC IMMUNE PATHOGENESIS OF BIPOLAR DISORDER

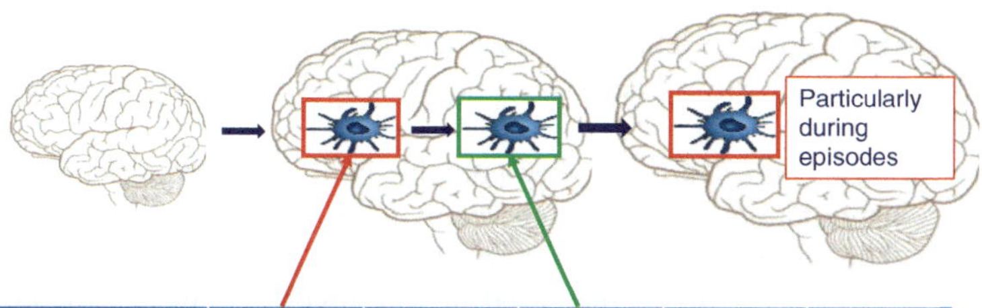

	17 years	21 years	28 years	30-50 years	> 50 years
	Euthymic children of a bipolar parent			Bipolar patients	
Tendency to monocytosis/lymphopenia, especially shortage of CD3+ T cells and CD3+CD4+T helper cells	+	+	+	+	+
CD3+ CD4+ CD25+ FOXP3+ T regulatory cells and serum sCD25 levels	decreased	normal	normal	increased in age >40 years	increased
CD3+ CD4+ IL17+ T cells	normal	decreased	normal	increased	increased
Pro-inflammatory monocyte genes	increased	slightly increased	normal	increased in episodes	decreased, increased in episodes
Serum CCL2 levels	normal	increased	increased	increased	not tested
Pro-inflammatory serum compounds (PTX3, hsCRP and IL-6)	increased	increased	not tested	increased, particularly in episodes	not tested

Fig. 15.1 The figure shows the immune aberrancies found in the peripheral blood mononuclear cell (PBMC) preparations of the bipolar or bipolar-related cohorts studied in the EU-MOODINFLAME studies. These cohorts comprise established bipolar patients, but also euthymic offspring of a bipolar parent who are at high risk to develop bipolar disorder. Remarkable are the dynamic changes over time in the cell-mediated immune system, and we assume that these changes are driven by inborn abnormalities, environmental (microbial, stress) influences, and aging of the immune system. See for details text and listed references. In all bipolar (related) subjects, we found a tendency to have reduced percentages of circulating lymphocytes, particularly of CD3+ T cells and CD3+ CD4+ T helper cells (with increased percentages of monocytes). In a twin study this reduced percentage of CD3+ T cells was found to be associated with the familial inborn liability to develop bipolar disorder. We assume that this minor T cell defect has an influence on hippocampal neogenesis and mood regulation, since T cells are known to be essential for these processes. Within the reduced T and T helper cell populations, we found in the offspring a proneness to have reduced T regulatory cells at adolescence. These low T regulatory cells correlated to a high pro-inflammatory state, as measured by a high expression of inflammatory genes in circulating monocytes and high serum inflammatory compounds at that age. We assume that at that time (adolescence) also the microglia is pro-inflammatory activated in the offspring, and has negative effects on hippocampal development and function. As time passes into adulthood in the offspring, the pro-inflammatory aberrancies largely disappear and normalize in the bipolar offspring, yet the CD3+ T cell lymphopenia remains. In episodic bipolar patients (and in postpartum mood disorders), pro-inflammatory aberrancies are clearly evident (monocyte gene expression, circulating serum inflammatory compounds), against the background of the minor CD3+ T cell lymphopenia. It is tempting to speculate that environmental microbial influences (alterations in the microbioma?) trigger the pro-inflammatory state in individuals with a proneness to develop bipolar disorder, such as the bipolar offspring. In the euthymic phases of bipolar patients the minor CD3+ T cell abnormalities stayed visible, while we found an abnormal apportioning of the T helper cell subsets (high T regulatory cells, high Th17 cells). We assume that the high T regulatory cells represent a controlled inflammatory state, and although high Th17 cells are present, pro-inflammatory monocytes were not present in the euthymic phase. Even an anti-inflammatory pro-angiogenic state of monocytes was found in senior bipolar patients with a high prevalence of the metabolic syndrome; we assume that this depended on the vascular problems occurring in these older bipolar patients

was hypothesized that an imbalance between the neurodegenerative and neuroprotective pathways leads to neurodegeneration and brings a person to a chronically depressive episode. This imbalance might either be due to a highly increased neurodegenerative pathway activity or due to a lack of sufficient neuroprotective factor activity [41].

Several studies have shown an involvement of the tryptophan to kynurenine pathway degradation in BD, which seems to be shifted toward its neurotoxic branch [42]. The plasma kynurenine/tryptophan ratio, defined as the tryptophan breakdown index, was found to be increased in BD, together with a reduction of the plasma kynurenic acid concentration, thus decreasing its neuroprotective effects [43]. More recently, similar data of decreased kynurenic acid levels were reported in a BD sample compared to healthy volunteers [44]. Finally, kynurenine breakdown has also been related to white matter microstructure in BD. In particular, BD patients show reduced concentrations of kynurenic acid and 5-Hydroxyindoleacetic acid (5-HIAA), a measure of serotonin levels. This was positively associated with diffusion tensor imaging (DTI) measures of white matter integrity [45].

15.4 Immune System and Glial Cell Aberrations

Neuroglia, consisting of glial cells, are the other predominant portion of the brain, next to neurons [46]. Glial cells were long thought to be mainly of use as structural supportive cells for the neurons, holding them in place, supplying them with nutrients and oxygen, and destroying pathogens. However, starting at the turn of the century, research demonstrated glial cells to have important functions in neurodevelopment and synaptic function [47, 48] and they are now known to be important regulators of neuroimmune interactions in the central nervous system [14, 49].

The glial cell population consists mainly of oligodendroglia, astrocytes, and microglia. In humans, astrocytes perform a multitude of functions such as, but not limited to, providing metabolic support as a lactate and glycogen energy buffer, vasomodulation by regulating blood flow [50], promoting myelinating activity of oligodendroglia [51, 52], regulating nervous system repair [53], facilitating long-term memory potentiation [54], and several kinds of signal transmission modulation, including modulation of synaptic transmission [55] and regulation of ion concentration in the extracellular space [56].

Microglia are the resident macrophages of the brain and spinal cord and thus act as the first and main form of active immune defense in the CNS, constantly scavenging the CNS for plaques, damaged neurons, and infectious agents. Besides functions relating to the immunoresponse, microglia play an important role in maintaining homeostasis. As with peripheral macrophages, microglial activation could be in an inflammatory sense (M1 macrophages), an anti-inflammatory sense (M2 macrophages), and a regenerating/tissue support sense (M2b macrophages). Animal models demonstrated that microglia are also involved in tissue regeneration and play an active role in neuronal support, i.e., the development of mature synapses during embryogenesis [57], pruning synapses postnatally [58], regulating neurogenesis [59], and inducing apoptosis [11]. It may well be the case that some microglial cells induce apoptosis, while others actively facilitate neurogenesis.

Activation of microglia has been studied in PET imaging studies, with tracers binding to the translocator protein (TSPO, previously known as peripheral benzodiazepine receptor (PBR)), since TSPO expression has been associated with a pro-inflammatory state [60]. Current tracers used to visualize TSPO expression are [^{11}C]PK11195, [^{11}C]-PBR28 and [^{18}F]-FEPPA.

In psychotic disorders, an increase in microglia activation was demonstrated after a first psychotic episode [61]. During a psychotic episode, this inflammation was found to "condense" in the hippocampus [62]. The first TSPO study in MDD, using [^{11}C]-PBR28, did not demonstrate an increase in binding between 10 MDD patients and 10 healthy controls [63]. However, subsequent studies, including studies with [^{11}C]-PBR28 and [^{18}F]-FEPPA, demonstrated microglia activation quite robustly in MDD patients, with varying duration of illness and age [64–66]. Interestingly, treatment with antidepressants and cognitive behavioral therapy had an ameliorating effect on this activation [67, 68].

With regard to BD, increased [^{11}C]PK11195 binding has been demonstrated in the hippocampus of 14 euthymic BD type I patients, compared to 11 healthy controls [69].

The immune system may also exert its effect on the brain via oligodendrocytes. Oligodendroglia create myelin sheaths around neuronal axons for support and to increase the axonal transmission speed. In addition they provide trophic support by producing glial cell line-derived neurotrophic factor (GDNF), brain-derived neurotrophic factor (BDNF), and insulin-like growth factor-1 (IGF-1) [70]. Oligodendrocyte function can be visualized in vivo using DTI. Using this technique, microstructural white matter aberrations involving all the major tracts have been demonstrated quite robustly in BD [71, 72]. Kynurenine catabolites, produced by cells of the immune system and derived from the serotonin precursor tryptophan, are known to affect oligodendrocyte function in vitro and inflammation-related cytokines, such as TNF-α, IFN-ɣ, and IL-10, have been found to be inversely associated with DTI-measured white matter microstructural integrity [73].

15.5 Potential Immune-Mediating Treatment Strategies

Randomized controlled trails (RCTs) investigating celecoxib, a cyclooxygenase-2 (COX-2) inhibiting non-steroidal anti-inflammatory drug (NSAID), demonstrated positive effects in BD. In BD, improvement of manic [74] and depressive symptoms was found [74–76]. In schizophrenia, treatment with this medication yielded improvement of positive symptomatology (hallucinations, delusions), negative symptomatology (passivity, apathy), and generally improved functioning [77]. These transdiagnostic and multi-dimensional effects of celecoxib support a common immune pathway model for severe mental illnesses and indicate that treatments, influencing the immune system, hold promise.

Omega-3 fatty acids have been extensively investigated for their antidepressant effects, but have failed to show overall treatment effectiveness in a meta-analysis [15]. Add-on treatment using N-acetyl cysteine, a glutathione precursor antioxidant, initially showed success for alleviating depression in BD [78]; however, a follow-up study failed to demonstrate a significant effect as maintenance treatment [79] and a recent replication study also was not able to show benefit over placebo [80].

Treatment with aspirin has also been suggested to be beneficial in BD. In a study testing the efficacy of aspirin and minocycline as an augmentation therapy for bipolar depression [81], a main effect of aspirin on depressive symptoms was observed. In a large pharmaco-epidemiological study related to BD [82], in which medication histories on subjects who had been prescribed lithium were collected using health care registry data, low-dose aspirin was found to be associated with a reduction in the relative risk of clinical deterioration in subjects, whereas other NSAIDs and glucocorticoids did not. In another study assessing the effect of 240 mg of aspirin on lithium-related sexual dysfunction [83], patients in the aspirin group showed significantly greater improvement in total sexual function scores than the placebo group (14.4% and 19.7% improvement respectively), while mood symptoms remained stable over the course of the study. However, to date no RCT has been performed investigating the direct effect of aspirin on mood symptoms or mood stability.

15.6 The Gut-Brain Axis

Recent investigations have pointed to the gut-brain axis as a new target for treatment to affect brain functioning in a significant subset of patients [84]. In this approach the chronic low-grade inflammation stems from increased intestinal permeability, associated with gut microbiome disturbances.

Recently, two papers elaborately reviewed the evidence for the contribution of increased intestinal permeability to the pathophysiology of BD in this rapidly developing field of research [84, 85]. Numerous studies have reported that BD patients have abnormal reactions to food-derived antigens, indicative of increased intestinal permeability. In support of this view, BD patients were also found to have elevated serum concentrations of immunoglobulin G (IgG) to gliadin and deamidated gliadin in comparison to controls [86]. In a follow-up study, patients with manic symptoms had increased baseline IgG to gliadin, which normalized after 6 months of treatment [87]. In the same study, re-hospitalized patients during a 6-month follow-up period were more likely to have increased IgG to gliadin at the beginning of the follow-up.

It has been hypothesized that BD can originate from early exposure to microbial infections, contributing to the etiology, through chronic neuro-inflammatory and autoimmune processes [88]. *Anti-Saccharomyces cervisiae* IgG antibodies (ASCA), typically increased in Crohn's disease or ulcerative colitis, is a marker of intestinal inflammation. Patients with BD were found to have increased levels of ASCA along with IgG to casein and gluten, and ASCA correlated with IgG to these food antigens compared to controls [89]. ASCA also correlated to IgG to *T. gondii* and measles in patients who experienced a recent onset of psychosis in the course of BD.

It is also interesting that an imbalance of the intestinal microbiota is associated with BD [90], as this may offer a non-invasive and relatively simple strategy to improve symptoms and the condition of the brain. One study found that a lower abundance of a strain of *Faecalibacterium* was associated with improved physical health, better depression scores, and sleep quality scores, thereby providing support for the hypothesis that targeting the microbiome may be an effective treatment paradigm for BD [91]. Another study also found a decrease in abundance of *Faecalibacterium* in the BD group in comparison to non-psychiatric subjects [92]. Besides this, investigators found a decrease in abundance in *Ruminococcaceae* and both the phylum *Actinobacteria* and the class *Coriobacteria* as significantly more abundant in BD patients as compared to healthy controls.

Coello et al. [93] found that not only the gut microbiota composition of BD patients but also that of their unaffected first-degree relatives differed from that of healthy controls. This observation is interesting in the light of the slight T cell deficiencies also found in unaffected first degree relatives of BD patients (see before) and the monocyte inflammatory gene activation in first degree relatives (twins) linked to common environmental influences [94].

As described above, increased intestinal permeability causes translocation of bacterial material and food-derived antigens. The translocation of these substances results in hyper-activation of the intestinal immune response through the interaction of, e.g., lipopolysaccharides (LPS), glycolipids derived from the outer membrane of gram-negative bacteria, with toll-like receptor 4 (TLR4) in immune cells, e.g., monocytes/macrophages. This interaction with the TLR4 activates the inflammatory NFkB pathway, over-production of pro-inflammatory cytokines, and disruption of the tryptophan catabolic pathway with a reduction of levels of serotonin [84]. Moreover, hyper-activation of the intestinal immune system may also result in the activation of the hypothalamic–pituitary–adrenal (HPA) axis, which in addition has a direct implication on BD [95].

In a large study in humans with schizophrenia and BD, *C. albicans* seropositivity was associated with gastro-intestinal (GI) disturbances as well as cognitive deficits [96]. In a study in patients with diabetes mellitus type 2, probiotics were found to cause a decrease in LPS and CRP, and a positive effect on cardiometabolic profile [97, 98]. In another study in postmenopausal women, a similar cardiometabolic effect was found [99].

Given the accumulating evidence for abnormal immune responses which are seen in BD patients, and the observation that the intestinal epithelial barrier and intestinal microbiota can play a role in both diseases, probiotic therapy can be viewed as a promising candidate for treatment in these patients [90, 100]. Probiotics were associated with a significantly lower rate of re-hospitalization in 66 patients [101]. The probiotic's effect was increased in individuals with elevated levels of systemic inflammation at baseline based on IgG class antibodies to the NR2 peptide fragment of the NMDA receptor, IgG class antibodies to gliadin, IgG class antibodies to the Mason-Pfizer monkey virus gag protein, and IgM class antibodies to

Toxoplasma gondii. In another recent study, a significant improvement in performance concerning attention and psychomotor processing speed was found in BD patients, supporting the hypothesis that probiotic might be beneficial to improve cognitive functioning [102].

Summarizing, in multiple studies increased intestinal permeability in BD has been demonstrated by translocation of food and bacterial antigens, as well as intestinal microbiome disturbances. These aberrancies are associated with a dysregulation of the immune system and the precipitation and exacerbation of psychiatric symptomatology, metabolic complications, and increased cognitive impairment.

15.7 Concluding Remarks

Over the last few decades, insight in the immune disturbances associated with BD has expanded greatly. Starting off with serological and epidemiological studies, molecular biological and imaging techniques have elucidated various aspects of the aberrant immune system, encompassing alterations in serum cytokines, chemokines, and tryptophan catabolites, alterations in the T cell and monocyte/macrophage-mediated immune reactions, and the cerebral processes linked to these immune and biochemical alterations. However, studies remain typically small in size and cross-sectional in design, complicating the exploration of these dynamic processes in detail and over time, and larger multi-modal longitudinal studies are needed.

New treatment approaches targeting the immune system directly or indirectly, via the gut, have also emerged, although limited in size and number, compared to pharmaceutical company–driven trials. Effect sizes of existing studies are typically not more than modest, and this is probably attenuated by general study methodologies on heterogeneous patient groups. A more personalized treatment approach toward the status of the immune state is a promising strategy to increase the impact of immune system targeting medication, while keeping adverse effects acceptable.

References

1. American Psychiatric Association. Diagnostic and statistical manual of mental disorders. 5th ed. Arlington, VA: American Psychiatric Publishing, Inc.; 2013.
2. Arts B, Jabben N, Krabbendam L, van Os J. Meta-analyses of cognitive functioning in euthymic bipolar patients and their first-degree relatives. Psychol Med. 2008;38:771–85.
3. Bora E, Yucel M, Pantelis C. Cognitive endophenotypes of bipolar disorder: a meta-analysis of neuropsychological deficits in euthymic patients and their first-degree relatives. J Affect Disord. 2009;113:1–20.
4. James SL, Abate D, Abate KH, Abay SM, Abbafati C, Abbasi N, et al. Global, regional, and national incidence, prevalence, and years lived with disability for 354 diseases and injuries for 195 countries and territories, 1990-2017: a systematic analysis for the global burden of disease study 2017. Lancet. 2018;392:1789–858.
5. Pini S, de Queiroz V, Pagnin D, Pezawas L, Angst J, Cassano GB, et al. Prevalence and burden of bipolar disorders in European countries. Eur Neuropsychopharmacol. 2005;15:425–34.

6. Merikangas KR, Jin R, He J-P, Kessler RC, Lee S, Sampson NA, et al. Prevalence and correlates of bipolar spectrum disorder in the world mental health survey initiative. Arch Gen Psychiatry. 2011;68:241.
7. World Health Organization. The world health report 2001: mental health : new understanding, new hope. Geneva, Switzerland: World Health; 2001.
8. Goodwin FK. Manic-depressive illness: bipolar disorders and recurrent depression. 2nd ed. New York: Oxford University Press; 2007.
9. Baldessarini RJ, Tondo L. Suicide risk and treatments for patients with bipolar disorder. JAMA. 2003;290:1517–9.
10. Begley CE, Annegers JF, Swann AC, Lewis C, Coan S, Schnapp WB, et al. The lifetime cost of bipolar disorder in the US: an estimate for new cases in 1998. PharmacoEconomics. 2001;19:483–95.
11. Beumer W, Gibney SM, Drexhage RC, Pont-Lezica L, Doorduin J, Klein HC, et al. The immune theory of psychiatric diseases: a key role for activated microglia and circulating monocytes. J Leukoc Biol. 2012;92:1–17.
12. Smith RSS. The macrophage theory of depression. Med Hypotheses. 1991;35:298–306.
13. Vonk R, van der Schot AC, Kahn RS. Nolen WA, Drexhage HA. Is autoimmune thyroiditis part of the genetic vulnerability (or an endophenotype) for bipolar disorder? Biol Psychiatry. 2007;62:135–40.
14. Haarman BCM, Riemersma-Van der Lek RF, Burger H, Drexhage HA, Nolen WA. The dysregulated brain: consequences of spatial and temporal brain complexity for bipolar disorder pathophysiology and diagnosis. Bipolar Disord. 2016;18:696–701.
15. Rosenblat JD, Cha DS, Mansur RB, McIntyre RS. Inflamed moods: a review of the interactions between inflammation and mood disorders. Prog Neuro-Psychopharmacol Biol Psychiatry. 2014;53:23–34.
16. Genedi M, Janmaat IE, Haarman BBCM, Sommer IEC. Dysregulation of the gut–brain axis in schizophrenia and bipolar disorder. Curr Opin Psychiatry. 2019;32:185–95.
17. O'Brien SM, Scully P, Scott LV, Dinan TG. Cytokine profiles in bipolar affective disorder: focus on acutely ill patients. J Affect Disord. 2006;90:263–7.
18. Hoekstra R, Fekkes D, Pepplinkhuizen L, Loonen AJM, Tuinier S, Verhoeven WMA. Nitric oxide and neopterin in bipolar affective disorder. Neuropsychobiology. 2006;54:75–81.
19. Rowland T, Perry BI, Upthegrove R, Barnes N, Chatterjee J, Gallacher D, Marwaha S. Neurotrophins, cytokines, oxidative stress mediators and mood state in bipolar disorder: systematic review and meta-analyses. Br J Psychiatry. 2018;213:514–25.
20. Goldsmith DR, Rapaport MH, Miller BJ. A meta-analysis of blood cytokine network alterations in psychiatric patients: comparisons between schizophrenia, bipolar disorder and depression. Mol Psychiatry. 2016;21:1696–709.
21. Bunevicius R, Peceliuniene J, Mickuviene N, Bunevicius A, Pop VJ, Girdler SS. Mood and thyroid immunity assessed by ultrasonographic imaging in a primary health care. J Affect Disord. 2007;97:85–90.
22. Carta MG, Loviselli A, Hardoy MC, Massa S, Cadeddu M, Sardu C, et al. The link between thyroid autoimmunity (antithyroid peroxidase autoantibodies) with anxiety and mood disorders in the community: a field of interest for public health in the future. BMC Psychiatry. 2004;4:25.
23. Benros ME, Waltoft BL, Nordentoft M, Ostergaard SD, Eaton WW, Krogh J, et al. Autoimmune diseases and severe infections as risk factors for mood disorders: a nationwide study. JAMA Psychiat. 2013;70:812–20.
24. Dayan CM, Daniels GH. Chronic autoimmune thyroiditis. N Engl J Med. 1996;335:99–107.
25. Hillegers MH, Reichart CG, Wals M, Verhulst FC, Ormel J, Nolen WA. Five-year prospective outcome of psychopathology in the adolescent offspring of bipolar parents. Bipolar Disord. 2005;7:344–50.
26. Padmos RC, Hillegers MHJ, Knijff EM, Vonk R, Bouvy A, Staal FJT, et al. A discriminating messenger RNA signature for bipolar disorder formed by an aberrant expression of inflammatory genes in monocytes. Arch Gen Psychiatry. 2008;65:395–407.

27. Becking K, Haarman BCM, van der Lek RFR, Grosse L, Nolen WA, Claes S, et al. Inflammatory monocyte gene expression: trait or state marker in bipolar disorder? Int J Bipolar Disord. 2015;3:20.
28. Haarman BCM, Riemersma-Van der Lek RF, Burger H, Netkova M, Drexhage RC, Bootsman F, et al. Relationship between clinical features and inflammation-related monocyte gene expression in bipolar disorder - towards a better understanding of psychoimmunological interactions. Bipolar Disord. 2014;16:137–50.
29. Vogels RJ, Koenders MA, van Rossum EFC, Spijker AT, Drexhage HA. T cell deficits and overexpression of hepatocyte growth factor in anti-inflammatory circulating monocytes of middle-aged patients with bipolar disorder characterized by a high prevalence of the metabolic syndrome. Front Psych. 2017;8:34.
30. Snijders G, Brouwer R, Kemner S, Bootsman F, Drexhage HA, Hillegers MHJ. Genetic and environmental influences on circulating NK and T cells and their relation to bipolar disorder. Int J Bipolar Disord. 2019;7:1–7.
31. Breunis MN, Kupka RW, Nolen WA, Suppes T, Denicoff KD, Leverich GS, et al. High numbers of circulating activated T cells and raised levels of serum IL-2 receptor in bipolar disorder. Biol Psychiatry. 2003;53:157–65.
32. Becking K, Haarman BCM, Grosse L, Nolen WA, Claes S, Arolt V, et al. The circulating levels of CD4+ t helper cells are higher in bipolar disorder as compared to major depressive disorder. J Neuroimmunol. 2018;319:28–36.
33. Mesman E, Hillegers MH, Ambree O, Arolt V, Nolen WA, Drexhage HA. Monocyte activation, brain-derived neurotrophic factor (BDNF), and S100B in bipolar offspring: a follow-up study from adolescence into adulthood. Bipolar Disord. 2014;17:39–49.
34. Barbosa IG, Machado-Vieira R, Soares JC, Teixeira AL. The immunology of bipolar disorder. Neuroimmunomodulation. 2014;21:117–22.
35. Hartmann do Prado C, Rizzo LB, Wieck A, Lopes RP, Teixeira AL, Grassi-Oliveira R, et al. Reduced regulatory T cells are associated with higher levels of Th1/TH17 cytokines and activated MAPK in type 1 bipolar disorder. Psychoneuroendocrinology. 2013;38:667–76.
36. Drexhage RC, Hoogenboezem TH, Versnel MA, Berghout A, Nolen WA, Drexhage HA. The activation of monocyte and T cell networks in patients with bipolar disorder. Brain Behav Immun. 2011;25:1206–13.
37. Babcock TA, Carlin JM. Transcriptional activation of indoleamine dioxygenase by interleukin 1 and tumor necrosis factor alpha in interferon-treated epithelial cells. Cytokine. 2000;12:588–94.
38. Bender DA, McCreanor GM. Kynurenine hydroxylase: a potential rate-limiting enzyme in tryptophan metabolism. Biochem Soc Trans. 1985;13:441–3.
39. Chiarugi A, Calvani M, Meli E, Traggiai E, Moroni F. Synthesis and release of neurotoxic kynurenine metabolites by human monocyte-derived macrophages. J Neuroimmunol. 2001;120:190–8.
40. Perkins MN, Stone TW. An iontophoretic investigation of the actions of convulsant kynurenines and their interaction with the endogenous excitant quinolinic acid. Brain Res. 1982;247:184–7.
41. Myint AM, Kim YK. Cytokine-serotonin interaction through IDO: a neurodegeneration hypothesis of depression. Med Hypotheses. 2003;61:519–25.
42. Erhardt S, Schwieler L, Imbeault S, Engberg G. The kynurenine pathway in schizophrenia and bipolar disorder. Neuropharmacology. 2017;112:297–306.
43. Myint AM, Kim Y-K, Verkerk R, Park SH, Scharpé S, Steinbusch HWM, et al. Tryptophan breakdown pathway in bipolar mania. J Affect Disord. 2007;102:65–72.
44. Birner A, Platzer M, Bengesser SA, Dalkner N, Fellendorf FT, Queissner R, et al. Increased breakdown of kynurenine towards its neurotoxic branch in bipolar disorder. PLoS One. 2017;12:e0172699.
45. Poletti S, Bollettini I, Melloni E, Dallaspezia S, Benedetti F. White matter microstructure in bipolar disorder changes after antidepressant treatment with total sleep deprivation. Eur Neuropsychopharmacol. 2015;25:S425.

46. Virchow R. Die cellularpathologie in ihrer begründung auf physiologische und pathologische gewebelehre. Berlin: Hirschwald; 1858.
47. Nadarajah B, Brunstrom JE, Grutzendler J, Wong RO, Pearlman AL. Two modes of radial migration in early development of the cerebral cortex. Nat Neurosci. 2001;4:143–50.
48. Araque A, Parpura V, Sanzgiri RP, Haydon PG. Tripartite synapses: glia, the unacknowledged partner. Trends Neurosci. 1999;22:208–15.
49. Antel JP, Becher B, Ludwin SK, Prat A, Quintana FJ. Glial cells as regulators of neuroimmune interactions in the central nervous system. J Immunol. 2020;204:251–5.
50. Parri R, Crunelli V. An astrocyte bridge from synapse to blood flow. Nat Neurosci. 2003;6:5–6.
51. Ishibashi T, Dakin KA, Stevens B, Lee PR, Kozlov SV, Stewart CL, et al. Astrocytes promote myelination in response to electrical impulses. Neuron. 2006;49:823–32.
52. Bartzokis G. Neuroglialpharmacology: myelination as a shared mechanism of action of psychotropic treatments. Neuropharmacology. 2012;62:2137–53.
53. Sofroniew MV. Reactive astrocytes in neural repair and protection. Neuroscientist. 2005;11:400–7.
54. Han X, Chen M, Wang F, Windrem M, Wang S, Shanz S, et al. Forebrain engraftment by human glial progenitor cells enhances synaptic plasticity and learning in adult mice. Cell Stem Cell. 2013;12:342–53.
55. Piet R, Vargová L, Syková E, Poulain DA, Oliet SHR. Physiological contribution of the astrocytic environment of neurons to intersynaptic crosstalk. Proc Natl Acad Sci U S A. 2004;101:2151–5.
56. Walz W. Role of astrocytes in the clearance of excess extracellular potassium. Neurochem Int. 2000;36:291–300.
57. Paolicelli RC, Bolasco G, Pagani F, Maggi L, Scianni M, Panzanelli P, et al. Synaptic pruning by microglia is necessary for normal brain development. Science. 2011;333:1456–8.
58. Schafer DP, Lehrman EK, Kautzman AG, Koyama R, Mardinly AR, Yamasaki R, et al. Microglia sculpt postnatal neural circuits in an activity and complement-dependent manner. Neuron. 2012;74:691–705.
59. Sierra A, Encinas JM, Deudero JJP, Chancey JH, Enikolopov G, Overstreet-Wadiche LS, et al. Microglia shape adult hippocampal neurogenesis through apoptosis-coupled phagocytosis. Cell Stem Cell. 2010;7:483–95.
60. Doorduin J, de Vries EFJ, Dierckx RA, Klein HC. PET imaging of the peripheral benzodiazepine receptor: monitoring disease progression and therapy response in neurodegenerative disorders. Curr Pharm Des. 2008;14:3297–315.
61. van Berckel BN, Bossong MG, Boellaard R, Kloet R, Schuitemaker A, Caspers E, et al. Microglia activation in recent-onset schizophrenia: a quantitative (R)-[11C]PK11195 positron emission tomography study. Biol Psychiatry. 2008;64:820–2.
62. Doorduin J, de Vries EFJ, Willemsen ATM, de Groot JC, Dierckx RA, Klein HC. Neuroinflammation in schizophrenia-related psychosis: a PET study. J Nucl Med. 2009;50:1801–7.
63. Hannestad J, DellaGioia N, Gallezot J-D, Lim K, Nabulsi N, Esterlis I, et al. The neuroinflammation marker translocator protein is not elevated in individuals with mild-to-moderate depression: a [^{11}C]PBR28 PET study. Brain Behav Immun. 2013;33:131–8.
64. Setiawan E, Wilson AA, Mizrahi R, Rusjan PM, Miler L, Rajkowska G, et al. Role of translocator protein density, a marker of neuroinflammation, in the brain during major depressive episodes. JAMA Psychiat. 2015;72:268–7.
65. Holmes SE, Hinz R, Conen S, Gregory CJ, Matthews JC, Anton-Rodriguez JM, et al. Elevated translocator protein in anterior cingulate in major depression and a role for inflammation in suicidal thinking: a positron emission tomography study. Biol Psychiatry. 2018;83:61–9.
66. Li H, Sagar AP, Kéri S. Microglial markers in the frontal cortex are related to cognitive dysfunctions in major depressive disorder. J Affect Disord. 2018;241:305–10.
67. Setiawan E, Attwells S, Wilson AA, Mizrahi R, Rusjan PM, Miler L, et al. Association of translocator protein total distribution volume with duration of untreated major depressive disorder: a cross-sectional study. Lancet Psychiatry. 2018;5:339–47.

68. Li H, Sagar AP, Kéri S. Translocator protein (18 kDa TSPO) binding, a marker of microglia, is reduced in major depression during cognitive-behavioral therapy. Prog Neuro-Psychopharmacol Biol Psychiatry. 2018;83:1–7.
69. Haarman BCMB, Riemersma-Van der Lek RF, de Groot JC, Ruhé HGE, Klein HC, Zandstra TE, et al. Neuroinflammation in bipolar disorder - a [(11)C]-(R)-PK11195 positron emission tomography study. Brain Behav Immun. 2014;40:219–25.
70. Bradl M, Lassmann H. Oligodendrocytes: biology and pathology. Acta Neuropathol. 2010;119:37–53.
71. Duarte JA, De Araújo e Silva JQ, Goldani AA, Massuda R, Gama CS. Neurobiological underpinnings of bipolar disorder focusing on findings of diffusion tensor imaging: a systematic review. Rev Bras Psiquiatr. 2016;38:167–75.
72. Haarman BCMB, Riemersma-Van Der Lek RF, Burger H, de Groot JC, Drexhage HA, Nolen WA, et al. Diffusion tensor imaging in euthymic bipolar disorder - a tract-based spatial statistics study. J Affect Disord. 2016;203:281–91.
73. Benedetti F, Poletti S, Hoogenboezem TA, Mazza E, Ambrée O, de Wit H, et al. Inflammatory cytokines influence measures of white matter integrity in bipolar disorder. J Affect Disord. 2016;202:1–9.
74. Mousavi SY, Khezri R, Karkhaneh-Yousefi M-A, Mohammadinejad P, Gholamian F, Mohammadi MR, et al. A randomized, double-blind placebo-controlled trial on effectiveness and safety of celecoxib adjunctive therapy in adolescents with acute bipolar mania. J Child Adolesc Psychopharmacol. 2017;27:494–500.
75. Nery FG, Monkul ES, Hatch JP, Fonseca M, Frey N, Bowden CL, et al. Celecoxib as an adjunct in the treatment of depressive or mixed episodes of bipolar disorder: a double-blind, randomized , placebo-controlled study. Hum Psychopharmacol Clin Exp. 2008;23:87–94.
76. Edberg D, Hoppensteadt D, Walborn A, Fareed J, Sinacore J, Halaris A. Plasma C-reactive protein levels in bipolar depression during cyclooxygenase-2 inhibitor combination treatment. J Psychiatr Res. 2018;102:1–7.
77. Zheng W, Cai D-B, Yang X-H, Ungvari GS, Ng CH, Müller N, et al. Adjunctive celecoxib for schizophrenia: a meta-analysis of randomized, double-blind, placebo-controlled trials. J Psychiatr Res. 2017;92:139–46.
78. Berk M, Copolov DL, Dean O, Lu K, Jeavons S, Schapkaitz I, et al. N-acetyl cysteine for depressive symptoms in bipolar disorder-A double-blind randomized placebo-controlled trial. Biol Psychiatry. 2008;64:468–75.
79. Berk M, Dean O, Cotton SM, Gama CS, Kapczinski F, Fernandes BS, et al. The efficacy of N-acetylcysteine as an adjunctive treatment in bipolar depression: an open label trial. J Affect Disord. 2011;135:389–94.
80. Ellegaard PK, Licht RW, Nielsen RE, Dean OM, Berk M, Poulsen HE, et al. The efficacy of adjunctive N-acetylcysteine in acute bipolar depression: a randomized placebo-controlled study. J Affect Disord. 2019;245:1043–51.
81. Savitz JB, Teague TK, Misaki M, Macaluso M, Wurfel BE, Meyer M, et al. Treatment of bipolar depression with minocycline and/or aspirin: an adaptive, 2×2 double-blind, randomized, placebo-controlled, phase IIA clinical trial. Transl Psychiatry. 2018;8:27.
82. Stolk P, Souverein PC, Wilting I, Leufkens HGM, Klein DF, Rapoport SI, et al. Is aspirin useful in patients on lithium? A pharmacoepidemiological study related to bipolar disorder. Prostaglandins Leukot Essent Fatty Acids. 2010;82:9–14.
83. Saroukhani S, Emami-Parsa M, Modabbernia A, Ashrafi M, Farokhnia M, Hajiaghaee R, et al. Aspirin for treatment of lithium-associated sexual dysfunction in men: randomized double-blind placebo-controlled study. Bipolar Disord. 2013;15:650–6.
84. Rudzki L, Szulc A. "Immune gate" of psychopathology-the role of gut derived immune activation in major psychiatric disorders. Front Psych. 2018;9:205.
85. Nguyen TT, Kosciolek T, Maldonado Y, Daly RE, Martin AS, Mcdonald D, et al. Differences in gut microbiome composition between persons with chronic schizophrenia and healthy comparison subjects. Schizophr Res. 2019;204:23–9.

86. Dickerson F, Stallings C, Origoni A, Vaughan C, Khushalani S, Alaedini A, et al. Markers of gluten sensitivity and celiac disease in bipolar disorder. Bipolar Disord. 2011;13:52–8.
87. Dickerson F, Stallings C, Origoni A, Vaughan C, Khushalani S, Yolken R. Markers of gluten sensitivity in acute mania: a longitudinal study. Psychiatry Res. 2012;196:68–71.
88. Yolken RH, Torrey EF. Are some cases of psychosis caused by microbial agents? A review of the evidence. Mol Psychiatry. 2008;13:470–9.
89. Severance EG, Gressitt KL, Yang S, Stallings CR, Origoni AE, Vaughan C, et al. Seroreactive marker for inflammatory bowel disease and associations with antibodies to dietary proteins in bipolar disorder. Bipolar Disord. 2014;16:230–40.
90. Dickerson F, Severance E, Yolken R. The microbiome, immunity, and schizophrenia and bipolar disorder. Brain Behav Immun. 2017;62:46–52.
91. Evans SJ, Bassis CM, Hein R, Assari S, Flowers SA, Kelly MB, et al. The gut microbiome composition associates with bipolar disorder and illness severity. J Psychiatr Res. 2017;87:23–9.
92. Painold A, Mörkl S, Kashofer K, Halwachs B, Dalkner N, Bengesser S, et al. A step ahead: exploring the gut microbiota in inpatients with bipolar disorder during a depressive episode. Bipolar Disord. 2019;21:40–9.
93. Coello K, Hansen TH, Sørensen N, Munkholm K, Kessing LV, Pedersen O, et al. Gut microbiota composition in patients with newly diagnosed bipolar disorder and their unaffected first-degree relatives. Brain Behav Immun. 2018;75:112–8.
94. Padmos RC, Van Baeal GCM, Vonk R, Wijkhuijs AJM, Kahn RS, Nolen WA, et al. Genetic and environmental influences on pro-inflammatory monocytes in bipolar disorder: a twin study. Arch Gen Psychiatry. 2009;66:957–65.
95. Belvederi Murri M, Prestia D, Mondelli V, Pariante C, Patti S, Olivieri B, et al. The HPA axis in bipolar disorder: systematic review and meta-analysis. Psychoneuroendocrinology. 2016;63:327–42.
96. Severance EG, Gressitt KL, Stallings CR, Katsafanas E, Schweinfurth LA, Savage CL, et al. Candida albicans exposures, sex specificity and cognitive deficits in schizophrenia and bipolar disorder. NPJ Schizophr. 2016;2:1–7.
97. Sabico S, Al-Mashharawi A, Al-Daghri NM, Yakout S, Alnaami AM, Alokail MS, et al. Effects of a multi-strain probiotic supplement for 12 weeks in circulating endotoxin levels and cardiometabolic profiles of medication naïve T2DM patients: a randomized clinical trial. J Transl Med. 2017;15:1–9.
98. Sabico S, Al-Mashharawi A, Al-Daghri NM, Wani K, Amer OE, Hussain DS, et al. Effects of a 6-month multi-strain probiotics supplementation in endotoxemic, inflammatory and cardiometabolic status of T2DM patients: a randomized, double-blind, placebo-controlled trial. Clin Nutr. 2018;38:1561–9.
99. Szulińska M, Łoniewski I, van Hemert S, Sobieska M, Bogdański P. Dose-dependent effects of multispecies probiotic supplementation on the lipopolysaccharide (LPS) level and cardiometabolic profile in obese postmenopausal women: a 12-week randomized clinical trial. Nutrients. 2018;10:773.
100. Nguyen TT, Kosciolek T, Eyler LT, Knight R, Jeste DV. Overview and systematic review of studies of microbiome in schizophrenia and bipolar disorder. J Psychiatr Res. 2018;99:50–61.
101. Dickerson F, Adamos M, Katsafanas E, Khushalani S, Origoni A, Savage C, et al. Adjunctive probiotic microorganisms to prevent rehospitalization in patients with acute mania: a randomized controlled trial. Bipolar Disord. 2018;20:1–8.
102. Reininghaus EZ, Wetzlmair L-C, Fellendorf FT, Platzer M, Queissner R, Birner A, et al. The impact of probiotic supplements on cognitive parameters in euthymic individuals with bipolar disorder: a pilot study. Neuropsychobiology. 2018;79:1–8.

Inflammation and Depression: Is Immunometabolism the Missing Link?

16

Robert Dantzer, Angela Casaril, and Elisabeth Vichaya

16.1 Introduction

The first experimental investigations of a role of inflammation in depression originated from the observation of the marked similarity between the clinical signs of sickness behavior and the symptoms of depression. The concept of sickness behavior encompasses how individuals sick with an infection behave. As pointed out by Yirmiya et al. at the time, "infectious illnesses are often associated with a range of depressive symptoms, including fatigue, psychomotor retardation, anorexia, somnolence, lethargy, muscle aches, cognitive disturbances and depressed mood" [1]. They went on to demonstrate that these behavioral alterations could be reproduced by administration of the cytokine inducer lipopolysaccharide (LPS) or pro-inflammatory cytokines such as interleukin (IL)-1. It was then observed that they are attenuated for some of them by chronic antidepressant treatment. It did not take long for the concept of depression as a brain inflammatory disease to emerge, encouraged by the observation of increased circulating levels of biomarkers of inflammation in depression, an observation originally reported by Maes et al. [2]. Twenty years later, the rest could be history except that the mechanisms by which inflammation induces depression have not yet revealed all their secrets. Preclinical studies conducted on rodent models of inflammation induced by the activation of the innate immune system or by stressors such as chronic unpredictable stress and repeated social defeat have vastly

R. Dantzer (✉)
Laboratories of Neuroimmunology, Department of Symptom Research, The University of Texas MD Anderson Cancer Center, Houston, TX, USA
e-mail: rdantzer@mdanderson.org

A. Casaril
Neurobiotechnology Research Group, Federal University of Pelotas, Pelotas, Rio Grande do Sul, Brazil

E. Vichaya
Department of Psychology & Neuroscience, Baylor University, Waco, TX, USA

M. Berk et al. (eds.), *Immuno-Psychiatry*, https://doi.org/10.1007/978-3-030-71229-7_16

contributed to our understanding of some of the pathways responsible for the development of depressive symptoms in the context of systemic or central inflammation. The multiple routes of communication involved in the propagation of inflammation from the periphery to the brain have been elucidated with a particular emphasis on neural afferents and endothelial cytokine receptors. At the behavioral level, it has been possible to identify the main features of inflammation-induced depressive symptoms and to show the relative importance of fatigue and reduced motivation in the behavioral phenotype of inflammation. At the cellular level, the pivotal role of reactive microglial cells in the brain inflammatory response to peripheral inflammation and their possible modulation by immune cells trafficking into the brain parenchyma in response to chronic stress have been evidenced. Further knowledge on the reciprocal interactions of microglia with other brain cell types including endothelial cells, astrocytes, oligodendrocytes, and neurons has been slowly emerging. At the molecular level, the main cytokines that induce depressive symptoms and their receptor signaling mechanisms have been identified. At the neurochemical level, inflammation has been demonstrated to interfere with brain neurotransmission and in particular to down-regulate dopaminergic neurotransmission and activate glutamatergic neurotransmission. However, all of this still has proven to be insufficient to drive novel drug therapies for inflammatory-liked depression, suggesting something—possibly in plain sight—is still missing.

Inflammation-induced depression does not develop *ex nihilo*. It slowly emerges on a background of symptoms of sickness represented by fatigue, sleep disorder, and reduced appetite [3]. These symptoms are still present in depressed patients with a low-grade inflammation and are part of the somatic symptoms of depression. In all the enthusiasm that has built up since the discovery of the profound behavioral effects of immune activation, we seem to have forgotten how inflammation-induced sickness behavior contributes to the reorganization of the organism's priorities in face of an infectious agent. The initial description of sickness behavior insisted on the adaptive value of this response to infection with regard to the necessity of sparing energy metabolism for allowing a full development of the fever response and meeting the energy requirements of immune cell proliferation [4]. The fitness-enhancing value of sickness behavior for the infected individual and the population in which it belongs has received considerable interest in the field of ecoimmunology [5–7]. However, with very rare exceptions [8] it has totally escaped the attention of biological psychiatrists who have been more interested in finding out how inflammation intersects with classical neurotransmitters, despite the limitations of the monoaminergic theory of depression.

An obvious question not sufficiently addressed by immunopsychiatry is: how does the energy-demanding process of inflammation affect brain function when this peripheral process propagates to the brain? In line with a Jacksonian perspective of brain functions during disease, the dissolution induced by the inflammatory process will first impact the higher mental processes before impacting the lower levels of sensory-motor processing [9]. Translated in the language of network analysis of human brain connectivity, highly structured brain hubs with rich elements of neural architecture that are characterized by expensive energy consumption will be more likely to be affected than less expensive "small world" networks in which information flows along short communication paths. How this corresponds to the major alterations in the brain connectome reported in major depressive disorder (MDD) remains to be determined. Based on a meta-analysis of resting-state functional connectivity [10], MDD appears to be characterized by hypoconnectivity within the frontoparietal network that is involved in cognitive control of attention and emotion, the dorsal attention network that is involved in attention to the external environment, the neural systems that are involved in processing emotional salience, and the midline cortical regions that mediate the top-down regulation of these functions. In contrast, there is hyperconnectivity within the default network that supports internally oriented and self-referential thought processes. These findings have been interpreted to suggest that MDD cognitive and affective symptoms are the result of an imbalanced connectivity among networks involved in regulating attention to the external versus the internal world together with a reduced connectivity between networks involved in regulating and responding to emotion or salience. It would certainly be interesting to determine whether this pattern of connectivity is a feature of a conserved mode of energy for the brain of an inflamed organism that has to process information arising from physiological changes within the body [11, 12] while having, at the same time, limited resources to do so. While all these issues remain to be addressed, important progress has been made at the mechanistic level as the reasons for the high metabolic cost associated with the inflammatory response have been elucidated at the molecular level. A new research field known as immunometabolism has emerged at the intersection between immunology and metabolism during the last decade, and it provides a new perspective on the relationship between inflammation and depression.

In this chapter we will first describe what we have learned from immunometabolism before examining the evidence for a relationship between immunometabolism and MDD and discussing possible neuronal networks involved in metabolic sensing and regulation of mood.

16.2 An Introduction to Immunometabolism

The field of inflammation has seen three successive waves of research. The first wave focused on the cellular aspects of inflammation. As inflammation is characterized by migration of leukocytes to the site of inflammation, it was important to understand (1) the mechanisms that allow this migration including vasodilatation and increased permeability of endothelial cells and (2) the characteristics of migratory leukocytes and their role at different stages of the inflammatory response. The second wave focused on the molecular events that are necessary to coordinate the different stages of the inflammatory response by allowing subsets of leukocytes to communicate between themselves and with other cell types, including endothelial cells. This second wave benefited from progress in molecular biology and the ability to produce relatively large quantities of recombinant proteins for in vitro and in vivo experiments using engineered strains of *Escherichia coli*. This research led to the functional characterization of cellular communication molecules and their receptors. The molecular factors allowing immune cells to communicate with each other within the immune system were initially labeled as interleukins. However, their pleiotropic activity and in particular their ability to act outside the immune system on non-immune cells quickly led to a shift to the more general term: cytokines. This wave of research is still very active as new cytokines are still being discovered and their signaling mechanisms are not yet fully elucidated. An important outcome of this second wave is the replacement of the morphological description of the different subsets of inflammatory cells by their functional profiling, which is based on the cytokines they produce. The third wave of research has emerged only recently. It builds on the observation that the proliferation of innate immune cells at the site of inflammation and their engagement in the production and release of multiple communication signals require a reprogramming of their energy metabolism from oxidative phosphorylation to aerobic glycolysis.

Oxidative phosphorylation is an important part of the cellular respiration process by which cells use oxygen to metabolize nutrients. This process takes place in the mitochondria and involves a series of multiple enzymatic steps allowing the transport of electrons across the inner mitochondrial membrane. Oxidative phosphorylation generates energy that is ultimately used by adenosine triphosphate (ATP) synthase to phosphorylate adenosine diphosphate (ADP) into ATP. The amount of energy released by oxidative phosphorylation is high in that it produces 36 molecules of ATP for one molecule of glucose converted to carbon dioxide and water and 14 ATP for each cycle of beta-oxidation of fatty acids.

This is in sharp contrast to glycolysis that occurs in the cytosol and converts one molecule of glucose into two molecules of pyruvate and H+. The amount of energy released by glycolysis generates only 2 ATP. Pyruvate needs to be decarboxylated to enter the Krebs cycle in the form of acetyl-coenzyme A. As the Krebs cycle takes place in the mitochondrial matrix, this requires the transport of pyruvate from the cytosol across the inner mitochondrial membrane. The problem with glycolysis is that it consumes NAD+ that is reduced into NADH. The easiest way to regenerate NAD+ is to oxidize NADH. However, this requires the conversion of pyruvate into lactate. This process produces 2 more ATP. The advantage of glycolysis is that it is much faster than oxidative phosphorylation. However, it cannot be sustained for long. This is what takes place for instance in skeletal muscles during a short, intense exercise. Lactate accumulation does not occur as the liver takes up excess lactate to convert it back into pyruvate and glucose via gluconeogenesis. Glucose can then be fed back to the muscles. The problem for this metabolic pathway is that it consumes 6 ATP for only 2 ATP gained from glycolysis, which results in a net consumption of 4 ATP per molecule of glucose.

Although glycolysis has mainly been studied in anaerobic conditions with reference to fermentation, interest in this metabolic pathway has surged recently in cancer biology based on the observation that glycolysis is the main metabolic pathway used by rapidly proliferating tumor cells. The German scientist Otto Warburg was the first to describe the ability of tumor cells to rely on glycolysis rather than on oxidative phosphorylation even in the presence of oxygen. He got the Nobel Prize in physiology in 1931 for his work. The so-called Warburg effect was originally proposed to be due to mitochondrial defect in cancer cells. The advantage of aerobic glycolysis over oxidative phosphorylation is that it facilitates the uptake and incorporation of nutrients (mainly glucose and glutamine) into the biomass, in a manner conducive to cell proliferation [13]. However, this is usually not ensured by mitochondrial deficiency as originally proposed by Warburg but by gain-of-function mutations in enzymes of the glycolytic pathway. Whether the Warburg effect takes place in cancer cells or in supporting cells of the tumor microenvironment such as stromal fibroblasts that can in this way feed lactate and other energy-rich nutrients directly to cancer cells leading to the reverse Warburg effect is still a matter of controversy.

Aerobic glycolysis is not restricted to cancer cells. Immune responses and wound repair also require a rapid proliferation of effector cells as the time factor becomes critical when microorganisms invade the body via breakage of the skin or epithelial barriers. The ability of immune stimuli to cause metabolic reprogramming of immune and non-immune cells has become a major focus of immunometabolism research [14]. Aerobic glycolysis has been found to be crucial for the ability of macrophages to engage in phagocytosis and production of pro-inflammatory cytokines. It is also necessary for the functioning of natural killer cells, Th1, Th2, and Th17 cells, as well as regulatory T cells. The link between metabolism and the phenotype of immune cells is so important that it is possible to switch macrophages from a pro-inflammatory phenotype to an anti-inflammatory phenotype just by blocking glycolysis and re-initiating the Krebs cycle. Like macrophages, microglia increase aerobic glycolysis and decrease oxidative phosphorylation when activated [15]. In both macrophages and microglia, the predominance of glycolysis over oxidative phosphorylation should not be seen as absolute. During macrophage activation the Krebs cycle is rewired rather than inhibited [16]. This results in the accumulation of the Krebs cycle intermediates succinate and citrate, and Krebs cycle-derived metabolite itaconate. These immunometabolites have important immune modulatory activities on their own. In addition, the electron transport chain becomes altered during macrophage activation and generates radical oxygen species from Complexes I and III.

The main limitation of these recent developments in immunometabolism is that they are based on the results of in vitro studies, which makes the generalization of these results to in vivo conditions difficult. A few ex vivo studies based on isolation of microglia from inflammatory brains of mice and humans have confirmed that microglia activation is associated with increased glycolysis [17, 18]. Conversely, attenuation of microglia activation by exercise in aged mice was found to decrease the glycolytic capacity of microglia [19]. Another important limitation is the absence of data on the impact of immunometabolism on neighboring organs. In the context of cancer, the metabolic reprogramming that fosters tumor cell proliferation has been proposed to extend to other organs including liver, fat tissue, and skeletal muscles as complementary sources of nutrients for rapidly developing tumors. This is at the origin of the cancer metabolism syndrome which culminates in cachexia [20]. Futile cycles that regulate handling of energy substrates between and within organs play an important role in this process [21]. For instance, the high levels of lactate produced by metabolically active tumors enter the hepatic Cori cycle for reconversion into glucose that is avidly taken up by tumor cells. This hepatic gluconeogenesis can also be fueled in part by amino acids derived from skeletal muscle protein degradation. Even when oxidative phosphorylation continues to take place, its efficacy can be compromised due to proton leak across the mitochondrial inner membrane caused by changes in content and fatty acid composition of the major phospholipid constituent of the mitochondrial inner membrane cardiolipin [22]. Recruitment of metabolically active organs by the tumor can take place via different modalities, including cancer metabolites such as lactate, cytokines (e.g., IL-6 and TNFα, but also MIC-1/GDF15, a transforming growth factor-beta superfamily cytokine), danger signals such as high-motility group box 1, and tumor produced factors such as activins and parathormone-related peptide. Similar mechanisms are likely to take place in the context of chronic inflammation with the important difference that the original inflammatory response can propagate from the initial organ or body site to other parts of the body including the brain, giving rise to systemic inflammation.

Although this section is focused on what is known concerning the metabolic aspects of inflammation, it is important to examine how the effects of inflammation are modulated by glucocorticoids in view of the potent metabolic effects of glucocorticoids and the intricate interactions between pro-inflammatory cytokines and the hypothalamic pituitary-adrenal (HPA) axis [23]. Pro-inflammatory cytokines activate the HPA axis by acting centrally whereas glucocorticoids released by the adrenal cortex are classically seen as having potent immunosuppressive properties. However, there is also evidence that glucocorticoids can enhance inflammation and immunity. Whether an immunosuppressive or an immunoenhancing effect is observed depends on both the levels of glucocorticoids—immunosuppressive effects are observed at high doses of glucocorticoids—and the temporal relation between the event that triggers HPA axis activation and the one at the origin of inflammation. In rodents, stress occurring before LPS enhances the inflammatory response whereas a decrease is observed when the glucocorticoid response takes place after the stressor. In terms of metabolism, the stress response is well known to be associated with a catecholamine-dependent increase in glucose production and use followed by a glucocorticoid-dependent increased gluconeogenesis from proteins and lipids. Glucocorticoids inhibit glucose uptake and utilization in peripheral tissues such as the liver and muscles [24] by inducing insulin resistance, allowing in this way more glucose to be available to the brain. In addition to these effects, non-genomic actions of glucocorticoids on mitochondrial respiration, calcium mobilization, and apoptosis have been described more recently in neurons [25]. These actions involve the translocation of glucocorticoid receptors into mitochondria and their modulation of mitochondrial genome. In response to acute stress, glucocorticoids enhance mitochondrial function to provide cells with more energy while the organism tries to cope with stressors. Glucocorticoid receptors form a complex with the anti-apoptotic protein B-cell-lymphoma (Bcl-2) and translocate into mitochondria of neurons [25]. This results in upregulation of mitochondrial calcium levels, membrane potential, and oxidation. In contrast, chronically elevated levels of glucocorticoids reduce expression of the glucocorticoid receptor and Bcl-2, with an opposite action to that of acute glucocorticoids on mitochondrial calcium levels, membrane potential, and oxidation.

At the whole organism level, the way the brain can efficiently compete for limited energy resources with the rest of the organism has been debated. According to the selfish brain theory, the brain maintains constant fluxes of large amounts of glucose to itself by regulating food intake and glucose allocation via ATP-sensitive potassium channels that function as "energy sensors" by coupling bioenergetic metabolism to membrane excitability [26]. The possibility that this trade-off between the brain energetic requirements and those of the rest of the body is so much compromised by chronic inflammation that it can result in the development of symptoms of depression has been presented already [27] at the same time as the metabolic programs associated with inflammation have been better delineated [28]. However, a critical assessment of this conceptualization requires both a minimum understanding of brain metabolism and the consideration of the evidence in favor of a role for metabolic dysfunction in depression. In the next section we will examine how the energy requirements of the brain are met and review the evidence for an involvement of metabolic dysregulation in depression.

16.3 Evidence for Metabolic Dysregulation in Major Depressive Disorder

16.3.1 Brain Metabolism

Glucose is the major oxidative fuel for the brain [29]. The brain is also able to oxidize fatty acids and amino acids, but these compounds make minor contribution to brain metabolism compared to glucose. In resting conditions, glucose oxidation provides most of the ATP consumed by the brain. However, when the brain is activated, glucose consumption increases much more than oxygen consumption, and this is made possible by a switch of brain metabolism from oxidative phosphorylation to aerobic glycolysis. Neuronal signaling accounts for most of the energy expense of the brain (about 70%) while nonsignaling activities account for the remainder. In particular, the ionic pump Na+,K + -ATPase consumes about 50% of the brain's ATP. Excitatory neurotransmission is much more expensive, accounting for 80–85% of brain ATP usage, compared to the expenses of inhibitory neurotransmission and baseline glial activity, which only account for a combined 15–20% of brain ATP. As such, gray matter has a much higher metabolic rate than white matter. Astrocytes have high oxidative capacity, similar to neurons, but their importance in glucose oxidation is limited due to their smaller volume fraction. Despite its high oxidative capacity, the brain preferentially uses glycolysis rather than oxygen consumption to sustain most of its function when activated. As pointed out by Dienel, "although the brain is a highly oxidative organ, it preferentially upregulates nonoxidative metabolism of glucose during activation" [29]. Not surprisingly the brain is highly sensitive to glucose availability as evidenced by the rapid degradation of brain functions that culminates in coma in response to hypoglycemia. Aerobic glycolysis involves three major pathways: (1) glycolysis with lactate production; (2) the pentose phosphate shunt which is an important pathway for the generation of NADPH, ribose-5-phosphate, a precursor for the synthesis of nucleotides, and erythrose-4-phospate, a precursor for the synthesis of aromatic amino acids. Increased pentose shunt activity is likely a response to oxidative stress; (3) astrocytic glycogen turnover made possible by the storage of glucose as glycogen in astrocytes. In the brain glycogen is not just a storage depot. Glycogen turnover plays an essential role in sensory processing, memory, and neurotransmission even in the presence of normal glucose levels. In particular, glycogen appears to be part of the carbohydrates consumed during neuronal activation.

There has been some controversy about the cellular site at which glycolysis takes place with brain activation. The astrocyte-to-neuron lactate shuttle proposes that glutamate released by neurons induces glycolysis in astrocytes that results in lactate shuttling to neurons where it is converted into pyruvate before entering the Krebs cycle [30]. However, this model has been challenged based on the observation that neurons upregulate glycolysis more than oxidation when activated and release lactate, rather than being fueled by extracellular lactate from astrocytic origin [31]. This increase in neuronal glycolysis would allow neurons to meet the increased energy demands of neuronal activation. Lactate produced by glycolytic neurons would then be taken up by astrocytes which help with dispersing and clearing it from the brain [32]. Of note, lactate is not a waste product as it has various signaling functions in the brain, including its ability to increase blood flow and to downregulate neuronal activity. Astrocytes have high oxidation capacity that is primarily used with the glutamate/GABA-glutamine shuttle which allows neurons to synthesize glutamate and GABA from astrocytic glutamate- and GABA-derived glutamine. This metabolic flux captures about 80% of glucose oxidation in glutamatergic neurons. The synthesis of glutamate in neurons requires the phosphate-activated glutaminase that is a mitochondrial enzyme. In addition, it requires cell-to-cell transfer of ammonia as the formation of glutamate from glutamine in neurons releases ammonium that is needed by astrocytes to form glutamine from glutamate [33, 34].

16.3.2 Preclinical Evidence for a Relationship Between Depression and Mitochondrial Dysfunction

A role for mitochondrial dysfunction in the pathophysiology of depression can be deduced from the examination of the negative impact of inflammation and stress on mitochondrial function and from intervention studies targeting metabolic factors. Most studies in the field are essentially correlative. For instance, mice treated with low doses of LPS display reduced maximum oxygen consumption in their hippocampus 3 h later and increased levels of the inhibitory neurotransmitter GABA, as measured by proton magnetic resonance spectroscopy [35]. In the same manner, induction of sickness behavior by the administration of LPS at the dose of 0.1 mg/kg increased glycolytic fluxes in the hippocampus 6 h later as measured by the mRNA expression of two key glycolytic enzymes (6-phosphofructo-2-kinase/fructose-2,6-biphosphatase 3 [*Pfkfb3*] and hexokinase 2 [*Hk2*]) in the hippocampus of mice and reduced levels of pyruvate and oxaloacetate [36].

Rats submitted to repeated immobilization stress for 21 days were found to display decreased activities of complexes I to III of the electron transport chain in the brain [37]. These alterations are not the same depending on the model and the brain areas under investigation. For instance, exposure of rats to chronic unpredictable stress for 40 days decreased complex I, III, and IV but had no effect on complex II [38]. In addition, these effects were observed in the cerebral cortex and cerebellum but not in the hippocampus, striatum, and prefrontal cortex. These earlier studies on the effects of stress on mitochondrial function did not try to relate the observed alterations to the most likely causal factor represented probably not by inflammation but by chronic activation of the hypothalamic pituitary-adrenal axis. As mentioned previously, there is evidence that chronic activation of the HPA axis or repeated administration of glucocorticoids induces similar signs of mitochondrial dysfunction in naïve rodents [39]. In addition, a complicating factor for the interpretation of chronic stress studies is that the brain mitochondrial alterations that are reported in chronic stress models might just represent another facet of the negative energy balance induced by stress, as evidenced by body weight loss, which is aggravated by stress-induced decreases in food intake.

More recent investigations are more mechanistic thanks in part to the progress in techniques for assessing mitochondrial function ex vivo and in vivo. Studies on inflammation-induced depression-like behavior have confirmed that the development of depression-like behavior is associated with mitochondrial dysfunction and decreased brain ATP levels. In addition, there is evidence that mitochondrial protectant agents can prevent inflammation-induced depression and, conversely, that mitochondrial toxicants can induce depression-like behavior in healthy naïve mice. As a typical example of this type of study, mice injected with the cytokine inducer lipopolysaccharide (LPS) at the dose of 0.8 mg/kg developed depression-like behavior measured 24 h later by increased immobility in the forced swim test and decreased sucrose preference [40]. These effects were associated with increased production of superoxide by mitochondria isolated from the hippocampus, reduced ATP levels, and decreased mitochondrial membrane potential. Intracerebroventricular administration of the mitochondrial targeted antioxidant Mito-Tempo blocked these effects in LPS-treated mice whereas administration by the same route of rotenone, an inhibitor of complex I of the mitochondrial respiratory chain, increased duration of immobility in the forced swim test and reduced sucrose preference in healthy naïve mice.

Similar approaches have been used for studies based on models of chronic stress. In one of these studies, mice that responded to chronic social defeat by social avoidance in a subsequent test of social exploration had lower levels of ATP in their hippocampus and prefrontal cortex than control mice or mice exposed to chronic social defeat but were not deficient in social exploration [41]. Repeated intraperitoneal administrations of ATP normalized the social behavior of mice susceptible to chronic social behavior. The same results were obtained on decreased sucrose preference of mice submitted to a model of chronic unpredictable stress.

At the cellular level, astrocytes have been investigated as the possible cell type involved in the effects of chronic stress. Genetic or pharmacological decrease of ATP release from astrocytes in naïve mice induced similar depression-like behavior as that produced by chronic social defeat stress and chronic unpredictable stress [41]. In addition, these effects could be corrected by stimulating ATP release from astrocytes. These findings were interpreted to mean that major depressive disorder is caused by the deficient release of ATP from astrocytes. Of note, the genetic deletion of Calhm2 which functions as an ATP-releasing channel in astrocytes resulted in the appearance of a depression-like phenotype in mice that was rescued by peripheral administration of ATP [42]. The interpretation of these two studies departs from the classical view of ATP as a neurotransmitter as it positions ATP as a communication signal between astrocytes and neurons. Microglial cells could play a role in this communication as they release small amounts of ATP within a few minutes in a toll-like receptor (TLR-)4-dependent manner when activated by LPS, and they do so independently of their ability to produce TNF or NO [43]. The release of ATP by microglia is amplified by astrocytes [43]. These findings point to a partnership between microglia and astrocytes in the modulation of excitatory neurotransmission. If these findings obtained in brain slices apply to in vivo conditions, any event leading to a decrease in the availability of ATP whether it is from astrocytic or from microglial origin will result in a deficient excitatory neurotransmission. This is likely to be the case when microglia undergo aerobic glycolysis to produce inflammatory cytokines. In vitro experiments confirm that LPS exposure is able to induce aerobic glycolysis in primary microglia [44]. This effect is associated with mitochondrial fragmentation as a consequence of increased mitochondrial fission. The addition of the mitochondrial fission inhibitor Mdivi-1 to primary microglia decreased the number of fragmented mitochondria, reduced glycolysis, and attenuated LPS-induced release of cytokines and chemokines, as well as LPS-induced succinate production. Of note, the accumulation of succinate caused by LPS could be responsible for reverse electron transport that would generate excessive mitochondrial radical oxygen species [45]. It is therefore not surprising that Mdivi-1 also inhibits mitochondrial ROS production and attenuates the LPS-induced increase in mitochondrial membrane potential [44].

A systematic study of the effects of stress on mitochondrial function reveals that in general chronic exposure to stress decreases mitochondrial energy production capacity and alters mitochondrial morphology [46]. In contrast, acute stress increases certain aspects of mitochondrial function. Some investigations have been conducted at the genetic level. Most of the mitochondrial proteins are encoded in the nuclear genome, but a few of them are encoded by the mitochondrial DNA (mtDNA) which lacks efficient repair mechanism and is therefore more susceptible to disruption. Mitochondrial DNA codes for a limited number of genes, 37, of which the product is involved in the electron transport chain and the ATP synthase complex, mitochondrial transfer RNAs, and ribosomal RNAs. It is inherited from the mother and it is present in 2 to 10 copies in mitochondria in contrast to nuclear DNA that is present only in 2 copies. Quantification of mtDNA copy number is carried out by quantitative real-time polymerase chain reaction (qPCR), and alterations in mtDNA copy numbers relative to nuclear DNA copy numbers have been associated with many phenotypes and diseases. In response to chronic stress mtDNA copy number is decreased in the brain but increased at the periphery, which would be due to upregulation of biogenesis and greater mtDNA replication in response to energy deficiency.

In order to determine whether mitochondrial function plays a pivotal role in the response to stress, Picard and his colleagues used mutations targeting either the mitochondrial DNA genes NADH dehydrogenase 6 (*Nd6*) and cytochrome c oxidase subunit 1 (*Coi*) to decrease electron transport chain and respiratory activity or the nuclear DNA genes *Ant1* or *Nnt* to reduce ATP/ADP transport across the inner mitochondrial membrane or reduce a major mitochondrial antioxidant system [47]. There was no evidence for an invariant pattern of response to mitochondrial defects as each mutation gave rise to specific alterations in the neuroendocrine and metabolic responses to a 30 min stress exposure. In particular, *Coi* and *Ant1* mutations were associated with a higher activation of the HPA axis in response to restraint whereas *Nnt* deficiency had the opposite effect. Stress-induced hyperglycemia was more marked in mice with mtDNA defects. However, it was blunted in *Ant1*-deficient mice. Plasma IL-6 reactivity was not significantly altered in mitochondrial mutants. In contrast, there was a tendency for mitochondrial mutations to attenuate the expression of pro-inflammatory genes in the hippocampus in response to restraint [47].

A few studies have investigated possible regional differences in the relationship between depression and mitochondrial activity. In a study carried out in mice submitted to chronic unpredictable stress for 6 weeks, mitochondria isolated from the cortex, hippocampus, and hypothalamus showed a decrease in respiratory rates and in mitochondrial membrane potential, together with the appearance of swollen and vacuolated mitochondria [48]. However, in a study carried out in rats submitted to 24 days of chronic mild stress, there was an indication of a higher rather than a lower mitochondrial activity in mitochondria isolated from the raphe nuclei of stressed rats compared to controls, as measured by respiratory rate, ATP production, superoxide dismutase activity, and glutathione peroxidase activity [49]. These findings indicate that mitochondrial dysfunction in animal models of depression could be region specific.

Non-pharmacological means can be used to improve mitochondrial function and to restore brain ATP levels. The beneficial effects of exercise on brain mitochondrial function have been less well studied than its effects on muscle mitochondria [50–52], but they appear to be robust enough to protect from depression-like behavior [53]. An entirely different approach is the use of low-level laser therapy [54]. Low-level laser therapy has antioxidant and anti-inflammatory properties and can preserve mitochondrial function by increasing cytochrome c oxidase activity and ATP synthesis. Applying low-level laser therapy to the head of mice for 30 min after each restraint session for a minimum of 14 days was sufficient to treat depression-like behavior. This effect was associated with a normalization of ATP levels and an increase in complex IV activity but only in the prefrontal cortex, not in the hippocampus and hypothalamus. Still another approach represented by deep brain stimulation targeting the nucleus accumbens was found to restore response to imipramine in rats chronically treated with ACTH, and this effect was associated with the normalization of mitochondrial respiration in mitochondria isolated from the prefrontal cortex [55].

Although the previous findings indicate that restoring mitochondrial function or normalizing ATP levels in the brain have beneficial effects on depression-like behavior induced by chronic stress or by inflammation, such a strategy is not without potential drawbacks. ATP is not only a metabolic marker but also an immunomodulator. It increases the production of pro-inflammatory cytokines, and this effect is mediated by the P2X7 purinergic receptor [56]. The pro-inflammatory activity of ATP is counterbalanced by the anti-inflammatory activity of adenosine. This means that it would certainly be counterproductive to increase brain ATP levels in conditions of brain inflammation unless this ATP can be quickly metabolized into adenosine.

Another approach for assessing the relationship between depression and ATP consists of investigating the processes that mediate the metabolism of ATP or those that are responsible for its consumption. CD39 also known as hydrolase ectonucleotide triphosphohydrolase is an important membrane enzyme present on several types of immune cells including macrophages, monocytes, and probably microglia. It regulates the level of extracellular ATP by metabolizing it into AMP that is further transformed into adenosine by CD73. Chronic social defeat was found to increase the hippocampal expression and activity of CD39 [57]. Administration of the CD39 analog, apyrase, mimicked the depression-like behavior induced by chronic social defeat, and this effect was reversed by replenishing hippocampal ATP levels. Conversely, genetic deletion of CD39 blocked the behavioral effects of chronic social defeat.

An article often cited as evidence for a negative relationship between depression and ATP is the study by Gamaro et al. [58]. The authors show that Na+,K + -ATPase activity in hippocampal synaptic membranes was decreased after 40 days of exposure of rats to chronic mild stress. The problem is that chronic administration of fluoxetine blocked this effect but did not normalize the decreased sweet food consumption induced by chronic mild stress.

If mitochondrial dysfunction plays a crucial role in the pathophysiology of depression, it should be possible to treat depression by replacing the deficient mitochondria by new ones. This possibility has been examined in a recent study conducted on LPS-induced depression-like behavior [59]. Mitochondrial transfer by intravenous injection of freshly isolated mitochondria from hippocampi of healthy mice either concomitantly to LPS or 16 h later was able to treat LPS-induced depression-like behavior. It also normalized LPS-induced oxidative stress and activation of microglia and astrocyte while at the same time increasing BDNF and restoring neurogenesis. Mitochondrial transfer was much more effective when administered concurrently with LPS rather than 16 h later. These results clearly need to be confirmed and expanded in order to determine in which compartment transplanted mitochondria are active, periphery or brain, and why they need to be injected before LPS.

Whether sex differences in the relationship between mitochondria dysfunction and depression could explain the prevalence of depression in females has given rise to some speculation [60, 61]. In general, males utilize mainly proteins and amino acids in mitochondria whereas females predominantly use fatty acids. Sex differences in oxidative/nitrosative stress, mitophagy, mitochondrial quality control, activation of the mitochondrial permeability transition pore, and cell death pathways have been described mainly in the context of brain injury but have not been given much consideration in the context of biological psychiatry.

16.3.3 Clinical Evidence for a Relationship Between MDD and Mitochondrial Dysfunction

Indirect evidence for a relationship between depression and alterations in energy metabolism comes from imaging studies of brain glucose metabolism and blood flow in MDD patients. Despite considerable heterogeneity in the results, depressed patients show a reduced blood flow and glucose metabolism in prefrontal cortex particularly when they exhibit psychomotor retardation. The same abnormalities are also found in anterior cingulate gyrus and basal ganglia whereas the parietal lobe shows increased blood flow and metabolism [62]. A more recent meta-analysis based on the activation likelihood estimate for each brain voxel and including studies carried out in Chinese patients showed that depressed patients have hypoactive glycose metabolism in insula, limbic system, and basal ganglia and an increased activity in the thalamus [63].

More focused studies on the relationship between MDD and mitochondrial dysfunction came originally from the investigation of neuropsychiatric disorders in patients with mitochondrial diseases due to either nuclear or mitochondrial DNA-encoded mutations [64]. As predicted based on the high energy requirements of the skeletal muscles and brain, this population is frequently afflicted with myopathy and neuropsychiatric symptomatology. The risk of comorbid depression is multiplied by 3.9 and the lifetime prevalence of depression is 54%. Of course, this is far from being sufficient to jump to the conclusion that MDD is a form of mitochondrial disease. Instead, the hypothesis proposed by several authors is that MDD could be due to suboptimal mitochondrial function making the energy produced by mitochondrial function unable to meet the metabolic cost of adaptation to psychosocial stressors [65]. Suboptimal mitochondrial function could be due to various genetic or acquired factors, including in this last case low-grade inflammation. If this hypothesis is correct, it should be possible to detect individuals at risk by measuring markers of mitochondrial function. The problem is that there is no gold standard of mitochondrial function and the methods that need to be deployed are fraught with the same pitfalls as those in other fields of biological psychiatry, e.g., the over-reliance on peripheral markers and the difficulty of running longitudinal studies in sufficiently sized samples unbiased by medication. The few available studies have measured by necessity mitochondrial function in peripheral blood mononuclear cells. In a study carried out in 22 women with MDD age-matched to 22 controls, mitochondrial respiration was assessed using a high-resolution respirometer [66]. MDD patients medicated for two thirds of them had decreased respiratory activity measured by baseline respiration, ATP turnover-related respiration, and spare respiratory capacity. The observed alterations suggested a lower ATP availability at baseline and a reduced efficiency of ATP production that were not related to a decrease in mitochondrial density as citrate synthase activity was not altered. These signs of mitochondrial dysfunction correlated negatively with depression severity measured by scores on the BDI and MADRS symptom scales. At the symptomatic level, items such as loss of energy, fatigue, disturbed sleep, and difficulties concentrating were associated with decreased respiratory activity, but it was also the case for sadness and irritability.

Much progress has been made during the last decade for assessing mitochondrial function thanks to the development of automated assays based on the continuous measurement of oxygen consumption rate of isolated mitochondria, cells, and even tissues exposed to various stress tests to separate the contribution of each complex of the electron transport chain to mitochondrial respiration. However, this specialized equipment is not easily accessible to psychiatrists. This has motivated a search for alternative approaches, including the measurement of mtDNA copy number. Contradictory results have been published, showing either an increase [67] or a decrease [68] as well as no change [69]. In a study carried out on white blood cells of 179 patients in primary health care with anxiety, depression, or stress and adjustment disorders compared to 320 healthy controls, patients were found to have a higher relative mtDNA copy number that correlated with Patient Health Questionnaire scores at baseline and decreased in response to treatment [70]. Complicating the picture, a few studies measured the levels of circulating cell-free mtDNA which comes from the release of mtDNA during cellular stress but does not reflect mitochondrial functional capacity. Cell-free mtDNA was found to be elevated in suicide attempters [71] but decreased in patients with MDD, with this decrease more marked during the depressive episode than during remittance [72]. A direct comparison of mtDNA copy number and cell free mtDNA in the same individuals revealed that MDD patients had higher cell-free mtDNA levels in the absence of any difference in mtDNA copy number measured in peripheral blood mononuclear cells [73]. There was no correlation between cell-free mtDNA and mtDNA copy number, confirming they represent different aspects of mitochondrial biology. Of note, antidepressant treatment normalized levels of cell-free mtDNA but only in patients who responded positively to the treatment. Similar studies on circulating cell-free DNA show that like cell-free mtDNA it is released in response to an acute bout of exercise or to the Trier social stress test in healthy individuals, with exercise being much more effective than the psychological stress [74]. The increase of cell-free mtDNA but not of cell-free DNA in response to psychological stress was confirmed independently [75].

16.3.4 Relationship Between Mitochondrial Dysfunction and Inflammation

From the experimental and clinical studies that examine the role of metabolic inefficiency in depression, it is obvious that there is still a strong tendency to consider inflammation and mitochondrial dysfunction as two separate entities. As we have seen, no more than a handful of studies have investigated the consequences of inflammation on mitochondrial function or the possibility of treating inflammation-induced depression like behavior by restoring energy balance. In most other cases, mitochondrial function is considered by itself, independently of any connection with either stress hormones or inflammation. This separation between inflammation and mitochondrial function is unfortunate as we know now that psychological stress can induce inflammation in addition to activating stress hormones and in addition that mitochondrial dysfunction can result in inflammation. Several excellent reviews have already been published on the influence of stress on inflammation [76–79]; therefore, there is no need to develop further this aspect. What is less commonly understood is the relationship between mitochondrial dysfunction and inflammation.

While we have learned much about the nature and mechanisms involved in LPS-induced depression, the emphasis on LPS as the inflammatory trigger has likely hindered our progress on the immunometabolic basis of depression. As LPS is derived from bacterial products, it is capable of directly activating inflammation via TLR4. Therefore, we have tended to neglect how other immune sensors and activators may uniquely contribute. In addition to the TLRs, there are numerous other pattern recognition receptors (PRRs), including the cytoplasmic retinoic acid-inducible gene 1 (RIG-1)-like receptors (RLRs) and nucleoid-binding oligomerization domain (NOD)-like receptors (NLRs) as well as the transmembrane C-type lectin receptors (CLRs).

While these receptors are often considered in the context of pathogen-associated molecular patterns (PAMPs), as in the case of viral DNA and RNA, they are also capable of responding to endogenous signals known as danger-associated molecular patterns (DAMPs). DAMPs, also known as "alarmins," are released by damaged or dying cells and can be actively released in response to cellular stress. Various mitochondrial components can serve as danger signals (mtDAMPS). Upon release, mtDAMPs can initiate inflammatory cytokine production and recruit immune cells to the site of damage through their interaction with PRRs [80, 81].

Mitochondrial-derived DNA (mtDNA) is one of the critical DAMPs tying mitochondrial dysfunction to inflammation. Mitochondria possess a circular, maternally inherited genome that consists of 37 genes that code for the 13 proteins. These proteins form the subunits of the electron transport chain, which is central to the process of oxidative phosphorylation. When mitochondria are damaged or stressed, they release mtDNA into the extracellular space and/or the cytosol. In the extracellular space, mtDNA is agonist of TLR9, which activates MAPK and NF-κB signaling cascades. Intracellular DNA has emerged as a critical activator of the immune response to sterile inflammation and has been shown to activate a number of various PRRs [81, 82]. The circular structure of mtDNA, which resembles that of bacteria and some viruses, may be what allows it to have such a potent effect on many of the PAMP pathways.

Absent in melanoma 2 (AIM2) is a cytosolic PRR and a component of the inflammasome that can be activated by mtDNA. When activated, AIM2 works in concert with other receptors of the inflammasome (e.g., NLRP1 and NLRP3) to activate caspase 1. Caspase-1 promotes the maturation of pro-IL-1β and pro-IL-18. Higher levels of both of these cytokines have been associated with depressive symptoms [83–85], but a possible role of AIM2 in inflammation-associated depression has not yet been investigated.

Another PRR that acts as a DNA sensor able to respond to cytosolic mtDNA is cyclic GMP-AMP synthase (cGAS) [81]. When cGAS binds mtDNA, it generates cGAMP, which acts as a second messenger to activate the Stimulator of Interferon Genes (STING). STING promotes the production of type I interferon (IFN) via the activation of the IRF3 transcription factor. There is strong history related to the ability of IFN to induce depressive symptoms. It is well accepted that treatment with IFN-α for cancer or infection with hepatitis C virus will increase depressive symptoms in patients [86]. Further, the activation of STING also appears to be capable of activating the NF-κB signaling pathway. However, this activation appears to be in a cGAS-independent fashion, instead relying on the DNA damage sensor ataxia telangiectasia mutated (ATM) [87].

Other mitochondrial-derived DAMPs that may play a role in inflammation-induced depression include cytochrome c (CytC) and mitochondrial transcription factor A (TFAM). Both CytC and TFAM are components of the mitochondrial intermembrane and can be released into the cytosol in response to cellular stress [88, 89]. When released by brain cells, CytC and TFAM can impact inflammation by activating glial cells [90]. As such, these DAMPs may serve a link between mitochondrial damage and neuroinflammation-induced depressive symptoms.

16.3.5 Summary

There is not much evidence yet available on the relationship between the consequences of immunometabolism on brain metabolism and their possible contribution to inflammation-induced depression. A handful of experimental studies support the hypothesis that inflammation-induced depression-like behavior is associated with signs of mitochondrial dysfunction. Conversely, restoration of mitochondrial dysfunction directly or indirectly treats depression-like behavior. Most studies on mitochondrial dysfunction have been carried out in the context of stress biology. There is still a strong disconnect in the literature as the relationship of depression to mitochondrial dysfunction has been studied independently of a possible involvement of inflammation either as a causal factor for mitochondrial damage or as a consequence of mitochondrial dysfunction.

16.4 Neuronal Networks Sensitive to Energy Metabolism Inefficiency

If the hypothesis that depression is caused by inefficient energy metabolism taking place at the periphery or in the brain has some validity, there should be *a minimum* some evidence of sensitivity to variations in energy metabolism within parts of the neuronal networks that mediate symptoms of depression. However, inflammation propagating from the periphery into the brain is a diffuse process that does not target any specific brain area or neuronal network. In contrast, in conditions of acute or chronic stress such as social defeat in which a mouse is defeated by an opponent, microglial activation preferentially occurs in those brain areas that are involved in the processing of the information relative to the dangerous situation, possibly because of a local weakening of the blood-brain barrier facilitating the brain trafficking of peripheral inflammatory monocytes. In the context of a peripheral inflammation relayed to the brain by the vagus nerves or spinal neurons, one could also imagine that neuronal activation in the projection areas of these nerves will be able to increase the level of local microglial activation. This would affect preferentially the insular cortex that substantializes feelings from the body and the cingulate cortex in which interoceptive information conjoins with homeostatic motivations to guide adaptive behavior [91]. Another possibility is represented by the exquisite sensitivity of a certain category of neurons to inflammation, oxidative stress, and mitochondrial dysfunction. This appears to be the case for dopaminergic neurons and more specifically those dopaminergic neurons that project from the *substantia nigra* to the striatum. Alteration of dopaminergic neurotransmission is usually not considered as a landmark of the neurochemical signature of MDD. However, there is much evidence that: (1) inflammation-associated depression is characterized by a predominance of symptoms reflecting hypoactivity of the dopaminergic system, including anergia and reduced motivation, and (2) inflammation impairs dopaminergic neurotransmission.

16.4.1 Inflammation and Motivational Alterations

Epidemiological studies in the general population consistently show an association of inflammation with somatic symptoms of depression, including reduced motivation, psychomotor retardation, and fatigue labeled as anergia in the context of depression, which are relatively resistant to usual antidepressant treatments [92–94]. This symptomatology reflects the consistent observations that innate immune activation preferentially affects midbrain dopamine [95]. The largest population of midbrain dopaminergic neurons are localized in the *substantia nigra pars compacta* (SNc) and the ventral tegmental area (VTA), which have different axonal projections to subcortical and cortical areas and encodes different aspects of motivated behavior [96]. Dopaminergic neurons projecting from the VTA and terminating in the ventral striatum (including the nucleus accumbens (NAc)) appear to play a key role in modulating effort-based decision-making [97–99]. Such observation is supported by preclinical studies demonstrating that effortful choices can be reduced by 6-hydroxydopamine (6-OHDA) lesions of the NAc and increased by blockade of dopamine uptake. Further, the effort expenditure for rewards can be modulated by increasing or decreasing dopaminergic signaling.

Regarding the impact of inflammation on effort valuation, preclinical studies in rodents and non-human primates demonstrate that administration of inflammatory cytokines (e.g., IL-1β, IL-6, or IFN-α) reduces willingness to work for highly palatable rewards without reducing consumption of freely available but less palatable food [100–102]. However, when both high and low rewards are available simultaneously in a concurrent choice task contrasting high effort/high reward and low effort/low reward options based on the same type of operant responding, LPS not only reduces incentive motivation but also shifts mice behavior toward the most valuable reward despite the higher effort it requires [103]. This effect is also apparent in humans [104, 105], suggesting that in an effort-based decision-making situation, inflammation shifts responding toward the reward that is perceived as most valuable, despite the higher effort it requires [106]. This indicates that inflammation does not just reduce motivation but increases sensitivity to the hedonic value of incentive stimuli, making less valuable incentive stimuli even less worth the effort. This extends to social situations as inflammation increases rejection of strangers' faces and favors positive responding to familiar faces [107].

16.4.2 Inflammation and Mitochondrial Dysfunction in Dopaminergic Neurons

The effects of inflammation on neurotransmission are usually explained in terms of interference with neurotransmitter synthesis, release, and reuptake. However, these effects are not specific to dopamine as they affect all monoaminergic neurotransmitters. In addition to these effects, it has been proposed that dopaminergic neurons receive information from the periphery via the hypothalamus about the metabolic state of the body to guide energy and effort allocation in the face of inflammation [108]. However, dopaminergic neurons have also the peculiarity of being under sustained oxidative stress due to the auto-oxidation of free cytosolic dopamine that results in the formation of dopamine-quinones and superoxide radicals. Dopamine quinones and superoxide radicals can damage the electron transport chain and oxidize mitochondrial proteins and lipids, leading to further generation of radical oxygen species, reduced ATP production, decreased mitochondrial membrane potential, and bioenergetic defects [109]. Importantly, mtDNA is particularly vulnerable to ROS because of its close proximity to the ETC and the lack of DNA repair mechanism. This means that any additional metabolic and bioenergetic burden, such as inflammation, might push dopaminergic neurons over the edge and impair their function if not their structure.

During inflammation, high levels of ROS are generated by activated microglia, which repurpose mitochondria from generating ATP to ROS production [110]. The midbrain dopaminergic pathway has an enriched microglial population as compared to other brain regions [111], which might contribute to the vulnerability of these neurons to inflammation. Inflammation occurring in the periphery or in the brain is well known to preferentially damage dopaminergic neurons in comparison to serotoninergic or noradrenergic neurons [112, 113], and this is associated with oxidative damage to mitochondrial components and decreased complex III and V respiration [112]. Both celecoxib (an inhibitor of cyclooxygenase-2 activity) and pioglitazone (an agonist of peroxisome proliferator-activated receptor gamma; PPAR-γ) prevented mitochondrial dysfunction, confirming that mitochondrial dysfunction is secondary to inflammation. Together, these data indicate that inflammation activates microglia to generate inflammatory mediators that, combined with the high oxidative burden of dopaminergic neurons, lead to mitochondrial dysfunction. Thus, inflammation, oxidative stress, and mitochondrial dysfunction have the potential to create a detrimental vicious cycle for negatively impacting dopaminergic neurotransmission in depression.

Because defective mitochondria not only produce more ROS but also fail to generate ATP and regulate calcium buffering, their removal by mitophagy is important to maintain cellular homeostasis and allow their replacement by healthier mitochondria. Mitophagy mediated by PTEN-induced kinase 1 (PINK1)/cytosolic E3 ubiquitin ligase (Parkin, PRKN) (PINK1/Parkin) plays a key role in the maintenance of mitochondrial fitness in dopaminergic neurons. *Pink1* or *prkn* gene mutations cause early-onset recessive familial forms of Parkinson's disease (PD) [114]. In damaged mitochondria, PINK1 accumulates on the outer mitochondrial membrane to recruit and phosphorylate Parkin and ubiquitin, leading to lysosomal degradation. Despite the increasing data pointing to mitochondrial dysfunction in depression, few studies have addressed the possibility of impaired or insufficient mitophagy leading to the accumulation of damaged mitochondria and decreased mitochondrial turnover in inflammation-associated depression.

There is evidence that mtDNA leakage into the cytosol and peripheral inflammation facilitate impairment in dopaminergic signaling. While mutations in *Pink1* and *Parkin* in PD patients lead to disease progression, *pink1−/−* and *prkn−/−* mice are healthy and display little motor impairment reminiscent of Parkinson's disease. This observation indicates that factors other than the loss of function of these proteins are required to impair dopaminergic signaling. In chronic models of mitochondrial stress with impaired mitophagy in dopaminergic neurons (double knock out of mutator mice that accumulate high levels of mtDNA mutations with either *pink1−/−* or *prkn−/−*), mtDNA that is released in the cytosol triggers the activation of the cgas-sting pathway to promote inflammation, neurodegeneration, and locomotor defects, while the loss of *sting* abrogates these alterations [115]. Thus, accumulation of mtDNA leading to sting activation creates the necessary condition for a positive feedback loop between inflammation and mitochondrial damage. In addition, intestinal infection of *pink1−/−* mice with Gram-negative bacteria transforms asymptomatic mice into mice with a full PD-like phenotype [116]. Besides their role in mitophagy, PINK1 and Parkin are involved in antigen presentation. They normally suppress antigen presentation derived from LPS-induced mitochondrial degradation. In the absence of PINK1, presentation of mitochondrial antigens to T cells results in the formation of mitochondria-specific cytotoxic CD8+ T cells. These T cells are able to traffic from the gut into the brain and to attack dopaminergic neurons expressing major histocompatibility complex class I (MCH-I) in an autoimmune manner.

Although mitochondrial dysfunction in inflammation-induced depression remains under-studied, it is likely to represent an important component of the relationship between inflammation, dopamine, and motivational alterations. This opens the possibility that inflammation-induced mitochondrial dysfunction is exacerbated in dopaminergic neurons because of their intrinsic susceptibility to metabolic damage due to sustained oxidative stress and high bioenergetic requirement. Further, inflammation-induced mitochondrial damage leads to cytosolic mtDNA accumulation that activates the cgas-sting pathway and increases the inflammatory insult on dopaminergic neurons. This could explain why reduced motivation and psychomotor slowing are the predominant symptoms in inflammation-associated depression.

16.4.3 Summary

Inflammation-associated depression is characterized by a predominance of somatic symptoms over cognitive and affective symptoms. This could be due to the exquisite sensitivity of dopaminergic neurons to mitochondrial dysfunction caused by the switch of brain innate immune cells from oxidative phosphorylation to aerobic glycolysis and the ensuing metabolic inefficiency it generates. Alterations in mitochondrial structure could lead to mtDNA leakage, which would induce the activation of the cgas-sting pathway and create the condition for a vicious cycle between inflammation and mitochondrial dysfunction. Although not examined in the present section, it can be proposed that the affective and cognitive symptoms of depression in inflamed individuals are a consequence of inflammation negatively affecting mitochondria function in the neurogenic niche, therefore impairing neurogenesis.

16.5 Conclusion and Perspectives

It should be apparent from the literature reviewed in this chapter that inflammation-associated depression is unlikely to be due solely to a direct effect of inflammatory mediators on neuronal function possibly relayed by mediators such as prostaglandins. We have made the case for an involvement of immunometabolism and its consequences on mitochondrial function and structure. This possibility has mainly been studied so far in the context of neurodegenerative diseases rather than psychiatric disorders. Even if there is no common measure between the level of inflammation that is necessary for the progressive loss of neurons in the central or peripheral nervous system and the level of inflammation that is observed in MDD, there is no reason for not accepting the possibility of a continuum in the mechanisms that are triggered by inflammation, with functional rather than structural alterations predominating in the case of inflammation-associated depression. In the assessment of the nature of this continuum, it is important to remember that in contrast to neurodegeneration that occurs primarily in the brain, the low-grade inflammation that is associated with MDD originates at the periphery before propagating to the brain. This means that the energy requirements of the peripheral immune response are already sufficient for compromising the amount of energy that is available to normal brain functions independently of the propagation of inflammation from the periphery to the brain. Although this has not been investigated specifically, there is evidence that in mice submitted to chronic social stress, the increased energy expenditure at the periphery is associated with a reduced glucose utilization by the brain [117] possibly because of insulin resistance. Not surprisingly, the ability of neurons to sustain the consequences of brain inflammation is reduced and their sensitivity to mitochondrial dysfunction exacerbated. This process is likely to affect preferentially the neurons that are the most sensitive to inflammation and oxidative stress, and we have described how this could explain the association of the somatic symptoms of depression with decreased dopaminergic neurotransmission in the fronto-striatal network. When considering mitochondrial dysfunction, it is important to keep in mind that mitochondria are very dynamic organelles with high motility within the cytoplasm. To increase their metabolic capacity in conditions of low energy they form networks by fusion of their outer and inner membranes. When damaged, they undergo fission to get rid of the damaged part. Damaged mitochondria are ultimately eliminated by mitophagy. Each of these processes involves specific processes orchestrated by GTPases including mitofusin (Mfn)1 and 2 and optic atrophy 1 (Opa1) for fusion and dynamin-related protein-1 (Drp1) for fission. The activation of innate immune cells by LPS biases the balance between fusion and fission toward fission [118]. A similar bias has been described in activated microglia [44, 119] with mitochondria fragmentation being associated with glycolytic shift and production of pro-inflammatory cytokines. This bias can be due to either activation of Drp1 or down-regulation of Mfn1/2 and, as expected, it is corrected by interventions targeting these factors. The same bias toward mitochondrial fission has been reported in neurons undergoing degeneration. Very surprisingly, overexpression of Mfn2 specifically in neurons prevented microglial activation induced by a septic dose of LPS in mice and reduced lethality in addition to protecting neuronal death [120].

Much work is still needed to improve our understating of how chronic low-grade inflammation impacts brain metabolism and mitochondrial function in specific brain networks to ultimately help the development of better approaches for treating symptoms of depression in inflamed individuals. A number of strategies for improving, preserving, or rescuing brain energetics are available [121]. They involve restoring oxidative phosphorylation and repairing the broken Krebs cycle, correcting mitochondrial dysfunction by mitochondrial protectants or mitochondrial transfer to repair damaged mitochondria, recourse to ketogenic strategies, administering hormones or hormone-like molecules that modulate cerebral energetics, and various other interventions that have been presented in this chapter and tested in experimental models. However, it is important to remember that strategies that provide promising results in preclinical studies do not always fulfill their premises when tested in the real world. A recent example is provided by the failed attempt to target the PI3kinase/Akt/mTOR pathway for the treatment of depression that was initially based on the preclinical observation that the fast-acting antidepressant activity of ketamine, a NMDA receptor antagonist, requires increased production of BDNF and activation of mTOR signaling [122]. This result agrees with the concept that recovery from depression requires the restoration of neuronal plasticity which itself is dependent on protein synthesis orchestrated by mTOR signaling. Blockade of mTOR activation by prior treatment with rapamycin, an antagonist of mTOR signaling, abrogated the antidepressant activity of ketamine in mice [122]. However, contrary to expectation, administration of rapamycin to depressed patients treated with ketamine prolonged instead of inhibited the antidepressant activity of ketamine [123].

In summary, the rapid advances in immunometabolism during the last decade have amply demonstrated that metabolic reprogramming at the cellular and organismic levels is a critical aspect of the host inflammatory response. The possibility that the depressive symptoms that are apparent in inflamed individuals are the outward expression of the response of the brain to this metabolic reprogramming amplified by the metabolic adjustments that take place in the inflamed brain cannot be ignored any longer. New targets for pathophysiology and treatment are emerging from the still sparse research taking place in this field. Their ultimate success will depend on a close cooperation between preclinical and clinical researchers.

Acknowledgments Funded by a graduate fellowship to AC (National Council for Scientific and Technological Development SWE 206541), a NARSAD Distinguished Investigator Award to RD, grants from the National Institutes of Health (R01 CA193522 and R01 NS073939), and an MD Anderson Cancer Support Grant (P30 CA016672).

References

1. Yirmiya R, Pollak Y, Morag M, Reichenberg A, Barak O, Avitsur R, Shavit Y, Ovadia H, Weidenfeld J, Morag A, Newman ME, Pollmacher T. Illness, cytokines, and depression. Ann N Y Acad Sci. 2000;917:478–87.
2. Maes M, Smith R, Scharpe S. The monocyte-T-lymphocyte hypothesis of major depression. Psychoneuroendocrinology. 1995;20:111–6.
3. Dantzer R, O'Connor JC, Freund GG, Johnson RW, Kelley KW. From inflammation to sickness and depression: when the immune system subjugates the brain. Nat Rev Neurosci. 2008;9:46–56.
4. Hart BL. Biological basis of the behavior of sick animals. Neurosci Biobehav Rev. 1988;12:123–37.
5. Adelman JS, Martin LB. Vertebrate sickness behaviors: adaptive and integrated neuroendocrine immune responses. Integr Comp Biol. 2009;49:202–14.
6. Demas GE, Carlton ED. Ecoimmunology for psychoneuroimmunologists: considering context in neuroendocrine-immune-behavior interactions. Brain Behav Immun. 2015;44:9–16.
7. Hawley DM, Etienne RS, Ezenwa VO, Jolles AE. Does animal behavior underlie covariation between hosts' exposure to infectious agents and susceptibility to infection? Implications for disease dynamics. Integr Comp Biol. 2011;51:528–39.

8. Miller AH, Raison CL. The role of inflammation in depression: from evolutionary imperative to modern treatment target. Nat Rev Immunol. 2016;16:22–34.
9. Franz EA, Gillett G. John Hughlings Jackson's evolutionary neurology: a unifying framework for cognitive neuroscience. Brain. 2011;134:3114–20.
10. Kaiser RH, Andrews-Hanna JR, Wager TD, Pizzagalli DA. Large-scale network dysfunction in major depressive disorder: a meta-analysis of resting-state functional connectivity. JAMA Psychiat. 2015;72:603–11.
11. Critchley HD, Harrison NA. Visceral influences on brain and behavior. Neuron. 2013;77:624–38.
12. Harrison NA, Brydon L, Walker C, Gray MA, Steptoe A, Dolan RJ, Critchley HD. Neural origins of human sickness in interoceptive responses to inflammation. Biol Psychiatry. 2009;66:415–22.
13. Vander Heiden MG, Cantley LC, Thompson CB. Understanding the Warburg effect: the metabolic requirements of cell proliferation. Science. 2009;324:1029–33.
14. O'Neill LA, Kishton RJ, Rathmell J. A guide to immunometabolism for immunologists. Nat Rev Immunol. 2016;16:553–65.
15. Ghosh S, Castillo E, Frias ES, Swanson RA. Bioenergetic regulation of microglia. Glia. 2018;66:1200–12.
16. Ryan DG, O'Neill LAJ. Krebs cycle reborn in macrophage immunometabolism. Annu Rev Immunol. 2020;38:289–313.
17. McIntosh A, Mela V, Harty C, Minogue AM, Costello DA, Kerskens C, Lynch MA. Iron accumulation in microglia triggers a cascade of events that leads to altered metabolism and compromised function in APP/PS1 mice. Brain Pathol. 2019;29:606–21.
18. van der Poel M, Ulas T, Mizee MR, Hsiao CC, Miedema SSM, Adelia, Schuurman KG, Helder B, Tas SW, Schultze JL, Hamann J, Huitinga I. Transcriptional profiling of human microglia reveals grey-white matter heterogeneity and multiple sclerosis-associated changes. Nat Commun. 2019;10:1139.
19. Mela V, Mota BC, Milner M, McGinley A, Mills KHG, Kelly AM, Lynch MA. Exercise-induced re-programming of age-related metabolic changes in microglia is accompanied by a reduction in senescent cells. Brain Behav Immun. 2020;87:413–28.
20. Porporato PE. Understanding cachexia as a cancer metabolism syndrome. Oncogenesis. 2016;5:e200.
21. Rohm M, Zeigerer A, Machado J, Herzig S. Energy metabolism in cachexia. EMBO Rep. 2019;20:e47258.
22. Dumas JF, Goupille C, Julienne CM, Pinault M, Chevalier S, Bougnoux P, Servais S, Couet C. Efficiency of oxidative phosphorylation in liver mitochondria is decreased in a rat model of peritoneal carcinosis. J Hepatol. 2011;54:320–7.
23. Cain DW, Cidlowski JA. Immune regulation by glucocorticoids. Nat Rev Immunol. 2017;17:233–47.
24. Munck A. Glucocorticoid inhibition of glucose uptake by peripheral tissues: old and new evidence, molecular mechanisms, and physiological significance. Perspect Biol Med. 1971;14:265–9.
25. Du J, McEwen B, Manji HK. Glucocorticoid receptors modulate mitochondrial function: a novel mechanism for neuroprotection. Commun Integr Biol. 2009;2:350–2.
26. Peters A, Schweiger U, Pellerin L, Hubold C, Oltmanns KM, Conrad M, Schultes B, Born J, Fehm HL. The selfish brain: competition for energy resources. Neurosci Biobehav Rev. 2004;28:143–80.
27. Straub RH. The brain and immune system prompt energy shortage in chronic inflammation and ageing. Nat Rev Rheumatol. 2017;13:743–51.
28. Wang A, Luan HH, Medzhitov R. An evolutionary perspective on immunometabolism. Science. 2019a;363:6423.
29. Dienel GA. Brain glucose metabolism: integration of energetics with function. Physiol Rev. 2019;99:949–1045.

30. Pellerin L, Magistretti PJ. Sweet sixteen for ANLS. J Cereb Blood Flow Metab. 2012;32:1152–66.
31. Diaz-Garcia CM, Mongeon R, Lahmann C, Koveal D, Zucker H, Yellen G. Neuronal stimulation triggers neuronal glycolysis and not lactate uptake. Cell Metab. 2017;26(361–374):e4.
32. Gandhi GK, Cruz NF, Ball KK, Dienel GA. Astrocytes are poised for lactate trafficking and release from activated brain and for supply of glucose to neurons. J Neurochem. 2009;111:522–36.
33. Bak LK, Schousboe A, Waagepetersen HS. The glutamate/GABA-glutamine cycle: aspects of transport, neurotransmitter homeostasis and ammonia transfer. J Neurochem. 2006;98:641–53.
34. Provent P, Kickler N, Barbier EL, Bergerot A, Farion R, Goury S, Marcaggi P, Segebarth C, Coles JA. The ammonium-induced increase in rat brain lactate concentration is rapid and reversible and is compatible with trafficking and signaling roles for ammonium. J Cereb Blood Flow Metab. 2007;27:1830–40.
35. Moshkin MP, Akulov AE, Petrovski DV, Saik OV, Petrovskiy ED, Savelov AA, Koptyug IV. Proton magnetic resonance spectroscopy of brain metabolic shifts induced by acute administration of 2-deoxy-d-glucose and lipopolysaccharides. NMR Biomed. 2014;27:399–405.
36. Verma M, Kipari TMJ, Zhang Z, Man TY, Forster T, Homer NZM, Seckl JR, Holmes MC, Chapman KE. 11beta-hydroxysteroid dehydrogenase-1 deficiency alters brain energy metabolism in acute systemic inflammation. Brain Behav Immun. 2018;69:223–34.
37. Madrigal JL, Olivenza R, Moro MA, Lizasoain I, Lorenzo P, Rodrigo J, Leza JC. Glutathione depletion, lipid peroxidation and mitochondrial dysfunction are induced by chronic stress in rat brain. Neuropsychopharmacology. 2001;24:420–9.
38. Rezin GT, Cardoso MR, Goncalves CL, Scaini G, Fraga DB, Riegel RE, Comim CM, Quevedo J, Streck EL. Inhibition of mitochondrial respiratory chain in brain of rats subjected to an experimental model of depression. Neurochem Int. 2008;53:395–400.
39. Liu W, Zhou C. Corticosterone reduces brain mitochondrial function and expression of mitofusin, BDNF in depression-like rodents regardless of exercise preconditioning. Psychoneuroendocrinology. 2012;37:1057–70.
40. Chen WJ, Du JK, Hu X, Yu Q, Li DX, Wang CN, Zhu XY, Liu YJ. Protective effects of resveratrol on mitochondrial function in the hippocampus improves inflammation-induced depressive-like behavior. Physiol Behav. 2017;182:54–61.
41. Cao X, Li LP, Wang Q, Wu Q, Hu HH, Zhang M, Fang YY, Zhang J, Li SJ, Xiong WC, Yan HC, Gao YB, Liu JH, Li XW, Sun LR, Zeng YN, Zhu XH, Gao TM. Astrocyte-derived ATP modulates depressive-like behaviors. Nat Med. 2013;19:773–7.
42. Jun M, Xiaolong Q, Chaojuan Y, Ruiyuan P, Shukun W, Junbing W, Li H, Hong C, Jinbo C, Rong W, Yajin L, Lanqun M, Fengchao W, Zhiying W, Jianxiong A, Yun W, Xia Z, Chen Z, Zengqiang Y. Calhm2 governs astrocytic ATP releasing in the development of depression-like behaviors. Mol Psychiatry. 2018;23:1091.
43. Pascual O, Ben Achour S, Rostaing P, Triller A, Bessis A. Microglia activation triggers astrocyte-mediated modulation of excitatory neurotransmission. Proc Natl Acad Sci U S A. 2012;109:E197–205.
44. Nair S, Sobotka KS, Joshi P, Gressens P, Fleiss B, Thornton C, Mallard C, Hagberg H. Lipopolysaccharide-induced alteration of mitochondrial morphology induces a metabolic shift in microglia modulating the inflammatory response in vitro and in vivo. Glia. 2019;67:1047–61.
45. Chouchani ET, Pell VR, Gaude E, Aksentijevic D, Sundier SY, Robb EL, Logan A, Nadtochiy SM, Ord ENJ, Smith AC, Eyassu F, Shirley R, Hu CH, Dare AJ, James AM, Rogatti S, Hartley RC, Eaton S, Costa ASH, Brookes PS, Davidson SM, Duchen MR, Saeb-Parsy K, Shattock MJ, Robinson AJ, Work LM, Frezza C, Krieg T, Murphy MP. Ischaemic accumulation of succinate controls reperfusion injury through mitochondrial ROS. Nature. 2014;515:431–5.
46. Picard M, McEwen BS. Psychological stress and mitochondria: a systematic review. Psychosom Med. 2018;80:141–53.

47. Picard M, McManus MJ, Gray JD, Nasca C, Moffat C, Kopinski PK, Seifert EL, McEwen BS, Wallace DC. Mitochondrial functions modulate neuroendocrine, metabolic, inflammatory, and transcriptional responses to acute psychological stress. Proc Natl Acad Sci U S A. 2015;112:E6614–23.
48. Gong Y, Chai Y, Ding JH, Sun XL, Hu G. Chronic mild stress damages mitochondrial ultrastructure and function in mouse brain. Neurosci Lett. 2011;488:76–80.
49. Wen L, Jin Y, Li L, Sun S, Cheng S, Zhang S, Zhang Y, Svenningsson P. Exercise prevents raphe nucleus mitochondrial overactivity in a rat depression model. Physiol Behav. 2014;132:57–65.
50. Gusdon AM, Callio J, Distefano G, O'Doherty RM, Goodpaster BH, Coen PM, Chu CT. Exercise increases mitochondrial complex I activity and DRP1 expression in the brains of aged mice. Exp Gerontol. 2017;90:1–13.
51. Memme JM, Erlich AT, Phukan G, Hood DA. Exercise and mitochondrial health. J Physiol. 2019;599:803–17.
52. Steiner JL, Murphy EA, McClellan JL, Carmichael MD, Davis JM. Exercise training increases mitochondrial biogenesis in the brain. J Appl Physiol (1985). 2011;111:1066–71.
53. Aguiar AS Jr, Stragier E, da Luz Scheffer D, Remor AP, Oliveira PA, Prediger RD, Latini A, Raisman-Vozari R, Mongeau R, Lanfumey L. Effects of exercise on mitochondrial function, neuroplasticity and anxio-depressive behavior of mice. Neuroscience. 2014;271:56–63.
54. Xu Z, Guo X, Yang Y, Tucker D, Lu Y, Xin N, Zhang G, Yang L, Li J, Du X, Zhang Q, Xu X. Low-level laser irradiation improves depression-like behaviors in mice. Mol Neurobiol. 2017;54:4551–9.
55. Kim Y, McGee S, Czeczor JK, Walker AJ, Kale RP, Kouzani AZ, Walder K, Berk M, Tye SJ. Nucleus accumbens deep-brain stimulation efficacy in ACTH-pretreated rats: alterations in mitochondrial function relate to antidepressant-like effects. Transl Psychiatry. 2016;6:e842.
56. Bhattacharya A, Jones DNC. Emerging role of the P2X7-NLRP3-IL1beta pathway in mood disorders. Psychoneuroendocrinology. 2018;98:95–100.
57. Cui QQ, Hu ZL, Hu YL, Chen X, Wang J, Mao L, Lu XJ, Ni M, Chen JG, Wang F. Hippocampal CD39/ENTPD1 promotes mouse depression-like behavior through hydrolyzing extracellular ATP. EMBO Rep. 2020;21:e47857.
58. Gamaro GD, Streck EL, Matte C, Prediger ME, Wyse AT, Dalmaz C. Reduction of hippocampal Na+, K+-ATPase activity in rats subjected to an experimental model of depression. Neurochem Res. 2003;28:1339–44.
59. Wang Y, Ni J, Gao C, Xie L, Zhai L, Cui G, Yin X. Mitochondrial transplantation attenuates lipopolysaccharide- induced depression-like behaviors. Prog Neuro-Psychopharmacol Biol Psychiatry. 2019b;93:240–9.
60. Demarest TG, McCarthy MM. Sex differences in mitochondrial (dys)function: implications for neuroprotection. J Bioenerg Biomembr. 2015;47:173–88.
61. Shimamoto A, Rappeneau V. Sex-dependent mental illnesses and mitochondria. Schizophr Res. 2017;187:38–46.
62. Videbech P. PET measurements of brain glucose metabolism and blood flow in major depressive disorder: a critical review. Acta Psychiatr Scand. 2000;101:11–20.
63. Su L, Cai Y, Xu Y, Dutt A, Shi S, Bramon E. Cerebral metabolism in major depressive disorder: a voxel-based meta-analysis of positron emission tomography studies. BMC Psychiatry. 2014;14:321.
64. Marin SE, Saneto RP. Neuropsychiatric features in primary mitochondrial disease. Neurol Clin. 2016;34:247–94.
65. Morava E, Kozicz T. Mitochondria and the economy of stress (mal)adaptation. Neurosci Biobehav Rev. 2013;37:668–80.
66. Karabatsiakis A, Bock C, Salinas-Manrique J, Kolassa S, Calzia E, Dietrich DE, Kolassa IT. Mitochondrial respiration in peripheral blood mononuclear cells correlates with depressive subsymptoms and severity of major depression. Transl Psychiatry. 2014;4:e397.
67. Cai N, Chang S, Li Y, Li Q, Hu J, Liang J, Song L, Kretzschmar W, Gan X, Nicod J, Rivera M, Deng H, Du B, Li K, Sang W, Gao J, Gao S, Ha B, Ho HY, Hu C, Hu J, Hu Z, Huang G,

Jiang G, Jiang T, Jin W, Li G, Li K, Li Y, Li Y, Li Y, Lin YT, Liu L, Liu T, Liu Y, Liu Y, Lu Y, Lv L, Meng H, Qian P, Sang H, Shen J, Shi J, Sun J, Tao M, Wang G, Wang G, Wang J, Wang L, Wang X, Wang X, Yang H, Yang L, Yin Y, Zhang J, Zhang K, Sun N, Zhang W, Zhang X, Zhang Z, Zhong H, Breen G, Wang J, Marchini J, Chen Y, Xu Q, Xu X, Mott R, Huang GJ, Kendler K, Flint J. Molecular signatures of major depression. Curr Biol. 2015;25:1146–56.
68. Kim MY, Lee JW, Kang HC, Kim E, Lee DC. Leukocyte mitochondrial DNA (mtDNA) content is associated with depression in old women. Arch Gerontol Geriatr. 2011;53:e218–21.
69. He Y, Tang J, Li Z, Li H, Liao Y, Tang Y, Tan L, Chen J, Xia K, Chen X. Leukocyte mitochondrial DNA copy number in blood is not associated with major depressive disorder in young adults. PLoS One. 2014;9:e96869.
70. Wang X, Sundquist K, Rastkhani H, Palmer K, Memon AA, Sundquist J. Association of mitochondrial DNA in peripheral blood with depression, anxiety and stress- and adjustment disorders in primary health care patients. Eur Neuropsychopharmacol. 2017;27:751–8.
71. Lindqvist D, Fernstrom J, Grudet C, Ljunggren L, Traskman-Bendz L, Ohlsson L, Westrin A. Increased plasma levels of circulating cell-free mitochondrial DNA in suicide attempters: associations with HPA-axis hyperactivity. Transl Psychiatry. 2016;6:e971.
72. Kageyama Y, Kasahara T, Kato M, Sakai S, Deguchi Y, Tani M, Kuroda K, Hattori K, Yoshida S, Goto Y, Kinoshita T, Inoue K, Kato T. The relationship between circulating mitochondrial DNA and inflammatory cytokines in patients with major depression. J Affect Disord. 2018;233:15–20.
73. Lindqvist D, Wolkowitz OM, Picard M, Ohlsson L, Bersani FS, Fernstrom J, Westrin A, Hough CM, Lin J, Reus VI, Epel ES, Mellon SH. Circulating cell-free mitochondrial DNA, but not leukocyte mitochondrial DNA copy number, is elevated in major depressive disorder. Neuropsychopharmacology. 2018;43:1557–64.
74. Hummel EM, Hessas E, Muller S, Beiter T, Fisch M, Eibl A, Wolf OT, Giebel B, Platen P, Kumsta R, Moser DA. Cell-free DNA release under psychosocial and physical stress conditions. Transl Psychiatry. 2018;8:236.
75. Trumpff C, Marsland AL, Basualto-Alarcon C, Martin JL, Carroll JE, Sturm G, Vincent AE, Mosharov EV, Gu Z, Kaufman BA, Picard M. Acute psychological stress increases serum circulating cell-free mitochondrial DNA. Psychoneuroendocrinology. 2019;106:268–76.
76. Kiecolt-Glaser JK, Derry HM, Fagundes CP. Inflammation: depression fans the flames and feasts on the heat. Am J Psychiatry. 2015;172:1075–91.
77. Marsland AL, Walsh C, Lockwood K, John-Henderson NA. The effects of acute psychological stress on circulating and stimulated inflammatory markers: a systematic review and meta-analysis. Brain Behav Immun. 2017;64:208–19.
78. Niraula A, Sheridan JF, Godbout JP. Microglia priming with aging and stress. Neuropsychopharmacology. 2017;42:318–33.
79. Slavich GM, Irwin MR. From stress to inflammation and major depressive disorder: a social signal transduction theory of depression. Psychol Bull. 2014;140:774–815.
80. Nakahira K, Hisata S, Choi AM. The roles of mitochondrial damage-associated molecular patterns in diseases. Antioxid Redox Signal. 2015;23:1329–50.
81. West AP. Mitochondrial dysfunction as a trigger of innate immune responses and inflammation. Toxicology. 2017;391:54–63.
82. Unterholzner L. The interferon response to intracellular DNA: why so many receptors? Immunobiology. 2013;218:1312–21.
83. Al-Hakeim HK, Al-Kufi SN, Al-Dujaili AH, Maes M. Serum interleukin levels and insulin resistance in major depressive disorder. CNS Neurol Disord Drug Targets. 2018;17:618–25.
84. Merendino RA, Di Rosa AE, Di Pasquale G, Minciullo PL, Mangraviti C, Costantino A, Ruello A, Gangemi S. Interleukin-18 and CD30 serum levels in patients with moderate-severe depression. Mediat Inflamm. 2002;11:265–7.
85. Swartz JR, Prather AA, Di Iorio CR, Bogdan R, Hariri AR. A functional Interleukin-18 haplotype predicts depression and anxiety through increased threat-related amygdala reactivity in women but not men. Neuropsychopharmacology. 2017;42:419–26.

86. Capuron L, Miller AH. Cytokines and psychopathology: lessons from interferon-alpha. Biol Psychiatry. 2004;56:819–24.
87. Dunphy G, Flannery SM, Almine JF, Connolly DJ, Paulus C, Jonsson KL, Jakobsen MR, Nevels MM, Bowie AG, Unterholzner L. Non-canonical activation of the DNA sensing adaptor STING by ATM and IFI16 mediates NF-kappaB signaling after nuclear DNA damage. Mol Cell. 2018;71(745–760):e5.
88. Julian MW, Shao G, Bao S, Knoell DL, Papenfuss TL, VanGundy ZC, Crouser ED. Mitochondrial transcription factor a serves as a danger signal by augmenting plasmacytoid dendritic cell responses to DNA. J Immunol. 2012;189:433–43.
89. Kagan VE, Tyurin VA, Jiang J, Tyurina YY, Ritov VB, Amoscato AA, Osipov AN, Belikova NA, Kapralov AA, Kini V, Vlasova II, Zhao Q, Zou M, Di P, Svistunenko DA, Kurnikov IV, Borisenko GG. Cytochrome c acts as a cardiolipin oxygenase required for release of proapoptotic factors. Nat Chem Biol. 2005;1:223–32.
90. Bajwa E, Pointer CB, Klegeris A. The role of mitochondrial damage-associated molecular patterns in chronic neuroinflammation. Mediat Inflamm. 2019;2019:4050796.
91. Strigo IA, Craig AD. Interoception, homeostatic emotions and sympathovagal balance. Philos Trans R Soc Lond Ser B Biol Sci. 2016;371:20160010.
92. Chu AL, Stochl J, Lewis G, Zammit S, Jones PB, Khandaker GM. Longitudinal association between inflammatory markers and specific symptoms of depression in a prospective birth cohort. Brain Behav Immun. 2019;76:74–81.
93. Jokela M, Virtanen M, Batty GD, Kivimaki M. Inflammation and specific symptoms of depression. JAMA Psychiat. 2016;73:87–8.
94. Kohler-Forsberg O, Buttenschon HN, Tansey KE, Maier W, Hauser J, Dernovsek MZ, Henigsberg N, Souery D, Farmer A, Rietschel M, McGuffin P, Aitchison KJ, Uher R, Mors O. Association between C-reactive protein (CRP) with depression symptom severity and specific depressive symptoms in major depression. Brain Behav Immun. 2017;62:344–50.
95. Felger JC, Treadway MT. Inflammation effects on motivation and motor activity: role of dopamine. Neuropsychopharmacology. 2017;42:216–41.
96. Bromberg-Martin ES, Matsumoto M, Hikosaka O. Dopamine in motivational control: rewarding, aversive, and alerting. Neuron. 2010;68:815–34.
97. Salamone JD, Correa M. The mysterious motivational functions of mesolimbic dopamine. Neuron. 2012;76:470–85.
98. Treadway MT, Zald DH. Parsing anhedonia: translational models of reward-processing deficits in psychopathology. Curr Dir Psychol Sci. 2013;22:244–9.
99. Tsutsui-Kimura I, Natsubori A, Mori M, Kobayashi K, Drew MR, de Kerchove d'Exaerde A, Mimura M, Tanaka KF. Distinct roles of ventromedial versus ventrolateral striatal medium spiny neurons in reward-oriented behavior. Curr Biol. 2017;27(3042–3048):e4.
100. Felger JC, Mun J, Kimmel HL, Nye JA, Drake DF, Hernandez CR, Freeman AA, Rye DB, Goodman MM, Howell LL, Miller AH. Chronic interferon-alpha decreases dopamine 2 receptor binding and striatal dopamine release in association with anhedonia-like behavior in nonhuman primates. Neuropsychopharmacology. 2013;38:2179–87.
101. Nunes EJ, Randall PA, Estrada A, Epling B, Hart EE, Lee CA, Baqi Y, Muller CE, Correa M, Salamone JD. Effort-related motivational effects of the pro-inflammatory cytokine interleukin 1-beta: studies with the concurrent fixed ratio 5/chow feeding choice task. Psychopharmacology. 2014;231:727–36.
102. Yohn SE, Arif Y, Haley A, Tripodi G, Baqi Y, Muller CE, Miguel NS, Correa M, Salamone JD. Effort-related motivational effects of the pro-inflammatory cytokine interleukin-6: pharmacological and neurochemical characterization. Psychopharmacology. 2016;233:3575–86.
103. Vichaya EG, Hunt SC, Dantzer R. Lipopolysaccharide reduces incentive motivation while boosting preference for high reward in mice. Neuropsychopharmacology. 2014;39:2884–90.
104. Harrison NA, Voon V, Cercignani M, Cooper EA, Pessiglione M, Critchley HD. A neurocomputational account of how inflammation enhances sensitivity to punishments versus rewards. Biol Psychiatry. 2016;80:73–81.

105. Lasselin J, Treadway MT, Lacourt TE, Soop A, Olsson MJ, Karshikoff B, Paues-Goranson S, Axelsson J, Dantzer R, Lekander M. Lipopolysaccharide alters motivated behavior in a monetary reward task: a randomized trial. Neuropsychopharmacology. 2017;42:801–10.
106. Vichaya EG, Dantzer R. Inflammation-induced motivational changes: perspective gained by evaluating positive and negative valence systems. Curr Opin Behav Sci. 2018;22:90–5.
107. Eisenberger NI, Moieni M, Inagaki TK, Muscatell KA, Irwin MR. In sickness and in health: the co-regulation of inflammation and social behavior. Neuropsychopharmacology. 2017;42:242–53.
108. Treadway MT, Cooper JA, Miller AH. Can't or Won't? Immunometabolic constraints on dopaminergic drive. Trends Cogn Sci. 2019;23:435–48.
109. Abou-Sleiman PM, Muqit MM, Wood NW. Expanding insights of mitochondrial dysfunction in Parkinson's disease. Nat Rev Neurosci. 2006;7:207–19.
110. Mills EL, Kelly B, Logan A, Costa ASH, Varma M, Bryant CE, Tourlomousis P, Dabritz JHM, Gottlieb E, Latorre I, Corr SC, McManus G, Ryan D, Jacobs HT, Szibor M, Xavier RJ, Braun T, Frezza C, Murphy MP, O'Neill LA. Succinate dehydrogenase supports metabolic repurposing of mitochondria to drive inflammatory macrophages. Cell. 2016;167(457–470):e13.
111. Lawson LJ, Perry VH, Dri P, Gordon S. Heterogeneity in the distribution and morphology of microglia in the normal adult mouse brain. Neuroscience. 1990;39:151–70.
112. Hunter RL, Dragicevic N, Seifert K, Choi DY, Liu M, Kim HC, Cass WA, Sullivan PG, Bing G. Inflammation induces mitochondrial dysfunction and dopaminergic neurodegeneration in the nigrostriatal system. J Neurochem. 2007;100:1375–86.
113. Qin L, Wu X, Block ML, Liu Y, Breese GR, Hong JS, Knapp DJ, Crews FT. Systemic LPS causes chronic neuroinflammation and progressive neurodegeneration. Glia. 2007;55:453–62.
114. Ryan BJ, Hoek S, Fon EA, Wade-Martins R. Mitochondrial dysfunction and mitophagy in Parkinson's: from familial to sporadic disease. Trends Biochem Sci. 2015;40:200–10.
115. Sliter DA, Martinez J, Hao L, Chen X, Sun N, Fischer TD, Burman JL, Li Y, Zhang Z, Narendra DP, Cai H, Borsche M, Klein C, Youle RJ. Parkin and PINK1 mitigate STING-induced inflammation. Nature. 2018;561:258–62.
116. Matheoud D, Cannon T, Voisin A, Penttinen AM, Ramet L, Fahmy AM, Ducrot C, Laplante A, Bourque MJ, Zhu L, Cayrol R, Le Campion A, McBride HM, Gruenheid S, Trudeau LE, Desjardins M. Intestinal infection triggers Parkinson's disease-like symptoms in Pink1(−/−) mice. Nature. 2019;571:565–9.
117. Carneiro-Nascimento S, Opacka-Juffry J, Costabile A, Boyle CN, Herde AM, Ametamey SM, Sigrist H, Pryce CR, Patterson M. Chronic social stress in mice alters energy status including higher glucose need but lower brain utilization. Psychoneuroendocrinology. 2020;119:104747.
118. Kapetanovic R, Afroz SF, Ramnath D, Lawrence GM, Okada T, Curson JE, de Bruin J, Fairlie DP, Schroder K, St John JC, Blumenthal A, Sweet MJ. Lipopolysaccharide promotes Drp1-dependent mitochondrial fission and associated inflammatory responses in macrophages. Immunol Cell Biol. 2020;98:528–39.
119. Katoh M, Wu B, Nguyen HB, Thai TQ, Yamasaki R, Lu H, Rietsch AM, Zorlu MM, Shinozaki Y, Saitoh Y, Saitoh S, Sakoh T, Ikenaka K, Koizumi S, Ransohoff RM, Ohno N. Polymorphic regulation of mitochondrial fission and fusion modifies phenotypes of microglia in neuroinflammation. Sci Rep. 2017;7:4942.
120. Harland M, Torres S, Liu J, Wang X. Neuronal mitochondria modulation of LPS-induced neuroinflammation. J Neurosci. 2020;40:1756–65.
121. Cunnane SC, Trushina E, Morland C, Prigione A, Casadesus G, Andrews ZB, Beal MF, Bergersen LH, Brinton RD, de la Monte S, Eckert A, Harvey J, Jeggo R, Jhamandas JH, Kann O, la Cour CM, Martin WF, Mithieux G, Moreira PI, Murphy MP, Nave KA, Nuriel T, Oliet SHR, Saudou F, Mattson MP, Swerdlow RH, Millan MJ. Brain energy rescue: an emerging therapeutic concept for neurodegenerative disorders of ageing. Nat Rev Drug Discov. 2020;19:609–33.

122. Li N, Lee B, Liu RJ, Banasr M, Dwyer JM, Iwata M, Li XY, Aghajanian G, Duman RS. mTOR-dependent synapse formation underlies the rapid antidepressant effects of NMDA antagonists. Science. 2010;329:959–64.
123. Abdallah CG, Averill LA, Gueorguieva R, Goktas S, Purohit P, Ranganathan M, Sherif M, Ahn KH, D'Souza DC, Formica R, Southwick SM, Duman RS, Sanacora G, Krystal JH. Modulation of the antidepressant effects of ketamine by the mTORC1 inhibitor rapamycin. Neuropsychopharmacology. 2020;45:990–7.

Immune Dysfunction in Obsessive-Compulsive Disorder: From Risk Factors to Multisystem Involvement

17

Ana Maia, Bernardo Barahona-Corrêa, Albino J. Oliveira-Maia, and José Oliveira

17.1 Introduction

Obsessive-compulsive disorder (OCD) is a frequent disorder, with a lifetime prevalence of 2.3% and a mean age at the onset of 19.5 years, characterized by recurrent and intrusive thoughts and/or compulsions [1, 2]. Clinical presentation is heterogeneous, varying along a spectrum of insight and a broad range of comorbid psychiatric and general medical disorders such as depression, bipolar disorder, psychotic disorders, eating disorders, allergies, migraine headaches, thyroid diseases, and metabolic syndrome [3–5]. Additionally, OCD symptoms spread across several diagnostic entities and many individuals present with seemingly subclinical forms of OCD [6]. The chronic course, early-onset, and nature of symptoms contribute to the negative impact of OCD on quality of life, including worse social functioning than patients with major depressive disorder (MDD) or schizophrenia [7]. Furthermore, while treatment, including cognitive-behavioral therapy (CBT) and

A. Maia · B. Barahona-Corrêa · A. J. Oliveira-Maia
Champalimaud Research and Clinical Centre, Champalimaud Centre for the Unknown, Lisbon, Portugal

Department of Psychiatry and Mental Health, Centro Hospitalar de Lisboa Ocidental, Lisbon, Portugal

NOVA Medical School | Faculdade de Ciências Médicas, Universidade Nova de Lisboa, Lisbon, Portugal
e-mail: ana.maia@neuro.fchampalimaud.org; bernardo.correa@research.fchampalimaud.org; albino.maia@neuro.fchampalimaud.org

J. Oliveira (✉)
Champalimaud Research and Clinical Centre, Champalimaud Centre for the Unknown, Lisbon, Portugal

NOVA Medical School | Faculdade de Ciências Médicas, Universidade Nova de Lisboa, Lisbon, Portugal
e-mail: jose.oliveira@neuro.fchampalimaud.org

M. Berk et al. (eds.), *Immuno-Psychiatry*, https://doi.org/10.1007/978-3-030-71229-7_17

pharmacotherapy, mainly with serotonin reuptake inhibitors (SSRIs), is available, approximately 40% of patients are resistant to medication [8], around 26% fail to initiate CBT, and 31% drop out before completing therapy [8, 9]. What is more, patients take an average of 10 years before searching for professional care and there is a mean 17 years lag before receiving appropriate treatment [10].

While the etiology and pathophysiology of OCD remain unknown, genetic, neurobiological, neurochemical, and psychological theories have been proposed. However, no consensus has been achieved, hindering advances in diagnosis and treatment [11–14]. Recently, immunopsychiatry has enhanced our understanding of the specific factors that mediate interactions between the brain, infectious agents, and the immune system, proposing new pathways of research and new integrative hypotheses for psychiatric disorders. Here we will review the literature of both human and animal studies supporting that OCD may be a systemic, rather than a pure brain disorder, progressing in a background of immune dysfunction. Regarding the latter, the available data suggests that early-life risk factors, such as childhood trauma and infectious events, may act cumulatively to disrupt immune homeostasis [15, 16]. Immune-induced changes of OCD-related circuits in the CNS can then trigger or modulate the psychopathological presentation in individuals that are vulnerable, while peripheral dysregulation of immune processes compromises physical health, resulting in low-grade chronic inflammation, oxidative damage, and a higher burden of comorbidity.

17.2 Obsessive-Compulsive Disorder as a Multisystem Disorder

Paul et al. (2014) proposed an integrative model suggesting that patients with OCD may have a genetic vulnerability to adverse environmental factors that dysregulate glutamatergic, serotoninergic, and dopaminergic neurotransmission [11]. Hypothetically, since this could reflect vulnerability to environmental risk factors rather than to the disorder itself, interindividual variability in gene-environment crosstalk may result in the expression of distinct psychiatric or non-psychiatric phenotypes, which may even co-occur. In fact, similarly to other psychiatric disorders, in OCD, a systemic involvement was initially suspected due to the association with several general medical disorders [17].

In fact, comorbidity between OCD and inflammation-associated disorders seems to occur more frequently than expected. Specifically, patients with auto-immune disorders (i.e. rheumatic fever, multiple sclerosis or systemic lupus erythematosus) have a higher prevalence of obsessive-compulsive symptoms, while patients with OCD have a higher prevalence of auto-immune disorders [18–20]. A population-based study including 30.082 patients with OCD found a 43% higher risk of any autoimmune disorder when compared with population controls [21]. Not surprisingly, the risk for several of these disorders was also significantly elevated in first-degree relatives, more than in second- and third-degree relatives, suggesting a shared heritability between OCD and autoimmune disorders [21]. Frequent comorbidity with other inflammation-related disorders, namely, allergies, migraine headaches, thyroid disorders, obesity, type 2 diabetes mellitus, and systemic circulatory disorders, has also been described [4, 22, 23]. Indeed, another population-based study including 25.415 patients with OCD found that these individuals have a 45% increased risk of metabolic and cardiovascular disorders [23]. These occurrences were higher when compared with unaffected siblings, suggesting that these comorbidities may be a consequence of OCD itself [23].

Increased prevalence of systemic comorbidities also seems to contribute to morbidity and mortality. Meier et al. (2016) evaluated data from 10,155 individuals with OCD in a prospective cohort study in Denmark and verified that these patients had twice the risk of premature death when compared with the general population, with 60% of deaths due to natural causes [24]. The authors found a strong contribution of comorbid anxiety disorders, depression, and, particularly, substance use disorders; but mortality remained higher even when excluding patients with such psychiatric comorbidities [24]. Overall, while disability due to OCD seems to be higher than disability due to physical diseases, individuals with both OCD and physical comorbidities are at the greatest risk of functional impairment [22]. Thus, these results not only support the multisystem character of OCD but also emphasize the need to carefully monitor and treat psychiatric and non-psychiatric comorbidities in individuals with OCD, underlining the need to understand their causes.

17.3 Immune-Related Risk Factors for Obsessive-Compulsive Disorder

In addition to systemic comorbidities, the identification of OCD risk factors that are closely related to inflammation also supports the hypothesis of an immune-based pathophysiology for the disorder. In OCD, as in other complex disorders, differential contributions of genetic and environmental factors to a global aetiopathogenic model of the disorder remain a research challenge and are far from being fully understood [25]. Immune dysfunction, acting as a cause or a consequence of genetic variability, environmental insults, or lifestyle, offers new research and clinical possibilities that are being integrated into the explicative models of OCD [19, 26].

17.3.1 Environmental Risk Factors

Brander et al. (2016) systematically reviewed the literature for case-control or cohort studies identifying environmental risk factors for OCD [27]. The authors identified nine main broad areas of risk factors, namely, (i) perinatal complications, parental age, family size, birth order, and season of birth; (ii) reproductive cycle events; (iii) stressful and traumatic life events; (iv) parental rearing styles; (v) socioeconomic status; (vi) brain injury; (vii) substance use disorders; (viii) vitamin deficiency; and (ix) infections. Although there is more evidence supporting the impact of the first three factors, the authors underline that evidence is limited due to the quantity and quality of studies, and suggest that all 9 of the identified risk factors should be equally considered. Importantly, while most of these factors are thought to induce inflammation, infection provides the most direct support for an immune-based hypothesis for the pathophysiology of OCD [28–33].

The hypothesis of immune dysregulation in OCD was first suggested by the observation that patients with Sydenham chorea frequently present obsessions and compulsions, leading to the description of a new clinical entity, designated as Pediatric Autoimmune Neuropsychiatric Disorders Associated with Streptococcus (PANDAS). PANDAS is defined by the presence of OCD and/or tic disorder with prepubertal onset, in association with neurological symptoms and with episodic exacerbations in temporal association with group A beta-hemolytic streptococcus (GABHS) infection [34]. Recently, Orlovska et al. (2017) performed a population-based cohort study in Denmark, with more than 600,000 children that received a rapid antigen diagnostic test for group A β-hemolytic streptococcal throat infection, and up to 17 years follow-up. While the authors found that those who had a positive test had an increased risk of any mental disorder, particularly OCD and tic disorders, they also described that the risk for any mental disorder was increased after nonstreptococcal throat infections [35].

Indeed, GABHS is not the only microorganism that has been associated with the onset or exacerbation of obsessive symptoms. Patients with OCD have significantly higher seropositivity for anti-*Toxoplasma gondii* IgG when compared with controls [36, 37], while seropositivity for *Toxoplasma gondii* is associated with obsessive-compulsive symptoms and a 2.5 times higher probability of an OCD diagnosis [38]. Interestingly, Strittmatter et al. (1992) in a *post-mortem* assessment of 204 brains with morphological evidence of toxoplasma encephalitis, collected from individuals that died from AIDS, concluded that the most frequently affected regions were the cerebral hemispheres and basal ganglia, in 91% and 78% of brains, respectively [39]. The latter are strongly implicated in the pathophysiology of OCD, further supporting a potential causal role for toxoplasma infection. Other studies also suggested a role for *Mycoplasma Pneumoniae* and *Borrelia burgdorferi* in the etiology of OCD [40, 41].

The description of case reports where obsessive-compulsive symptoms followed viral encephalitis suggested that OCD can also be triggered by a viral infection [42, 43]. Khanna and colleagues (1997) measured blood IgG antibodies in 76 patients with OCD and found an increase in antibodies against *herpes simplex virus* type 1 (HSV-1) and the *Mumps orthorubulavirus*, when compared with controls [44]. The authors also measured IgG antibodies for the same viruses in the cerebral spinal fluid (CSF) and found a statistically significant increase in anti-HSV-1, with a serum to CSF ratio indicating CNS antibody production [45]. In a study that measured event-related potentials during performance of a visual Go/No-Go reaction time task in patients with OCD and healthy controls, Dietrich et al. (2005) found that OCD patients with higher number of Borna Disease Virus (BDV)-specific circulating immune complexes had higher amplitude event-related brain potentials in temporo-parietal sites, suggesting that BDV infection could promote striato-thalamo-cortical hyperactivity and contribute to OCD psychopathology [46]. Overall, while an association between infections and OCD seems likely, future studies are needed in order to better understand the interaction between microorganisms and the dysregulation of CNS circuits, potentially contributing to the development of new forms of prevention, diagnosis, and treatment.

17.3.2 Immunogenetic Risk

Family and twin studies have provided strong evidence supporting the importance of genetic factors in OCD [47]. Mataix-Cols et al. (2013) with data from 24,768 patients with OCD, as well as their first- to third-degree relatives, found that the risk of OCD among relatives increases proportionally to the degree of genetic relatedness, with less effect attributed to shared environmental influences [21]. Regarding potential immunogenetic risk, tic disorder and OCD are more prevalent among first-degree relatives of children with PANDAS, suggesting that they may have increased genetic vulnerability to the effects of GABHS [48]. Also, there is an increased risk of obsessive-compulsive spectrum disorders in family members of patients with rheumatic fever, an infectious and autoimmune disease with high hereditability [49–51]. Cappi et al. (2016) sequenced all the coding regions from the entire genome of 20 sporadic OCD cases and their unaffected parents and detected 19 de novo single-nucleotide variants conferring risk for the development of OCD [52]. Interestingly, several of the genes have important functions in the immune system, such as the WW domain-containing E3 ubiquitin-protein ligase 1 (*WWP1*), which inhibits TGF-β-induced transcription, SMAD family member 4 (*SMAD4*), a signal transduction protein that is activated by TGF-β, and complement component (3b/4b) receptor 1 (*CR1*), an important regulator of complement activation and mediator of innate immunity [53–55].

The dense and polymorphic human-leukocyte antigen (*HLA*) genetic cluster, located within the major histocompatibility complex (*MHC*) on chromosome 6 (6p21.3–22.1), has also been proposed as a candidate region for OCD. It has a role in immune responses and it is classically divided into two gene clusters, HLA class I, that encodes HLA-A, HLA-B and HLA-C, and HLA class II that encodes HLA-DR, HLA-DQ, and HLA-DP, each including an α and β chain. HLA I proteins, which have an important role in detecting viruses or defective intracellular proteins and presenting them to CD8+ T cells or natural killer cells, are expressed in the surface of all nucleated cells and platelets. On the other hand, HLA II proteins are expressed only in active immune cells, including B cells, monocytes/macrophages, dendritic cells, and Langerhans cells, and are important in the recognition of extracellular exogenous proteins and presenting them to CD4+ T cells [56, 57]. HLA class II genes have been associated not only to auto-immune disorders such as rheumatoid arthritis, multiple sclerosis, or type 1 diabetes but also to psychiatric disorders such as schizophrenia, autism, and severe bipolar disorder [58–64]. Early-onset OCD patients also have a higher prevalence of HLA-DRβ1*04:01, *04:04, and *04:05 alleles (10.8%) when compared to a reference sample (6.8%), suggesting that the association between immune dysregulation and OCD could be mediated by allele variability in *HLA* class II genes [65].

Two specific genes within the *HLA* cluster have been specifically proposed for OCD, namely, *Myelin Oligodendrocyte Glycoprotein* (*MOG*), and *Tumour Necrosis Factor* (*TNF*) gene. *MOG* codes for a protein that is part of the myelin sheath and acts as a mediator between myelin and the immune system, mainly through complement activation or modulation [66]. *MOG* has been implicated in the pathophysiology of auto-immune demyelinating disorders, such as multiple sclerosis, and has also been studied in some neuropsychiatric disorders, such as MDD [67–69]. Patients with OCD seem to have a higher prevalence of the *MOG4* allele 2, which was associated with higher Y-BOCS severity scores, both in the obsession and compulsion subscales [68]. *TNF* encodes a pro-inflammatory cytokine that is mainly produced by macrophages and has an important role in synaptic plasticity and in inflammatory responses [70]. Several studies have assessed the potential relation between *TNF* polymorphisms and OCD, with promising results [71–73]. In a recent meta-analysis including a total of 435 OCD patients and 1,073 controls, Jiang et al. (2018) found that the *TNF rs*361525 (−238G/A) polymorphism was associated with a reduced risk of OCD, suggesting that this specific polymorphism could act as a protective factor [74]. However, the quantitative analysis only included 3 studies, and only one reported statistically significant results [71].

In order to assess the involvement of other immune-related genes on the pathophysiology of OCD, additional case-control association studies investigated polymorphisms in NFKB inhibitor like 1 (*NFKBIL1*, *rs*2071592), interleukin 12B (*IL12B*, *rs*3212227), and C-C motif chemokine ligand 2 (*CCL2*, *rs*1024611), but results were not statistically significant [75–77]. Thus, while the existing evidence suggests immunogenetic risk in OCD, further studies are needed to support this possibility, including more robust case-control, family-based, and genome sequencing studies. In addition to identifying risk-modulating polymorphisms, such studies should also test associations with illness characteristics, potential interactions with environmental risk factors, and their contribution to immune dysfunction and oxidative stress.

17.4 Evidence of Immune-Related Dysfunction in Obsessive-Compulsive Disorder

17.4.1 Inflammation and Autoimmunity

Several case-control studies measured peripheral inflammatory markers in OCD patients and healthy controls, namely, cytokines, lymphocytes subsets, anti-basal ganglia antibodies (ABGA), reactivity to D8/17 antibody, and C-reactive protein [78–95]. While results among studies were often inconsistent, variability between individual studies does not exclude the existence of immune dysregulation and alternative explanations have been proposed to explain non-significant results. First, markers of immune function can be elevated only transiently during illness exacerbations, with non-significant results resulting from measurements performed during periods of remission [96]. While pharmacological treatment has also been proposed to affect immune and inflammatory markers, studies testing this hypothesis were often inconsistent [85, 87–89, 97, 98]. Methodological approaches with variable sensitivities and specificities may also lead to discrepancies among studies [99, 100]. Lack of consideration of age at onset in subgroup analyses can also have an impact given that the pathophysiology of OCD can differ among child and adult populations [19]. Finally, we also hypothesize that OCD patients presenting with immune system dysregulation may represent a subgroup of patients with specific pathophysiology, with differences resulting from the varying representation of this subgroup between studies.

Variability in individual studies motivated the development of meta-analyses for joint consideration of quantitative evidence. Gray et al. (2012) found a statistically significant reduction in IL-1β levels in OCD, with non-significant differences in plasma IL-6 or TNF-α [97]. By performing subgroup analyses, the authors also found that studies evaluating children or adults on psychoactive medication found significantly lower levels of IL-6 than studies evaluating adults without current medication. Furthermore, studies including individuals with comorbid depression found significantly higher levels of TNF-α than studies including OCD patients without comorbid depression [97]. However, a recent meta-analysis including a higher number of studies and participants did not find a statistically significant difference in any of the evaluated cytokines (i.e. TNF-α, IL-6, IL-1β, IL-4, IL-10, and interferon-γ) between OCD patients and healthy controls [101]. Pearlman et al. (2014) described an increase of plasma ABGA in OCD patients and referred one study reporting a statistically significant increase in CSF ABGA in 23 patients with OCD when compared to controls [102, 103]. More recently, other peripheral markers of immune function have been explored in the context of the disorder. For example, child and adolescent-onset OCD patients present with higher levels of the pro-inflammatory Th17 cells, which control extracellular bacterial and fungal infections and lower levels of the anti-inflammatory Treg cells, suggesting a dysregulated immune response [104].

However, nearly all of these markers were measured in peripheral blood, and neuroinflammation has only recently been suggested in purely OCD patients. Attwells et al. (2017) evaluated brain inflammation in patients with OCD *in vivo*, by using translocator protein (TSPO) positron emission tomography (PET) imaging as a proxy of microglial activation. In this case-control-study, the authors verified that patients with OCD had an increased TSPO VT in the cortico-striato-thalamo-cortical circuits [105]. Furthermore, distress associated with preventing compulsions was correlated with TSPO VT expression in the orbitofrontal cortex [105].

Immune dysfunction in OCD has also been selected as a therapeutic target in some clinical trials testing the effect of anti-inflammatory molecules. Minocycline is a tetracycline antibiotic that passes the blood-brain barrier and is thought to have a neuroprotective effect by the suppression of the upregulation of pro-inflammatory agents (i.e., nitric oxide, IL-1β, and TNF-α) and inhibition of microglial activation [106]. Two clinical trials, one of them open-label and the other one a randomized controlled, evaluated the effect of combined treatment with SSRI + minocycline or placebo in the treatment of OCD [107, 108]. While the former included only nine patients and did not find statistically significant results, the latter included 126 patients and found a significantly greater rate of response in the minocycline group, suggesting that minocycline might be an effective adjuvant option in the treatment of OCD.

17.4.2 Oxidative and Nitrosative Stress

Free radicals, also known as reactive oxygen species (ROS) or reactive nitrogen species (RNS), are molecules derived from oxygen or nitrogen that have an unpaired electron in their outer orbital and tend to oxidize other molecules. Free radicals are constantly formed as products of normal metabolic pathways, and in physiological conditions, they are balanced with antioxidant defenses that reduce ROS/RNS, preventing them from reacting with the surrounding substances. However, in pathological conditions, the generation of ROS/RNS may overcome the capacity of antioxidant defenses, inducing damage to cellular constituents, with irreversible modifications to DNA, proteins, lipids, or sugars [109]. Such imbalance is called oxidative stress and has been demonstrated to occur in several non-psychiatric and psychiatric illnesses [110, 111], such as MDD, bipolar disorder, and schizophrenia [112–117]. We recently performed a systematic review and meta-analysis evaluating O&NS markers in OCD, including a total of 433 OCD patients and 459 healthy controls, and found evidence supporting elevated oxidative stress in OCD, without consistent evidence for an adequate antioxidant response, suggesting that patients with OCD have a systemic oxidative imbalance that is not adequately buffered by the antioxidant system [118].

It is important to underline that oxidative balance is critical for immune system physiology. In fact, immune cells have a high percentage of polyunsaturated fatty acids in their plasma membranes, making them extremely sensitive to oxidative stress. Moreover, signal transduction and gene expression events, which are critical to the normal function of immune cells, are extremely sensitive to oxidation. Finally, immune reactions produce high quantities of free radicals, further increasing the risk of oxidation. Nevertheless, in physiological conditions immune cells have high levels of antioxidant defense and their maintenance in optimal levels is critical to immune function. However, in pathological conditions, oxidant molecules might overcome the antioxidant capacity and oxidative stress might occur, affecting immune function, mainly through the decline of T cell responses [119, 120]. Oxidative and immune systems are intimately correlated and both seem to be dysregulated in OCD. The integration of these two systems is crucial to the understanding of OCD and to the development of new treatment options.

In this context, several clinical trials have tested the pharmacological use of N-acetylcysteine (NAC) in the treatment of OCD [121, 122]. NAC, mostly known for its anti-inflammatory, mucolytic, and hepatoprotective activity, is also an antioxidant precursor to cysteine, which is used as a substrate for the synthesis of one of the major antioxidant molecules in the brain, glutathione [121, 123]. Two recent systematic reviews summarized the evidence for NAC as monotherapy or adjunctive treatment in OCD or OCD-related disorders, suggesting its potential use as an augmentation strategy [121, 122]. Moreover, one controlled clinical trial randomized 48 OCD patients failing to respond to a course of SSRI treatment, to 12-week augmentation with NAC or placebo, with 52.6% of patients in the active treatment group achieving clinical response, compared with only 15% in the control group [124]. These encouraging results strengthen the importance of oxidative dysregulation in OCD and encourage the development of new clinical trials that might reinforce the evidence for the use of antioxidants in the treatment of psychiatric disorders. Assuming that oxidative dysregulation may be restricted to a specific subgroup of patients, it would be interesting to develop such trials stratifying according to levels of O&NS markers.

17.5 Research in Animal Models

Animal studies in psychiatry are limited by the difficulties in representing and interpreting complex human psychopathology in nonhuman species. For OCD animal models, despite the limitations in the study of obsessions, compulsion-like behaviors are easily observed and measured in the form of stereotypic/repetitive, grooming, or collecting/hoarding behaviors. These studies may allow a more controlled and detailed comprehension of the association between immune dysregulation and OCD.

Microglia are macrophage-lineage cells derived from myeloid progenitors. While, in the past, they were considered to be phagocytic cells quiescent under physiological conditions [125], current evidence supports that microglia are constantly active and have important physiologic functions for the development of mature synapses during embryogenesis, as well as for neurogenesis and synaptic pruning during adulthood [126–128]. Animal models have contributed to a better understanding of the relationship between microglia and behavior, with *Hoxb8* knockout (KO) mice as an example of particular interest. *Hox* genes code for transcription factors with roles in embryo development across different tissues and organs, including the hematopoietic system, where *Hoxb8* is responsible for the maintenance and differentiation of myeloid progenitor cells [129]. Importantly, *Hoxb8* KO mice show excessive grooming behavior, characterized by excessive hair removal and self-inflicted wounds, which was thought to be related to strong *Hoxb8* expression in the cortico-striato-thalamo-cortical circuit, namely, the basal ganglia and cortex, as well as in the olfactory bulb, hippocampus, and cerebellum [130, 131]. Importantly, the only brain cells derived from *Hoxb8* lineage are microglia that have reduced numbers in *Hoxb8* KO [132], which may underlie synaptic dysfunction within the corticostriatal circuit, namely, synaptic expansion in the frontal cortex, and synaptic contraction in the striatum, which has been described in these animals [133, 134]. Furthermore, *Hoxb8* KO mice develop autoimmune processes driven by autoantibodies against different self-tissues, including brain, kidney, and liver [133, 134]. Notably, Chen et al. (2010) demonstrated that the compulsive-like behavioral dysfunction expressed by these mice is reversible after bone marrow transplantation from control mice [132].

Progranulin KO mice (*Grn*$^{-/-}$) have also raised great interest in the field of OCD pathophysiology. Progranulin is a glycoprotein with many different roles both outside and within the brain, acting, namely, as a neuroprotective agent and in the regulation of neuroinflammation and neuronal lysosome function regulation [135]. Autosomal dominant mutations in the human progranulin gene are associated to a drastic reduction in progranulin levels and contribute to frontotemporal lobar degeneration, the second most common form of early-onset dementia after Alzheimer's disease [136, 137]. Lui et al. (2016) demonstrated that *Grn*$^{-/-}$ mice show an age-dependent up-regulation of lysosomal and innate immunity genes in microglia, with an increase in microglia infiltration and neuronal loss [138]. Specifically, microglia-driven elimination of inhibitory synapses occurs preferentially in the ventral thalamus, with hyperactivity in the thalamocortical circuit and, not surprisingly, development of compulsive-like grooming behaviors. Notably, after observing that C1qa and C3 mRNA levels were much higher in *Grn*$^{-/-}$ mice microglia, and considering the roles of complement in innate immunity and synaptic pruning, the authors deleted C1qa gene in *Grn*$^{-/-}$ mice and observed a reduction in synaptic pruning with increased synaptic density around microglia and an amelioration in grooming behaviors [127, 138]. This study supports the idea that progranulin is required for the inhibition of excessive microglia activation and that blocking complement activation might ameliorate grooming behaviors.

Mice lacking fractalkine chemokine receptor (*Cx3cr1* KO) have a significant reduction in microglia density and reduced synaptic pruning [128]. Zhan et al. (2014) demonstrated that *Cx3cr1* KO mice have reduced number of synapses per axonal input (i.e., synaptic multiplicity), reduced functional connectivity between the right and left dorsal hippocampus and the medial prefrontal cortex, compromised social interaction and excessive grooming behavior when exposed to novelty [139]. While the authors interpreted this behavior pattern as representative of an autism-like phenotype, they also support the hypothesis for microglia dysregulation in OCD pathophysiology, eventually through synaptic pruning.

Animal studies have also been important in elucidating the pathophysiology of PANDAS. In mice, GABHS are predominantly found in nasal-associated lymphoid tissue (NALT), a functional equivalent to human palatine tonsils, and recurrent GABHS infection in mice, similar to what occurs in human tonsils, induces a dominant Th17 response in NALT with cytokine shift to an IL-17A^{+}IFN-γ^{+} profile [140–142]. Dileepan et al. (2016) demonstrated that immunization by multiple GABHS infections promotes migration of specific Th17 cells from NALT to the olfactory tube and then to different brain regions. This migration is associated with a blood-brain barrier breakdown that consequently allows the entry of circulating IgG and additional CD4^{+} T cells, promoting microglia activation and altered synaptic connectivity [142]. Furthermore, passive transfer of serum with streptococcus-induced antibodies from PANDAS mice reproduced the donor behavioral pattern in naïve mice. Importantly, this effect was not observed after the depletion of IgG from

GABHS donor sera before injection [143]. However, these results were not replicated in subsequent studies and the mechanisms by which antibodies cross the blood-brain barrier remain unknown.

17.6 Conclusions and Future Challenges

The existing evidence suggests that OCD is a multisystem disorder, developing in a background of immune dysfunction. The origin of such immune dysfunction is thought to be multifactorial, with both constitutive and environmental elements, contributing to illness development, clinical presentation, and multisystem impact (Fig. 17.1). In fact, we believe the available evidence is suggestive that early-life risk factors may disrupt immune balance and induce dysfunction in OCD-specific circuitry, inducing psychopathology in genetically vulnerable individuals. Chronic dysregulation of the immune system may also promote low-grade inflammation, oxidative damage, and the development of psychiatric and non-psychiatric comorbidities. Moreover, the behavioral and social impact of the disorder can promote additional pro-inflammatory insults, further disrupting immune homeostasis. Nevertheless, evidence remains controversial and future studies are needed in order to further explore these hypotheses and translate findings into clinical practice, namely, regarding the identification of genetic or environmental biomarkers of OCD vulnerability and of response to treatment.

The sparsity of longitudinal studies represents a significant additional barrier to integrate immune dysfunction in OCD pathophysiology since this might contribute to the development of OCD, as well as be a consequence of OCD impact over behavior and physical health, or an adaptive physiological response to illness. Longitudinal studies are crucial to better understand causal relations between immune markers and relevant clinical characteristics. It is also important to

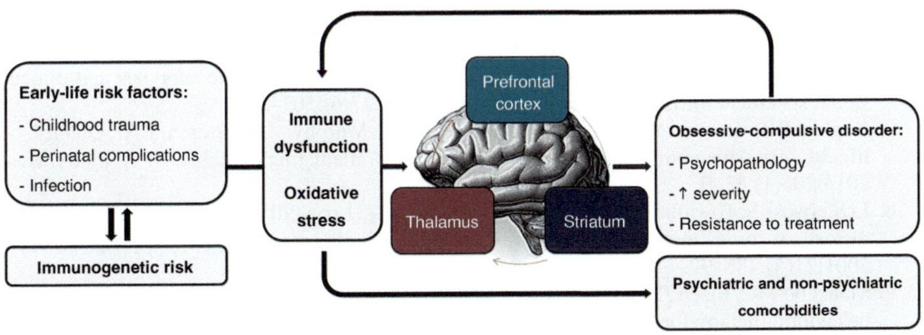

Fig. 17.1 Integrative model of obsessive-compulsive disorder pathophysiology. In vulnerable individuals, environmental risk factors induce low-grade inflammation and disrupt immune and oxidative homeostasis, promoting immune-induced dysfunction in the cortico-striatal-thalamic-cortical circuit and OCD psychopathology. Additionally, systemic dysfunction may also promote non-psychiatric comorbidities and, by affecting different brain regions, also psychiatric comorbidities. *O&NS* Oxidative & Nitrosative Stress

underline that immune dysfunction seems to be unspecific, occurring in several other psychiatric illnesses [144]. In fact, OCD may have shared immunogenetic heritability with other psychiatric illnesses, with different psychopathological patterns resulting from additional brain-related susceptibility factors. However, to our knowledge, so far no study has compared immune dysfunction between different psychiatric illnesses. Finally, few clinical trials have assessed the use of anti-inflammatory or anti-oxidative substances in the treatment of OCD, but data remains controversial. We propose that immune dysfunction may be a predominant pathophysiological mechanism in a subgroup of patients, which would potentially justify the limited robustness of results. Consequently, we consider that pre-treatment measurement of immune markers in future clinical trials could allow for correlation of baseline immune dysfunction with treatment outcomes, with potential validation of relevant treatments as well as biomarkers. Ultimately, enhanced comprehension over the genesis and characteristics of immune dysfunction in OCD could promote the development of better prevention, diagnostic, and treatment methods, paving the path toward enhanced care and improvements in quality of life.

References

1. Ruscio AM, Stein DJ, Chiu WT, Kessler RC. The epidemiology of obsessive-compulsive disorder in the National Comorbidity Survey Replication. Mol Psychiatry. 2010;15(1):53–63.
2. American Psychiatric Association. Diagnostic and statistical manual of mental disorders (DSM-V). 5th ed; 2013.
3. Brady CF. Obsessive-compulsive disorder and common comorbidities. J Clin Psychiatry. 2014;75(1):e02.
4. Albert U, Aguglia A, Chiarle A, Bogetto F, Maina G. Metabolic syndrome and obsessive-compulsive disorder: a naturalistic Italian study. Gen Hosp Psychiatry. 2013;35(2):154–9.
5. Lochner C, Fineberg NA, Zohar J, van Ameringen M, Juven-Wetzler A, Altamura AC, et al. Comorbidity in obsessive-compulsive disorder (OCD): a report from the International College of Obsessive-Compulsive Spectrum Disorders (ICOCS). Compr Psychiatry. 2014;55(7):1513–9.
6. Leckman JF, Denys D, Simpson HB, Mataix-Cols D, Hollander E, Saxena S, et al. Obsessive-compulsive disorder: a review of the diagnostic criteria and possible subtypes and dimensional specifiers for DSM-V. Depress Anxiety. 2010;27(6):507–27.
7. Kugler BB, Lewin AB, Phares V, Geffken GR, Murphy TK, Storch EA. Quality of life in obsessive-compulsive disorder: the role of mediating variables. Psychiatry Res. 2013;206(1):43–9.
8. Erzegovesi S, Cavallini MC, Cavedini P, Diaferia G, Locatelli M, Bellodi L. Clinical predictors of drug response in obsessive-compulsive disorder. J Clin Psychopharmacol. 2001;21(5):488–92.
9. Mancebo MC, Eisen JL, Sibrava N, Dyck IR, Rasmussen SA. Patient utilization of cognitive-behavioral therapy for OCD. Behav Ther. 2011;42(3):399–412.
10. Hollander E, Stein DJ, Kwon JH, Rowland C, Wong CM, Broatch J, et al. Psychosocial function and economic costs of obsessive-compulsive disorder. CNS Spectr. 1997;2(10):16–25.
11. Pauls DL, Abramovitch A, Rauch SL, Geller DA. Obsessive-compulsive disorder: an integrative genetic and neurobiological perspective. Nat Rev Neurosci. 2014;15(6):410–24.
12. Rotge JY, Aouizerate B, Tignol J, Bioulac B, Burbaud P, Guehl D. The glutamate-based genetic immune hypothesis in obsessive-compulsive disorder. An integrative approach from genes to symptoms. Neuroscience. 2010;165(2):408–17.

13. Nakao T, Okada K, Kanba S. Neurobiological model of obsessive-compulsive disorder: evidence from recent neuropsychological and neuroimaging findings. Psychiatry Clin Neurosci. 2014;68(8):587–605.
14. Zohar J, Greenberg B, Denys D. Obsessive-compulsive disorder. Handb Clin Neurol. 2012;106:375–90.
15. Gerentes M, Pelissolo A, Rajagopal K, Tamouza R, Hamdani N. Obsessive-compulsive disorder: autoimmunity and neuroinflammation. Curr Psychiatry Rep. 2019;21(8):78.
16. Lamothe H, Baleyte J-M, Smith P, Pelissolo A, Mallet L. Individualized immunological data for precise classification of OCD patients. Brain Sci. 2018;8(8)
17. Leboyer M, Oliveira J, Tamouza R, Groc L. Is it time for immunopsychiatry in psychotic disorders? Psychopharmacology. 2016;233(9).1651–60.
18. Dinn WM, Harris CL, McGonigal KM, Raynard RC. Obsessive-compulsive disorder and immunocompetence. Int J Psychiatry Med. 2001;31(3):311–20.
19. Marazziti D, Mucci F, Fontenelle LF. Immune system and obsessive-compulsive disorder. Psychoneuroendocrinology. 2018;93:39–44.
20. Pérez-Vigil A, Fernández de la Cruz L, Brander G, Isomura K, Gromark C, Mataix-Cols D. The link between autoimmune diseases and obsessive-compulsive and tic disorders: a systematic review. Neurosci Biobehav Rev. 2016;71:542–62.
21. Mataix-Cols D, Frans E, Pérez-Vigil A, Kuja-Halkola R, Gromark C, Isomura K, et al. A total-population multigenerational family clustering study of autoimmune diseases in obsessive-compulsive disorder and Tourette's/chronic tic disorders. Mol Psychiatry. 2018;23(7): 1652–8.
22. Witthauer CT, Gloster A, Meyer AH, Lieb R. Physical diseases among persons with obsessive compulsive symptoms and disorder: a general population study. Soc Psychiatry Psychiatr Epidemiol. 2014;49(12):2013–22.
23. Isomura K, Brander G, Chang Z, Kuja-Halkola R, Rück C, Hellner C, et al. Metabolic and cardiovascular complications in obsessive-compulsive disorder: a total population, sibling comparison study with long-term follow-up. Biol Psychiatry. 2018;84(5): 324–31.
24. Meier SM, Mattheisen M, Mors O, Schendel DE, Mortensen PB, Plessen KJ. Mortality among persons with obsessive-compulsive disorder in Denmark. JAMA Psychiat. 2016;73(3):268–74.
25. Zammit S, Owen MJ, Lewis G. Misconceptions about gene-environment interactions in psychiatry. Evid Based Ment Health. 2010;13(3):65–8.
26. Murphy TK, Sajid MW, Goodman WK. Immunology of obsessive-compulsive disorder. Psychiatr Clin North Am. 2006;29(2):445–69.
27. Brander G, Pérez-Vigil A, Larsson H, Mataix-Cols D. Systematic review of environmental risk factors for obsessive-compulsive disorder: a proposed roadmap from association to causation. Neurosci Biobehav Rev. 2016;65:36–62.
28. Baumeister D, Akhtar R, Ciufolini S, Pariante CM, Mondelli V. Childhood trauma and adulthood inflammation: a meta-analysis of peripheral C-reactive protein, interleukin-6 and tumour necrosis factor-α. Mol Psychiatry. 2016;21(5):642–9.
29. Depino AM. Perinatal inflammation and adult psychopathology: from preclinical models to humans. Semin Cell Dev Biol. 2018;77:104–14.
30. Muscatell KA, Brosso SN, Humphreys KL. Socioeconomic status and inflammation: a meta-analysis. Mol Psychiatry. 2018;1
31. Glaus J, Vandeleur CL, von Känel R, Lasserre AM, Strippoli M-PF, Gholam-Rezaee M, et al. Associations between mood, anxiety or substance use disorders and inflammatory markers after adjustment for multiple covariates in a population-based study. J Psychiatr Res. 2014;58:36–45.
32. Corps KN, Roth TL, McGavern DB. Inflammation and neuroprotection in traumatic brain injury. JAMA Neurol. 2015;72(3):355–62.
33. Calton EK, Keane KN, Newsholme P, Soares MJ. The impact of vitamin D levels on inflammatory status: a systematic review of immune cell studies. PLoS One. 2015;10(11)

34. Swedo SE, Leonard HL, Garvey M, Mittleman B, Allen AJ, Perlmutter S, et al. Pediatric autoimmune neuropsychiatric disorders associated with streptococcal infections: clinical description of the first 50 cases. Am J Psychiatry. 1998;155(2):264–71.
35. Orlovska S, Vestergaard CH, Bech BH, Nordentoft M, Vestergaard M, Benros ME. Association of streptococcal throat infection with mental disorders: testing key aspects of the PANDAS hypothesis in a nationwide study. JAMA Psychiat. 2017;74(7):740–6.
36. Miman O, Mutlu EA, Ozcan O, Atambay M, Karlidag R, Unal S. Is there any role of toxoplasma gondii in the etiology of obsessive-compulsive disorder? Psychiatry Res. 2010;177(1–2):263–5.
37. Akaltun İ, Kara SS, Kara T. The relationship between toxoplasma gondii IgG antibodies and generalized anxiety disorder and obsessive-compulsive disorder in children and adolescents: a new approach. Nord J Psychiatry. 2018;72(1):57–62.
38. Flegr J, Horáček J. Toxoplasma-infected subjects report an obsessive-compulsive disorder diagnosis more often and score higher in obsessive-compulsive inventory. Eur Psychiatry. 2017;40:82–7.
39. Strittmatter C, Lang W, Wiestler OD, Kleihues P. The changing pattern of human immunodeficiency virus-associated cerebral toxoplasmosis: a study of 46 postmortem cases. Acta Neuropathol (Berl). 1992;83(5):475–81.
40. Johnco C, Kugler BB, Murphy TK, Storch EA. Obsessive-compulsive symptoms in adults with Lyme disease. Gen Hosp Psychiatry. 2018;51:85–9.
41. Ercan TE, Ercan G, Severge B, Arpaozu M, Karasu G. Mycoplasma pneumoniae infection and obsessive-compulsive disease: a case report. J Child Neurol. 2008;23(3):338–40.
42. Johnson J, Lucey PA. Encephalitis lethargica, a contemporary cause of catatonic stupor. A report of two cases. Br J Psychiatry. 1987;151:550–2.
43. Laplane D, Levasseur M, Pillon B, Dubois B, Baulac M, Mazoyer B, et al. Obsessive-compulsive and other behavioural changes with bilateral basal ganglia lesions. A neuropsychological, magnetic resonance imaging and positron tomography study. Brain. 1989;112(3):699–725.
44. Khanna S, Ravi V, Shenoy PK, Chandramukhi A, Channabasavanna SM. Viral antibodies in blood in obsessive compulsive disorder. Indian J Psychiatry. 1997;39(3):190–5.
45. Khanna S, Ravi V, Shenoy PK, Chandramukhi A, Channabasavanna SM. Cerebrospinal fluid viral antibodies in obsessive-compulsive disorder in an Indian population. Biol Psychiatry. 1997;41(8):883–90.
46. Dietrich DE, Zhang Y, Bode L, Münte TF, Hauser U, Schmorl P, et al. Brain potential amplitude varies as a function of Borna disease virus-specific immune complexes in obsessive–compulsive disorder. Mol Psychiatry. 2005;10(6):515.
47. Pauls DL. The genetics of obsessive-compulsive disorder: a review. Dialogues Clin Neurosci. 2010;12(2):149–63.
48. Lougee L, Perlmutter SJ, Nicolson R, Garvey MA, Swedo SE. Psychiatric disorders in first-degree relatives of children with pediatric autoimmune neuropsychiatric disorders associated with streptococcal infections (PANDAS). J Am Acad Child Adolesc Psychiatry. 2000;39(9):1120–6.
49. Seixas AAA, Hounie AG, Fossaluza V, Curi M, Alvarenga PG, De Mathis MA, et al. Anxiety disorders and rheumatic fever: is there an association? CNS Spectr. 2008;13(12):1039–46.
50. Hounie AG, Pauls DL, do Rosario-Campos MC, Mercadante MT, Diniz JB, De Mathis MA, et al. Obsessive-compulsive spectrum disorders and rheumatic fever: a family study. Biol Psychiatry. 2007;61(3):266–72.
51. Engel ME, Stander R, Vogel J, Adeyemo AA, Mayosi BM. Genetic susceptibility to acute rheumatic fever: a systematic review and meta-analysis of twin studies. PLoS One. 2011;6(9):e25326.
52. Cappi C, Brentani H, Lima L, Sanders SJ, Zai G, Diniz BJ, et al. Whole-exome sequencing in obsessive-compulsive disorder identifies rare mutations in immunological and neurodevelopmental pathways. Transl Psychiatry. 2016;6(3):e764.

53. Komuro A, Imamura T, Saitoh M, Yoshida Y, Yamori T, Miyazono K, et al. Negative regulation of transforming growth factor-beta (TGF-beta) signaling by WW domain-containing protein 1 (WWP1). Oncogene. 2004;23(41):6914–23.
54. ten Dijke P, Hill CS. New insights into TGF-beta-Smad signalling. Trends Biochem Sci. 2004;29(5):265–73.
55. Noris M, Remuzzi G. Overview of complement activation and regulation. Semin Nephrol. 2013;33(6):479–92.
56. Mosaad YM. Clinical role of human leukocyte antigen in health and disease. Scand J Immunol. 2015;82(4):283–306.
57. Choo SY, The HLA. System: genetics, immunology, clinical testing, and clinical implications. Yonsei Med J. 2007;48(1):11–23.
58. Needleman LA, McAllister AK. The major histocompatibility complex and autism spectrum disorder. Dev Neurobiol. 2012;72(10):1288–301.
59. Mokhtari R, Lachman HM. The major histocompatibility complex (MHC) in schizophrenia: a review. J Clin Cell Immunol. 2016;7(6)
60. Thomson G, Valdes AM, Noble JA, Kockum I, Grote MN, Najman J, et al. Relative predispositional effects of HLA class II DRB1-DQB1 haplotypes and genotypes on type 1 diabetes: a meta-analysis. Tissue Antigens. 2007;70(2):110–27.
61. Fogdell-Hahn A, Ligers A, Grønning M, Hillert J, Olerup O. Multiple sclerosis: a modifying influence of HLA class I genes in an HLA class II associated autoimmune disease. Tissue Antigens. 2000;55(2):140–8.
62. Kampstra ASB, Toes REM. HLA class II and rheumatoid arthritis: the bumpy road of revelation. Immunogenetics. 2017;69(8–9):597–603.
63. Miyadera H, Tokunaga K. Associations of human leukocyte antigens with autoimmune diseases: challenges in identifying the mechanism. J Hum Genet. 2015;60(11):697–702.
64. Tamouza R, Oliveira J, Etain B, Bengoufa D, Hamdani N, Manier C, et al. HLA genetics in bipolar disorder. Acta Psychiatr Scand. 2018;138(5):464–71.
65. Rodriguez N, Morer A, González-Navarro EA, Gassó P, Boloc D, Serra-Pagès C, et al. Human-leukocyte antigen class II genes in early-onset obsessive-compulsive disorder. World J Biol Psychiatry. 2017:1–7.
66. Johns TG, Bernard CC. The structure and function of myelin oligodendrocyte glycoprotein. J Neurochem. 1999;72(1):1–9.
67. Peschl P, Bradl M, Höftberger R, Berger T, Reindl M. Myelin oligodendrocyte glycoprotein: deciphering a target in inflammatory demyelinating diseases. Front Immunol. 2017;8
68. Zai G, Bezchlibnyk YB, Richter MA, Arnold P, Burroughs E, Barr CL, et al. Myelin oligodendrocyte glycoprotein (MOG) gene is associated with obsessive-compulsive disorder. Am J Med Genet Part B Neuropsychiatr Genet. 2004;129B(1):64–8.
69. Wu F, Kong L, Zhu Y, Zhou Q, Jiang X, Chang M, et al. The influence of myelin oligodendrocyte glycoprotein on white matter abnormalities in different onset age of drug-Naïve depression. Front Psych. 2018;9
70. Parameswaran N, Patial S. Tumor necrosis factor-α signaling in macrophages. Crit Rev Eukaryot Gene Expr. 2010;20(2):87–103.
71. Hounie AG, Cappi C, Cordeiro Q, Sampaio AS, Moraes I, Rosário MC, do Rosario MC, et al. TNF-alpha polymorphisms are associated with obsessive-compulsive disorder. Neurosci Lett. 2008;442(2):86–90.
72. Cappi C, Muniz RK, Sampaio AS, Cordeiro Q, Brentani H, Palácios SA, et al. Association study between functional polymorphisms in the TNF-alpha gene and obsessive-compulsive disorder. Arq Neuropsiquiatr. 2012;70(2):87–90.
73. Lüleyap H, Onatoğlu D, Tahiroğlu A, Alptekin D, Yılmaz M, Cetiner S, et al. Association between obsessive compulsive disorder and tumor necrosis factor-α gene −308 (G>a) and −850 (C>T) polymorphisms in Turkish children. Balk J Med Genet. 2012;15(2): 61–6.
74. Jiang C, Ma X, Qi S, Han G, Li Y, Liu Y, et al. Association between TNF-α-238G/A gene polymorphism and OCD susceptibility. Medicine (Baltimore). 2018;97(5)

75. Zhag X, Yin W, Liu S, Ma X. A case-control association study between obsessive-compulsive disorder (OCD) and the MCP-1 -2518G/a polymorphism in a Chinese sample. Braz J Psychiatry. 2012;34(4):451–3.
76. Liu S, Liu Y, Yin Y, Zhang X, Ma X. A case-control study of interleukin-12 1188A/C polymorphism in obsessive-compulsive disorder in Chinese population. Acta Neuropsychiatr. 2012;24(3):172–5.
77. Cordeiro Q, Cappi C, Sampaio AS, Palácios SA, Pereira CA, de B, Shavitt RG, et al. Association study between the -62A/T NFKBIL1 polymorphism and obsessive-compulsive disorder. Braz J Psychiatry. 2009;31(2):131–5.
78. Murphy TK, Goodman WK, Fudge MW, Williams RC, Ayoub EM, Dalal M, et al. B lymphocyte antigen D8/17: a peripheral marker for childhood-onset obsessive-compulsive disorder and Tourette's syndrome? Am J Psychiatry. 1997;154(3):402–7.
79. Swedo SE, Leonard HL, Mittleman BB, Allen AJ, Rapoport JL, Dow SP, et al. Identification of children with pediatric autoimmune neuropsychiatric disorders associated with streptococcal infections by a marker associated with rheumatic fever. Am J Psychiatry. 1997;154(1):110–2.
80. Luo F, Leckman JF, Katsovich L, Findley D, Grantz H, Tucker DM, et al. Prospective longitudinal study of children with tic disorders and/or obsessive-compulsive disorder: relationship of symptom exacerbations to newly acquired streptococcal infections. Pediatrics. 2004;113(6):e578–85.
81. Kiessling LS, Marcotte AC, Culpepper L. Antineuronal antibodies: tics and obsessive-compulsive symptoms. J Dev Behav Pediatr. 1994;15(6):421–5.
82. Peterson BS, Leckman JF, Tucker D, Scahill L, Staib L, Zhang H, et al. Preliminary findings of antistreptococcal antibody titers and basal ganglia volumes in tic, obsessive-compulsive, and attention deficit/hyperactivity disorders. Arch Gen Psychiatry. 2000;57(4):364–72.
83. Pavone P, Bianchini R, Parano E, Incorpora G, Rizzo R, Mazzone L, et al. Anti-brain antibodies in PANDAS versus uncomplicated streptococcal infection. Pediatr Neurol. 2004;30(2):107–10.
84. Dale RC, Heyman I, Giovannoni G, Church AJ. Incidence of anti-brain antibodies in children with obsessive–compulsive disorder. Br J Psychiatry. 2005;187(4):314–9.
85. Barber Y, Toren P, Achiron A, Noy S, Wolmer L, Weizman R, et al. T cell subsets in obsessive-compulsive disorder. Neuropsychobiology. 1996;34(2):63–6.
86. Marazziti D, Presta S, Pfanner C, Gemignani A, Rossi A, Sbrana S, et al. Immunological alterations in adult obsessive-compulsive disorder. Biol Psychiatry. 1999;46(6):810–4.
87. Ravindran AV, Griffiths J, Merali Z, Anisman H. Circulating lymphocyte subsets in obsessive compulsive disorder, major depression and normal controls. J Affect Disord. 1999;52(1–3):1–10.
88. Weizman R, Laor N, Barber Y, Hermesh H, Notti I, Djaldetti M, et al. Cytokine production in obsessive-compulsive disorder. Biol Psychiatry. 1996;40(9):908–12.
89. Brambilla F, Perna G, Bellodi L, Arancio C, Bertani A, Perini G, et al. Plasma interleukin-1 beta and tumor necrosis factor concentrations in obsessive-compulsive disorders. Biol Psychiatry. 1997;42(11):976–81.
90. Maes M, Meltzer HY, Bosmans E. Psychoimmune investigation in obsessive-compulsive disorder: assays of plasma transferrin, IL-2 and IL-6 receptor, and IL-1 beta and IL-6 concentrations. Neuropsychobiology. 1994;30(2–3):57–60.
91. Monteleone P, Catapano F, Fabrazzo M, Tortorella A, Maj M. Decreased blood levels of tumor necrosis factor-alpha in patients with obsessive-compulsive disorder. Neuropsychobiology. 1998;37(4):182–5.
92. Carpenter LL, Heninger GR, McDougle CJ, Tyrka AR, Epperson CN, Price LH. Cerebrospinal fluid interleukin-6 in obsessive-compulsive disorder and trichotillomania. Psychiatry Res. 2002;112(3):257–62.
93. Denys D, Fluitman S, Kavelaars A, Heijnen C, Westenberg H. Decreased TNF-alpha and NK activity in obsessive-compulsive disorder. Psychoneuroendocrinology. 2004;29(7):945–52.

94. Konuk N, Tekin IO, Ozturk U, Atik L, Atasoy N, Bektas S, et al. Plasma levels of tumor necrosis factor-alpha and interleukin-6 in obsessive compulsive disorder. Mediat Inflamm. 2007;65704
95. Ekinci A, Ekinci O. The relationships between low grade inflammation, demographic and clinical characteristics in patients with obsessive compulsive disorder. Anatolian J Psychiatry. 2017;18(5):438–45.
96. da Rocha F, Correa H, Lucio TA. Obsessive-compulsive disorder and immunology: a review. Prog Neuro-Psychopharmacol Biol Psychiatry. 2008;32(5):1139–46.
97. Gray SM, Bloch MH. Systematic review of proinflammatory cytokines in obsessive-compulsive disorder. Curr Psychiatry Rep. 14(3):220–8.
98. Denys D, Fluitman S, Kavelaars A, Heijnen C, Westenberg HGM. Effects of paroxetine and venlafaxine on immune parameters in patients with obsessive compulsive disorder. Psychoneuroendocrinology. 31(3):355–60.
99. Murphy T, Goodman W. Genetics of childhood disorders: XXXIV. Autoimmune disorders, part 7: D8/17 reactivity as an immunological marker of susceptibility to neuropsychiatric disorders. J Am Acad Child Adolesc Psychiatry. 2002;41(1):98–100.
100. Church AJ, Cardoso F, Dale RC, Lees AJ, Thompson EJ, Giovannoni G. Anti-basal ganglia antibodies in acute and persistent Sydenham's chorea. Neurology. 2002;59(2):227–31.
101. Cosco TD, Pillinger T, Emam H, Solmi M, Budhdeo S, Matthew Prina A, et al. Immune aberrations in obsessive-compulsive disorder: a systematic review and meta-analysis. Mol Neurobiol. 2019;56(7):4751–9.
102. Pearlman DM, Vora HS, Marquis BG, Najjar S, Dudley LA. Anti-basal ganglia antibodies in primary obsessive-compulsive disorder: systematic review and meta-analysis. Br J Psychiatry. 2014;205(1):8–16.
103. Bhattacharyya S, Khanna S, Chakrabarty K, Mahadevan A, Christopher R, Shankar SK. Anti-brain autoantibodies and altered excitatory neurotransmitters in obsessive-compulsive disorder. Neuropsychopharmacology. 2009;34(12):2489–96.
104. Rodríguez N, Morer A, González-Navarro EA, Serra-Pages C, Boloc D, Torres T, et al. Altered frequencies of Th17 and Treg cells in children and adolescents with obsessive-compulsive disorder. Brain Behav Immun. 2019 Oct;81:608–16.
105. Attwells S, Setiawan E, Wilson AA, Rusjan PM, Mizrahi R, Miler L, et al. Inflammation in the neurocircuitry of obsessive-compulsive disorder. JAMA Psychiat. 2017;74(8):833–40.
106. Lai AY, Todd KG. Hypoxia-activated microglial mediators of neuronal survival are differentially regulated by tetracyclines. Glia. 2006;53(8):809–16.
107. Esalatmanesh S, Abrishami Z, Zeinoddini A, Rahiminejad F, Sadeghi M, Najarzadegan M-R, et al. Minocycline combination therapy with fluvoxamine in moderate-to-severe obsessive-compulsive disorder: a placebo-controlled, double-blind, randomized trial. Psychiatry Clin Neurosci. 2016;70(11):517–26.
108. Rodriguez CI, Bender J, Marcus SM, Snape M, Rynn M, Simpson HB. Minocycline augmentation of pharmacotherapy in obsessive-compulsive disorder: an open-label trial. J Clin Psychiatry. 2010;71(9):1247.
109. Birben E, Sahiner UM, Sackesen C, Erzurum S, Kalayci O. Oxidative stress and antioxidant defense. World Allergy Organ J. 2012;5(1):9–19.
110. Pisoschi AM, Pop A. The role of antioxidants in the chemistry of oxidative stress: a review. Eur J Med Chem. 2015;97:55–74.
111. Hassan W, Noreen H, Castro-Gomes V, Mohammadzai I, da Rocha JBT, Landeira-Fernandez J. Association of oxidative stress with psychiatric disorders. Curr Pharm Des. 2016;22(20):2960–74.
112. Brown NC, Andreazza AC, Young LT. An updated meta-analysis of oxidative stress markers in bipolar disorder. Psychiatry Res. 2014;218(1–2):61–8.
113. Flatow J, Buckley P, Miller BJ. Meta-analysis of oxidative stress in schizophrenia. Biol Psychiatry. 2013;74(6):400–9.
114. Jiménez-Fernández S, Gurpegui M, Díaz-Atienza F, Pérez-Costillas L, Gerstenberg M, Correll CU. Oxidative stress and antioxidant parameters in patients with major depressive

disorder compared to healthy controls before and after antidepressant treatment: results from a meta-analysis. J Clin Psychiatry. 2015;76(12):1658–67.
115. Black CN, Bot M, Scheffer PG, Cuijpers P, Penninx BWJH. Is depression associated with increased oxidative stress? A systematic review and meta-analysis. Psychoneuroendocrinology. 2015;51:164–75.
116. Liu T, Zhong S, Liao X, Chen J, He T, Lai S, et al. A meta-analysis of oxidative stress markers in depression. PLoS One. 2015;10(10):e0138904.
117. Andreazza AC, Kauer-Sant'anna M, Frey BN, Bond DJ, Kapczinski F, Young LT, et al. Oxidative stress markers in bipolar disorder: a meta-analysis. J Affect Disord. 2008;111(2–3):135–44.
118. Maia A, Oliveira J, Lajnef M, Mallet L, Tamouza R, Leboyer M, et al. Oxidative and nitrosative stress markers in obsessive-compulsive disorder: a systematic review and meta-analysis. Acta Psychiatr Scand. 2019;139(5):420–33.
119. Knight JA. Review: free radicals, antioxidants, and the immune system. Ann Clin Lab Sci. 2000;30(2):145–58.
120. Meydani SN, Wu D, Santos MS, Hayek MG. Antioxidants and immune response in aged persons: overview of present evidence. Am J Clin Nutr. 1995;62(6 Suppl):1462S–76S.
121. Oliver G, Dean O, Camfield D, Blair-West S, Ng C, Berk M, et al. N-acetyl cysteine in the treatment of obsessive compulsive and related disorders: a systematic review. Clin Psychopharmacol Neurosci. 2015;13(1):12–24.
122. Smith L, Tracy DK, Giaroli G. What future role might N-acetyl-cysteine have in the treatment of obsessive compulsive and grooming disorders?: a systematic review. J Clin Psychopharmacol. 2016;36(1):57–62.
123. Berk M, Malhi GS, Gray LJ, Dean OM. The promise of N-acetylcysteine in neuropsychiatry. Trends Pharmacol Sci. 2013;34(3):167–77.
124. Afshar H, Roohafza H, Mohammad-Beigi H, Haghighi M, Jahangard L, Shokouh P, et al. N-acetylcysteine add-on treatment in refractory obsessive-compulsive disorder: a randomized, double-blind, placebo-controlled trial. J Clin Psychopharmacol. 2012;32(6):797–803.
125. Gehrmann J, Matsumoto Y, Kreutzberg GW. Microglia: intrinsic immuneffector cell of the brain. Brain Res Brain Res Rev. 1995;20(3):269–87.
126. Sierra A, Encinas JM, Deudero JJP, Chancey JH, Enikolopov G, Overstreet-Wadiche LS, et al. Microglia shape adult hippocampal neurogenesis through apoptosis-coupled phagocytosis. Cell Stem Cell. 2010;7(4):483–95.
127. Schafer DP, Lehrman EK, Kautzman AG, Koyama R, Mardinly AR, Yamasaki R, et al. Microglia sculpt postnatal neural circuits in an activity and complement-dependent manner. Neuron. 2012;74(4):691–705.
128. Paolicelli RC, Bolasco G, Pagani F, Maggi L, Scianni M, Panzanelli P, et al. Synaptic pruning by microglia is necessary for normal brain development. Science. 2011;333(6048):1456–8.
129. Tay TL, Savage JC, Hui CW, Bisht K, Tremblay M. Microglia across the lifespan: from origin to function in brain development, plasticity and cognition. J Physiol. 2017;595(6):1929–45.
130. Greer JM, Capecchi MR. Hoxb8 is required for normal grooming behavior in mice. Neuron. 2002;33(1):23–34.
131. Holstege JC, de Graaff W, Hossaini M, Cardona Cano S, Jaarsma D, van den Akker E, et al. Loss of Hoxb8 alters spinal dorsal laminae and sensory responses in mice. Proc Natl Acad Sci U S A. 2008;105(17):6338–43.
132. Chen S-K, Tvrdik P, Peden E, Cho S, Wu S, Spangrude G, et al. Hematopoietic origin of pathological grooming in Hoxb8 mutant mice. Cell. 2010;141(5):775–85.
133. Nagarajan N, Jones BW, West PJ, Marc RE, Capecchi MR. Corticostriatal circuit defects in Hoxb8 mutant mice. Mol Psychiatry. 2018;23(9):1.
134. Chen SK, He X, Hu D, Jensen P, Capecchi M. Autoimmunity developed in Hoxb8 knock-out mice (P4082). J Immunol. 2013;190(1 Supplement):51.7.
135. Toh H, Chitramuthu BP, Bennett HPJ, Bateman A. Structure, function, and mechanism of progranulin; the brain and beyond. J Mol Neurosci. 2011;45(3):538–48.

136. Sleegers K, Brouwers N, Van Damme P, Engelborghs S, Gijselinck I, van der Zee J, et al. Serum biomarker for progranulin-associated frontotemporal lobar degeneration. Ann Neurol. 2009;65(5):603–9.
137. Finch N, Baker M, Crook R, Swanson K, Kuntz K, Surtees R, et al. Plasma progranulin levels predict progranulin mutation status in frontotemporal dementia patients and asymptomatic family members. Brain. 2009;132(3):583–91.
138. Lui H, Zhang J, Makinson SR, Cahill MK, Kelley KW, Huang H-Y, et al. Progranulin deficiency promotes circuit-specific synaptic pruning by microglia via complement activation. Cell. 2016;165(4):921–35.
139. Zhan Y, Paolicelli RC, Sforazzini F, Weinhard L, Bolasco G, Pagani F, et al. Deficient neuron-microglia signaling results in impaired functional brain connectivity and social behavior. Nat Neurosci. 2014;17(3):400–6.
140. Park H-S, Francis KP, Yu J, Cleary PP. Membranous cells in nasal-associated lymphoid tissue: a portal of entry for the respiratory mucosal pathogen group A streptococcus. J Immunol. 2003;171(5):2532–7.
141. Wang B, Dileepan T, Briscoe S, Hyland KA, Kang J, Khoruts A, et al. Induction of TGF-beta1 and TGF-beta1-dependent predominant Th17 differentiation by group A streptococcal infection. Proc Natl Acad Sci U S A. 2010;107(13):5937–42.
142. Dileepan T, Smith ED, Knowland D, Hsu M, Platt M, Bittner-Eddy P, et al. Group A Streptococcus intranasal infection promotes CNS infiltration by streptococcal-specific Th17 cells. J Clin Invest. 2016;126(1):303–17.
143. Yaddanapudi K, Hornig M, Serge R, De Miranda J, Baghban A, Villar G, et al. Passive transfer of streptococcus-induced antibodies reproduces behavioral disturbances in a mouse model of pediatric autoimmune neuropsychiatric disorders associated with streptococcal infection. Mol Psychiatry. 2010;15(7):712–26.
144. Oliveira J, Tabouy L, Leboyer M. Immune dysfunction: a common feature of major psychiatric disorders? In: Teixeira AL, Bauer ME, editors. Immunopsychiatry a Clinician's introduction to the immune basis of mental disorders. Oxford: Oxford University Press; 2018. p. 141–64.

Immune Dysfunction and Catatonia

18

Jonathan Rogers and Thomas Pollak

18.1 An Introduction to Catatonia

Catatonia is a disorder that occupies a mysterious hinterland between psychiatry and general medicine. First described in print by Karl Ludwig Kahlbaum in 1874, [1] it has attracted the interest of psychiatrists and neurologists alike.

Catatonia features numerous signs and symptoms, the variety of which often generates some confusion. It may exist in stuporous and excited forms, which themselves may alternate [2]. The stupor consists of hypomobility, mutism, withdrawal and staring, but catatonia is distinctive for several more bizarre features, including echophenomena, posturing, automatic obedience, stereotypies, *Gegenhalten* and *Mitmachen* [3]. Catatonia may also be conceived as a movement disorder with spontaneous features (such as posturing) and induced features (such as waxy flexibility) [4].

In terms of diagnosis, both DSM-5 and ICD-11 now permit the presence of catatonia in a range of psychiatric and non-psychiatric disorders [5, 6].

In 1974, the British psychiatrist Mahendra wrote a now famous editorial in *Psychological Medicine*, in which he argued that catatonia had largely disappeared because it was an epiphenomenon and may have represented a psychomotor response to a particular infective agent that was no longer prevalent [7]. The idea that catatonia is practically extinct is common but is not supported by the available

J. Rogers
Division of Psychiatry, University College London, London, UK

South London and Maudsley NHS Foundation Trust, London, UK
e-mail: jonathan.rogers@ucl.ac.uk

T. Pollak (✉)
South London and Maudsley NHS Foundation Trust, London, UK

Institute of Psychiatry, Psychology and Neuroscience, King's College London, London, UK
e-mail: thomas.pollak@kcl.ac.uk

M. Berk et al. (eds.), *Immuno-Psychiatry*, https://doi.org/10.1007/978-3-030-71229-7_18

evidence. In fact, examining six studies since 1977, Daniels found that the prevalence of catatonia among psychiatric inpatients ranged from 7 to 31% [8]. The idea that catatonia is rare seems to come from poor recognition of the syndrome, with one study showing rates of catatonia rose from 2% to 18% when patients underwent systematic clinical assessment for catatonia [9].

Originally conceived as a subtype of schizophrenia, we now regard catatonia as being caused by a large range of psychiatric, neurological and general medical disorders [8]. The most commonly associated psychiatric disorder is actually depression. Other mental disorders linked to catatonia include mania, autism, Tourette's syndrome and learning disability [10–12]. However, one curious aspect of catatonia is that it also features in numerous infective, inflammatory, metabolic, drug-induced and degenerative disorders [11]. For instance, more than 50 cases of systemic lupus erythematosus in association with catatonia have been reported [13] and several in association with various thyroid disorders [14–16]. It is therefore critical that psychiatrists are aware of the possibility of an underlying organic disorder and investigate accordingly.

Due to poor identification of the syndrome and difficulties conducting randomised controlled trials with small numbers, research has mostly been confined to case reports and series with small unblinded clinical trials [17]. Moreover, until recently, the best animal model for catatonia (bulbocapnine-induced catalepsy) was a poor match of aetiology and treatment compared to the disorder itself [18]. Despite these methodological difficulties, the importance of studying catatonia is underlined by its significant physical morbidity in the form of venous thromboembolism, infection, aspiration and contractures as well as a mortality of 9% in its most severe form, malignant catatonia [8]. Furthermore, by understanding one of the most severe psychomotor disorders, we may be able to apply our knowledge to the psychomotor abnormalities observed in other neuropsychiatric disorders.

Current theories of catatonia pathogenesis rely on concepts of antagonism of GABA, dopamine or glutamate receptors [19]. Traditional treatment uses the GABA-A receptor non-competitive agonists benzodiazepines with success rates of up to 80%, a practice which has a theoretical basis in findings of reduced GABA-A receptor density in the motor cortex of catatonic patients [20, 21]. However, more recent evidence has supported the use of memantine and amantadine, both antagonists at the NMDA receptor (NMDAR), achieving success in patients refractory to benzodiazepines [17]. Electroconvulsive therapy (ECT) – for poorly understood reasons – is also very effective and is often the treatment of choice in critically unwell patients, such as those with autonomic dysregulation, severe dehydration or venous thromboembolism [22]. Optimal management involves both symptomatic treatment of the catatonia and correction of the underlying cause, as well as supportive therapy with venous thromboembolism prophylaxis, urinary catheterisation and artificial rehydration and feeding as indicated [23].

The presence of these medical comorbidities reminds us that catatonia may also be seen as a form of extreme illness behaviour, just as depression has been likened to the psychomotor response to infection (reduced social interaction, oral intake and activity) [24].

18.2 Autoimmune Movement Disorders

What distinguishes catatonia from most other psychiatric syndromes is its status as a movement disorder. In recent years, increasing numbers of neurological diseases have been shown to have autoimmune causes, or at least an inflammatory component to pathogenesis (see Table 18.1). Several of these feature prominent movement disorders and altered mental status is common as well. Some bear marked similarities to catatonia, for instance, emotional triggers in narcolepsy, anxiety in stiff person syndrome and choreiform movements in various disorders [25–27].

18.3 Infective Causes of Catatonia

In our recent systematic review, we found 124 cases of catatonia in the context of infective illness [13]. Notably, 45 out of 47 cases of specific viral infection involved viruses that affect the central nervous system, but it is unclear what the causal mechanism of catatonia may be. Our findings are shown in Table 18.2.

18.4 Inflammatory Causes of Catatonia

The results of a recent systematic review of autoimmune causes of catatonia are presented in Table 18.3. The most striking finding is that the vast majority of cases were due to autoimmune encephalitis, specifically NMDA receptor encephalitis. In fact, in one case series of NMDA receptor encephalitis, 88% of patients developed catatonia at some point in their illness, with features including negativism, echophenomena, grimacing and alternating stupor and excitement [34]. A recent study

Table 18.1 Autoimmune disorders affecting the central nervous system [28–33]

Autoimmune CNS disorders
• Brainstem encephalitis • Cerebellar ataxia in coeliac disease • Chorea associated with SLE • Encephalomyelitis • Multiple sclerosis • Narcolepsy • Neuromyelitis optica • Neuromyotonia • NMDAR encephalitis • Opsoclonus-myoclonus ataxia • Paraneoplastic cerebellar degeneration • Progressive encephalomyelitis with rigidity and myoclonus (PERM) • Rasmussen's encephalitis • Sensory neuronopathy • Sjögren's syndrome • Stiff person syndrome • Sydenham's chorea

Table 18.2 Infective causes of catatonia. Rogers JP, Pollak TA, Blackman G, David AS. Catatonia and the immune system: a review. Lancet Psychiatry 6 (7):620–630. Copyright © Elsevier 2019. doi: https://doi.org/10.1016/S2215-0366(19)30190-7

Infective cause	*n*	Suspected organisms	*n* with laboratory evidence of specific organism
Bacterial meningitis/ encephalitis	5	*Borrelia burgdorferi* (4), unspecified (1)	4
Viral meningitis / encephalitis	26	*Adenovirus* (1), *Cytomegalovirus* (1), *Coronavirus* (1), *Epstein Barr virus* (1), *HHV6* (1), *Herpes simplex virus* (8), *Japanese encephalitis virus* (1), *Measles virus* (2), *Tick-borne encephalitis virus* (1), *Varicella zoster virus* (1), unspecified (9)	14
Cerebral malaria	2	*Plasmodium falciparum* (1), unspecified (1)	1
CNS infection unspecified	3	Unspecified (3)	0
Respiratory tract infection	10	*Influenza* (1), Group A *Streptococcus* (2), *Mycoplasma* (1), *Klebsiella* (1), *Epstein Barr Virus* (1), unspecified (4)	2
HIV-related	22	HIV (20), HIV and *John Cunningham (JC) virus* (2)	22
Syphilis	3	*Treponema pallidum* (2)	2
Systemic bacterial infection	31	*Coxiella burnetti* (1), *Salmonella typhi* (29), unspecified (2)	28
Systemic viral infection	4	*Cytomegalovirus* (2), *Epstein Barr virus* (1), *Flavivirus* (1)	3
Prion-related disorders	7	*PrP* (7)	7
Other	11	*Flavivirus* vaccination (1), *Tropheryma whipplei* (1), *E. coli* (1), *Mycobacterium tuberculosis* (1), *Taenia solium* (1), *Chlamydia trachomatis* (1), *Trypanosoma cruzi* (1), unspecified (4)	2
Total	124	–	85

systematically assessed 58 inpatients with NMDA receptor encephalitis, using a rigorous threshold of DSM-5 criteria or the presence of four items on the Bush-Francis Catatonia Screening Instrument to define catatonia [35]. They found that 41 individuals (71%) had catatonia and the full spectrum of catatonic features was present, including motor signs, disordered speech and alternating stupor and excitement. Benzodiazepines and electroconvulsive therapy (ECT) were not curative on their own, but in some cases were useful to treat catatonia alongside immunotherapy. While catatonia is poorly recognised, a systematic review of the psychiatric presentation of all reported cases of NMDA receptor encephalitis found catatonia to be present in 32.7% of cases [36].

Table 18.3 Autoimmune causes of catatonia. Rogers JP, Pollak TA, Blackman G, David AS. Catatonia and the immune system: a review. Lancet Psychiatry 6(7):620–630. Copyright © Elsevier 2019. doi: https://doi.org/10.1016/S2215-0366(19)30190-7

Category of autoimmunity	*n*	Specific disorder	*n*
Autoimmune thyroid disorders	13	Hyperthyroid state	3
		Hypothyroid state	4
		Euthyroid state with thyroid antibodies	4
		Thyroid state not stated	2
Autoimmune encephalitis	259	GABA-AR encephalitis	2
		NMDAR encephalitis	249
		Progressive encephalomyelitis with rigidity and myoclonus (PERM)	1
		'Voltage-gated potassium channel (VGKC) complex' encephalitis	4
		Unspecified	3
Demyelinating disorders	13	Acute disseminated encephalomyelitis	2
		Multiple sclerosis	10
		Neuromyelitis optica	1
Pernicious anaemia	4	Pernicious anaemia	4
Systemic lupus erythematosus (SLE) and related	53	Antiphospholipid syndrome	2
		SLE	51
Other	4	Addison's disease	1
		Crohn's disease	1
		MOG antibody disease	1
		Paediatric autoimmune neuropsychiatric disorders associated with streptococcal infections (PANDAS)	1
Total	346		

Case series of other forms of encephalitis have not been systematically evaluated for the presence of catatonic features, although there is some evidence that catatonia may be more common in patients with antibodies to the NMDA receptor than in those with antibodies to the voltage-gated potassium channel or calcium channel [37]. Antibodies to the GABA-A receptor would fit with a theoretical GABA-ergic hypofunction in catatonia [18].

18.5 Catatonia Variants

Encephalitis lethargica, as vividly described in Oliver Sacks' memoir *Awakenings*, was a cryptogenic disorder that frequently presented with catatonia or had catatonia as a sequela [38]. Although encephalitis lethargica has often been linked to pandemic influenza, it appeared before the 1918 outbreak, no contemporary investigators found evidence of an infective cause and there was no convincing contagion [39]. Moreover, modern investigators have found no viral antigens present, while benefit has been noted from immunotherapies [40]. A post-infective immune response has been proposed [41] and one study found that of twenty contemporary paediatric patients with CSF samples available, ten tested positive for antibodies to the NMDA receptor, four of whom had convincing catatonic features [40]. Another two cases of NMDAR positivity have since been reported in encephalitis lethargica, while several children have been found to have antibodies to the dopamine D_2 receptor [42, 43]. This suggests it is possible that a number of the cases formerly identified as encephalitis lethargica may be catatonia due to autoimmune encephalitis.

Neuroleptic malignant syndrome is a more recent disorder, recognised since the advent of dopamine D_2 receptor antagonists in the 1960s. It is characterised by rigidity, altered mental status, hyperthermia and autonomic instability [44]. Some have suggested that neuroleptic malignant syndrome represents a form of medication-induced catatonia; certainly, the syndrome is more common in patients who have already shown signs of catatonia [45, 46]. Interestingly, it appears to be common in patients with NMDAR encephalitis [47]. Raised creatine kinase is a recognised hallmark of neuroleptic malignant syndrome, [48] but it has also been noted that raised counts of leukocytes and platelets are common, suggesting that an inflammatory component may be central [49, 50]. These studies also highlight low serum iron in neuroleptic malignant syndrome and – since iron is a negative acute phase marker – use this to point to further evidence of immune activation.

18.6 Laboratory Markers in Catatonia

Low serum iron is also the most commonly reported laboratory finding in catatonia. This was first hypothesised based on the similarity between NMS and catatonia, given the ferropenia present in NMS. A small initial study found low serum iron in three of twelve catatonic episodes, occurring in eleven patients [51]. In two of these episodes, the patient developed NMS, suggesting that low serum iron may identify a subgroup of catatonic patients at high risk of NMS. Lee performed a larger study, which sought to replicate this with 39 patients with catatonia admitted to a psychiatric intensive care unit, 17 of whom developed low serum iron [52]. Of the ferropenic patients in this study, 7 developed malignant catatonia, of whom 5 developed NMS. There was an association between low serum iron and non-response to benzodiazepines. None of the patients with normal serum iron developed malignant catatonia or NMS. Ferropenia appears to be relatively specific to catatonia, since one study found rates of ferropenia to be 35% in catatonia and only 7.5% in non-catatonic patients with psychosis [53]. A more recent study found a trend towards low serum iron in catatonia, but no statistically significant difference when compared to a psychiatric control group, although the sample size was smaller than the Peralta study [54]. This ferropenia is, in our view, unlikely to represent an acute phase response due to a primary muscular pathology as part of developing NMS. This is because, firstly, many of the patients with low serum iron in these studies did not in fact develop NMS and some had not been treated with antipsychotics. Secondly, in one case where the authors managed to perform serial venipuncture, ferropenia predated the rise in CPK in what was thought to be developing NMS by four days [55].

The place of ferropenia in the acute phase response is well established. It is caused by the up-regulation of ferritin and hepcidin production by the actions of TNF-α and IL-1 on the liver, resulting in reduced absorption and increased binding of free iron [56]. Its adaptive function appears to be the deprivation of pathogens of the iron they require for growth [57]. In catatonia – or a subgroup of catatonia, it may be a maladaptive response to extreme stress, mediated by the acute phase response.

One study also demonstrated raised creatine kinase in catatonia compared to healthy controls, [58] but another group did not replicate this [54] and it is questionable as to whether any rise in creatine kinase is a consequence of rigidity rather than part of the pathogenesis. D-dimer and hsCRP have also been found to be raised compared to other psychiatric patients in single studies, [54, 59] but these findings have not been repeated.

18.7 Conclusions

Catatonia has a heterogeneous presentation with an extremely diverse list of possible aetiological factors. It is therefore likely that the pathophysiology will not be uniform, although the existence of effective treatments suggests there may exist a final common pathway.

Given the crude measurements available in studies to date for activation of the innate immune system, there does not appear to be evidence that all cases of catatonia demonstrate systemic inflammation. The findings of low iron, raised D-dimer and raised hsCRP, however, do hold out the possibility that a sub-group of patients with catatonia have an inflammatory pathology.

More promising is the evidence for specific autoimmune causes of catatonia, notably autoimmune encephalitis and systemic lupus erythematosus. Catatonic features in NMDA receptor encephalitis have been systematically studied, but it is possible that other forms of autoimmune encephalitis also feature catatonia prominently.

18.8 Future Directions

Synthesis of existing studies of laboratory markers in catatonia into a meta-analysis would clarify some of the ambiguities in the current literature. It will also be necessary to conduct larger studies where patients with catatonia are compared against non-catatonic psychiatric patients in terms of inflammatory markers. Priority should be given to research that examines more subtle indicators for activation of the humoral immune system (such as cytokines). Moreover, forms of autoimmune encephalitis other than NMDARE need to be systematically studied for the presence of catatonic features, while conversely patients with catatonia should be screened for known encephalitis-causing antibodies.

References

1. Kahlbaum KL. Die Katatonie : oder das Spannungsirresein, eine klinische Form psychischer Krankheit [Internet]. 1874 [cited 2017 Aug 18]. https://archive.org/details/39002079238854.med.yale.edu
2. Shorter E, Fink M. The madness of fear: a history of catatonia. Oxford: Oxford University Press; 2018.
3. Bush G, Fink M, Petrides G, Dowling F, Francis A, Catatonia I. Rating scale and standardized examination. Acta Psychiatr Scand. 1996;93(2):129–36. [cited 2018 Apr 18]. http://www.ncbi.nlm.nih.gov/pubmed/8686483
4. Wijemanne S, Jankovic J. Movement disorders in catatonia. J Neurol Neurosurg Psychiatry. 2015;86(8):825–32. [cited 2017 Oct 25]. http://www.ncbi.nlm.nih.gov/pubmed/25411548
5. World Health Organization. The ICD-11 classification of mental and behavioural disorders: Clinical descriptions and diagnostic guidelines. Geneva; 2018.
6. American Psychiatric Association. Diagnostic and statistical manual of mental disorders: Dsm-5. American Psychiatric Pub Incorporated; 2013p. 991. [cited 2013 Aug 6]. http://books.google.com/books?id=EIbMlwEACAAJ&pgis=1
7. Mahendra B. Where have all the catatonics gone? Psychol Med. 1981;11(4):669–71. [cited 2018 Jan 18]. http://www.ncbi.nlm.nih.gov/pubmed/7323228
8. Daniels J. Catatonia: clinical aspects and neurobiological correlates. J Neuropsychiatry Clin Neurosci. 2009;21(4):371–80. [cited 2017 Aug 22]. http://psychiatryonline.org/doi/abs/10.1176/jnp.2009.21.4.371
9. van der Heijden FMMA, Tuinier S, Arts NJM, Hoogendoorn MLC, Kahn RS, Verhoeven WMA. Catatonia: disappeared or under-diagnosed? Psychopathology. 2005;38(1):3–8. [cited 2018 Apr 18]. http://www.ncbi.nlm.nih.gov/pubmed/15714008
10. Rasmussen SA, Mazurek MF, Rosebush PI. Catatonia: our current understanding of its diagnosis, treatment and pathophysiology. World J Psychiatry. 2016;6(4):391. [cited 2017 Aug 18]. http://www.ncbi.nlm.nih.gov/pubmed/28078203
11. Fink M, Taylor MA. Catatonia: a clinician's guide to diagnosis and treatment. Cambridge: Cambridge University Press; 2006.
12. Dhossche DM. Catatonia in autism spectrum disorders. Elsevier; San Diego, CA, 2006. p. 314. [cited 2017 Nov 8]. https://books.google.co.uk/books?hl=en&lr=&id=v9FvvOxzZAwC&oi=fnd&pg=PR7&dq=Dhossche+DM,+Wing+L,+Ohta+M,+Neumärker+K-J,+eds.+Catatonia+in+Autism+Spec-trum+Disorders.+Int+Rev+Biol+72.+Amsterdam,+the+Netherlands:+Academic+Press%3B+2006.&ots=CCv2J4QBPI&sig=iCVSQF6Ae5jVRw3Bh1JIeNolw3c&redir_esc=y#v=onepage&q=retardation&f=false.
13. Rogers JP, Pollak TA, Blackman G, David AS. Catatonia and the immune system: a review. Lancet Psychiatry. 2019;6(7):620–30. [cited 2019 Aug 22]. https://www.sciencedirect.com/science/article/pii/S2215036619301907?via%3Dihub
14. Lee SW, Donlon S, Caplan JP. Steroid responsive encephalopathy associated with autoimmune thyroiditis (SREAT) or Hashimoto's encephalopathy: a case and review. Psychosomatics. 2011;52(2):99–108. [cited 2017 Jun 21] http://www.sciencedirect.com/science/article/pii/S0033318210000332
15. Bharadwaj B, Sugaparaneetharan A, Rajkumar RP. Graves' disease presenting with catatonia: A probable case of encephalopathy associated with autoimmune thyroid disease. Acta Neuropsychiatr. 2012;24(6):374–9.
16. Lalanne L, Meriot M-E, Ruppert E, Zimmermann M-A, Danion J-M, Vidailhet P. Attempted infanticide and suicide inaugurating catatonia associated with Hashimoto's encephalopathy: a case report. BMC Psychiatry. 2016;16(1):13. [cited 2018 Feb 7]. http://www.biomedcentral.com/1471-244X/16/13
17. Carroll BT, Goforth HW, Thomas C, Ahuja N, McDaniel WW, Kraus MF, et al. Review of adjunctive glutamate antagonist therapy in the treatment of catatonic syndromes. J

Neuropsychiatry Clin Neurosci. 2007;19(4):406–12. [cited 2017 Nov 8]. http://psychiatryonline.org/doi/abs/10.1176/jnp.2007.19.4.406
18. Northoff G. What catatonia can tell us about "top-down modulation": a neuropsychiatric hypothesis. Behav Brain Sci. 2002;25(05):555–77. [cited 2017 Nov 8]. http://www.journals.cambridge.org/abstract_S0140525X02000109
19. Walther S, Strik W. Catatonia. CNS Spectr. 2016;21(04):341–8. [cited 2017 Aug 18]. http://www.ncbi.nlm.nih.gov/pubmed/27255726
20. Sienaert P, van Harten P, Rhebergen D. The psychopharmacology of catatonia, neuroleptic malignant syndrome, akathisia, tardive dyskinesia, and dystonia. Handb Clin Neurol. 2019;165:415–28. [cited 2020 Jan 31]. https://www.sciencedirect.com/science/article/pii/B9780444640123000253?via%3Dihub#bb0505
21. Northoff G, Steinke R, Czcervenka C, Krause R, Ulrich S, Danos P, et al. Decreased density of GABA-A receptors in the left sensorimotor cortex in akinetic catatonia: investigation of in vivo benzodiazepine receptor binding. J Neurol Neurosurg Psychiatry. 1999;67(4):445–50. [cited 2017 Oct 25]. http://www.ncbi.nlm.nih.gov/pubmed/10486389.
22. Pelzer AC, van der Heijden FM, den Boer E. Systematic review of catatonia treatment. Neuropsychiatr Dis Treat. 2018;14:317–26. [cited 2018 Mar 5]. http://www.ncbi.nlm.nih.gov/pubmed/29398916
23. Clinebell K, Azzam PN, Gopalan P, Haskett R. Guidelines for preventing common medical complications of catatonia. J Clin Psychiatry. 2014;75(06):644–51. [cited 2018 Jun 11]. http://www.ncbi.nlm.nih.gov/pubmed/25004188
24. Wohleb ES, Franklin T, Iwata M, Duman RS. Integrating neuroimmune systems in the neurobiology of depression. Nat Rev Neurosci. 2016;17(8):497–511. [cited 2017 Sep 20]. http://www.nature.com/doifinder/10.1038/nrn.2016.69
25. Dalakas MC. Stiff person syndrome: Advances in pathogenesis and therapeutic interventions. Curr Treat Options Neurol. 2009;11(2):102–10. [cited 2020 Feb 27]. http://link.springer.com/10.1007/s11940-009-0013-9
26. Siegel JM, Boehmer LN. Narcolepsy and the hypocretin system—where motion meets emotion. Nat Clin Pract Neurol. 2006;2(10):548–56. [cited 2020 Feb 27]. http://www.nature.com/articles/ncpneuro0300
27. Wild EJ, Tabrizi SJ. The differential diagnosis of chorea. Pract Neurol. 2007;7(6):360–73. [cited 2020 Feb 27]. http://www.ncbi.nlm.nih.gov/pubmed/18024776
28. Panzer J, Dalmau J. Movement disorders in paraneoplastic and autoimmune disease. Curr Opin Neurol. 2011;24(4):346–53. [cited 2018 Feb 26]. http://www.ncbi.nlm.nih.gov/pubmed/21577108
29. Baizabal-Carvallo JF, Jankovic J. Movement disorders in autoimmune diseases. Mov Disord. 2012;27(8):935–46. [cited 2018 Feb 26]. http://www.ncbi.nlm.nih.gov/pubmed/22555904
30. Reich DS, Lucchinetti CF, Calabresi PA. Multiple sclerosis. Longo DL, editor. N Engl J Med. 2018;378(2):169–80. [cited 2018 Feb 26]. http://www.nejm.org/doi/10.1056/NEJMra1401483
31. Scammell TE. Narcolepsy. Campion EW, editor. N Engl J Med. 2015;373(27):2654–62. [cited 2018 Feb 7]. http://www.ncbi.nlm.nih.gov/pubmed/26716917
32. Hardy TA, Reddel SW, Barnett MH, Palace J, Lucchinetti CF, Weinshenker BG. Atypical inflammatory demyelinating syndromes of the CNS. Lancet Neurol. 2016;15(9):967–81. [cited 2018 Feb 26]. http://linkinghub.elsevier.com/retrieve/pii/S1474442216300436
33. Honorat JA, McKeon A. Autoimmune movement disorders: a clinical and laboratory approach. Curr Neurol Neurosci Rep. 2017;17, 4(1). [cited 2018 Feb 26]. http://www.ncbi.nlm.nih.gov/pubmed/28120141
34. Dalmau J, Gleichman AJ, Hughes EG, Rossi JE, Peng X, Lai M, et al. Anti-NMDA-receptor encephalitis: case series and analysis of the effects of antibodies. Lancet Neurol. 2008;7(12):1091–8. [cited 2017 Oct 25]. http://www.ncbi.nlm.nih.gov/pubmed/18851928
35. Espinola-Nadurille M, Flores-Rivera J, Rivas-Alonso V, Vargas-Cañas S, Fricchione GL, Bayliss L, et al. Catatonia in patients with anti-NMDA receptor encephalitis. Psychiatry Clin Neurosci 2019;73(9):574–580. [cited 2020 Mar 10]. https://onlinelibrary.wiley.com/doi/abs/10.1111/pcn.12867

36. Warren N, Siskind D, O'Gorman C. Refining the psychiatric syndrome of anti-N-methyl-d-aspartate receptor encephalitis. Acta Psychiatr Scand. 2018;138:401–8.
37. Kruse JL, Lapid MI, Lennon VA, Klein CJ, Toole OO, Pittock SJ, et al. Psychiatric autoimmunity: N-methyl-D-aspartate receptor IgG and beyond. Psychosomatics. 2015;56(3):227–41. [cited 2017 Nov 1]. http://www.ncbi.nlm.nih.gov/pubmed/25975857
38. Sacks O. Awakenings. Picador; 1973.
39. Reid AH, McCall S, Henry JM, Taubenberger JK. Experimenting on the past: the enigma of von Economo's encephalitis lethargica. J Neuropathol Exp Neurol. 2001;60(7):663–70. [cited 2018 Feb 14]. http://www.ncbi.nlm.nih.gov/pubmed/11444794
40. Dale RC, Irani SR, Brilot F, Pillai S, Webster R, Gill D, et al. N-methyl-D-aspartate receptor antibodies in pediatric dyskinetic encephalitis lethargica. Ann Neurol. 2009;66(5):704–9. [cited 2018 Feb 14]. http://www.ncbi.nlm.nih.gov/pubmed/19938173
41. Dale RC, Church AJ, Surtees RAH, Lees AJ, Adcock JE, Harding B, et al. Encephalitis lethargica syndrome: 20 new cases and evidence of basal ganglia autoimmunity. Brain. 2004;127(1):21–33. [cited 2018 Jan 9]. https://academic.oup.com/brain/article-lookup/doi/10.1093/brain/awh008
42. Tan A, Shuey N, Bladin C. A modern perspective on the differential diagnosis between encephalitis lethargica or anti-NMDA-receptor encephalitis. J Clin Neurosci. 2010;17(9):1204–6. [cited 2018 Feb 14]. http://www.ncbi.nlm.nih.gov/pubmed/20605463
43. Dale RC, Merheb V, Pillai S, Wang D, Cantrill L, Murphy TK, et al. Antibodies to surface dopamine-2 receptor in autoimmune movement and psychiatric disorders. Brain. 2012;135(11):3453–68. [cited 2019 Dec 20]. https://academic.oup.com/brain/article-lookup/doi/10.1093/brain/aws256
44. Pileggi DJ, Cook AM. Neuroleptic malignant syndrome. Ann Pharmacother. 2016;50(11):973–81. [cited 2017 Oct 9]. http://www.ncbi.nlm.nih.gov/pubmed/27423483
45. Carroll BT, Taylor RE. The nondichotomy between lethal catatonia and neuroleptic malignant syndrome. J Clin Psychopharmacol. 1981;17(3):235–6. [cited 2017 Oct 9]. http://ovidsp.uk.ovid.com/sp-3.26.1a/ovidweb.cgi?QS2=434f4e1a73d37e8c4c7d6b65ba1a76f1838575f686c142ac9a227268a5cf55e122333e9358a6109919d81c7d11a7aae623a3a864fb19fbca15f184ce781b3b1347a435c1d9e08cbd6102635c5b7709243c21d804c331c1b367147d333c6f132bb6f6c615b5
46. Fink M. Recognizing NMS as a type of catatonia. Neuropsychiatry, Neuropsychol Behav Neurol. 1995;8(1):75–6. [cited 2018 Mar 14]. http://psycnet.apa.org/record/1995-40529-001
47. Lejuste F, Thomas L, Picard G, Desestret V, Ducray F, Rogemond V, et al. Neuroleptic intolerance in patients with anti-NMDAR encephalitis. Neurol Neuroimmunol neuroinflammation. 2016;3(5):e280. [cited 2018 Feb 21]. http://www.ncbi.nlm.nih.gov/pubmed/27606355
48. Tse L, Barr AM, Scarapicchia V, Vila-Rodriguez F. Neuroleptic malignant syndrome: a review from a clinically oriented perspective. Curr Neuropharmacol. 2015;13(3):395–406. [cited 2017 Sep 6]. http://www.ncbi.nlm.nih.gov/pubmed/26411967
49. Rosebush P, Stewart T. A prospective analysis of 24 episodes of neuroleptic malignant syndrome. Am J Psychiatry. 1989;146(6):717–25. [cited 2018 Jan 10]. http://psychiatryonline.org/doi/abs/10.1176/ajp.146.6.717
50. Anglin RE, Rosebush PI, Mazurek MF. Neuroleptic malignant syndrome: a neuroimmunologic hypothesis. CMAJ. 2010;182(18):E834–8. [cited 2017 Sep 6]. http://www.ncbi.nlm.nih.gov/pubmed/20696799
51. Carroll BT, Goforth HW. Serum iron in catatonia. Biol Psychiatry. 1995;38(11):776–7.
52. Lee J. Serum iron in catatonia and neuroleptic malignant syndrome. Biol Psychiatry. 1998;44(6):499–507. [cited 2017 Nov 8]. http://www.sciencedirect.com/science/article/pii/S0006322398001097
53. Peralta V, Cuesta MJ, Mata I, Serrano JF, Perez-Nievas F, Natividad MC. Serum iron in catatonic and noncatatonic psychotic patients. Biol Psychiatry. 1999;45(6):788–90. [cited 2018 Jan 10]. http://www.ncbi.nlm.nih.gov/pubmed/10188010

54. Haouzir S, Lemoine X, Desbordes M, Follet M, Meunier C, Baarir Z, et al. The role of coagulation marker fibrin D-dimer in early diagnosis of catatonia. Psychiatry Res. 2009;168(1):78–85. [cited 2018 Jan 10]. http://linkinghub.elsevier.com/retrieve/pii/S0165178108000413
55. Raja M, Altavista MC, Cavallari S, Lubich L. Neuroleptic malignant syndrome and catatonia. A report of three cases. Eur Arch Psychiatry Clin Neurosci. 1994;243(6):299–303.
56. Northrop-Clewes CA. Interpreting indicators of iron status during an acute phase response – lessons from malaria and human immunodeficiency virus. Ann Clin Biochem. 2008;45(1):18–32. [cited 2018 Jan 31]. http://acb.sagepub.com/lookup/doi/10.1258/acb.2007.007167
57. Gruys E, Toussaint MJM, Niewold TA, Koopmans SJ. Acute phase reaction and acute phase proteins. J Zhejiang Univ Sci B. 2005;6(11):1045–56. [cited 2018 Jan 31]. http://www.ncbi.nlm.nih.gov/pubmed/16252337
58. Northoff G, Wenke J, Pflug B. Increase of serum creatine phosphokinase in catatonia: an investigation in 32 acute catatonic patients. Psychol Med. 1996;26(03):547. [cited 2018 Jan 10]. http://www.journals.cambridge.org/abstract_S0033291700035625
59. Akanji AO, Ohaeri JU, Al-Shammri S, Fatania HR. Association of blood levels of C-reactive protein with clinical phenotypes in Arab schizophrenic patients. Psychiatry Res. 2009;169(1):56–61.

Suicide as a Systemic Disorder

19

Aiste Lengvenyte, Emilie Olié, and Philippe Courtet

19.1 Introduction

Suicide, broadly defined as the intentional termination of one's own life, is a complex phenomenon, which affects human societies worldwide. Despite increasing efforts to reduce this burden, suicide rates remain as high as ever, and in some Western countries are even growing. Suicide transcends common disciplines. It is driven by intricate interactions between genetic predisposition and environment. Accumulating evidence indicates that the alteration of the immune system is of paramount importance to the pathophysiology of suicidal behaviours (SB) [1]. In this chapter, we will overview the current evidence for the role of inflammation in the pathway from health to suicide.

19.2 Suicide and Inflammation: Epidemiological and Clinical Findings

Recent analyses of large-scale registry data contributed significantly to the increasing appreciation of the innate immunity involvement in the pathway from health to suicide. Data from Danish registries showed the dose-dependent long-term increase in SB risk following infections treated with anti-infective agents for up to 5 years. Moreover, the risk was the highest for individuals treated with broad-spectrum antibiotics and requiring hospitalization [2]. Another large-scale sero-epidemiological case-control study from Denmark also showed a specific association between

A. Lengvenyte · E. Olié · P. Courtet (✉)
Department of Emergency Psychiatry and Acute Care, CHU Montpellier, Montpellier, France

University of Montpellier, Montpellier, France

FondaMental Foundation, Créteil, France
e-mail: e-olie@chu-montpellier.fr; philippe.courtet@umontpellier.fr

M. Berk et al. (eds.), *Immuno-Psychiatry*, https://doi.org/10.1007/978-3-030-71229-7_19

herpes simplex virus type 1 infection and suicide attempt or suicide in an otherwise healthy population [3].

Accordingly, medical conditions whose core feature is immune system dysfunction, such as systemic lupus erythematosus [4], multiple sclerosis [5], and asthma [6] have also been consistently associated with SB. An inflammatory response to increased air pollen counts in sensitized individuals could also serve as a putative explanation for increased suicide occurrence in spring season [7]. Indeed, intranasal corticosteroids have been shown to reduce suicide risk [8]. Though allergic conditions consist of various immune responses in the periphery with unknown effects on the central nervous system (CNS), supporting evidence for the peripheral inflammation and CNS function has been provided by tumour necrosis factor (TNF)-α inhibitors trials. Apart for some studies demonstrating the causal relationship between the induced inflammation and subsequent onset of depression [9], suicidal ideation and attempts have also been documented in previously psychiatrically healthy patients with multiple sclerosis following treatment with interferon-β [10]. Seasonal changes in vitamin D, which contributes to immune function via T-helper system promotion, concentration might also add to this connection, as deficiency in vitamin D has been associated with both higher levels of inflammatory cytokines in blood and suicide attempt history [11].

Substantial evidence also links the presence of infectious agents in the CNS with SB risk, very likely at least partly via increased neuroinflammation. Studies have consistently confirmed the association between seropositivity to *Toxoplasma gondii* and cytomegalovirus, common conditions in worldwide populations causing chronic low-grade inflammation and increased SB risk [12].

19.3 Peripheral Inflammation Markers and Suicide

A mounting number of studies detected inflammatory marker changes in the blood of suicidal subjects. Suicide attempt history in psychiatric patients has been related to higher neutrophil to lymphocyte ratio [13]. Furthermore, meta-analytical evidence demonstrated increased interleukin (IL)-1β and IL-6 in in-vivo blood levels and decreased in-vitro IL-2 levels in suicidal patients compared to both non-suicidal patients and healthy controls [14]. Another meta-analysis confirmed lower IL-2 plasma levels in suicidal patients, also adding that these subjects had lower IL-4 and higher TNF-β plasma levels than healthy controls, but not psychiatric patients [15].

Contrary to cytokines, C-reactive protein (CRP) has a sufficiently long half-life and is widely measured in everyday clinical practice, supporting its applicability in clinical research. A study that measured fasting high sensitivity CRP (hs-CRP) in depressed patients found a direct dose-dependent relationship between hs-CRP and suicide attempt history, and low-grade inflammation (hs-CRP > 3 mg/L) compared to those with low levels of hs-CRP (<1 mg/L), even after exclusion of patients with chronic diseases and high CRP levels (>10 mg/L). Meanwhile, suicidal ideation was not related to hs-CRP levels in this study, suggesting that inflammatory changes may serve as a trait, but not state, markers for suicidal vulnerability in depressed patients [16]. Accordingly, two recent studies with bipolar disorder and unipolar depression patients reported a positive link between high serum CRP levels (>3 mg/L) and suicide attempt history compared to those with low levels of CRP [17, 18], though the study in depressed people found that the existence of physical illness could explain this relationship [18]. A study in youth observed distinct inflammatory profiles in suicide attempters compared to suicide ideators and healthy controls, as suicide attempters had higher CRP, TNF-α mRNA, and lower glucocorticoid receptor mRNA levels [19]. In a study of women with depression and anxiety diagnoses, the biological profile of patients assessed to be at increased suicide risk, the biological cluster containing increased levels of IL-6, lymphocytes, monocytes, white blood cell count, and polymorphonuclear leukocyte count significantly impacted suicide risk, while the cytokine IL-8 was independently and negatively associated with increased suicide risk [20].

19.4 From Systemic Inflammation to Central Nervous System Changes

Several lines of evidence converge on the link between peripheral and central inflammation and its effects on brain structure and function. Possibly due to their short half-life, cytokine levels in the periphery do not reflect their levels in the CNS. Peripheral and central inflammation are nevertheless tightly linked. In a study with depressed patients, plasma CRP levels were related to cerebrospinal fluid (CSF) CRP levels, which, in turn, were linked to CSF cytokine receptors [21]. Different mechanisms have been proposed to link immune system and brain function changes that can mediate suicidal behaviours. Firstly, systemic inflammation and neuroinflammation cause blood-brain barrier (BBB) lesions, including changes of BBB permeability [22]. An increase in blood-brain barrier (BBB) permeability impairs synaptic transmission and neuronal functioning [23]. Interestingly, changes in blood levels of S100B, a protein biomarker of BBB permeability, were found in adolescents with suicidal ideation in comparison to healthy controls [24]. Altogether, it is hypothesized that BBB permeability may have an impact on the communication between peripheral inflammation and the brain [25], and may play a role in suicidal physiopathology.

Systemic inflammation is also proposed to affect the body's interoceptive systems. Following the immune activation, circulating inflammatory mediators activate visceral autonomic afferents, humoral, and cellular interoceptive pathways in parallel that then communicate the changes in immune state to the brain. When inflammation is severe, chronic, occurs during critical developmental period, or on a background of other chronic brain exposures, prolonged activation of interoceptive pathways can precipitate long-standing maladaptive neurobiological and behavioural changes [26]. Systemic inflammation has been demonstrated to alter the microstructure of the insular cortex, which is implicated in representing internal physiologic states including inflammation, also linking it to subjective fatigue [27]. Moreover, in accordance with the stress-diathesis model of suicide, interoceptive pathways activation has been linked to the stress sensitization. For example, direct monocyte trafficking to brain, a cellular interoceptive pathway, increases significantly following severe stress, and possibly serves as a mechanism for amplifying behavioural stress responses when stress is repetitive or prolonged [28]. Self-reported interoceptive deficits, or the inability to effectively and accurately monitor the physiological state of the body, have been linked to both suicidal ideation and suicide attempts [29, 30], and are more pronounced in the extreme end of the suicidal continuum [30]. Indeed, in a large multiple sample study, self-reported interoceptive deficits in adult participants were associated with suicide attempts history, but not suicidal ideation [31].

19.5 Central Inflammation and Suicide

While normal brain function requires low levels of inflammatory cytokines, when inflammation surpasses brain adaptive capacity, elevated cytokine levels result in anatomical and functional damage, entailing maladaptive neurobiological and behavioural changes. Cerebrospinal fluid (CSF) levels of IL-6 are increased in suicide attempters regardless of their psychiatric diagnosis [32], and IL-1β and IL-6 levels in both CSF and post-mortem brain samples have been linked to suicidality in patients with psychiatric disorders [14]. Consistently, a human post-mortem study found a significant increase in the complement system, which plays a critical role in inflammation, component 3 expression in the prefrontal cortex of depressed suicide subjects [33]. Another putative neuroinflammation marker found in patients with suicidal ideation, the translocator protein (TSPO), reflecting microglial activation. A post-hoc analysis of a small sample of depressed patients demonstrated that TSPO was increased in individuals with suicidal thoughts compared to those without suicidal thoughts, who were not different from healthy controls, most robustly in the anterior cingulate cortex and insula [34].

Compelling evidence comes from studies examining the relationship between conditions directly causing neuroinflammation and glial activation in the brain, such as traumatic brain injury [35] and concussion [36], and SB. Microglia and macrophages belong to the innate immune system and are highly reactive to alterations in homeostasis. Upon the recognition of environmental stressors, they morph into active phenotypes and induce the transcription of the inflammasome [37]. In the face of repetitive environmental challenges, microglia and macrophages are primed for amplified and persistent inflammatory responses. This chronic neuroinflammation might increase susceptibility to new stressors, serving as a neurobiological mediator within the stress-diathesis model of suicide. Indeed, individuals with traumatic brain injury history have been demonstrated to have significantly higher TNF-α levels than healthy controls, which were associated both with disinhibition and suicidal ideation up to 12 months after the injury [38]. Several post-mortem studies found higher microglia priming, demonstrated by overactive de-ramification, in the anterior cingulate cortex of suicide descendants compared to subjects that died from other causes [39, 40].

A study has demonstrated that, within the default mode network, which is crucial for the self-referential processes, IL-6 covaried positively with the connectivity of the subgenual anterior cingulate cortex and negatively with a region of the dorsal medial prefrontal cortex [41]. Increased default mode network activity has been observed in suicide attempters, especially in recent attempters [42]. Salience network, which is involved in coordinating the activation of executive control and default mode networks coherence, has been demonstrated to decrease in functional connectivity in response to increased plasma IL-6 and TNF-α concentration [43], and reduction in suicidal ideation is associated with increased salience network coherence [44].

Genetic and epigenetic changes have been proposed to take part in this complex relationship between inflammation and SB. A family-based analysis revealed a genetic overlap between IL-8 and risk for suicide attempt in females [45]. Postmortem studies demonstrated increased mRNA and protein levels of IL-1β, IL-6, TNF-α, lymphotoxin A, and certain Toll-like receptors, as well as decreased anti-inflammatory cytokine IL-10, and IL-1 receptor antagonist levels in the prefrontal cortex of depressed individuals who died by suicide compared with controls [46, 47]. In accordance, a study that used two different cohorts of brain samples revealed consistently increased TNF-α expression in the dorsolateral prefrontal cortex of all individuals who died by suicide regardless of psychiatric diagnosis [48].

19.6 Kynurenine Pathway

A growing body of evidence suggests that a putative pathway linking inflammation and SB is the dysregulation of the kynurenine pathway of tryptophan metabolism. Under normal circumstances, around 90% of tryptophan is metabolized via this pathway, raising the levels of cellular energy, while a fraction of tryptophan is converted to 5-HT and, subsequently, melatonin. In the brain, where tryptophan is transported via the BBB, the kynurenine pathway produces several neuroactive compounds, of which quinolinic acid and kynurenic acid are of particular importance. Increased levels of pro-inflammatory cytokines due to the inflammation induce the kynurenine pathway, preferentially generating cellular energy, in disadvantage of 5-HT production [49]. Chronic excess of pro-inflammatory cytokines continually up-regulates the expression of the enzymes that launch the kynurenine pathway hepatic tryptophan-2,3-dioxygenase (TDO) and extrahepatic indoleamine-2,3-dioxygenase (IDO), while in the brain-activated microglia and infiltrating monocytes and macrophages convert kynurenine into quinolinic acid. Quinolinic acid, synthesized mainly by activated microglia and brain-infiltrating macrophages, selectively agonizes *N*-methyl-*D*-aspartate (NMDA) receptors, inhibits glutamate uptake by astrocytes, and stimulates glutamate release, resulting in decreased brain-derived neurotrophic factor (BDNF) expression and ecotoxicity [50]. Moreover, it has pro-inflammatory and immunoregulatory properties. Meanwhile, astrocytes express the enzyme kynurenine aminotransferase essential to produce kynurenic acid, which, in contrast to quinolinic acid, exerts neuroprotective properties via antagonism of NMDA and cholinergic α7 nicotinic receptors [51]. Preclinical evidence shows that chronic mild stress leads to increased IDO expression and increased levels of quinolinic acid in rats. Interestingly, antidepressants restored these effects [52].

Plasma level of kynurenine, the first metabolite produced along the kynurenine pathway, has been reported to be significantly elevated in depressed suicide attempters compared to non-suicidal patients [53]. Another study found a net decrease in plasma tryptophan levels and an increase in kynurenine/tryptophan ratio in suicidal adolescents with major depressive disorder, compared to non-suicidal individuals with major depressive disorder and healthy controls. Moreover, the kynurenine/tryptophan ratio was correlated with the severity of suicidal ideation [54]. Quinolinic acid levels in CSF have been demonstrated to be two to three times in suicide attempters compared to controls [55]. Moreover, in accordance with the inflammatory hypothesis, they positively correlated with IL-6 levels in CSF. Notably, quinolinic acid levels, though decreasing, remained increased at almost 2 years after the suicide attempt, and the magnitude of suicidal symptoms during the follow-up was related to fluctuations in cytokines and kynurenic acid, with direct relationship with the former and inverse with the latter, showing sustained dysregulation of the tryptophan-kynurenine pathway [56]. Post-mortem study demonstrated increased counts of quinolinic acid-reactive microglia cells in the subgenual anterior cingulate cortex and anterior midcingulate cortex in depressed suicide completers [57]. Moreover, the deficient activity of one kynurenine pathway enzyme has been linked to increased suicidal vulnerability [58]. Accordingly, a post-mortem study has demonstrated decreased 5-HT transporter and increased 5-HT1A and 5-HT2A binding in the neocortex of depressed suicide victims compared to healthy controls [59], suggestive of an adaptive response to low 5-HT availability in the brain, which could result from the kynurenine pathway hyperactivation. Involvement of the kynurenine pathway in the pathophysiology of suicide might also explain the specific rapid anti-suicidal effect of ketamine, an NMDA-antagonist [60].

19.7 Inflammation as a Mediator Between Stress and Suicidal Behaviour

Stress, broadly referred to as the disruption of homeostatic balance by a stressor has been proposed to play a crucial role in increased SB susceptibility. Glucocorticoids, the end-products of the stress-response pathway, execute rapid anti-inflammatory action via a plethora of mechanisms, such as altered gene expression of pro-inflammatory cytokines [61], and protective action on the BBB [62]. Notably, glucocorticoids have a direct action on the brain, as their receptors are expressed by microglia [63]. However, this tight relationship between the stress-immune axes is highly susceptible to dysfunction, and excessive glucocorticoid release can contribute to increased inflammation by stimulating the release of IL-1β from microglia, which further contributes to activation of microglia and recruitment of monocytes into the brain.

Glucocorticoids and peripheral catecholamines facilitate inflammatory responses to future stimuli by stimulating monocytes to leave the bone marrow, down-regulating inhibitory receptors on microglia, and priming inflammatory responses mediated by peripheral monocytes or macrophages [64]. Pre-clinical studies show that stressors significantly increase microglial reactivity in the brains of experimental rodent models, which then contributes to altered behavioural responses [65]. Pro-inflammatory stress effects are also seen in clinical populations, as stress significantly increases the levels of circulating pro-inflammatory cytokines [66], possibly contributing to increased vulnerability when facing life challenges. Conversely, baseline peripheral inflammation modifies the prefrontal activity during social stress in patients having a history of depression but independently of suicidal status [67].

Inflammatory immune system dysregulation has also been proposed to act as a biological mediator linking SB and early life adversity. Solid evidence proves that early life adversity increases SB risk [68]. Early-life exposure to stress can trigger dysfunctional immune reprogramming, altering brain development, and increasing reactivity to stressors later in life. Pro-inflammatory state in adults, demonstrated by increased levels of such peripheral inflammation markers like CRP, IL-6, TNF-α [69], and soluble urokinase plasminogen activator receptor [70], has been consistently linked to early life adversity history. In accordance with the stress-diathesis model, unfavourable childhood environment has been associated with larger IL-6 stress responses in adulthood [71]. Increased levels of pro-inflammatory cytokines in depressed adolescent subjects with a childhood trauma history have been linked to inhibitory control deficits [72], behaviourally translating to impulsivity, which is linked to suicidality [73]. Interestingly, lithium, a proven anti-suicidal agent, is an inhibitor of the glycogen synthase kinase-3, which is activated in the brain by stress and promotes inflammation, as well as aggressive and depression-like behaviours in rodents [74].

19.8 Inflammation, Intermediate Phenotypes and Suicide

The increasing interest in the dimensional approach has led to a better understanding of certain behavioural dimensions that are implicated in suicidality. Anhedonia, a transdiagnostic positive valence symptom dimension, defined as the loss of pleasure or interest in previously rewarding stimuli, is independently related to increased suicidal ideation risk [75]. Convergent evidence suggests that inflammatory activation in response to physical, psychological or immunological stress disrupts mesolimbic reward functioning by interfering with dopamine synthesis, or via kynurenine-induced oxidative stress [76]. In animal models, chronic social stress led to immune activation and reduced the functioning of the ventral tegmental area-nucleus accumbens dopaminergic pathway, resulting in reduced reward-directed behaviours [77]. In humans, inflammation has been repeatedly linked to anhedonia [78] and related brain changes, such as the activation of the posterior cingulate cortex, prefrontal cortex, and basal ganglia regions, during reward processing [79].

Both increased glutamate levels in the basal ganglia and dorsal anterior cingulate cortex and anhedonia have been noted in depressed patients with serum CRP levels of 3 mg/L or higher, relative to those with CRP < 3 mg/L [80]. Another study identified that patients presenting a combination of elevated plasma CRP, basal ganglia glutamate levels, and greater severity of anhedonia also demonstrated lower regional homogeneity and impaired network integrity in the brain, supporting the link between peripheral inflammation, increased glutamate toxicity, and altered brain functionality [81]. Inflammation-induced neural responses to reward may provide insight into the sex gaps in suicide. For example, a functional magnetic resonance study that used an experimental inflammatory challenge found that endotoxin led to a reduced reward-related ventral striatum activity in anticipation of reward only in female participants [82]. Interestingly, anhedonia has also been linked to the ketamine's anti-suicidal effect [83].

Another intermediate phenotype, possibly linking inflammation and SB, is impulsivity. It has been linked to SB, especially the recent ones [73]. Increased anger and hostility have been observed in patients with hepatitis C that underwent IFN-α treatment [84]. In a sample with psychiatric inpatients, admitted because of suicide attempt or suicidal ideation, and healthy controls, TNF-α mRNA was associated with impulsivity and hopelessness [85]. Trait aggression and impulsivity have been proposed to mediate the relationship between *T.Gondii* infection and SB [86]. However, while some studies link immune system dysfunction to maladaptive decision-making patterns, characterized by impulsivity, present focus, and inability to delay gratification that can result in SB [87], other studies suggested that inflammatory profile and impulsivity both increase SB risk independently [88].

19.9 Conclusion

The current suicide prevention, prediction, and treatment strategies, vastly based on heterogenous categorical constructs of mental disorders, are both overwhelmingly unspecific and unsatisfactory in their outcomes. In light of strengthening position of dimensional approach to mental disorders in medicine, reflected by the rise of such frameworks as the Research Domain Criteria, inflammation may be regarded as a transdiagnostic phenomenon, conferring to increased suicide risk. As described in this chapter, inflammatory changes are the common denominator in suicidal behaviours occurring throughout a range of ailments of varying severity. Peripherally, increased cytokines and CRP levels are detected in suicide attempters and completers, while microglia activation and kynurenine pathway activation seem to be involved centrally. Multiple biological bodily systems are implicated in this intricate relationship, spanning from subtle molecular to overt neuroanatomical alterations. Addressing the inflammatory pathways is a viable way to complement clinical and research practices by both serving as the heuristic in the assessment and intervention in suicidal behaviour risk, stratifying intervention options for susceptible individuals, and facilitating the development of novel specific therapeutic targets in suicide.

References

1. Courtet P, Giner L, Seneque M, Guillaume S, Olie E, Ducasse D. Neuroinflammation in suicide: toward a comprehensive model. World J Biol Psychiatry. 2016;17:564–86.
2. Gjervig Hansen H, Köhler-Forsberg O, Petersen L, Nordentoft M, Postolache TT, Erlangsen A, et al. Infections, anti-infective agents, and risk of deliberate self-harm and suicide in a young cohort: a Nationwide study. Biol Psychiatry. 2019;85:744–51.
3. Nissen J, Trabjerg B, Pedersen M, Banasik K, Pedersen OB, Sørensen E, et al. Herpes simplex virus type 1 infection is associated with suicidal behavior and first registered psychiatric diagnosis in a healthy population. Psychoneuroendocrinology. 2019;108:150–4.
4. Xie L-F, Chen P-L, Pan H-F, Tao J-H, Li X-P, Zhang Y-J, et al. Prevalence and correlates of suicidal ideation in SLE inpatients: Chinese experience. Rheumatol Int. 2012;32:2707–14.
5. Fredrikson S, Cheng Q, Jiang G-X, Wasserman D. Elevated suicide risk among patients with multiple sclerosis in Sweden. Neuroepidemiology. 2003;22:146–52.
6. Barker E, Kãlves K, De Leo D. The relationship between asthma and suicidal behaviours: a systematic literature review. Eur Respir J. 2015;46:96–106.
7. Qin P, Waltoft BL, Mortensen PB, Postolache TT. Suicide risk in relation to air pollen counts: a study based on data from Danish registers. BMJ Open. 2013;3:e002462.
8. Woo J-M, Gibbons RD, Qin P, Komarow H, Kim JB, Rogers CA, et al. Suicide and prescription rates of intranasal corticosteroids and nonsedating antihistamines for allergic rhinitis. J Clin Psychiatry. 2011;72:1423–8.
9. Raison CL, Borisov AS, Majer M, Drake DF, Pagnoni G, Woolwine BJ, et al. Activation of central nervous system inflammatory pathways by interferon-alpha: relationship to monoamines and depression. Biol Psychiatry. 2009;65:296–303.
10. Fragoso YD, Frota ERC, Lopes JS, Noal JS, Giacomo MC, Gomes S, et al. Severe depression, suicide attempts, and ideation during the use of interferon Beta by patients with multiple sclerosis. Clin Neuropharmacol. 2010;33:312–6.
11. Grudet C, Malm J, Westrin Å, Brundin L. Suicidal patients are deficient in vitamin D, associated with a pro-inflammatory status in the blood. Psychoneuroendocrinology. 2014;50:210–9.
12. Dickerson F, Adamos M, Katsafanas E, Khushalani S, Origoni A, Savage C, et al. The association between immune markers and recent suicide attempts in patients with serious mental illness: a pilot study. Psychiatry Res. 2017;255:8–12.
13. Ekinci O, Ekinci A. The connections among suicidal behavior, lipid profile and low-grade inflammation in patients with major depressive disorder: a specific relationship with the neutrophil-to-lymphocyte ratio. Nord J Psychiatry. 2017;71:574–80.
14. Black C, Miller BJ. Meta-analysis of cytokines and chemokines in suicidality: distinguishing suicidal versus nonsuicidal patients. Biol Psychiatry. 2015;78:28–37.
15. Ducasse D, Olié E, Guillaume S, Artéro S, Courtet P. A meta-analysis of cytokines in suicidal behavior. Brain Behav Immun. 2015;46:203–11.
16. Courtet P, Jaussent I, Genty C, Dupuy AM, Guillaume S, Ducasse D, et al. Increased CRP levels may be a trait marker of suicidal attempt. Eur Neuropsychopharmacol. 2015;25:1824–31.
17. Gan Z, Wu X, Liao Y, Wu Y, He Z, Yang Z, et al. The association between low-grade inflammation and the clinical features of bipolar disorder in Han Chinese population. Psychoneuroendocrinology. 2019;101:286–94.
18. Oh KY, Van Dam NT, Doucette JT, Murrough JW. Effects of chronic physical disease and systemic inflammation on suicide risk in patients with depression: a hospital-based case-control study. Psychol Med. 2019:1–9.
19. Melhem NM, Munroe S, Marsland A, Gray K, Brent D, Porta G, et al. Blunted HPA axis activity prior to suicide attempt and increased inflammation in attempters. Psychoneuroendocrinology. 2017;77:284–94.
20. Keaton SA, Madaj ZB, Heilman P, Smart L, Grit J, Gibbons R, et al. An inflammatory profile linked to increased suicide risk. J Affect Disord. 2019;247:57–65.

21. Felger JC, Haroon E, Patel TA, Goldsmith DR, Wommack EC, Woolwine BJ, et al. What does plasma CRP tell us about peripheral and central inflammation in depression? Mol Psychiatry. 2018;17:1310–4.
22. Varatharaj A, Galea I. The blood-brain barrier in systemic inflammation. Brain Behav Immun. 2017;60:1–12.
23. Librizzi L, de Cutis M, Janigro D, Runtz L, de Bock F, Barbier EL, et al. Cerebrovascular heterogeneity and neuronal excitability. Neurosci Lett. 2018;667:75–83.
24. Falcone T, Fazio V, Lee C, Simon B, Franco K, Marchi N, et al. Serum S100B: a potential biomarker for suicidality in adolescents? PLoS One. 2010;5:e11089.
25. Bargerstock E, Puvenna V, Iffland P, Falcone T, Hossain M, Vetter S, et al. Is peripheral immunity regulated by blood-brain barrier permeability changes? PLoS One. 2014;9:e101477.
26. Savitz J, Harrison NA. Interoception and inflammation in psychiatric disorders. Biol Psychiatry Cogn Neurosci Neuroimaging. 2018;3:514–24.
27. Harrison NA, Cooper E, Dowell NG, Keramida G, Voon V, Critchley HD, et al. Quantitative magnetization transfer imaging as a biomarker for effects of systemic inflammation on the brain. Biol Psychiatry. 2015;78:49–57.
28. Wohleb ES, McKim DB, Sheridan JF, Godbout JP. Monocyte trafficking to the brain with stress and inflammation: a novel axis of immune-to-brain communication that influences mood and behavior. Front Neurosci. 2015;8:447.
29. Dodd DR, Smith AR, Forrest LN, Witte TK, Bodell L, Bartlett M, et al. Interoceptive deficits, nonsuicidal self-injury, and suicide attempts among women with eating disorders. Suicide Life-Threatening Behav. 2018;48:438–48.
30. Rogers ML, Hagan CR, Joiner TE. Examination of interoception along the suicidality continuum. J Clin Psychol. 2018;74:1004–16.
31. Hagan CR, Rogers ML, Brausch AM, Muehlenkamp JJ, Joiner TE. Interoceptive deficits, nonsuicidal self-injury, and suicide risk: a multi-sample study of indirect effects. Psychol Med. 2019:1–12.
32. Enache D, Pariante CM, Mondelli V. Markers of central inflammation in major depressive disorder: a systematic review and meta-analysis of studies examining cerebrospinal fluid, positron emission tomography and post-mortem brain tissue. Brain Behav Immun. 2019;
33. Crider A, Feng T, Pandya CD, Davis T, Nair A, Ahmed AO, et al. Complement component 3a receptor deficiency attenuates chronic stress-induced monocyte infiltration and depressive-like behavior. Brain Behav Immun. 2018;70:246–56.
34. Holmes SE, Hinz R, Conen S, Gregory CJ, Matthews JC, Anton-Rodriguez JM, et al. Elevated translocator protein in anterior cingulate in major depression and a role for inflammation in suicidal thinking: a positron emission tomography study. Biol Psychiatry. 2018;83:61–9.
35. Madsen T, Erlangsen A, Orlovska S, Mofaddy R, Nordentoft M, Benros ME. Association between traumatic brain injury and risk of suicide. JAMA. 2018;320:580.
36. Fralick M, Sy E, Hassan A, Burke MJ, Mostofsky E, Karsies T. Association of Concussion with the risk of suicide. JAMA Neurol. 2019;76:144.
37. Herman FJ, Pasinetti GM. Principles of inflammasome priming and inhibition: implications for psychiatric disorders. Brain Behav Immun. 2018;73:66–84.
38. Juengst SB, Kumar RG, Arenth PM, Wagner AK. Exploratory associations with tumor necrosis factor-α, disinhibition and suicidal endorsement after traumatic brain injury. Brain Behav Immun. 2014;41:134–43.
39. Torres-Platas SG, Cruceanu C, Chen GG, Turecki G, Mechawar N. Evidence for increased microglial priming and macrophage recruitment in the dorsal anterior cingulate white matter of depressed suicides. Brain Behav Immun. 2014;42:50–9.
40. Schnieder TP, Trencevska I, Rosoklija G, Stankov A, Mann JJ, Smiley J, et al. Microglia of prefrontal white matter in suicide. J Neuropathol Exp Neurol. 2014;73:880–90.
41. Marsland AL, Kuan DC-H, Sheu LK, Krajina K, Kraynak TE, Manuck SB, et al. Systemic inflammation and resting state connectivity of the default mode network. Brain Behav Immun. 2017;62:162–70.

42. Malhi GS, Das P, Outhred T, Bryant RA, Calhoun V, Mann JJ. Default mode dysfunction underpins suicidal activity in mood disorders. Psychol Med. 2019:1–10.
43. Labrenz F, Ferri F, Wrede K, Forsting M, Schedlowski M, Engler H, et al. Altered temporal variance and functional connectivity of BOLD signal is associated with state anxiety during acute systemic inflammation. NeuroImage. 2019;184:916–24.
44. Schwartz J, Ordaz SJ, Ho TC, Gotlib IH. Longitudinal decreases in suicidal ideation are associated with increases in salience network coherence in depressed adolescents. J Affect Disord. 2019;245:545–52.
45. Knowles EEM, Curran JE, Göring HHH, Mathias SR, Mollon J, Rodrigue A, et al. Family-based analyses reveal novel genetic overlap between cytokine interleukin-8 and risk for suicide attempt. Brain Behav Immun. 2019;
46. Pandey GN, Rizavi HS, Zhang H, Bhaumik R, Ren X. Abnormal protein and mRNA expression of inflammatory cytokines in the prefrontal cortex of depressed individuals who died by suicide. J Psychiatry Neurosci. 2018;43:376–85.
47. Pandey GN, Rizavi HS, Bhaumik R, Ren X. Innate immunity in the postmortem brain of depressed and suicide subjects: role of toll-like receptors. Brain Behav Immun. 2019;75:101–11.
48. Wang Q, Roy B, Turecki G, Shelton RC, Dwivedi Y. Role of complex epigenetic switching in tumor necrosis factor-α upregulation in the prefrontal cortex of suicide subjects. Am J Psychiatry. 2018;175:262–74.
49. Schwieler L, Larsson MK, Skogh E, Kegel ME, Orhan F, Abdelmoaty S, et al. Increased levels of IL-6 in the cerebrospinal fluid of patients with chronic schizophrenia--significance for activation of the kynurenine pathway. J Psychiatry Neurosci. 2015;40:126–33.
50. Tavares RG, Tasca CI, Santos CES, Alves LB, Porciúncula LO, Emanuelli T, et al. Quinolinic acid stimulates synaptosomal glutamate release and inhibits glutamate uptake into astrocytes. Neurochem Int. 2002;40:621–7.
51. Borsini A, Zunszain PA, Thuret S, Pariante CM. The role of inflammatory cytokines as key modulators of neurogenesis. Trends Neurosci. 2015;38:145–57.
52. Martín-Hernández D, Tendilla-Beltrán H, Madrigal JLM, García-Bueno B, Leza JC, Caso JR. Chronic mild stress alters kynurenine pathways changing the glutamate neurotransmission in frontal cortex of rats. Mol Neurobiol. 2019;56:490–501.
53. Sublette ME, Galfalvy HC, Fuchs D, Lapidus M, Grunebaum MF, Oquendo MA, et al. Plasma kynurenine levels are elevated in suicide attempters with major depressive disorder. Brain Behav Immun. 2011;25:1272–8.
54. Bradley KAL, Case JAC, Khan O, Ricart T, Hanna A, Alonso CM, et al. The role of the kynurenine pathway in suicidality in adolescent major depressive disorder. Psychiatry Res. 2015;227:206–12.
55. Erhardt S, Lim CK, Linderholm KR, Janelidze S, Lindqvist D, Samuelsson M, et al. Connecting inflammation with glutamate agonism in suicidality. Neuropsychopharmacology. 2013;38:743–52.
56. Bay-Richter C, Linderholm KR, Lim CK, Samuelsson M, Träskman-Bendz L, Guillemin GJ, et al. A role for inflammatory metabolites as modulators of the glutamate N-methyl-d-aspartate receptor in depression and suicidality. Brain Behav Immun. 2015;43:110–7.
57. Steiner J, Walter M, Gos T, Guillemin GJ, Bernstein H-G, Sarnyai Z, et al. Severe depression is associated with increased microglial quinolinic acid in subregions of the anterior cingulate gyrus: evidence for an immune-modulated glutamatergic neurotransmission? J Neuroinflammation. 2011;8:94.
58. Brundin L, Sellgren CM, Lim CK, Grit J, Pålsson E, Landén M, et al. An enzyme in the kynurenine pathway that governs vulnerability to suicidal behavior by regulating excitotoxicity and neuroinflammation. Transl Psychiatry. 2016;6:e865.
59. Underwood MD, Kassir SA, Bakalian MJ, Galfalvy H, Dwork AJ, Mann JJ, et al. Serotonin receptors and suicide, major depression, alcohol use disorder and reported early life adversity. Transl Psychiatry. 2018;8:279.

60. Wilkinson ST, Ballard ED, Bloch MH, Mathew SJ, Murrough JW, Feder A, et al. The effect of a single dose of intravenous ketamine on suicidal ideation: a systematic review and individual participant data meta-analysis. Am J Psychiatry. 2018;175:150–8.
61. Sorrells SF, Sapolsky RM. An inflammatory review of glucocorticoid actions in the CNS. Brain Behav Immun. 2007;21:259–72.
62. Salvador E, Shityakov S, Förster C. Glucocorticoids and endothelial cell barrier function. Cell Tissue Res. 2014;355:597–605.
63. Sierra A, Gottfried-Blackmore A, Milner TA, McEwen BS, Bulloch K. Steroid hormone receptor expression and function in microglia. Glia. 2008;56:659–74.
64. Johnson JD, Barnard DF, Kulp AC, Mehta DM. Neuroendocrine regulation of brain cytokines after psychological stress. J Endocr Soc. 2019;3:1302–20.
65. Calcia MA, Bonsall DR, Bloomfield PS, Selvaraj S, Barichello T, Howes OD. Stress and neuroinflammation: a systematic review of the effects of stress on microglia and the implications for mental illness. Psychopharmacology. 2016;233:1637–50.
66. Marsland AL, Walsh C, Lockwood K, John-Henderson NA. The effects of acute psychological stress on circulating and stimulated inflammatory markers: a systematic review and meta-analysis. Brain Behav Immun. 2017;64:208–19.
67. Conejero I, Jaussent I, Cazals A, Thouvenot E, Mura T, Le Bars E, et al. Association between baseline pro-inflammatory cytokines and brain activation during social exclusion in patients with vulnerability to suicide and depressive disorder. Psychoneuroendocrinology. 2019;99:236–42.
68. Angelakis I, Gillespie EL, Panagioti M. Childhood maltreatment and adult suicidality: a comprehensive systematic review with meta-analysis. Psychol Med. 2019;46:1–22.
69. Baumeister D, Akhtar R, Ciufolini S, Pariante CM, Mondelli V. Childhood trauma and adulthood inflammation: a meta-analysis of peripheral C-reactive protein, interleukin-6 and tumour necrosis factor-α. Mol Psychiatry. 2016;21:642–9.
70. Rasmussen LJH, Moffitt TE, Eugen-Olsen J, Belsky DW, Danese A, Harrington H, et al. Cumulative childhood risk is associated with a new measure of chronic inflammation in adulthood. J Child Psychol Psychiatry. 2019;60:199–208.
71. Lockwood KG, John-Henderson NA, Marsland AL. Early life socioeconomic status associates with interleukin-6 responses to acute laboratory stress in adulthood. Physiol Behav. 2018;188:212–20.
72. Peters AT, Ren X, Bessette KL, Goldstein BI, West AE, Langenecker SA, et al. Interplay between pro-inflammatory cytokines, childhood trauma, and executive function in depressed adolescents. J Psychiatr Res. 2019;114:1–10.
73. Liu RT, Trout ZM, Hernandez EM, Cheek SM, Gerlus N. A behavioral and cognitive neuroscience perspective on impulsivity, suicide, and non-suicidal self-injury: meta-analysis and recommendations for future research. Neurosci Biobehav Rev. 2017;83:440–50.
74. Beurel E, Jope RS. Inflammation and lithium: clues to mechanisms contributing to suicide-linked traits. Transl Psychiatry. 2014;4:e488.
75. Ducasse D, Loas G, Dassa D, Gramaglia C, Zeppegno P, Guillaume S, et al. Anhedonia is associated with suicidal ideation independently of depression: a meta-analysis. Depress Anxiety. 2018;35:382–92.
76. Stanton CH, Holmes AJ, Chang SWC, Joormann J. From stress to anhedonia: molecular processes through functional circuits. Trends Neurosci. 2019;42:23–42.
77. Bergamini G, Mechtersheimer J, Azzinnari D, Sigrist H, Buerge M, Dallmann R, et al. Chronic social stress induces peripheral and central immune activation, blunted mesolimbic dopamine function, and reduced reward-directed behaviour in mice. Neurobiol Stress. 2018;8:42–56.
78. Freed RD, Mehra LM, Laor D, Patel M, Alonso CM, Kim-Schulze S, et al. Anhedonia as a clinical correlate of inflammation in adolescents across psychiatric conditions. World J Biol Psychiatry. 2018:1–11.
79. Bradley KA. Stern ER. Xie H, Kim-Schulze S, Gabbay V. Relationships between neural activation during a reward task and peripheral cytokine levels in youth with diverse psychiatric symptoms. Brain Behav Immun: Alonso CM; 2019.

80. Haroon E, Woolwine BJ, Chen X, Pace TW, Parekh S, Spivey JR, et al. IFN-alpha-induced cortical and subcortical glutamate changes assessed by magnetic resonance spectroscopy. Neuropsychopharmacology. 2014;39:1777–85.
81. Haroon E, Chen X, Li Z, Patel T, Woolwine BJ, Hu XP, et al. Increased inflammation and brain glutamate define a subtype of depression with decreased regional homogeneity, impaired network integrity, and anhedonia. Transl Psychiatry. 2018;8:189.
82. Moieni M, Tan KM, Inagaki TK, Muscatell KA, Dutcher JM, Jevtic I, et al. Sex differences in the relationship between inflammation and reward sensitivity: a randomized controlled trial of endotoxin. Biol Psychiatry Cogn Neurosci Neuroimaging. 2019;4:619–26.
83. Ballard ED, Wills K, Lally N, Richards EM, Luckenbaugh DA, Walls T, et al. Anhedonia as a clinical correlate of suicidal thoughts in clinical ketamine trials. J Affect Disord. 2017;218:195–200.
84. Bezemer G, Van Gool AR, Fekkes D, Vrolijk JM, Hansen BE, Janssen HLA, et al. Psychiatric side effects and fluctuations in serotonergic parameters in the treatment of chronic hepatitis C infection. Neuropsychobiology. 2012;65:126–32.
85. Chang HB, Munroe S, Gray K, Porta G, Douaihy A, Marsland A, et al. The role of substance use, smoking, and inflammation in risk for suicidal behavior. J Affect Disord. 2019;243:33–41.
86. Cook TB, Brenner LA, Cloninger CR, Langenberg P, Igbide A, Giegling I, et al. "Latent" infection with toxoplasma gondii: association with trait aggression and impulsivity in healthy adults. J Psychiatr Res. 2015;60:87–94.
87. Gassen J, Prokosch ML, Eimerbrink MJ, Proffitt Leyva RP, White JD, Peterman JL, et al. Inflammation predicts decision-making characterized by impulsivity, present focus, and an inability to delay gratification. Sci Rep. 2019;9:4928.
88. Cáceda R, Griffin WST, Delgado PL. A probe in the connection between inflammation, cognition and suicide. J Psychopharmacol. 2018;32:482–8.

Inflammatory Bases of Neuropsychiatric Symptom Domains: Mechanisms and Specificity

20

Bruno Aouizerate, Sylvie Vancassel, Nathalie Castanon, and Lucile Capuron

20.1 Introduction

Psychiatric disorders are frequent in the general population, with an estimated lifetime prevalence of 30% [1]. Generally characterized by symptoms of severe intensity and recurrent/chronic course, they substantially impact the patient's daily functioning and quality of life and are responsible for life-years lost due to premature deaths, including suicide. Their socioeconomic repercussions are high, with substantial indirect costs, primarily related to the high rate of workplace absenteeism and loss of productivity at work, as well as direct medical costs mainly attributable to medical consultations, medications, and hospital admission. Based on data from the Global Burden of Disease Study, major depression is the most common mental disorder, representing one of the top leading causes of years lived with disability (YLDs) [2, 3].

Over the last five decades, significant advances in the development of pharmacological strategies have modified the poor prognosis of psychiatric diseases, notably in major depression. Controlled research has provided high-level evidence for the efficacy of a large panel of medications sharing common mechanisms of action primarily targeting monoamine systems in the management of mental disorders. However, a significant number of psychiatric patients still fail to respond successfully to these pharmacological treatments, experiencing insufficient clinical

B. Aouizerate
University of Bordeaux, INRAE, Bordeaux INP, NutriNeuro, UMR 1286, Bordeaux, France

CH Charles Perrens, Pôle de Psychiatrie Générale et Universitaire, Centre de référence régional des pathologies anxieuses et dépressives, Bordeaux, France
e-mail: bruno.aouizerate@u-bordeaux.fr

S. Vancassel · N. Castanon · L. Capuron (✉)
University of Bordeaux, INRAE, Bordeaux INP, NutriNeuro, UMR 1286, Bordeaux, France
e-mail: sylvie.vancassel@inrae.fr; nathalie.castanon@inrae.fr; lucile.capuron@inrae.fr

M. Berk et al. (eds.), *Immuno-Psychiatry*, https://doi.org/10.1007/978-3-030-71229-7_20

improvement after several weeks or months of administration. Side effects may also occur, therefore limiting the gradually increasing dosage regimen classically recommended until optimal therapeutic response is obtained. These issues highlight the necessity to improve current knowledge on the biological determinants of psychiatric diseases. Such a scientific approach is expected to ensure the promotion and use of innovative therapeutic alternatives that can be particularly helpful in psychiatric patients who are unresponsive to conventional treatments. This implies a better phenotyping of patients in order to match specific clinical profiles to biomarkers in the perspective to propose more adapted treatments targeting the biological substrates intimately related to clinical symptoms. This research strategy is in line with the Research Domain Criteria (RDoC) project introducing a conceptual and methodological breakthrough in mental health by emphasizing the need for a "*biosignature*" of clinical symptomatology enabling to define distinct and homogenous patient subgroups so as to improve therapeutic management [4, 5]. In this context, a growing attention has been paid to the critical role of the immune system in the emergence of neuropsychiatric symptoms with the aim of establishing close relationships between identified inflammatory pathways and key clinical symptom dimensions for the further development of appropriate and individualized therapies.

20.1.1 The Role of Inflammation in the Development of Neuropsychiatric Symptom Dimensions

Compelling evidence for a role of inflammation in the development of neuropsychiatric symptoms comes from preclinical and clinical findings indicating that treatment with inflammatory agents, including proinflammatory cytokines and endotoxins, induces behavioral alterations that resemble symptoms of major depression [6, 7]. The model of interferon (IFN)-alpha-induced depression in clinical settings has contributed significantly to demonstrate the causal role of cytokines in the pathophysiology of major depression in vulnerable subjects [7, 8]. In addition, several clinical observations have indicated that chronic inflammatory conditions, such as rheumatoid arthritis, ankylosing spondylitis, systemic lupus erythematosus, obesity, diabetes, or cardiovascular diseases, are frequently characterized by depressive symptoms that can be relieved by pharmacological anti-inflammatory or anticytokine interventions [7, 9]. Similarly, basal and stimulated-levels of inflammatory markers, including the acute phase protein, C-reactive protein (CRP), or the proinflammatory cytokine, Interleukin (IL)-6, have been associated with an increased risk for the development and persistence of depressive symptoms [10–15]. Four recently published meta-analyses based on 20 to 80 studies examining peripheral cytokine profile reported concordant results, with circulating concentrations of the proinflammatory cytokines IL-6 and Tumor Necrosis Factor (TNF)-alpha found to be higher in depressed subjects [16–19]. Increased levels of IL-6 were also found in the cerebrospinal fluid (CSF) of depressed patients [20].

Strong relationships have been established between markers of inflammation and the clinical severity of neuropsychiatric symptoms. Accordingly, peripheral concentrations of high-sensitive (hs) CRP were found to correlate with the intensity of depressive manifestations [21–25]. Interestingly, correlations were the strongest with the dimensions of anhedonia, loss of interest, apparent sadness, cognitive disturbances and suicidality [22]. Similarly, higher levels of IL-6 were associated with more severe symptoms of anhedonia [26], slowness of thought and movement [27], and cognitive impairment on sustained attention in depressed patients [28]. In large cohort studies of nonpathological populations, relationships between hsCRP and symptom dimensions were also established, but rather with nonspecific symptoms including fatigue, reduced appetite and sleep alterations [29].

Semiological, temporal, and clinical specificities were reported regarding the relationships between systemic inflammation and neuropsychiatric dimensions, allowing deconstructing inflammation-driven symptom dimensions based on their phenomenological aspects. This relies on clinical evidence showing that IFN-alpha treatment in medically ill patients induced two distinct sets of symptoms that differed by their time-course and responsiveness to classical antidepressant treatment [7, 30]. The first set, characterized by symptoms of fatigue, lassitude, decreased motivation, motor slowing, and changes in appetite and sleep, developed at early stages of IFN-alpha treatment in almost every patient. In contrast, the second set of symptoms, which included sadness, depressed mood, anhedonia, and cognitive alteration, developed at later stages of treatment in a subpopulation of patients (30–50%), suggesting vulnerability factors. This second set of symptoms was prevented by the prophylactic administration of paroxetine, a selective serotonin reuptake inhibitor (SSRI), in contrast to the first set of symptoms that did not respond to the antidepressant [30]. The differences between these two symptom dimensions in terms of temporal dynamics and antidepressant responsiveness suggested that they likely involved distinct underlying neurobiological mechanisms. This assumption was supported by preclinical studies performed in rodent models of inflammation developed to experimentally dissociate sickness behavior (appearing early after the immune stimulation) from protracted depressive-like behaviors [31–34]. These models showed that depressive-like symptoms, assessed in behavioral tests modeling despair/resignation, anhedonia, anxiety, or measuring cognitive performance, were still present while sickness behavior and increased circulating cytokines levels were no longer detectable [32–38]. Further supporting the implication of distinct underlying mechanisms, neuroanatomical dissociations were found to correlate with the time-course dissociation between lipopolysaccharide (LPS)-induced sickness and depressive-like behaviors in mice [31]. Since then, the use of preclinical models together with clinical studies helped decipher the mechanisms differentially involved in the development of inflammation-driven specific symptom dimensions and likely to be common to multiple neuropsychiatric conditions in which increased inflammatory markers have been reported. These studies particularly focused on the potential role of neurobiological systems known to be involved in mood regulation and targeted by inflammatory cytokines [6, 7, 39, 40].

20.1.2 Mechanisms Differentially Involved in the Development of Inflammation-Induced Specific Symptom Dimensions

Among the mechanisms that are likely to underlie the association of inflammation with neuropsychiatric symptoms, one of the most relevant refers to the impact of inflammatory factors on neurotransmitter metabolism and function. Consistent with this notion, a large database substantiates the differential contribution of inflammation-induced alterations in monoamine and glutamate systems, respectively (through effects on amino-acid metabolism and related enzymatic pathways) in the development of specific neuropsychiatric symptom dimensions.

20.1.2.1 Inflammation-Induced Alterations in Tryptophan Metabolism: Relevance to Serotonin/Glutamate Functions and Related Mood, Emotional and Cognitive Symptoms

Peripheral cytokines are able to impact serotonin (5-HT) and glutamate functions through the induction of the enzyme, indoleamine-2,3-dioxygenase (IDO). The activation of IDO by inflammatory factors leads to the transformation of tryptophan (TRP), the essential amino-acid precursor of 5-HT, in kynurenine (KYN) instead of 5-HT, contributing presumably to 5-HT deficit. KYN is then converted into neurotoxic derivatives such as quinolinic acid in microglia at the expense of the neuroprotective compound kynurenic acid in astrocytes [7, 41, 42]. In line with this, treatment with IFN-alpha in medically ill patients was found to induce significant reductions in circulating levels of TRP together with increases in KYN and in the ratio of KYN/TRP, indicative of augmented IDO activity [43]. Interestingly, these alterations correlated with depressive, anxious and cognitive symptoms [8, 43, 44]. Similar findings were reported in elderly subjects with elevated markers of inflammation, where inflammation-associated TRP catabolism correlated with depressive symptoms including pessimistic thoughts, reduced appetite, sleep disturbances, and lassitude [45]. These findings were corroborated by the observation that an elevated KYN/TRP ratio was linked to depressive symptom severity in patients with mastocytosis [46] and by data showing that depressed patients exhibit increased KYN/TRP ratio [47] together with lowered kynurenic acid/quinolinic acid ratio [48–50] correlating with severe anhedonia [48].

IDO-driven degradation of TRP along the KYN pathway leads to the production of neuroactive metabolites, including quinolinic acid, which exerts neurotoxic effects by stimulating glutamate transmission through activation of NMDA receptors, elevation of glutamate release, and inhibition of glutamate reuptake by astrocytes [7, 41, 42]. Consistent with this, elevated CSF concentrations of KYN and quinolinic acid were reported in patients treated with IFN-alpha and were associated with increased depressive symptoms [51]. Similarly, a postmortem brain analysis of depressed patients showed greater quinolinic acid-microglial cell immunoreactivity within both ventral and dorsal portions of anterior cingulate cortex [52], known to be involved in the regulation of emotional processes [53, 54]. Besides, a recent study using magnetic resonance spectroscopy in IFN-alpha-treated patients indicated that treatment-induced increased glutamate levels in the dorsal anterior cingulate cortex, which is intimately connected to basal ganglia, and is correlated with reduced motivation [55]. Similar findings were found in depressed patients who exhibited increased inflammation correlating with higher levels of glutamate in the basal ganglia that were in turn associated with greater anhedonia and motor retardation [56].

Strong support for a role of inflammation-induced IDO activation and related modulation of 5-HT/glutamate functions in depressive symptoms was also provided by preclinical studies. Rodent models of inflammation have shown that IDO activation, which occurs after the induction of cytokine production in immune-challenged animals [57, 58], coincides with the development of depressive-like symptoms [31, 34, 36, 37, 59, 60]. Concomitance between protracted brain IDO expression and depressive-like behaviors was also reported in aged mice [61, 62] and in medical conditions associated with chronic inflammation [63–67]. In addition, cytokine-induced IDO activation also paralleled the development of anxiety-like behaviors and/or cognitive alterations in animals treated with cytokine inducers [38, 64, 68–70], as well as in rodent models of chronic inflammatory diseases [67, 71–74]. Importantly, pharmacological or genetic inhibition of IDO activation in these inflammatory conditions abolished the induction of emotional and cognitive alterations without impacting sickness behavior [36–38, 59, 64, 67, 71–73], highlighting the causal role of IDO in the induction of these symptom dimensions.

While impaired 5-HT synthesis was initially thought to represent the main pathway by which cytokine-induced IDO activation promotes behavioral alterations, the lack of detectable impact on 5-HT turnover reported in several preclinical studies weakened this hypothesis [59, 61, 70, 75]. Nevertheless, it is worth mentioning that these findings do not necessarily discard the involvement of inflammation-related alterations of 5-HT neurotransmission in associated depressive symptoms. In support of this, cytokines were shown to increase expression of the 5-HT transporter [76], a mechanism that may be responsible for worsened disruptions in 5-HT neurotransmission contributing in turn to depressive symptoms. Mounting evidence rather supports the key role of neurotoxic KYN metabolites (e.g., quinolinic acid, 3-hydroxykynurenine [3-HK]), in the development of inflammation-related depressive symptoms [75, 77, 78]. In line with this, direct peripheral administration of KYN or 3-HK in rodents induces depressive-like behaviors, anxiety-like behaviors and/or cognitive impairments in a dose-dependent manner [38, 59, 75, 77, 79, 80]. In contrast, inhibition of the enzymes synthetizing the NMDA receptor agonist quinolinic acid [77, 78], or direct blockade of these glutamate receptors [81] abrogates cytokine-induced depressive-like behaviors. Interestingly, the efficiency of this effect was shown to differ according to symptoms, with behavioral changes modeling anhedonia being less impacted [77]. This agrees with a recent study reporting that inflammation-induced impairment of motivation-driven behaviors persists in IDO deficient mice [82]. While the dissociation between activation of the KYN pathway and specific depressive symptoms may rely on regional brain differences [75, 77, 78], it may also reflect the involvement of other metabolic pathways and/or neurotransmission systems.

20.1.2.2 Inflammation-Induced Alterations in Tyrosine Metabolism: Relevance to Dopamine Function and Related Symptom Dimensions

In addition to their effects on IDO and related monoamine pathways, proinflammatory cytokines are able to modulate the activity of GTP-cyclohydrolase I (GCH-I), a key enzyme for tetrahydrobiopterin (BH4) synthesis [83]. BH4 is an essential cofactor for aromatic amino acid hydroxylases, including phenylalanine hydroxylase (PAH), tyrosine hydroxylase (TH), TRP-hydroxylase (TPH), and nitrite oxide synthases (NOS). It is then crucial for the synthesis of noradrenaline, dopamine (DA), 5-HT, and nitric oxide from their respective precursors, the essential amino acids tyrosine, TRP, and arginine [84–87]. BH4 synthesis results from the sequential action of three complementary enzymes, GCH-I, 6-pyruvoyl tetrahydrobiopterin synthase (PTPS), and sepiapterin reductase (SPR) [88]. In human, the induction of GCH-I in macrophages and monocytes is not relayed by the activation of PTPS under inflammatory challenge, leading to accumulation of neopterin, a peripheral early marker of immune activation, at the expense of BH4 [87, 89]. Moreover, proinflammatory cytokines, such as IFN-gamma, trigger formation of large amounts of reactive oxygen species that can also destroy the oxidation-labile BH4 and then contribute to the substantial reductions in BH4 levels [90]. Consistent with this notion, elevated plasma levels of neopterin [43] together with reduced BH4, reflected in increased phenylalanine/tyrosine ratio [91], were reported in patients treated with IFN-alpha and in multiple inflammatory conditions [89].

Due to its crucial role as cofactor in the activity of TH and TPH, the oxidation and reduced production of BH4 during inflammatory conditions may lead to significant disruptions in monoamine biosynthesis and neurotransmission [83, 89, 92]. In line with this, inflammatory cytokines have been shown to strongly affect DA and DA-relevant neurocircuitry [93–96]. Interestingly, IFN-alpha-induced reductions in BH4, as indicated by increased phenylalanine/tyrosine ratio, correlated with increased levels of systemic markers of inflammation together with reduced CSF levels of DA and its metabolite, homovanillic acid [91]. In the same study, the oxidized form of BH4, BH2, was also increased in the CSF of IFN-alpha treated patients. Measurements of monoamine levels in murine models of partial deficiencies in BH4 have confirmed its important role in monoamine synthesis [97]. Accordingly, reduced levels of 5-HT and DA were described in the brain of *hph-1* mouse, which are genetically deficient for BH4 [98–102]. Interestingly, those mice exhibited anxiety and depressive-like behavior when compared to wild-type control mice [101]. Similarly, mice deficient in the SPR gene (*Spr−/−*), which catalyzes the final step of BH4 synthesis, displayed reductions in brain BH4 and monoamine levels, including DA and 5HT, together with disruption in brain maturation, severe growth retardation, and locomotor deficits at adulthood [103–105]. Interestingly, oral supplementation with tyrosine or BH4 and neurotransmitter precursors improved body weight and motor alterations, and restored phenylalanine metabolism in these animals [103, 106].

Impairments in DA activity and related neurocircuitry have been repeatedly documented during inflammatory conditions. Inflammatory challenges (e.g., IFN-alpha or endotoxin administration, typhoid vaccine) in clinical populations lead to significant alterations in the activity of the basal ganglia and substantia nigra that correlate with symptoms of fatigue, reduced motivation, anhedonia, and psychomotor slowing [94, 107–110]. Similarly, increased phenylalanine/tyrosine ratio was shown to correlate with reduced motivation, fatigue, and motor symptoms in elderly subjects with low-grade inflammation [45]. Moreover, dietary depletion of DA precursors, including phenylalanine and tyrosine, was found to decrease neural activation of the ventral striatum to hedonic reward [111], similar to that observed following administration of IFN-alpha or endotoxin [94, 107]. Interestingly, the phenylalanine/tyrosine ratio was shown to be lower in depressed patients who responded to electroconvulsive therapy [112] whereas reduced BH4 levels were found in *postmortem* brains of subjects with a history of severe depression [113, 114].

Animal studies have confirmed the role of inflammatory processes in the occurrence of alterations in DA function and neurocircuitry and their repercussions on the development of DA-related symptoms. Accordingly, nonhuman primates treated with IFN-alpha were found to exhibit lower D2/D3 DA receptor density and reduced striatum DA release in response to amphetamine that correlated with low motivation for food-related rewarding stimulus [115]. Interestingly, reduction in DA was restored by L-DOPA administration via reverse in vivo microdialysis, suggesting a specific effect of IFN-alpha treatment on impaired DA synthesis [116], consistent with the clinical findings documenting disrupted presynaptic DA function in IFN-alpha-treated patients [94]. In line with these data, studies in rodents have indicated that acute peripheral administration of TNF-alpha induces anhedonia and increases the catabolism of monoamines in the nucleus accumbens [117]. Similarly, treatment with IL1-beta or IL6 was found to reduce motivation for food in rats and to significantly lower extracellular DA release in the nucleus accumbens at high dose of IL6 [118, 119].

Administration of BH4 has been tested in depressed patients with contrasting results, inducing either improvement in depressive symptoms [120, 121] or no effect [122]. At the preclinical level, peripheral BH4 injection was found to increase hyper-locomotion induced by methamphetamine challenge in mice [123]. A prolocomotor effect of repeated BH4 administration was also reported in a rat model of neonatal serotoninergic lesion [124]. More recently, acute peripheral injection of BH4 in mice was shown to enhance amphetamine-stimulated DA release in the nucleus accumbens and to increase motivation [125]. However, it remains unclear whether BH4-mediated enhancement of DA release is due to an increase in DA synthesis or to a direct prorelease effect independently of its cofactor action on TH.

20.1.2.3 Inflammation-Induced Alterations in Brain Circuitry

Chronic inflammation has been linked to functional brain abnormalities in numerous neuroimaging studies. In particular, inflammatory stimuli were found to disrupt frontal-subcortical loops, involving the anterior cingulate cortex and the basal ganglia. In medically ill patients, treatment with IFN-alpha was found to increase activity of the dorsal anterior cingulate cortex during an attention-demanding task. This activation was highly correlated with the number of errors made during the task in

IFN-alpha treated patients, albeit task performance of these patients was similar to that measured in control subjects [126]. The dorsal anterior cingulate cortex is highly implicated in error detection and conflict monitoring [127–130]. Accordingly, overactivation within this cortical area may reflect an aberrant error processing, possibly source of automatic negative thoughts as shown in patients with obsessive-compulsive disorders [126, 131–134]. Increased activity of the anterior cingulate cortex was also found to be part of the response to peer rejection and was considered a predictive marker of the development of depressive symptomatology [135, 136]. Interestingly, studies investigating social exclusion and associated negative affect in healthy subjects reported significant associations between greater activity in the dorsal anterior cingulate cortex and insula and increased peripheral concentrations of inflammatory markers in response to acute social stress [137]. The activity of the ventral anterior cingulate cortex, which is specifically involved in the regulation of emotional responses [127, 128] is also highly modulated by inflammation. Accordingly, acute inflammatory challenge (typhoid vaccination) in healthy subjects was found to produce an inflammatory response that was associated with mood deterioration, which correlated with increased activity of the subgenual anterior cingulate cortex during the processing and recognition of facial emotions [138].

The basal ganglia were found to represent privileged targets for inflammatory processes. Neuroimaging studies in patients treated with IFN-alpha have contributed to reveal changes in basal ganglia activity, notably in the striatum and globus pallidus, during the first weeks of treatment [108]. Interestingly, these brain alterations were associated with the intensity of fatigue experienced by patients at early stages of treatment. In another study, lowered activation of the ventral striatum in response to monetary rewards was found to correlate with IFN-alpha-induced reduced motivation, depression, and fatigue [94]. Midbrain DA neurons projecting to the striatum have been extensively demonstrated to encode a reward prediction error rule and provide information about the predictability of reward, which is essential during reward-directed learning [139–141]. An error signal is therefore generated when differences are perceived between reward expectation and reality. Increases in plasma levels of IL-6 after acute stress in healthy volunteers were recently coupled to blunted reward prediction error signals within the ventral striatum during reinforcement learning [142]. Interestingly, reduced prediction errors in the striatum and midbrain were documented in depressed patients and this reduction was inversely correlated with severity of anhedonia [143]. Increased levels of hsCRP were also found to be associated with decreased functional connectivity between the medial prefrontal cortex and ventral striatum, which in turn correlated with anhedonia and motor slowing in depressed subjects [96].

Because of their neurotoxic effects, IDO-related KYN derivatives, including quinolinic acid, may also contribute, at least in part, to structural brain abnormalities. In support of this notion, a decreased kynurenic acid/quinolinic acid ratio, which correlated with severity of anhedonia [48], was found to be associated with reduced thickness of the pregenual cingulate cortex in a sample of depressed patients [49]. In line with this, elevated levels of hsCRP or IL-6 were linked to reduced volume of multiple brain regions, including the prefrontal cortex, amygdala, striatum, and hippocampus [144–147], found to be involved in disrupted emotional behaviors and cognitive aspects mediating the expression of neuropsychiatric symptoms [53, 148].

20.1.3 Towards the Promotion of a Phenotype-Guided Medicine

The discovery that inflammatory processes play a crucial role in the development of various neuropsychiatric symptom dimensions that are common to multiple psychiatric conditions places these processes as prime targets for the implementation of new therapeutic strategies. Inflammatory factors significantly impact the functionality of two distinct enzymatic pathways, IDO and GCH-I, thereby contributing to monoamine deficits contrasting with the excessive production of compounds with neurotoxic properties related to overactivation of the glutamate system (Fig. 20.1). Disruptions in these pathways were found to lead to profound structural abnormalities along with significant changes in the functional activity and connectivity of brain circuits regulating cognition, emotion, arousal, and motivational aspects, and encompassing key brain regions such as the anterior cingulate cortex, basal ganglia, amygdala, and hippocampus. Close relationships were established with specific clinical dimensions ranging from depressive symptoms (sadness, anhedonia, suicidal thoughts) to cognitive (memory/attention/concentration deficit) and neurovegetative symptoms (fatigue/anergia, abnormal sleep, psychomotor retardation). Noteworthy, the activation of GCH-I and IDO pathways by inflammatory processes, and the related alterations in monoamine and glutamate function, are not exclusive and may share common paths since both monoamines and glutamate are critically involved in basal ganglia function where they are highly interconnected [149–151]. In line with this, data obtained in clinical and preclinical models of IFN-alpha-induced neuropsychiatric symptoms indicate that inflammation-induced anhedonia relies on alterations in both DA and glutamate systems [56, 94, 115, 152].

This type of research is particularly relevant to the area of integrative and translational neurosciences interconnecting biomarkers, mainly referring to inflammatory mechanisms, executive function, emotional processing, reward, and behavior-related neurocircuitry, to particular clinical symptom domains. Increasing knowledge regarding immune-to-brain interactions is expected to facilitate the development and implementation of novel and innovative therapeutic interventions against inflammation targeting, at distinct levels of integration, mechanisms, processes, and brain circuits underlying the expression of specific clinical profiles. This will help to prevent or interrupt the cascade of biological events associated with inflammation leading to psychiatric illnesses. Overall, this research approach is a necessary step for the promotion of a precision medicine as a medical procedure intending to better determine "which therapeutics for which patients" [4, 5, 153]. Precise characterization of clinical phenotypes based on the patient's inflammatory profile should contribute to further guide decision toward adapted and personalized strategies in everyday practice, thereby enabling improvement in the poor treatment outcomes in Psychiatry.

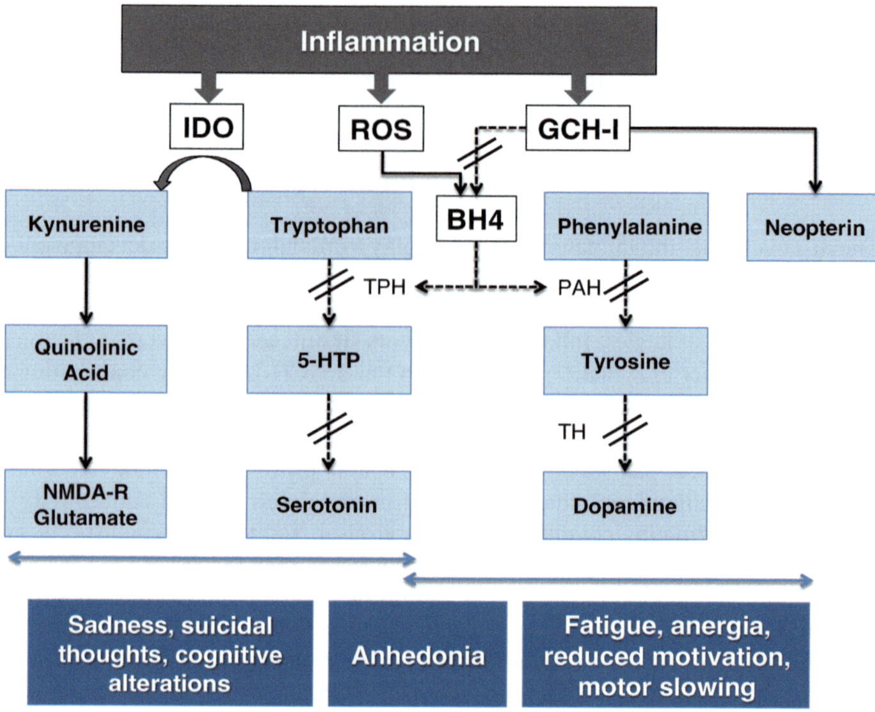

Fig. 20.1 Inflammation-induced alterations in indoleamine-2,3-dioxygenase (IDO) and GTP-cyclohydrolase 1 (GCH-I) pathways and associations with neuropsychiatric symptom dimensions. Inflammatory factors activate the enzymes IDO and GCH-I that are involved in the biosynthesis of serotonin, dopamine, and glutamate. Inflammation-induced IDO activation leads to the degradation of tryptophan, the essential amino acid precursor of serotonin, along the kynurenine pathway, contributing presumably to serotonin deficit. Kynurenine is further degraded in glutamatergic neuroactive compounds, including quinolinic acid that stimulates NMDA receptors (NMDA-R) and promotes oxidative stress. This pathway is believed to contribute to the development of inflammation-related mood and cognitive symptoms, including sadness, suicidal thoughts, cognitive alterations, and anhedonia. The activation of GCH-I under inflammatory condition leads to the formation of neopterin to the detriment of tetrahydrobiopterin (BH4), an essential co-factor for phenylalanine hydroxylase (PAH)/tyrosine hydroxylase (TH), tryptophan hydroxylase (TPH), and nitric oxide synthases involved in the synthesis of serotonin, dopamine, and nitric oxide, respectively. Inflammatory factors also trigger formation of high amounts of reactive oxygen species (ROS) that destroy the oxidation-labile BH4 and then amplify BH4 deficit. Inflammation-driven alterations in GCH-I/BH4 pathway were found to contribute to the development of fatigue, anergia, reduced motivation, motor slowing, and anhedonia. *Abbreviations*: *BH4* tetrahydrobiopterin, *GCH-I* GTP-cyclohydrolase I, *5-HTP* 5-hydroxytryptophan, *IDO* indoleamine-2,3-dioxygenase, *NMDA-R* NMDA receptors, *PAH* phenylalanine hydroxylase, *ROS* reactive oxygen species, *TH* tyrosine hydroxylase, *TPH* tryptophan hydroxylase

Conflict of Interest The authors have no conflicts of interest to declare.

References

1. Steel Z, Marnane C, Iranpour C, Chey T, Jackson JW, Patel V, et al. The global prevalence of common mental disorders: a systematic review and meta-analysis 1980-2013. Int J Epidemiol. 2014;43(2):476–93.
2. Whiteford HA, Degenhardt L, Rehm J, Baxter AJ, Ferrari AJ, Erskine HE, et al. Global burden of disease attributable to mental and substance use disorders: findings from the global burden of disease study 2010. Lancet. 2013;382(9904):1575–86.
3. Disease GBD, Injury I, Prevalence C. Global, regional, and national incidence, prevalence, and years lived with disability for 354 diseases and injuries for 195 countries and territories, 1990-2017: a systematic analysis for the global burden of disease study 2017. Lancet. 2018;392(10159):1789–858.
4. Insel TR, Cuthbert BN. Medicine. Brain disorders? Precisely. Science. 2015;348(6234):499–500.
5. Insel T, Cuthbert B, Garvey M, Heinssen R, Pine DS, Quinn K, et al. Research domain criteria (RDoC): toward a new classification framework for research on mental disorders. Am J Psychiatry. 2010;167(7):748–51.
6. Dantzer R, O'Connor JC, Freund GG, Johnson RW, Kelley KW. From inflammation to sickness and depression: when the immune system subjugates the brain. Nat Rev Neurosci. 2008;9(1):46–56.
7. Capuron L, Miller AH. Immune system to brain signaling: neuropsychopharmacological implications. Pharmacol Ther. 2011;130(2):226–38.
8. Capuron L, Miller AH. Cytokines and psychopathology: lessons from interferon-alpha. Biol Psychiatry. 2004;56(11):819–24.
9. Kappelmann N, Lewis G, Dantzer R, Jones PB, Khandaker GM. Antidepressant activity of anti-cytokine treatment: a systematic review and meta-analysis of clinical trials of chronic inflammatory conditions. Mol Psychiatry. 2018;23(2):335–43.
10. Valkanova V, Ebmeier KP, Allan CL. CRP, IL-6 and depression: a systematic review and meta-analysis of longitudinal studies. J Affect Disord. 2013;150(3):736–44.
11. Wium-Andersen MK, Orsted DD, Nielsen SF, Nordestgaard BG. Elevated C-reactive protein levels, psychological distress, and depression in 73, 131 individuals. JAMA Psychiat. 2013;70(2):176–84.
12. Vogelzangs N, de Jonge P, Smit JH, Bahn S, Penninx BW. Cytokine production capacity in depression and anxiety. Transl Psychiatry. 2016;6(5):e825.
13. Zalli A, Jovanova O, Hoogendijk WJ, Tiemeier H, Carvalho LA. Low-grade inflammation predicts persistence of depressive symptoms. Psychopharmacology. 2016;233(9):1669–78.
14. Huang M, Su S, Goldberg J, Miller AH, Levantsevych OM, Shallenberger L, et al. Longitudinal association of inflammation with depressive symptoms: a 7-year cross-lagged twin difference study. Brain Behav Immun. 2019;75:200–7.
15. Lamers F, Milaneschi Y, Smit JH, Schoevers RA, Wittenberg G, Penninx B. Longitudinal association between depression and inflammatory markers: results from the Netherlands study of depression and anxiety. Biol Psychiatry. 2019;85(10):829–37.
16. Dowlati Y, Herrmann N, Swardfager W, Liu H, Sham L, Reim EK, et al. A meta-analysis of cytokines in major depression. Biol Psychiatry. 2010;67(5):446–57.

17. Goldsmith DR, Rapaport MH, Miller BJ. A meta-analysis of blood cytokine network alterations in psychiatric patients: comparisons between schizophrenia, bipolar disorder and depression. Mol Psychiatry. 2016;21(12):1696–709.
18. Kohler CA, Freitas TH, Maes M, de Andrade NQ, Liu CS, Fernandes BS, et al. Peripheral cytokine and chemokine alterations in depression: a meta-analysis of 82 studies. Acta Psychiatr Scand. 2017;135(5):373–87.
19. Yuan N, Chen Y, Xia Y, Dai J, Liu C. Inflammation-related biomarkers in major psychiatric disorders: a cross-disorder assessment of reproducibility and specificity in 43 meta-analyses. Transl Psychiatry. 2019;9(1):233.
20. Wang AK, Miller BJ. Meta-analysis of cerebrospinal fluid cytokine and tryptophan catabolite alterations in psychiatric patients: comparisons between schizophrenia, bipolar disorder, and depression. Schizophr Bull. 2018;44(1):75–83.
21. Vetter ML, Wadden TA, Vinnard C, Moore RH, Khan Z, Volger S, et al. Gender differences in the relationship between symptoms of depression and high-sensitivity CRP. Int J Obes. 2013;37(Suppl 1):S38–43.
22. Kohler-Forsberg O, Buttenschon HN, Tansey KE, Maier W, Hauser J, Dernovsek MZ, et al. Association between C-reactive protein (CRP) with depression symptom severity and specific depressive symptoms in major depression. Brain Behav Immun. 2017;62:344–50.
23. Ambrosio G, Kaufmann FN, Manosso L, Platt N, Ghisleni G, Rodrigues ALS, et al. Depression and peripheral inflammatory profile of patients with obesity. Psychoneuroendocrinology. 2018;91:132–41.
24. Delgado I, Huet L, Dexpert S, Beau C, Forestier D, Ledaguenel P, et al. Depressive symptoms in obesity: relative contribution of low-grade inflammation and metabolic health. Psychoneuroendocrinology. 2018;91:55–61.
25. Schmidt FM, Sander C, Minkwitz J, Mergl R, Dalton B, Holdt LM, et al. Serum markers of inflammation mediate the positive association between neuroticism and depression. Front Psych. 2018;9:609.
26. Jha MK, Miller AH, Minhajuddin A, Trivedi MH. Association of T and non-T cell cytokines with anhedonia: role of gender differences. Psychoneuroendocrinology. 2018;95:1–7.
27. Goldsmith DR, Haroon E, Woolwine BJ, Jung MY, Wommack EC, Harvey PD, et al. Inflammatory markers are associated with decreased psychomotor speed in patients with major depressive disorder. Brain Behav Immun. 2016;56:281–8.
28. Ye G, Yin GZ, Tang Z, Fu JL, Chen J, Chen SS, et al. Association between increased serum interleukin-6 levels and sustained attention deficits in patients with major depressive disorder. Psychol Med. 2018;48(15):2508–14.
29. Jokela M, Virtanen M, Batty GD, Kivimaki M. Inflammation and specific symptoms of depression. JAMA Psychiat. 2016;73(1):87–8.
30. Capuron L, Gumnick JF, Musselman DL, Lawson DH, Reemsnyder A, Nemeroff CB, et al. Neurobehavioral effects of interferon-alpha in cancer patients: phenomenology and paroxetine responsiveness of symptom dimensions. Neuropsychopharmacology. 2002;26(5):643–52.
31. Frenois F, Moreau M, O'Connor J, Lawson M, Micon C, Lestage J, et al. Lipopolysaccharide induces delayed FosB/DeltaFosB immunostaining within the mouse extended amygdala, hippocampus and hypothalamus, that parallel the expression of depressive-like behavior. Psychoneuroendocrinology. 2007;32(5):516–31.
32. Klaus F, Paterna JC, Marzorati E, Sigrist H, Gotze L, Schwendener S, et al. Differential effects of peripheral and brain tumor necrosis factor on inflammation, sickness, emotional behavior and memory in mice. Brain Behav Immun. 2016;58:310–26.
33. Merali Z, Brennan K, Brau P, Anisman H. Dissociating anorexia and anhedonia elicited by interleukin-1beta: antidepressant and gender effects on responding for "free chow" and "earned" sucrose intake. Psychopharmacology. 2003;165(4):413–8.
34. Moreau M, Andre C, O'Connor JC, Dumich SA, Woods JA, Kelley KW, et al. Inoculation of Bacillus Calmette-Guerin to mice induces an acute episode of sickness behavior followed by chronic depressive-like behavior. Brain Behav Immun. 2008;22(7):1087–95.

35. Noble F, Rubira E, Boulanouar M, Palmier B, Plotkine M, Warnet JM, et al. Acute systemic inflammation induces central mitochondrial damage and mnesic deficit in adult Swiss mice. Neurosci Lett. 2007;424(2):106–10.
36. O'Connor JC, Andre C, Wang Y, Lawson MA, Szegedi SS, Lestage J, et al. Interferon-gamma and tumor necrosis factor-alpha mediate the up-regulation of indoleamine 2,3-dioxygenase and the induction of depressive-like behavior in mice in response to bacillus Calmette-Guerin. J Neurosci. 2009;29(13):4200–9.
37. O'Connor JC, Lawson MA, Andre C, Briley EM, Szegedi SS, Lestage J, et al. Induction of IDO by bacille Calmette-Guerin is responsible for development of murine depressive-like behavior. J Immunol. 2009;182(5):3202–12.
38. Salazar A, Gonzalez Rivera BL, Redus L, Parrott JM, O'Connor JC. Indoleamine 2,3-dioxygenase mediates anhedonia and anxiety-like behaviors caused by peripheral lipopolysaccharide immune challenge. Horm Behav. 2012;62(3):202–9.
39. Capuron L, Castanon N. Role of inflammation in the development of neuropsychiatric symptom domains: evidence and mechanisms. Curr Top Behav Neurosci. 2017;31:31–44.
40. Haroon E, Miller AH, Sanacora G. Inflammation, glutamate, and glia: a trio of trouble in mood disorders. Neuropsychopharmacology. 2017;42(1):193–215.
41. Miller AH, Maletic V, Raison CL. Inflammation and its discontents: the role of cytokines in the pathophysiology of major depression. Biol Psychiatry. 2009;65(9):732–41.
42. Miller AH, Raison CL. The role of inflammation in depression: from evolutionary imperative to modern treatment target. Nat Rev Immunol. 2016;16(1):22–34.
43. Capuron L, Neurauter G, Musselman DL, Lawson DH, Nemeroff CB, Fuchs D, et al. Interferon-alpha-induced changes in tryptophan metabolism. Relationship to depression and paroxetine treatment. Biol Psychiatry. 2003;54(9):906–14.
44. Capuron L, Ravaud A, Neveu PJ, Miller AH, Maes M, Dantzer R. Association between decreased serum tryptophan concentrations and depressive symptoms in cancer patients undergoing cytokine therapy. Mol Psychiatry. 2002;7(5):468–73.
45. Capuron L, Schroecksnadel S, Feart C, Aubert A, Higueret D, Barberger-Gateau P, et al. Chronic low-grade inflammation in elderly persons is associated with altered tryptophan and tyrosine metabolism: role in neuropsychiatric symptoms. Biol Psychiatry. 2011;70(2):175–82.
46. Georgin-Lavialle S, Moura DS, Salvador A, Chauvet-Gelinier JC, Launay JM, Damaj G, et al. Mast cells' involvement in inflammation pathways linked to depression: evidence in mastocytosis. Mol Psychiatry. 2016;21(11):1511–6.
47. Zoga M, Oulis P, Chatzipanagiotou S, Masdrakis VG, Pliatsika P, Boufidou F, et al. Indoleamine 2,3-dioxygenase and immune changes under antidepressive treatment in major depression in females. In Vivo. 2014;28(4):633–8.
48. Savitz J, Drevets WC, Wurfel BE, Ford BN, Bellgowan PS, Victor TA, et al. Reduction of kynurenic acid to quinolinic acid ratio in both the depressed and remitted phases of major depressive disorder. Brain Behav Immun. 2015;46:55–9.
49. Meier TB, Drevets WC, Wurfel BE, Ford BN, Morris HM, Victor TA, et al. Relationship between neurotoxic kynurenine metabolites and reductions in right medial prefrontal cortical thickness in major depressive disorder. Brain Behav Immun. 2016;53:39–48.
50. Wurfel BE, Drevets WC, Bliss SA, McMillin JR, Suzuki H, Ford BN, et al. Serum kynurenic acid is reduced in affective psychosis. Transl Psychiatry. 2017;7(5):e1115.
51. Raison CL, Dantzer R, Kelley KW, Lawson MA, Woolwine BJ, Vogt G, et al. CSF concentrations of brain tryptophan and kynurenines during immune stimulation with IFN-alpha: relationship to CNS immune responses and depression. Mol Psychiatry. 2010;15(4):393–403.
52. Steiner J, Walter M, Gos T, Guillemin GJ, Bernstein HG, Sarnyai Z, et al. Severe depression is associated with increased microglial quinolinic acid in subregions of the anterior cingulate gyrus: evidence for an immune-modulated glutamatergic neurotransmission? J Neuroinflammation. 2011;8:94.
53. Phillips ML, Ladouceur CD, Drevets WC. A neural model of voluntary and automatic emotion regulation: implications for understanding the pathophysiology and neurodevelopment of bipolar disorder. Mol Psychiatry. 2008;13(9):829. 33-57

54. Phillips ML, Drevets WC, Rauch SL, Lane R. Neurobiology of emotion perception I: the neural basis of normal emotion perception. Biol Psychiatry. 2003;54(5):504–14.
55. Haroon E, Woolwine BJ, Chen X, Pace TW, Parekh S, Spivey JR, et al. IFN-alpha-induced cortical and subcortical glutamate changes assessed by magnetic resonance spectroscopy. Neuropsychopharmacology. 2014;39(7):1777–85.
56. Haroon E, Fleischer CC, Felger JC, Chen X, Woolwine BJ, Patel T, et al. Conceptual convergence: increased inflammation is associated with increased basal ganglia glutamate in patients with major depression. Mol Psychiatry. 2016;21(10):1351–7.
57. Andre C, O'Connor JC, Kelley KW, Lestage J, Dantzer R, Castanon N. Spatio-temporal differences in the profile of murine brain expression of proinflammatory cytokines and indoleamine 2,3-dioxygenase in response to peripheral lipopolysaccharide administration. J Neuroimmunol. 2008;200(1–2):90–9.
58. Moreau M, Lestage J, Verrier D, Mormede C, Kelley KW, Dantzer R, et al. Bacille Calmette-Guerin inoculation induces chronic activation of peripheral and brain indoleamine 2,3-dioxygenase in mice. J Infect Dis. 2005;192(3):537–44.
59. O'Connor JC, Lawson MA, Andre C, Moreau M, Lestage J, Castanon N, et al. Lipopolysaccharide-induced depressive-like behavior is mediated by indoleamine 2,3-dioxygenase activation in mice. Mol Psychiatry. 2009;14(5):511–22.
60. Lawson MA, McCusker RH, Kelley KW. Interleukin-1 beta converting enzyme is necessary for development of depression-like behavior following intracerebroventricular administration of lipopolysaccharide to mice. J Neuroinflammation. 2013;10:54.
61. Godbout JP, Moreau M, Lestage J, Chen J, Sparkman NL, O'Connor J, et al. Aging exacerbates depressive-like behavior in mice in response to activation of the peripheral innate immune system. Neuropsychopharmacology. 2008;33(10):2341–51.
62. Kelley KW, O'Connor JC, Lawson MA, Dantzer R, Rodriguez-Zas SL, McCusker RH. Aging leads to prolonged duration of inflammation-induced depression-like behavior caused by Bacillus Calmette-Guerin. Brain Behav Immun. 2013;32:63–9.
63. Andre C, Dinel AL, Ferreira G, Laye S, Castanon N. Diet-induced obesity progressively alters cognition, anxiety-like behavior and lipopolysaccharide-induced depressive-like behavior: focus on brain indoleamine 2,3-dioxygenase activation. Brain Behav Immun. 2014;41:10–21.
64. Corona AW, Norden DM, Skendelas JP, Huang Y, O'Connor JC, Lawson M, et al. Indoleamine 2,3-dioxygenase inhibition attenuates lipopolysaccharide induced persistent microglial activation and depressive-like complications in fractalkine receptor (CX(3)CR1)-deficient mice. Brain Behav Immun. 2013;31:134–42.
65. Du HX, Chen XG, Zhang L, Liu Y, Zhan CS, Chen J, et al. Microglial activation and neurobiological alterations in experimental autoimmune prostatitis-induced depressive-like behavior in mice. Neuropsychiatr Dis Treat. 2019;15:2231–45.
66. Lawson MA, Kelley KW, Dantzer R. Intracerebroventricular administration of HIV-1 tat induces brain cytokine and indoleamine 2,3-dioxygenase expression: a possible mechanism for AIDS comorbid depression. Brain Behav Immun. 2011;25(8):1569–75.
67. Souza LC, Jesse CR, de Gomes MG, Del Fabbro L, Goes ATR, Donato F, et al. Activation of brain indoleamine-2,3-dioxygenase contributes to depressive-like behavior induced by an Intracerebroventricular injection of Streptozotocin in mice. Neurochem Res. 2017;42(10):2982–95.
68. Casaril AM, Domingues M, de Andrade LD, Birmann PT, Padilha N, Vieira B, et al. Depression- and anxiogenic-like behaviors induced by lipopolysaccharide in mice are reversed by a selenium-containing indolyl compound: behavioral, neurochemical and computational insights involving the serotonergic system. J Psychiatr Res. 2019;115:1–12.
69. Heisler JM, O'Connor JC. Indoleamine 2,3-dioxygenase-dependent neurotoxic kynurenine metabolism mediates inflammation-induced deficit in recognition memory. Brain Behav Immun. 2015;50:115–24.
70. Gibney SM, McGuinness B, Prendergast C, Harkin A, Connor TJ. Poly I:C-induced activation of the immune response is accompanied by depression and anxiety-like behav-

iours, kynurenine pathway activation and reduced BDNF expression. Brain Behav Immun. 2013;28:170–81.
71. Barichello T, Generoso JS, Simoes LR, Elias SG, Tashiro MH, Dominguini D, et al. Inhibition of indoleamine 2,3-dioxygenase prevented cognitive impairment in adult Wistar rats subjected to pneumococcal meningitis. Transl Res. 2013;162(6):390–7.
72. Fertan E, Stover KRJ, Brant MG, Stafford PM, Kelly B, Diez-Cecilia E, et al. Effects of the novel IDO inhibitor DWG-1036 on the behavior of male and female 3xTg-AD mice. Front Pharmacol. 2019;10:1044.
73. Souza LC, Jesse CR, Antunes MS, Ruff JR, de Oliveira ED, Gomes NS, et al. Indoleamine-2,3-dioxygenase mediates neurobehavioral alterations induced by an intracerebroventricular injection of amyloid-beta1-42 peptide in mice. Brain Behav Immun. 2016;56:363–77.
74. Xie W, Cai L, Yu Y, Gao L, Xiao L, He Q, et al. Activation of brain indoleamine 2,3-dioxygenase contributes to epilepsy-associated depressive-like behavior in rats with chronic temporal lobe epilepsy. J Neuroinflammation. 2014;11:41.
75. Parrott JM, Redus L, O'Connor JC. Kynurenine metabolic balance is disrupted in the hippocampus following peripheral lipopolysaccharide challenge. J Neuroinflammation. 2016;13(1):124.
76. Baganz NL, Lindler KM, Zhu CB, Smith JT, Robson MJ, Iwamoto H, et al. A requirement of serotonergic p38alpha mitogen-activated protein kinase for peripheral immune system activation of CNS serotonin uptake and serotonin-linked behaviors. Transl Psychiatry. 2015;5:e671.
77. Parrott JM, Redus L, Santana-Coelho D, Morales J, Gao X, O'Connor JC. Neurotoxic kynurenine metabolism is increased in the dorsal hippocampus and drives distinct depressive behaviors during inflammation. Transl Psychiatry. 2016;6(10):e918.
78. Laumet G, Zhou W, Dantzer R, Edralin JD, Huo X, Budac DP, et al. Up-regulation of neuronal kynurenine 3-monooxygenase mediates depression-like behavior in a mouse model of neuropathic pain. Brain Behav Immun. 2017;66:94–102.
79. Agudelo LZ, Femenia T, Orhan F, Porsmyr-Palmertz M, Goiny M, Martinez-Redondo V, et al. Skeletal muscle PGC-1alpha1 modulates kynurenine metabolism and mediates resilience to stress-induced depression. Cell. 2014;159(1):33–45.
80. Chess AC, Landers AM, Bucci DJ. L-kynurenine treatment alters contextual fear conditioning and context discrimination but not cue-specific fear conditioning. Behav Brain Res. 2009;201(2):325–31.
81. Walker AK, Budac DP, Bisulco S, Lee AW, Smith RA, Beenders B, et al. NMDA receptor blockade by ketamine abrogates lipopolysaccharide-induced depressive-like behavior in C57BL/6J mice. Neuropsychopharmacology. 2013;38(9):1609–16.
82. Vichaya EG, Laumet G, Christian DL, Grossberg AJ, Estrada DJ, Heijnen CJ, et al. Motivational changes that develop in a mouse model of inflammation-induced depression are independent of indoleamine 2,3 dioxygenase. Neuropsychopharmacology. 2019;44(2):364–71.
83. Vancassel S, Capuron L, Castanon N. Brain kynurenine and BH4 pathways: relevance to the pathophysiology and treatment of inflammation-driven depressive symptoms. Front Neurosci. 2018;12:499.
84. Huang A, Zhang YY, Chen K, Hatakeyama K, Keaney JF Jr. Cytokine-stimulated GTP cyclohydrolase I expression in endothelial cells requires coordinated activation of nuclear factor-kappaB and Stat1/Stat3. Circ Res. 2005;96(2):164–71.
85. Lazarus RA, Wallick DE, Dietrich RF, Gottschall DW, Benkovic SJ, Gaffney BJ, et al. The mechanism of phenylalanine hydroxylase. Fed Proc. 1982;41(9):2605–7.
86. Sakai N, Kaufman S, Milstien S. Parallel induction of nitric oxide and tetrahydrobiopterin synthesis by cytokines in rat glial cells. J Neurochem. 1995;65(2):895–902.
87. Werner ER, Werner-Felmayer G, Fuchs D, Hausen A, Reibnegger G, Yim JJ, et al. Tetrahydrobiopterin biosynthetic activities in human macrophages, fibroblasts, THP-1, and T 24 cells. GTP-cyclohydrolase I is stimulated by interferon-gamma, and 6-pyruvoyl tetrahydropterin synthase and sepiapterin reductase are constitutively present. J Biol Chem. 1990;265(6):3189–92.

88. Werner ER, Blau N, Thony B. Tetrahydrobiopterin: biochemistry and pathophysiology. Biochem J. 2011;438(3):397–414.
89. Neurauter G, Schrocksnadel K, Scholl-Burgi S, Sperner-Unterweger B, Schubert C, Ledochowski M, et al. Chronic immune stimulation correlates with reduced phenylalanine turnover. Curr Drug Metab. 2008;9(7):622–7.
90. Kirsch M, Korth HG, Stenert V, Sustmann R, de Groot H. The autoxidation of tetrahydrobiopterin revisited. Proof of superoxide formation from reaction of tetrahydrobiopterin with molecular oxygen. J Biol Chem. 2003;278(27):24481–90.
91. Felger JC, Li L, Marvar PJ, Woolwine BJ, Harrison DG, Raison CL, et al. Tyrosine metabolism during interferon-alpha administration: association with fatigue and CSF dopamine concentrations. Brain Behav Immun. 2013;31:153–60.
92. Felger JC, Lotrich FE. Inflammatory cytokines in depression: neurobiological mechanisms and therapeutic implications. Neuroscience. 2013;246:199–229.
93. Felger JC, Miller AH. Cytokine effects on the basal ganglia and dopamine function: the subcortical source of inflammatory malaise. Front Neuroendocrinol. 2012;33(3):315–27.
94. Capuron L, Pagnoni G, Drake DF, Woolwine BJ, Spivey JR, Crowe RJ, et al. Dopaminergic mechanisms of reduced basal ganglia responses to hedonic reward during interferon alfa administration. Arch Gen Psychiatry. 2012;69(10):1044–53.
95. Miller AH, Haroon E, Raison CL, Felger JC. Cytokine targets in the brain: impact on neurotransmitters and neurocircuits. Depress Anxiety. 2013;30(4):297–306.
96. Felger JC, Li Z, Haroon E, Woolwine BJ, Jung MY, Hu X, et al. Inflammation is associated with decreased functional connectivity within corticostriatal reward circuitry in depression. Mol Psychiatry. 2016;21(10):1358–65.
97. Longo N. Disorders of biopterin metabolism. J Inherit Metab Dis. 2009;32(3):333–42.
98. Barker JE, Strangward HM, Brand MP, Hurst RD, Land JM, Clark JB, et al. Increased inducible nitric oxide synthase protein but limited nitric oxide formation occurs in astrocytes of the hph-1 (tetrahydrobiopterin deficient) mouse. Brain Res. 1998;804(1):1–6.
99. Brand MP, Hyland K, Engle T, Smith I, Heales SJ. Neurochemical effects following peripheral administration of tetrahydropterin derivatives to the hph-1 mouse. J Neurochem. 1996;66(3):1150–6.
100. Lam AA, Hyland K, Heales SJ. Tetrahydrobiopterin availability, nitric oxide metabolism and glutathione status in the hph-1 mouse; implications for the pathogenesis and treatment of tetrahydrobiopterin deficiency states. J Inherit Metab Dis. 2007;30(2):256–62.
101. Nasser A, Moller LB, Olesen JH, Konradsen Refsgaard L, Andreasen JT. Anxiety- and depression-like phenotype of hph-1 mice deficient in tetrahydrobiopterin. Neurosci Res. 2014;89:44–53.
102. Zeng BY, Heales SJ, Canevari L, Rose S, Jenner P. Alterations in expression of dopamine receptors and neuropeptides in the striatum of GTP cyclohydrolase-deficient mice. Exp Neurol. 2004;190(2):515–24.
103. Yang S, Lee YJ, Kim JM, Park S, Peris J, Laipis P, et al. A murine model for human sepiapterin-reductase deficiency. Am J Hum Genet. 2006;78(4):575–87.
104. Homma D, Katoh S, Tokuoka H, Ichinose H. The role of tetrahydrobiopterin and catecholamines in the developmental regulation of tyrosine hydroxylase level in the brain. J Neurochem. 2013;126(1):70–81.
105. Homma D, Sumi-Ichinose C, Tokuoka H, Ikemoto K, Nomura T, Kondo K, et al. Partial biopterin deficiency disturbs postnatal development of the dopaminergic system in the brain. J Biol Chem. 2011;286(2):1445–52.
106. Kwak SS, Jeong M, Choi JH, Kim D, Min H, Yoon Y, et al. Amelioration of behavioral abnormalities in BH(4)-deficient mice by dietary supplementation of tyrosine. PLoS One. 2013;8(4):e60803.
107. Eisenberger NI, Berkman ET, Inagaki TK, Rameson LT, Mashal NM, Irwin MR. Inflammation-induced anhedonia: endotoxin reduces ventral striatum responses to reward. Biol Psychiatry. 2010;68(8):748–54.

108. Capuron L, Pagnoni G, Demetrashvili MF, Lawson DH, Fornwalt FB, Woolwine B, et al. Basal ganglia hypermetabolism and symptoms of fatigue during interferon-alpha therapy. Neuropsychopharmacology. 2007;32(11):2384–92.
109. Felger JC, Treadway MT. Inflammation effects on motivation and motor activity: role of dopamine. Neuropsychopharmacology. 2017;42(1):216–41.
110. Brydon L, Harrison NA, Walker C, Steptoe A, Critchley HD. Peripheral inflammation is associated with altered substantia nigra activity and psychomotor slowing in humans. Biol Psychiatry. 2008;63(11):1022–9.
111. Bjork JM, Grant SJ, Chen G, Hommer DW. Dietary tyrosine/phenylalanine depletion effects on behavioral and brain signatures of human motivational processing. Neuropsychopharmacology. 2014;39(3):595–604.
112. Anderson DN, Wilkinson AM, Abou-Saleh MT, Blair JA. Recovery from depression after electroconvulsive therapy is accompanied by evidence of increased tetrahydrobiopterin-dependent hydroxylation. Acta Psychiatr Scand. 1994;90(1):10–3.
113. Blair JA, Barford PA, Morar C, Pheasant AE, Hamon CG, Whitburn SB, et al. Tetrahydrobiopterin metabolism in depression. Lancet. 1984;2(8395):163.
114. Knapp S, Irwin M. Plasma levels of tetrahydrobiopterin and folate in major depression. Biol Psychiatry. 1989;26(2):156–62.
115. Felger JC, Mun J, Kimmel HL, Nye JA, Drake DF, Hernandez CR, et al. Chronic interferon-alpha decreases dopamine 2 receptor binding and striatal dopamine release in association with anhedonia-like behavior in nonhuman primates. Neuropsychopharmacology. 2013;38(11):2179–87.
116. Felger JC, Hernandez CR, Miller AH. Levodopa reverses cytokine-induced reductions in striatal dopamine release. Int J Neuropsychopharmacol. 2015;18(4).
117. van Heesch F, Prins J, Korte-Bouws GA, Westphal KG, Lemstra S, Olivier B, et al. Systemic tumor necrosis factor-alpha decreases brain stimulation reward and increases metabolites of serotonin and dopamine in the nucleus accumbens of mice. Behav Brain Res. 2013;253:191–5.
118. Nunes EJ, Randall PA, Estrada A, Epling B, Hart EE, Lee CA, et al. Effort-related motivational effects of the pro-inflammatory cytokine interleukin 1-beta: studies with the concurrent fixed ratio 5/ chow feeding choice task. Psychopharmacology. 2014;231(4):727–36.
119. Yohn SE, Arif Y, Haley A, Tripodi G, Baqi Y, Muller CE, et al. Effort-related motivational effects of the pro-inflammatory cytokine interleukin-6: pharmacological and neurochemical characterization. Psychopharmacology. 2016;233(19–20):3575–86.
120. Curtius HC, Niederwieser A, Levine RA, Lovenberg W, Woggon B, Angst J. Successful treatment of depression with tetrahydrobiopterin. Lancet. 1983;1(8325):657–8.
121. Pan L, McKain BW, Madan-Khetarpal S, McGuire M, Diler RS, Perel JM, et al. GTP-cyclohydrolase deficiency responsive to sapropterin and 5-HTP supplementation: relief of treatment-refractory depression and suicidal behaviour. BMJ Case Rep. 2011;2011
122. Woggon B, Angst J, Curtius HC, Niederwieser A. Unsuccessful treatment of depression with tetrahydrobiopterin. Lancet. 1984;2(8417–8418):1463.
123. Asami T, Kuribara H. Enhancement of ambulation-increasing effect of methamphetamine by peripherally-administered 6R-L-erythro-5,6,7,8-tetrahydrobiopterin (R-THBP) in mice. Jpn J Pharmacol. 1989;50(2):175–84.
124. Mizuma H, Mizutani M, Nozaki S, Iizuka H, Tohyama H, Nishimura N, et al. Improvement by repeated administration of 6R-tetrahydrobiopterin of 5,7-dihydroxytryptamine-induced abnormal behaviors in immature rats. Biochem Biophys Res Commun. 2003;302(1):156–61.
125. Fanet H, Ducrocq F, Tournissac M, Oummadi A, Lo A, Bourrassa P, et al. Tetrahydrobiopterin administration facilitates amphetamine-induced dopamine release and motivation in mice. Behav Brain Res. 2020;379:112348.
126. Capuron L, Pagnoni G, Demetrashvili M, Woolwine BJ, Nemeroff CB, Berns GS, et al. Anterior cingulate activation and error processing during interferon-alpha treatment. Biol Psychiatry. 2005;58(3):190–6.
127. Devinsky O, Morrell MJ, Vogt BA. Contributions of anterior cingulate cortex to behaviour. Brain. 1995;118(Pt 1):279–306.

128. Bush G, Luu P, Posner MI. Cognitive and emotional influences in anterior cingulate cortex. Trends Cogn Sci. 2000;4(6):215–22.
129. Botvinick MM, Cohen JD, Carter CS. Conflict monitoring and anterior cingulate cortex: an update. Trends Cogn Sci. 2004;8(12):539–46.
130. Carter CS, Braver TS, Barch DM, Botvinick MM, Noll D, Cohen JD. Anterior cingulate cortex, error detection, and the online monitoring of performance. Science. 1998;280(5364):747–9.
131. Aouizerate B, Guehl D, Cuny E, Rougier A, Bioulac B, Tignol J, et al. Pathophysiology of obsessive-compulsive disorder: a necessary link between phenomenology, neuropsychology, imagery and physiology. Prog Neurobiol. 2004;72(3):195–221.
132. Maltby N, Tolin DF, Worhunsky P, O'Keefe TM, Kiehl KA. Dysfunctional action monitoring hyperactivates frontal-striatal circuits in obsessive-compulsive disorder: an event-related fMRI study. NeuroImage. 2005;24(2):495–503.
133. Riesel A, Endrass T, Kaufmann C, Kathmann N. Overactive error-related brain activity as a candidate endophenotype for obsessive-compulsive disorder: evidence from unaffected first-degree relatives. Am J Psychiatry. 2011;168(3):317–24.
134. Agam Y, Greenberg JL, Isom M, Falkenstein MJ, Jenike E, Wilhelm S, et al. Aberrant error processing in relation to symptom severity in obsessive-compulsive disorder: a multimodal neuroimaging study. Neuroimage Clin. 2014;5:141–51.
135. Masten CL, Colich NL, Rudie JD, Bookheimer SY, Eisenberger NI, Dapretto M. An fMRI investigation of responses to peer rejection in adolescents with autism spectrum disorders. Dev Cogn Neurosci. 2011;1(3):260–70.
136. Hamilton JP, Farmer M, Fogelman P, Gotlib IH. Depressive rumination, the default-mode network, and the dark matter of clinical neuroscience. Biol Psychiatry. 2015;78(4):224–30.
137. Slavich GM, Way BM, Eisenberger NI, Taylor SE. Neural sensitivity to social rejection is associated with inflammatory responses to social stress. Proc Natl Acad Sci U S A. 2010;107(33):14817–22.
138. Harrison NA, Brydon L, Walker C, Gray MA, Steptoe A, Critchley HD. Inflammation causes mood changes through alterations in subgenual cingulate activity and mesolimbic connectivity. Biol Psychiatry. 2009;66(5):407–14.
139. Schultz W. Predictive reward signal of dopamine neurons. J Neurophysiol. 1998;80(1):1–27.
140. Schultz W. Getting formal with dopamine and reward. Neuron. 2002;36(2):241–63.
141. Schultz W, Dickinson A. Neuronal coding of prediction errors. Annu Rev Neurosci. 2000;23:473–500.
142. Treadway MT, Admon R, Arulpragasam AR, Mehta M, Douglas S, Vitaliano G, et al. Association between Interleukin-6 and striatal prediction-error signals following acute stress in healthy female participants. Biol Psychiatry. 2017;82(8):570–7.
143. Gradin VB, Kumar P, Waiter G, Ahearn T, Stickle C, Milders M, et al. Expected value and prediction error abnormalities in depression and schizophrenia. Brain. 2011;134(Pt 6):1751–64.
144. Savitz J, Dantzer R, Wurfel BE, Victor TA, Ford BN, Bodurka J, et al. Neuroprotective kynurenine metabolite indices are abnormally reduced and positively associated with hippocampal and amygdalar volume in bipolar disorder. Psychoneuroendocrinology. 2015;52:200–11.
145. Doolin K, Allers KA, Pleiner S, Liesener A, Farrell C, Tozzi L, et al. Altered tryptophan catabolite concentrations in major depressive disorder and associated changes in hippocampal subfield volumes. Psychoneuroendocrinology. 2018;95:8–17.
146. Opel N, Cearns M, Clark S, Toben C, Grotegerd D, Heindel W, et al. Large-scale evidence for an association between low-grade peripheral inflammation and brain structural alterations in major depression in the BiDirect study. J Psychiatry Neurosci. 2019;44(6):423–31.
147. Ironside M, Admon R, Maddox SA, Mehta M, Douglas S, Olson DP, et al. Inflammation and depressive phenotypes: evidence from medical records from over 12 000 patients and brain morphology. Psychol Med. 2019:1–9.
148. Phillips ML, Chase HW, Sheline YI, Etkin A, Almeida JR, Deckersbach T, et al. Identifying predictors, moderators, and mediators of antidepressant response in major depressive disorder: neuroimaging approaches. Am J Psychiatry. 2015;172(2):124–38.

149. Pralong E, Magistretti P, Stoop R. Cellular perspectives on the glutamate-monoamine interactions in limbic lobe structures and their relevance for some psychiatric disorders. Prog Neurobiol. 2002;67(3):173–202.
150. Schmidt WJ. Dopamine-glutamate interactions in the basal ganglia. Amino Acids. 1998;14(1–3):5–10.
151. Wang M, Wong AH, Liu F. Interactions between NMDA and dopamine receptors: a potential therapeutic target. Brain Res. 2012;1476:154–63.
152. Haroon E, Chen X, Li Z, Patel T, Woolwine BJ, Hu XP, et al. Increased inflammation and brain glutamate define a subtype of depression with decreased regional homogeneity, impaired network integrity, and anhedonia. Transl Psychiatry. 2018;8(1):189.
153. Vogenberg FR, Isaacson Barash C, Pursel M. Personalized medicine: part 1: evolution and development into theranostics. Pharm Ther. 2010;35(10):560–76.

Autoimmune Psychosis

21

Karl Bechter

21.1 Introduction

Years ago the mild encephalitis (ME) hypothesis of severe mental disorders (SMDs), (especially relevant when presenting with psychotic syndromes of the affective or schizophrenia spectrum) was proposed [1]. ME was defined as a type of low-grade neuroinflammation that was not diagnosed using available clinical methods. Nevertheless it was thought to be the underlying cause of the observed psychiatric syndrome. The idea of ME hypothesis was based on findings in natural Bornavirus (a highly neurotropic virus) infection, including meningoencephalitis, on models of Bornavirus infection in animals, and especially on the findings about the prevalence of antibodies against Bornavirus in SMD cohorts and own clinical studies in Bornavirus seropositive SMD cohorts [2–4]. Based on the clinical studies including CSF investigations and on general considerations [5, 6], a Bornavirus infection-triggered autoimmune ME appeared a plausible concept and explanation of observed clinical syndromes in therapy-resistant patients of the schizophrenia and affective spectra and might justify rather aggressive immune modulating therapy. At that time, CSF filtration was a promising therapy, which was successfully used in the (typically infection-triggered) autoimmune neurological disorder Guillain-Barre-Syndrome (GBS) [7, 8]. Although CSF filtration was strikingly successful in about two-third of the overall few cases treated with this method (see below), the technical difficulties were considerable, and better alternative therapies in GBS were developed. Nevertheless, the case of successful CSF filtration in cases of SMDs supported the principal idea of undetected low-grade encephalitis prevailing in SMD cohorts.

K. Bechter (✉)
University of Ulm, Ulm, Germany

Department Psychiatry and Psychotherapy 2, Bezirkskrankenhaus Guenzburg, Guenzburg, Germany
e-mail: Karl.bechter@bkh-guenzburg.de

M. Berk et al. (eds.), *Immuno-Psychiatry*, https://doi.org/10.1007/978-3-030-71229-7_21

Meanwhile, evidence supports the plausibility that low-grade neuroinflammation may be involved in the pathogenesis of SMDs, reflecting a relevant subgroup of unknown size [9–26]. However, the difficulty of defining the exact type of the actual underlying pathological process in the individual SMD patient is still a major research question. These clinical challenges of defining and diagnosing autoimmune psychosis (AP) were recently outlined in the notion of precision medicine [27]. An example is the discovery of N-Methyl-D-aspartate-receptor autoantibodies (NMDAR abs) and respective autoimmune encephalitis (AE) [28]. The new diagnosis of AE in neurology revived the plausibility of analogous pathological relevance of autoimmunity in a subgroup of SMDs [27]: the challenges of a diagnosis of AP ranged from genetics and environmental risk factors to clinical presentation and treatment. Others voiced possible autoimmune pathology related to previously unknown antibodies [29], from neurovascular and blood brain barrier dysfunction [30] and, more speculatively though based on brain biopsy findings, from cellular immunity [31]. Apparently, the time was ripe for, and the clinical field required, a consensus definition of AP.

21.2 The Recent Consensus Definition of Autoimmune Psychosis (AP)

After nearly 2 years of discussion, a large international group of clinicians and researchers proposed detailed criteria for the diagnosis, differential diagnosis, and management of AP, designed for use in SMD cohorts and in general psychiatry [32]. The evidence linking inflammation, immune dysregulation, and autoimmunity to psychotic disorders (lastly the consensus definition of AP) and AE was evaluated and was both convincing and rather similar. The consensus criteria may eventually allow one to diagnose "definite" or "probable" AP. The criteria were chosen rather conservatively, thus AP diagnosis by consensus criteria was rather close to consensus criteria of AE diagnosis. But compared to AE diagnosis, "definite" and "probable" AP diagnosis was focusing on cases with pure psychiatric syndromes. A third diagnosis of "possible" AP was reserved for specialized research groups only, involved in research projects in the psycho-neuro-immunology field. Of notice, the AP case as defined by these consensus criteria would match the previous ME criteria. Beyond the importance of clinical signs (red flags), the paraclinical methods of CNS antibody testing, neuroimaging, EEG, and CSF examination are prominent in AP diagnosis in multimodal approaches. Treatments of AP include a panel of potentially escalating options, similar to what is being used in treatment of AE. But it should be mentioned that no controlled studies in AP are available yet, representing a primary research requirement for now.

Some criticism was raised against this position paper and the proposed consensus diagnosis of AP, to which we replied [33]. The criticisms raised from two renowned neurological research groups included aspects of terminology, although there was contradiction between them about the use of the terms of "autoimmune epilepsy" and "autoimmune dementia" (as compared to AP), illustrating the problem of accepted consensus terminology/nosology prevailing also in neurology. Indeed, terminological and nosological principles are in some way competitive terms in clinical use that need typically some compromise in different principles. But terminology apparently needs to be checked with regard to theories and emerging insights [34]. The best choice of a clinical term may be defined by the best clinical practice effect: e.g., although the term ME might theoretically better describe and (by respective diagnostic approach) pick up a case of SMD caused by low-grade neuroinflammation, including options for differing etiologies of ME (infectious or autoimmune ME), the term AP might more directly point to the possibility of autoimmune ME as a differential diagnosis of SMD, thus focusing on the awareness of the psychiatrist to such differential diagnoses bound to important differing treatment consequences. The situation is analogous to the criticisms raised contra or pro the terms autoimmune epilepsy and autoimmune dementia. The predominant clinical utility of terms will eventually depend on practicability, not least shortness, and also the overall epidemiological prevalence of respective types of pathology within the cohort of special interest. In an epilepsy and dementia cohort of neurological patients, a term specifically addressing the option of autoimmune etiology may heighten the awareness of clinicians to a rare possibility with specific treatment options, when AE represented a rare type of pathophysiology; but such a term would be unnecessary when most epilepsy or dementia cases were of autoimmune etiology. Terms also have their history, for example, related to predominant clinical relevance and/or to ease of diagnostics: the historic template for definition of encephalitis was infectious encephalitis [35]; for schizophrenia it may have been the predominant psychopathological appearance, which may include important compensatory aspects on the psychopathological level, which in a historical perspective may be somehow similar to (scientific) misinterpretations of predominant signs in diabetes mellitus [36].

The difficulties to represent and the inevitable need to (partially) neglect potentially relevant aspects of disease etiology and pathophysiology in categorical clinical terms, are illustrated in Fig. 21.1, sorted by general principles and detailed in various aspects of potential relevance for best practice use:

21.3 AP/ME and Expected Difficulties of Future Research

The hypothesis that mild neuroinflammation may potentially represent the core of pathology (in certain stages/subgroups of SMDs) but may remain undetected due to limitations of available clinical methods, was raised by various arguments including the epidemiology and the age of onset of major SMDs, eg. a similarity of age-related variance of pathogenicity of infections (depending on age-related variance of immunological resistance factors), and when compared with animal models of Bornavirus and with findings in natural Bornavirus infection [1]. Bornavirus was known as the most frequent cause of meningoencephalitis in horses and sheep in Middle Europe. When BDV-specific antibodies were found also in humans, the possibility of human cases of Bornavirus encephalitis was raised, and the possibility of

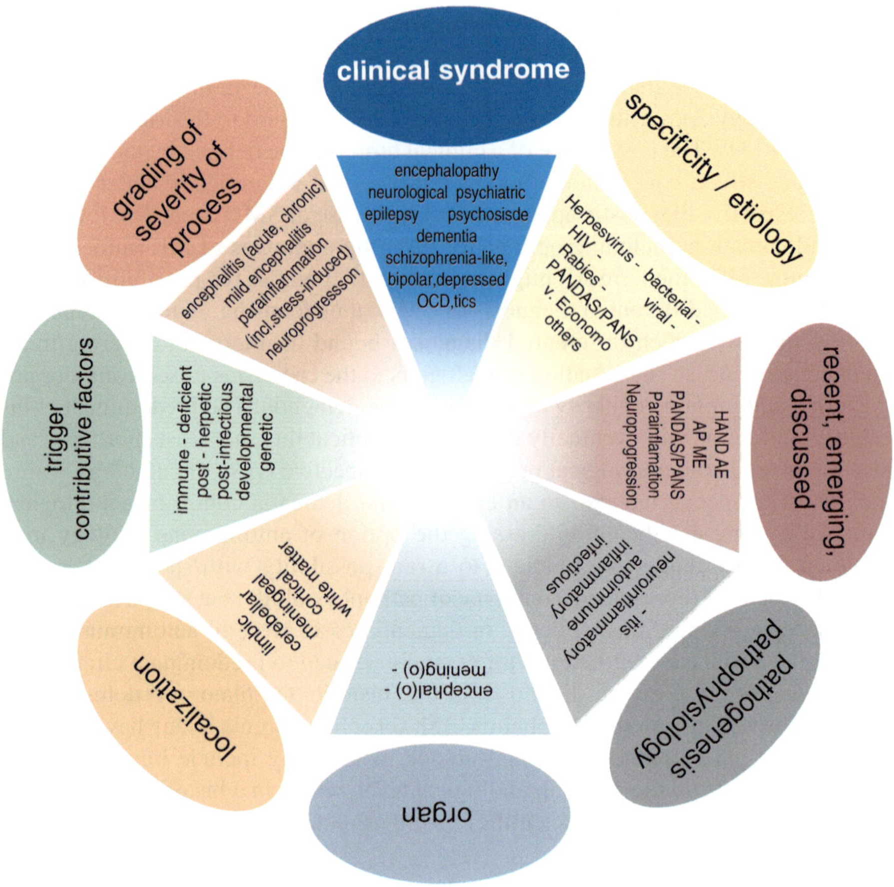

Fig. 21.1 Panel of a multitude of aspects, which may be or may not be represented in clinical terms, which may represent important aspects of etiology or pathophysiology or risk factors or something else. Terms in clinical use are preferably short for apparent reasons and therefore typically selective in one way or another. Abbreviations: *PANDAS/PANS* pediatric autoimmune neuropsychiatric disorders associated with streptococcal infections/pediatric acute-onset neuropsychiatric syndrome, *HAND* HIV-associated neurocognitive disorder, *AE* autoimmune encephalitis, *AP* autoimmune psychosis, *ME* mild encephalitis

formes frustes presenting with pure psychiatric syndromes lacking neurological hard signs represented a serious concern [2–4]. Clinical data in cohorts of Bornavirus seropositive psychiatric patients, compared with patients from neurology and surgery, suggested the prevalence of a small subgroup of neurological patients suffering from classical lymphocytic meningoencephalitis caused by Bornavirus infection. Clinical data also suggested that a considerable subgroup of psychiatric patients suffering from various SMDs that were potentially caused by mild form of Bornavirus encephalitis [37–39]. Clearly, Bornavirus infection may represent only a rare cause of SMD in our hospital which is located in an endemic region with a maximum 3% of cases (compare [40]). When assuming a potential role of Bornavirus in the etiology of a subgroup of SMDs, two main pathological scenarios appeared to be potentially relevant [1] either acute infectious ME or infection-triggered autoimmune ME. The term mild encephalitis (ME) was proposed for cases that were not suffering from neurological hard signs nor presenting any other established signs/findings of classical encephalitis. Instead, cases presented only psychiatric syndromes (potentially associated with neurological soft signs). Both ME types (or models) were compatible with findings in Bornavirus infection and with animal models of Bornavirus infection. The ME hypothesis was thought to potentially provide a generalizable model for the role of infections and infection-triggered CNS autoimmunity in SMD subgroups by other infectious agents and from a number of circumstantial aspects and arguments [40].

Proof of any type of Bornavirus ME or triggered autoimmune ME in SMD subgroups remained challenging [40]. This was not surprising, as a non-deadly meningoencephalitis, could be represented by both suspected types of ME and remains difficult to prove in humans. Even in human malaria, burdened with a considerable number of deaths and frequently associated with severe brain involvement, cerebral malaria was evaluated "understudied" mainly for ethical reasons [41]. In the Bornavirus research field considerable confusion arose from the erroneous methodology used in several studies [42]. The human strain (Bornavirus 1) recently caused three deadly cases of encephalitis in Germany, one spontaneous case of classical encephalitis [43], and three cases (two of these cases ending fatally) occurred after organ transplant from a neurologically healthy organ donor [44].

Bornavirus meningoencephalitis presenting with classical neurological syndrome has been proven as a rare disease. This may support the view, that cases of Bornavirus ME presenting with pure psychiatric syndromes may rarely prevail and/or Bornavirus-infection-triggered autoimmune ME may occur (compare [45]), but remain difficult to prove. Nevertheless, Bornavirus infection is discussed in detail here, as it may represent a recent example of the difficulties faced in psycho-immunological research and the respective interplay with infections and independent environmental factors (compare also with [40]).

21.4 Conclusion

The recent consensus criteria of AP diagnosis and treatment represents an important step to a differential diagnosis with consequent new potential treatment options in an emerging autoimmune research field. The consensus-defined AP group represents only a small subgroup of SMDs, but the new AP concept appears rather relevant clinically offering improved treatment options for this subgroup. AP criteria match the proposed ME criteria, which remains preliminary, requiring further improvements to defining ME, e.g. by more sensitive diagnostic methods, including newly discovered CNS autoantibodies and others. The ME category will require refined differentiation between sub-categories of low-grade immune-inflammatory pathologies involved in SMDs, like parainflammation [46] and neuroprogression [47–49]. Clinical terminology is important to guide the diagnostic approach and select the best available treatments, but will be possible only from emerging insights into the most relevant pathophysiological processes involved in SMDs. Therefore, it is important to further discuss and sharpen the defining criteria of mild neuroinflammatory processes, to achieve a well-balanced consensus based on improved diagnostic methods and inform better clinical decisions.

References

1. Bechter K. Mild encephalitis underlying psychiatric disorders-a reconsideration and hypothesis exemplified on Borna disease. Neurol Psychiatry Brain Res. 2001;9:55–70.
2. Rott R, Herzog S, Bechter K, Frese K. Borna disease, a possible hazard for man? Arch Virol. 1991;118:143–9.
3. Herzog S. Molecular characterization of Borna disease virus from naturally infected animals and possible links to human disorders. Arch Virol. 1997;13(Suppl):183–90.
4. Richt JA. Borna disease virus infection in animals and humans. Em Infect Dis. 1997;3:343–52.
5. Bechter K. Research strategies in 'slow' infections in psychiatry. Hist Psychiatry. 1995;6:503–11.
6. Bechter K, Herzog S, Behr W, Schüttler R. Investigations of cerebrospinal fluid in Borna disease virus seropositive psychiatric patients. Eur Psychiatry. 1995;10(5):250–8. https://doi.org/10.1016/0924-9338(96)80302-6.
7. Wollinsky KH. CSF filtration is an effective treatment of Guillain-Barre syndrome: a randomized clinical trial. Neurology. 2001;57:774–80.
8. Bechter K, Herzog S, Schreiner V, Wollinsky KH, Schüttler R. Cerebrospinal fluid filtration in Borna-disease-virus-encephalitis-related schizophrenia: a new therapeutic perspective? Neurology. Psychiatry and Brain Res. 1998;6:85–6.
9. Bechter K, Deisenhammer F. Psychiatric syndromes other than dementia. Handb Clin Neurol. 2017;146:285–96. https://doi.org/10.1016/B978-0-12-804279-3.00017-4.
10. Müller N. Neuroprogression in schizophrenia and psychotic disorders: the possible role of inflammation. Mod Trends Pharmacopsychiatry. 2017;31:1–9. https://doi.org/10.1159/000470802.
11. Anderson G, Berk M, Dodd S, et al. Immuno-inflammatory, oxidative and nitrosative stress, and neuroprogressive pathways in the etiology, course and treatment of schizophrenia. Prog Neuro-Psychopharmacol Biol Psychiatry. 2013;42:1–4. https://doi.org/10.1016/j.pnpbp.2012.10.008.
12. Meyer U. New serological evidence points toward an infectious route to bipolar disorder. Am J Psychiatry. 2014;171(5):485–8. https://doi.org/10.1176/appi.ajp.2014.14010095.
13. Meyer U. Developmental neuroinflammation and schizophrenia. Prog Neuropsychopharmacol Biol Psychiatry. 2013;42:20–34. https://doi.org/10.1016/j.pnpbp.2011.11.003.
14. van Kesteren CFMG, Gremmels H, de Witte LD, et al. Immune involvement in the pathogenesis of schizophrenia: a meta-analysis on postmortem brain studies. Transl Psychiatry. 2017;7(3):e1075. https://doi.org/10.1038/tp.2017.4.
15. Pollak TA, Lennox BR. Time for a change of practice: the real-world value of testing for neuronal autoantibodies in acute first-episode psychosis. BJPsych Open. 2018;4(4):262–4. https://doi.org/10.1192/bjo.2018.27.
16. Pollak TA, McCormack R, Peakman M, Nicholson TR, David AS. Prevalence of anti-N-methyl-D-aspartate (NMDA) receptor corrected antibodies in patients with schizophrenia and related psychoses: a systematic review and meta-analysis. Psychol Med. 2014;44(12):2475–87. https://doi.org/10.1017/S003329171300295X.

17. Al-Diwani A, Pollak TA, Langford AE, Lennox BR. Synaptic and neuronal autoantibody-associated psychiatric syndromes: controversies and hypotheses. Front Psych. 2017;8 https://doi.org/10.3389/fpsyt.2017.00013.
18. Berk M, Williams LJ, Jacka FN, et al. So depression is an inflammatory disease, but where does the inflammation come from? BMC Med. 2013;11:200. https://doi.org/10.1186/1741-7015-11-200.
19. Berk M, Kapczinski F, Andreazza AC, et al. Pathways underlying neuroprogression in bipolar disorder: focus on inflammation, oxidative stress and neurotrophic factors. Neurosci Biobehav Rev. 2011;35(3):804–17. https://doi.org/10.1016/j.neubiorev.2010.10.001.
20. Fillman SG, Sinclair D, Fung SJ, Webster MJ, Shannon WC. Markers of inflammation and stress distinguish subsets of individuals with schizophrenia and bipolar disorder. Transl Psychiatry. 2014;4:e365. https://doi.org/10.1038/tp.2014.8.
21. Yolken RH, Torrey EF, Lieberman JA, Yang S, Dickerson FB. Serological evidence of exposure to herpes simplex virus type 1 is associated with cognitive deficits in the CATIE schizophrenia sample. Schizophr Res. 2011;128(1–3):61–5. https://doi.org/10.1016/j.schres.2011.01.020.
22. Severance EG, Gressitt KL, Stallings CR, et al. Discordant patterns of bacterial translocation markers and implications for innate immune imbalances in schizophrenia. Schizophr Res. 2013;148(1–3):130–7. https://doi.org/10.1016/j.schres.2013.05.018.
23. Severance EG, Dickerson FB, Viscidi RP, et al. Coronavirus immunoreactivity in individuals with a recent onset of psychotic symptoms. Schizophr Bull. 2011;37(1):101–7. https://doi.org/10.1093/schbul/sbp052.
24. Dickerson F, Katsafanas E, Schweinfurth LAB, et al. Immune alterations in acute bipolar depression. Acta Psychiatr Scand. 2015;132(3):204–10. https://doi.org/10.1111/acps.12451][
25. Cai HQ, Catts VS, Webster MJ, et al. Increased macrophages and changed brain endothelial cell gene expression in the frontal cortex of people with schizophrenia displaying inflammation. Mol Psychiatry. 2020;25(4):761–75. https://doi.org/10.1038/s41380-018-0235-x.
26. Halaris A, Bechter K, Haroon E, et al. The future of psychoneuroimmunology: promises and challenges. In: Javed A, Fountoulakis KN, editors. Advances in psychiatry. Cham: Springer International Publishing; 2019. p. 235–66.
27. Ellul P, Groc L, Tamouza R, Leboyer M. The clinical challenge of autoimmune psychosis: learning from anti-NMDA receptor autoantibodies. Front Psych. 2017;8 https://doi.org/10.3389/fpsyt.2017.00054.
28. Graus F, Titulaer MJ, Balu R, et al. A clinical approach to diagnosis of autoimmune encephalitis. Lancet Neurol. 2016;15(4):391–404. https://doi.org/10.1016/S1474-4422(15)00401-9.
29. Najjar S, Pearlman D, Zagzag D, Golfinos J, Devinsky O. Glutamic acid decarboxylase autoantibody syndrome presenting as schizophrenia. Neurologist. 2012;18(2):88–91. https://doi.org/10.1097/NRL.0b013e318247b87d.
30. Najjar S, Pearlman DM. Neuroinflammation and white matter pathology in schizophrenia: systematic review. Schizophr Res. 2015;161(1):102–12. https://doi.org/10.1016/j.schres.2014.04.041.
31. Najjar S, Steiner J, Najjar A, Bechter K. A clinical approach to new-onset psychosis associated with immune dysregulation: the concept of autoimmune psychosis. J Neuroinflammation. 2018;15(1):40. https://doi.org/10.1186/s12974-018-1067-y.
32. Pollak TA, Lennox BR, Müller S, et al. Autoimmune psychosis: an international consensus on an approach to the diagnosis and management of psychosis of suspected autoimmune origin. Lancet Psychiatry. 2019;7(1):93–108. https://doi.org/10.1016/S2215-0366(19)30290-1.
33. Pollak TA. Reply to McKeon et al. and Martinez-Martinez and Titulaer. Lancet Psychiatry 2020; (in press).
34. Bechter K. Encephalitis, mild encephalitis, Neuroprogression, or encephalopathy-not merely a question of terminology. Front Psych. 2018;9:782. https://doi.org/10.3389/fpsyt.2018.00782.
35. Venkatesan A, Tunkel AR, Bloch KC, et al. Case definitions, diagnostic algorithms, and priorities in encephalitis: consensus statement of the international encephalitis consortium. Clin Infect Dis. 2013;57(8):1114–28. https://doi.org/10.1093/cid/cit458.

36. Bechter K, van Tebartz Elst L. Schizophrenia, schizophrenic syndrome or what? The pros and cons of a term and concept under pressure with a look back to diabetes mellitus. Neurol Psychiatry Brain Res. 2018;29:1–3. https://doi.org/10.1016/j.npbr.2018.01.051].
37. Bechter K, Herzog S, Fleischer B, Schüttler R, Rott R. Magnetic resonance imaging in psychiatric patients with and without serum antibodies against Borna disease. Nervenarzt. 1987;58:617–24.
38. Bechter K, Herzog S, Schuettler R. Case of neurological and behavioral abnormalities: due to Borna disease virus encephalitis ? Psychiatry Res. 1992;42:193–6.
39. Bechter K, Herzog S, Schuettler R. Borna disease virus- possible causal agent in psychiatric and neurological disorders in two families. Psychiatry Res. 1992;42:291–4.
40. Bechter K. Updating the mild encephalitis hypothesis of schizophrenia. Prog Neuro-Psychopharmacol Biol Psychiatry. 2013;42:71–91. https://doi.org/10.1016/j.pnpbp.2012.06.019.
41. Kurup SP, Butler NS, Harty JT. T cell-mediated immunity to malaria. Nat Rev Immunol. 2019;19(7):457–71. https://doi.org/10.1038/s41577-019-0158-z].
42. Ralf D. Meta-analysis of putative human bornavirus sequences fails to provide evidence implicating Borna disease virus in mental illness. Rev Med Virol. 2007;17:181–203.
43. Coras R, Korn K, Kuerten S, Huttner HB, Ensser A. Severe bornavirus-encephalitis presenting as Guillain–Barré-syndrome. Acta Neuropathol. 2019;137(6):1017–9.
44. Schlottau K, Forth L, Angstwurm K, et al. Fatal encephalitic Borna disease virus 1 in solid-organ transplant recipients. N Engl J Med. 2018;379(14):1377–9. https://doi.org/10.1056/NEJMc1803115.
45. Karl B. Borna Disease Virus: Mögliche Ursache neurologischer und psychiatrischer Störungen des Menschen. Steinkopff: Darmstadt; 1998.
46. Medzhitov R. Origin and physiological roles of inflammation. Nature. 2008;454(7203):428–35. https://doi.org/10.1038/nature07201.
47. Halaris A. Neuroinflammation and neurotoxicity contribute to neuroprogression in neurological and psychiatric disorders. Future Neurol. 2018;13(2):59–69. https://doi.org/10.2217/fnl-2017-0039].
48. Davis J, Moylan S, Harvey BH, Maes M, Berk M. Neuroprogression in schizophrenia: pathways underpinning clinical staging and therapeutic corollaries. Aust N Z J Psychiatry. 2014;48(6):512–29. https://doi.org/10.1177/0004867414533012.
49. Berk M. Neuroprogression: pathways to progressive brain changes in bipolar disorder. Int J Neuropsychopharmacol. 2009;12(4):441–5. https://doi.org/10.1017/S1461145708009498.

Part III

Immunotherapies for Major Psychiatric Disorders

Anti-inflammatory Agents for Patients with Schizophrenia

22

Nico J. M. van Beveren, Nuray Çakici, and Iris E. Sommer

22.1 Introduction

The last decade has seen increasing evidence for dysregulations of the immune system as one of the contributing factors to the schizophrenia syndrome. Genetic associations show that people with schizophrenia on average have an immune system subtly more prone to activation. This is expressed in major histocompatibility complex molecules [1, 2], its enhancers [3], complement factor 4 [4] and environmental circumstances that naturally activate the immune system, such as prenatal infection, trauma, and stress. This may put components of the immune system (i.e., microglia) in an altered state of activity [5, 6]. Under such circumstances, microglia and other glia may reduce their neurotrophic function and produce less growth factors, such as brain-derived neurotrophic factor (BDNF), leading to decreased proliferation of neurons, resulting in reduced connectivity and, finally, brain tissue degradation. In addition, pruning may be increased by opsonization of synaptic buds with activated complement [7, 8]. Glutamatergic and dopaminergic neurotransmissions are particularly vulnerable for an increased activation of microglia,

N. J. M. van Beveren
Antes Center for Mental Health Care, Poortugaal, The Netherlands

Department of Psychiatry, Erasmus Medical Center, Rotterdam, The Netherlands

Department of Neuroscience, Erasmus Medical Center, Rotterdam, The Netherlands
e-mail: N.Beveren@parnassiagroep.nl

N. Çakici
Department of Psychiatry and Amsterdam Neuroscience, Academic Medical Center, Amsterdam, The Netherlands
e-mail: cakici@amsterdamumc.nl

I. E. Sommer (✉)
Department of Psychiatry and Biomedical Sciences of Cells and Systems, University Medical Center Groningen, Groningen, The Netherlands
e-mail: i.e.c.sommer@umcg.nl

M. Berk et al. (eds.), *Immuno-Psychiatry*, https://doi.org/10.1007/978-3-030-71229-7_22

which can induce or exacerbate positive, negative, and cognitive symptoms of schizophrenia [9, 10].

Over the years, many studies have presented evidence to support this theory. A schizophrenia genome-wide association study found associations between schizophrenia and certain genes that are involved in immune processes [11]. Peripheral blood markers, such as BDNF, interleukin (IL)-10, and C-reactive protein (CRP), are associated with cognitive decline in schizophrenia [12–14]. Interestingly, a recent study identified macrophages in the brain side of the endothelial wall in a subgroup of patients with schizophrenia but not in controls, demonstrating an influx of peripheral immune cells [15].

The immune hypothesis readily suggests a possible treatment for those patients with schizophrenia in which the underlying pathophysiology is related to a subtle increase in the activation of microglia. Many medications can decrease the production of pro-inflammatory factors; however, it is not certain whether these agents can induce microglia, astrocytes, and other cells to resume their normal neurotrophic functions [16, 17]. For one frequently used anti-inflammatory drug, minocycline, Sellgren et al. showed that this drug was indeed able to reduce microglia engulfment of complement opsonized synapses in a stem cell model derived from patients [18]. This finding suggests that at least minocycline, but perhaps also other anti-inflammatory drugs, can correct one of the basic mechanisms underlying schizophrenia. Yet, components that work in vitro do not always work in vivo.

In two previous meta-analyses on augmentation with anti-inflammatory medications [17, 19], we investigated the efficacy of immune modulatory compounds on symptoms of schizophrenia. The data we present here are based on the findings in these two meta-analyses. We discuss those compounds of which meta-analytic data showed a significant effect.

22.2 Immunomodulatory Strategies

22.2.1 General Considerations When Interpreting the Data

It should be stressed that the schizophrenia syndrome is a heterogeneous disorder both with respect to the underlying etiology and to the clinical expression. This is of importance when interpreting the presented data. First, we could not identify studies that selected patients with evidence of immune dysfunction (i.e. altered cytokine status at baseline). Therefore, the effect sizes of the compounds presented reflect the efficacy in patient groups which are diagnosed according to DSM or ICD criteria, as is at present the common practice in psychiatric research. In patient groups selected for altered immune status, the effect sizes might be attenuated. Moreover, the efficacy of compounds that showed no significant effect might reach the level of significance in subgroups with baseline altered immune status. Second, as schizophrenia is by and large a chronic disorder, the phase of the disorder (either first-episode or later multi-episode) may affect results, and should be taken into account. Third, the clinical expression of schizophrenia consists of three broad domains: positive symptoms (delusions and hallucinations), negative symptoms (affective blunting and loss of social responsivity), and cognitive disorders (i.e. disorders of attention and working memory). The effects of immune modulation may vary between these symptom domains.

Therefore, Table 22.1 presents the mean weighted effects sizes [ES] for the main analyses as reported by Cakici et al. [19] as well as the ES for the positive- and negative symptom domains, when available.

22.2.2 Aspirin

Aspirin is an NSAID that modifies cyclooxygenase-2 (COX-2) activity and irreversibly inhibits cyclooxygenase-1 (COX-1), thereby suppressing the production of prostaglandins and thromboxanes, which are involved in the inflammatory process [20, 21]. Aspirin also reduces hypothalamic-pituitary-adrenal axis response [22]. The BBB is not readily crossed by aspirin, and aspirin levels in the central nervous system are lower than in peripheral blood [23]. Two studies provided 1000 mg aspirin daily to schizophrenia patients in addition to their regular treatment for 3 [24] or 4 months [25]. A significant positive influence on total symptom severity was observed (ES: 0.3, $p = 0.014$).

22.2.3 Fatty Acids

Fatty acids, especially EPA (Eicosapentaenoic Acid) and DHA (Docosahexaenoic Acid), have several mild anti-inflammatory effects, such as decreasing levels of serum IL-1β, tumor necrosis factor alpha (TNF-α) and interferon-γ levels, and neuroprotective effects [26, 27]. Fatty acids also enhance synaptic plasticity and membrane fluidity and affect dopaminergic, serotonergic, and glutamatergic neurotransmission [26, 28]. Eleven studies were included, of which seven studies added EPA, one study added DHA, and four studies added omega-3 fatty acids (i.e., combination of EPA and DHA) to antipsychotic treatment for patients with schizophrenia [29–39]. Daily treatment doses of fatty acids varied (EPA 0.5 to 4 g, DHA 2 g, omega-3 0.4 g to 2.2 g) as did treatment duration across the studies (8 weeks to 2 years). We observed a trend toward beneficial results for treatment with EPA and/or DHA fatty acids (ES; 0.19, $p = 0.075$). One study reported a large negative ES of −0.64 and was regarded as an outlier in an additional analysis [29]. Exclusion of this outlier yielded a mean weighted ES of 0.23, which was significant (CI, 0.05 to 0.41; $p = 0.012$). Subgroup analysis showed a trend toward beneficial effects for FEP patients (ES: 0.31; CI, −0.02 to 0.64; $p = 0.064$).

Table 22.1 Baseline characteristics of the included studies

Study	Type of treatment	Treatment N	Placebo N	Treatment N males/N females	Placebo N males/N females	Treatment age mean (SD)	Placebo age mean (SD)	Treatment duration of illness	Placebo duration of illness	Daily treatment dose	Duration of treatment	FEP	Treatment baseline PANSS total mean (SD)	Placebo baseline PANSS total mean (SD)
Laan et al. (2010)	Aspirin	33	37	25/8	33/4	31.6 (8.9)	30.6 (9.2)	4.1 (3.0) years	3.4 (2.5) years	1000 mg	3 months	No	71.1 (10.6)	73.1 (10.3)
Weiser et al. (2012)	Aspirin	100	100	n/a	n/a	43.2 (10.5)	41.4 (10.4)	n/a	n/a	n/a	12 weeks	n/a	n/a	n/a
Lerner et al. (2013)	Bexarotene	45	45	41/4	40/5	41.2 (12.4)	41.7 (10.0)	n/a	n/a	75 mg	6 weeks	No	73.2 (18.9)	74.9 (24.0)
Akhondzadeh et al. (2007)	Celecoxib	30	30	18/12	17/13	33.10 (7.29)	34.30 (7.21)	7.79 (5.87) years	7.98 (5.87) years	400 mg	6 weeks	No	n/a	n/a
Müller et al. (2002)	Celecoxib	25	25	14/11	11/14	35.9 (12.8)	35.5(13.6)	n/a	n/a	400 mg	5 weeks	No	n/a	n/a
Müller et al. (2010)	Celecoxib	25	25	14/11	16/9	26.2 (7.7)	30.9 (8.1)	16.0 (5.0) months	14.9 (4.6) months	400 mg	6 weeks	Yes	94.5 (16.2)	95.9 (19.1)
Rapaport et al. (2005)	Celecoxib	18	17	16/2	13/4	44.1 (9.2)	47.3 (11.4)	n/a	n/a	400 mg	8 weeks	No	84.1 (11.4)	84.2 (12.9)
Rappard and Müller (2004)	Celecoxib	138	132	n/a	n/a	n/a	n/a	n/a	n/a	400 mg	11 weeks	No	n/a	n/a
Javitt et al. (2012) (30 mg)[a]	Davunetide	21	22	n/a	n/a	n/a	n/a	n/a	n/a	30 mg	12 weeks	No	BPRS: 29.1 (6.1)	BPRS: 29.3 (7.6)
Javitt et al. (2012) (5 mg)[a]	Davunetide	20	22	n/a	n/a	45.2 (8.2)	41.4 (10.4)	n/a	n/a	5 mg	12 weeks	No	BPRS: 31.2 (5.5)	BPRS: 29.3 (7.6)
Lee et al. (2015)	Dextro-methorphan	74	75	44/30	46/29	30.6 (8.2)	30.0 (7.2)	n/a	n/a	60 mg	11 weeks	No	86.3 (12.6)	86.9 (14.9)
Akhondzadeh et al. (2003)	Estrogen (ethinyl estradiol)	16	16	0/16	0/16	32.128 (6.31)	33.37 (6.72)	96.87 (90.52) months	87.37 (49.13) months	0.5 mg	8 weeks	No	n/a	n/a

Ghafari et al. (2013)	Estrogen (conjugated estrogen)	15	15	0/15	0/15	34.2 (9.1)	34.8 (8.3)	n/a	n/a	0.625 mg	4 weeks	No	n/a	n/a
Khodaie-Ardakani et al. (2015)	Estrogen (raloxifene)	21	21	21/0	21/0	31.4 (5.9)	32.4 (7.8)	89.3 (70.9) months	96.2 (45.9) months	120 mg	8 weeks	No	101.6 (13.5)	100.7 (15.5)
Kianimehr et al. (2014)	Estrogen (raloxifene)	25	25	0/25	0/25	61.96 (4.49)	60.44 (5.28)	17.24 (12.03)[b]	13.64 (12.41)[b]	120 mg	8 weeks	No	105.52 (16.96)	105.00 (11.68)
Kulkarni et al. (2001) (0.05 mg)[a]	Estrogen (transdermal estradiol)	12	12	0/12	0/12	34.00 (9.2)	34.91 (7.6)	5.5 (5.3) years	10.33 (8.7) years	0.05 mg every 4 days	4 weeks	Yes	68.17 (10.8)	67.58 (14.5)
Kulkarni et al. (2001) (10 mg)[a]	Estrogen (transdermal estradiol)	12	12	0/12	0/12	32.83 (8.6)	34.91 (7.6)	7.38 (7.1) years	10.33 (8.7) years	0.10 mg every 4 days	4 weeks	Yes	75.83 (18.8)	67.58 (14.5)
Kulkarni et al. (2008)	Estrogen (transdermal estradiol)	56	46	0/56	0/46	33.5 (8.8)	33.8 (7.7)	n/a	n/a	0.10 mg every 3.5 days	28 days	No	77.48 (20.0)	73.40 (12.5)
Kulkarni et al. (2011) (only men included)	Estrogen (estradiol valerate)	26	27	26/0	27/0	32.9 (10.2)	31.2 (12.4)	7.6 (7.7) years	6.1 (7.1) years	2 mg	14 days	No	72.6 (10.7)	73.5 (9.2)
Kulkarni et al. (2016)	Estrogen (raloxifene)	26	30	0/26	0/30	52.92 (8.07)	53.07 (7.43)	24 (11) years[c]	24 (11) years[c]	120 mg	12 weeks	No	79.96 (15.91)	77.03 (14.85)
Louzã et al. (2004)	Estrogen (conjugated estrogen)	21	19	0/21	0/19	34.1 (7.9)	30.4 (8.3)	n/a	n/a	0.625 mg	4 weeks	No	n/a	n/a
Usall et al. (2016)	Estrogen (raloxifene)	38	32	0/38	0/32	62.03 (9.39)	61.34 (10.41)	n/a	n/a	60 mg	24 weeks	No	80.47 (14.30)	74.66 (13.26)
Weiser et al. (2017)	Estrogen (raloxifene)	100	100	0/100	0/100	56.6 (4.6)	55.8 (4.7)	n/a	n/a	120 mg	16 weeks	No	101.7 (18.5)	101.2 (18.1)
Berger et al. (2007)	Fatty acids (EPA)	35	34	25/10	28/7	20.5 (3.8)	20.6 (3.7)	7.2 (10) months	10.0 (13.1) months	2 g	12 weeks	Yes	BPRS: 61.6 (9.6)	BPRS: 62.8 (13.8)

(continued)

Table 22.1 (continued)

Study	Type of treatment	Treatment N	Placebo N	Treatment N males/N females	Placebo N males/N females	Treatment age mean (SD)	Placebo age mean (SD)	Treatment duration of illness	Placebo duration of illness	Daily treatment dose	Duration of treatment	FEP	Treatment baseline PANSS total mean (SD)	Placebo baseline PANSS total mean (SD)
Boskovic et al. (2016)	Fatty acids (omega-3: EPA, DHA, ALA, OE)	9	11	4/5	4/7	53.6 (8.7)	45.6 (8.7)	201 (94) months	190 (116) months	Omega-3 (EPA 132 mg, DHA 88 mg, ALA 94 mg, and OE 52 mg)	4 months	No	58 .9 (21.5)	57.8(14.2)
Emsley et al. (2002)	Fatty acids (EPA)	20	20	n/a	n/a	46.2 (10.6)	43.6 years (13.9)	23.1 years	22.2 years	3 g	12 weeks	No	n/a	n/a
Emsley et al. (2006)	Fatty acids (EPA)	39	38	27/12	24/14	42.4 (10.3)	43.4 (10.9)	16.0 (10.5) years	16.8 (10.4) years	2 g	12 weeks	No	59.2 (13.0)	57.5 (11.8)
Emsley et al. (2014)	Fatty acids (omega-3)	21	12	16/5	8/4	30.6 (7.4)	28.1 (8.9)	n/a	n/a	Omega-3 (EA 2 g and DHA 1 g)	2 years or until relapse	Yes	36.1 (4.2)	38.2 (4.0)
Fenton et al. (2001)	Fatty acids (EPA)	43	44	53/34[c]	53/34[c]	40 years (10)[c]		n/a	n/a	3 g	16 weeks	No	74 (16)	76 (18)
Jamilian et al. (2017)	Fatty acids (omega-3)	30	30	16/14	15/15	32.01 (7.13)	31.01 (8.81)	n/a	n/a	1 g	8 weeks	No	96.13 (9.61)	98.26 (4.51)
Pawełczyk et al. (2016)	Fatty acids (omega-3: EPA and DHA)	36	35	23.2 (4.8)	23.3 (4.8)	19/17	23/12	3.1 (4.2) months	2.7 (3.5) months	Omega-3 2.2 g (EPA 1.32 g and DHA 0.88 g)	26 weeks	Yes	98.4 (13.22)	96.8 (12.01)
Peet et al. (2001) (DHA)[a]	Fatty acids (DHA)	16	14	12/4	8/6	42.0 (10.6)	43.8 (10.8)	n/a	n/a	2 gr DHA	12 weeks	Yes	73.4 (17.9)	76.2 (20.6)

Peet et al. (2001) (EPA)[a]	Fatty acids (EPA)	15	14	10/5	8/6	44.2 (11.3)	43.8 (10.8)	n/a	n/a	2 gr EPA	12 weeks	Yes	69.9 (12.9)	76.2 (20.6)
Peet and Horobin (2002) (1 gr)[a]	Fatty acids (EPA)	29	31	19/10	20/11	mean: 38, range: 20–60	mean: 39, range: 22–61	n/a	n/a	4 g	12 weeks	No	mean: 75, range: 50–96	mean: 78, range: 51–132
Peet and Horobin (2002) (2 gr)[a]	Fatty acids (EPA)	28	31	20/8	20/11	mean: 34, range: 20–62	mean: 39, range: 22–61	n/a	n/a	4 g	12 weeks	No	mean: 83, range: 50–124	mean: 78, range: 51–132
Peet and Horobin et al. (2002) (4 gr)[a]	Fatty acids (EPA)	27	31	17/10	20/11	mean: 37, range: 20–56	mean: 39, range: 22–61	n/a	n/a	4 g	12 weeks	No	mean: 79, range: 55–109	mean: 78, range: 51–132
Modabbernia et al. (2014)	Melatonin	18	18	13/5	12/6	32.7 (7.3)	32.8 (8.2)	n/a	n/a	3 mg	8 weeks	Yes	113.5 (12.7)	103.5 (18.0)
Chaudhry et al. (2012) (Brazil)	Minocycline	15	15	41/30	45/28	25.87 (7.07)[c]	26.59 (8.26)[c]	<5 years[c]	<5 years[c]	start dose: 50 mg; end dose: 200 mg	8 weeks	Yes	63.00 (17.19)	57.87 (13.25)
Chaudhry et al. (2012) (Pakistan)	Minocycline	56	58	41/30	45/28	25.87 (7.07)[c]	26.59 (8.26)[c]	<5 years[c]	<5 years[c]	start dose: 50 mg; end dose: 200 mg	8 weeks	Yes	82.24 (21.55)	83.84 (20.64)
Chaves et al. (2015)	Minocycline	16	14	13/3	11/3	24 (5.02)	25 (6.37)	31.8 (21.98 (months)	29.1 (17.9) months	200 mg	12 months	Yes	n/a	n/a
Deakin et al. (2018)	Minocycline	104	103	77/27	73/30	25.5(5.2)	25.7(5.1)	<5 years[c]	<5 years[c]	start dose: 200 mg; end dose: 300 mg	12 months	Yes	67.1 (13.2)	69.3 (15.4)
Ghanizadeh et al. (2014)	Minocycline	21	22	15/6	19/3	31.0 (7.6)	30.2 (8.9)	3.8 (1.7) years	3.2 (1.6) years	200 mg	8 weeks	No	43.9 (14.9)	40.3 (10.8)
Kelly et al. (2015)	Minocycline	29	23	20/8	18/5	42.9 (14.2)	42.3 (11.0)	24.4 years	23 years	200 mg	10 weeks	No	BPRS: 44.9 (8.7)	BPRS: 44.0 (7.9)

(continued)

Table 22.1 (continued)

Study	Type of treatment	Treatment N	Placebo N	Treatment N males/N females	Placebo N males/N females	Treatment age mean (SD)	Placebo age mean (SD)	Treatment duration of illness	Placebo duration of illness	Daily treatment dose	Duration of treatment	FEP	Treatment baseline PANSS total mean (SD)	Placebo baseline PANSS total mean (SD)
Khodaie-Ardakani et al. (2014)	Minocycline	20	20	14/6	15/5	41.05 (7.47)	38.95 (7.78)	20.90 (8.02) years	18.75 (7.55) years	start dose: 100 mg; end dose: 200 mg	8 weeks	No	71.35 (4.54)	71.90 (7.14)
Levkovitz et al. (2010)	Minocycline	13	8	3/10	3/15	24.8 (4.01)	25.5 (4.06)			200 mg	6 months	Yes	80.37 (12.77)	82.86 (13.90)
Liu et al. (2014)	Minocycline	39	40	25/14	24/16	27.05 (5.68)	27.70 (7.27)	21.00 (13.84) months	27.45 (14.25) months	200 mg	16 weeks	No	81.28 (12.88)	83.35 (10.65)
Weiser et al. (in press)	Minocycline	100	100	n/a	n/a	43.4 (10.5)	43.5 (9.7)	n/a	n/a	200 mg	16 weeks	No	94.6 (14.3)	96.5 (16.0)
Zhang et al. (2018) (100 mg minocycline)[a]	Minocycline	25	25	13/12	12/13	33.04 (7.78)	33.68 (6.18)	6.28 (1.82) years	6.27 (1.71) years	100 mg	3 months	No	79.04 (5.04)	78.08 (4.71)
Zhang et al. (2018) (200 mg minocycline)[a]	Minocycline	25	25	12/13	12/13	33.24 (6.48)	33.68 (6.18)	5.98 (1.78) years	6.27 (1.71) years	200 mg	3 months	No	78.52 (4.58)	78.08 (4.71)
Berk et al. (2008)	*N*-acetylcysteine	69	71	48/21	50/21	37.2 (10.1)	36.1 (11.7)	12.4 (8.2) years	12.1 (9.6) years	2000 mg	24 weeks	No	64.0 (15.4)	64.4 (16.3)
Breier et al. (2018)	*N*-acetylcysteine	30	30	23/7	24/6	22.2 (4.2)	25.0 (5.2)	1.3 (1.2) years	1.4 (1.1) years	3600 mg	52 weeks	No	56.7 (15.0)	56.4 (12.0)
Farokhnia et al. (2013)	*N*-acetylcysteine	21	21	9/12	11/10	32.23 (6.12)	33.38 (6.97)	83.23 (41.02) months	88.95 (44.66) months	2000 mg	8 weeks	No	113.42 (9.05)	114.61 (10.09)

Sepehrmanesh et al. (2018)	*N*-acetylcysteine	40	39	22/18	19/20	38.7 (1.9)	39.4 (2.2)	13.8 (9.9) years	17(11.6) years	1200 mg	12 weeks	No	104.0 (27.0)	87.7 (17.4)
Zhang et al. (2015)	*N*-acetylcysteine	61	60	32/29[c]	32/29[c]	34.6 (8.4)[c]	34.6 (8.4)[c]	6.6 (5.1)[c] months	6.6 (5.1)[c] months	600 mg	8 weeks	Yes	113.87 (3.57)	113.67 (4.36)
Iranpour et al. (2016)	Pioglitazone	21	21	14/7	15/6	38 (8.99)	37 (7.69)	16.25 (8.94) years	13.60 (8.21) years	30 mg	8 weeks	No	70.45 (5.54)	68.50 (5.46)
Noorbala et al. (1999)	Piracetam	14	16	18/16[c]	n/a	n/a	n/a	n/a	n/a	3200 mg	8 weeks	No	n/a	n/a
Ritsner et al. (2014)	Pregnenolone	25	27	22/3	23/4	26.9 (5.2)	27.8 (6.0)	2.5 (1.4) years	2.8 (1.5) years	50 mg	8 weeks	Yes	58.2 (11.9)	63.7 (10.5)
Tajik-Esmaeeli et al. (2016)	Statin (Simvastatin)	33	33	31/2	28/5	43.18 (8.89)	44.64 (9.11)	20.55 (10.79) years	19.60 (10.23) years	40 mg	8 weeks	No	47.09 (7.60)	48.18 (7.70)
Vincenzi et al. (2014)	Statin (Pravastatin)	30	30	22/8	16/14	42.57 (11)	44.53 (12.55)	20.89 (13.13)[b]	22.03 (6.74)[b]	40 mg	12 weeks	No	75.16 (21.87)	79.93 (18.53)
Hong et al. (2011)	Varenicline	32	32	20/12	22/10	44.03 (SE: 1.82)	41.57 (SE: 193)	n/a	n/a	1 mg	8 weeks	No	BPRS: 34.13 (1.44)	BPRS: 34.69 (1.52)
Smith et al. (2016)	Varenicline	42	45	35/7	39/6	46.6 (8.9)	43.6 (10.6)	n/a	n/a	2 mg	8 weeks	No	56.2 (14.9)	58.8 (15.7)
Chengappa et al. (2018)	Withania somnifera extract	34	34	21/13	14/20	45.18 (12.90)	47.38 (11.37)	20.85 (12.26) years	23.38 (11.61) years	1000 mg	12 weeks	No	69.88 (8)	69.48 (8.45)

ALA α-linolenic acid, *BPRS* brief psychiatric rating scale, *EPA* eicosapentaenoic acid, *DHA* docosahexaenoic acid, *FEP* first-episode, *OA* oleic acid, *n/a* not available, *PANSS* positive and negative syndrome scale, *SD* standard deviation, *SE* standard error

[a]Different treatment doses were applied within the same study

[b]Time unit not specified

[c]Total study population

22.2.4 Estrogens

Estrogens, especially 17β-estradiol, have immunomodulatory effects by, for example, regulating innate immune signaling pathways and modulating inflammatory elements such as cytokines [40]. Other properties of estrogens include reducing antioxidative stress, controlling energy balance and glucose homeostasis, and influencing dopaminergic neurotransmission [41]. Eleven studies provided estrogen as augmentation therapy for patients with schizophrenia [42–52]. Nine studies included only females and two studies included only males [44, 45]. Four studies applied (ethinyl) estradiol [42, 46, 47, 49], two studies applied conjugated estrogen [43, 50], and five studies applied raloxifene, a selective estrogen receptor modulator [44, 45, 48, 51, 52]. Estrogen doses ranged from 0.05 mg per day (patch) to 2 mg per day (orally), and raloxifene doses varied from 60 to 120 mg per day (orally). A significant positive effect of estrogen was observed (ES; 0.78, $p < 0.001$). One study reported a large ES of 3.7 [43]. Exclusion of this outlier yielded a mean weighted ES of 0.57, which was still significant (CI, 0.25 to 0.90; $p = 0.001$). A significant ES was also found when analyses were restricted to female studies only (ES: 0.52; CI, 0.18 to 0.87; $p = 0.003$; I2 = 72%).

22.2.5 Melatonin

Melatonin is a multifunctional hormone, best known for its role in regulation of day–night cycle. It is also an antioxidant and a widespread anti-inflammatory molecule, modulating both pro- and anti-inflammatory cytokines, which can easily pass the BBB [53]. One study ($N = 18$) investigated the effects of adding 3 mg melatonin daily to regular antipsychotic treatment for patients with schizophrenia for 8 weeks [54]. This single small study reported significant beneficial results on decreasing symptom severity in schizophrenia (ES: 2.82; $p < 0.001$).

22.2.6 Minocycline

Minocycline is a broad-spectrum tetracycline antibiotic that has strong inhibitory effects on microglia cells and can easily cross the BBB [55]. Ten studies assessed the effect of minocycline augmentation therapy for schizophrenia patients [56–65]. The daily treatments doses varied from 100 to 300 mg, and the duration of treatment was relatively long, ranging from 2 to 12 months. Minocycline treatment in addition to regular antipsychotic treatment showed significantly beneficial results on symptom severity (ES: 0.4; $p = 0.007$).. It should however be mentioned that one, well-conducted study, reported a large negative ES of −0.24 [58]. Excluding this study from the analysis yielded a mean weighted ES of 0.47 (CI, 0.18 to 0.76; $p = 0.002$). Subgroup analysis for patients with early-phase schizophrenia (retaining Deakin et al. [58]) showed a trend toward positive effects (ES: 0.38; CI −0.02 to 0.78; $p = 0.060$).

22.2.7 *N*-Acetylcysteine

NAC has evident anti-inflammatory properties and can modulate immune functions during the inflammatory response by inhibiting TNF-α, IL-1β, and IL-6 [66]. NAC can also easily pass the BBB [67]. Five studies investigated the effects of NAC augmentation therapy on symptom severity of patients with schizophrenia [68–72]. One of those studies restricted inclusion to FEP patients only [72]. Treatment doses varied from 600 mg to 3600 mg, and duration of treatment varied from 8 to 52 weeks. NAC as augmentation therapy had significantly beneficial effects on decreasing symptom severity in patients with schizophrenia compared with controls (ES: 1.00; $p < 0.001$). Subgroup analysis showed that augmentation therapy with NAC is beneficial in all illness stages, including FEP which yielded the largest ES (ES: 1.42; CI, 1.02 to 1.81; $p < 0.001$), early-phase schizophrenia (ES: 0.98; CI, 0.45 to 1.51; $p < 0.001$), and chronic schizophrenia (ES: 0.44; CI, 0.11 to 0.77; $p = 0.010$).

22.2.8 Pioglitazone

Pioglitazone is an antidiabetic agent with antioxidant and anti-inflammatory actions [73], and it can cross the BBB [74]. One study ($N = 21$) provided 30 mg pioglitazone daily in addition to standard treatment for 8 weeks to patients with schizophrenia [73]. This single small study showed significant beneficial results on reducing symptom severity (ES: 0.79; $p = 0.012$).

22.2.9 Piracetam

Piracetam is a nootropic analgesic agent and has anti-inflammatory effects. It can reduce TNF-α, IL-1β, and myeloperoxidase. There is some evidence that piracetam can cross the BBB [75]. One study ($N = 14$) provided 3200 mg piracetam in addition to regular antipsychotic treatment for 8 weeks to schizophrenia patients [76]. A significant positive influence on total symptom severity was observed in this single small study (ES: 0.77; $p = 0.014$) (Table 22.2).

22.2.10 *Withania somnifera* Extract

WSE, mostly used as a medicinal herb in Ayurvedic medicine, has anti-inflammatory actions (i.e., inhibition of NF-κβ inflammatory signaling pathways and COX-2) [77, 78]. WSE consists of various phytochemicals, of which the effects of 1000 mg withaferin A on symptom severity was investigated in one study for 12 weeks [79]. WSE with drug ligand withaferin A can readily cross the BBB [80]. A significant positive influence on total symptom severity was observed (ES: 0.81; CI, 0.32 to 1.30; $p = 0.001$; I2 = 0%).

Table 22.2 Meta-analysis of RCTs with aspirin, fatty acids, estrogen, minocycline, and NAC in schizophrenia: efficacy signal

Anti-inflammatory component	Positive symptoms	Negative symptoms	Cognition[a]
Aspirin	ES = 0.23; $p = 0.34$	n/a	–
Fatty acids	ES = −0.11; $p = 0.48$	ES = 0.20; $p = 0.47$	–
Estrogen	ES = 0.43; $p = 0.01$[b]	ES = 0.35; $p = 0.02$[b]	–
Minocycline	ES = 0.19; $p < 0.01$	ES = 0.51; $p < 0.01$	±
NAC	ES = 0.57; $p = 0.04$	ES = 0.69; $p < 0.01$	±

ES effect size (Hedges' *g*), *FEP* first-episode studies, *n/a* not available, *NAC N*-acetylcysteine, *p* *p*-value, *RCTs* randomized controlled trials, – probably no effects, ± probably some effects
[a]Heterogeneity of the used cognitive tests across the studies was too great to make a quantitative review of these effects
[b]One outlier was excluded from analysis

22.2.11 Effects of Moderators

Meta-regression analysis showed that illness duration, treatment duration, treatment dose, and baseline severity were insignificant predictors of the ES estimates for the effects of augmentation with EPA and/or DHA fatty acids, estrogen, and minocycline (Table 22.3). Study quality was not a significant moderator for the celecoxib, EPA and/or DHA fatty acids, minocycline, and NAC studies. For the estrogen studies, we observed that the beneficial effects of estrogen were mainly seen in good quality studies.

22.2.12 Effects on Negative Symptoms and Cognition

It is increasingly acknowledged that the prognosis of the schizophrenia syndrome is greatly influenced by the presence of negative symptoms, which include apathy and social withdrawal [81]. Similarly, recent considerations recognize cognitive deficits as the core component of the disorder, which may well be present years before psychotic phenomena emerge [82]. Anti-inflammatory agents may have additional effects on these symptom domains as compared to regular treatment strategies.

Augmentation therapy with minocycline (ES: 0.51; 95% CI, 0.17 to 0.84; $p = 0.003$), NAC (ES: 0.75; 95% CI, 0.19 to 1.32; $p = 0.009$), and estrogen (ES: 0.45; 95% CI, 0.13 to 0.77; $p = 0.006$) showed positive results on improving negative symptoms.

The heterogeneity of the cognitive tests used across studies was too great to make a quantitative review of cognitive effects. Notwithstanding, it seemed that minocycline improved attention, executive functions, and memory [62, 63]; NAC [71] improved attention, memory, and executive functions. However, other studies did not observe any beneficial effects on cognition for minocycline [56, 58, 60, 64] and NAC [69]. For the anti-inflammatory components bexarotene, celecoxib,

Table 22.3 Effects of anti-inflammatory agents on cognitive domains

	Aspirin	Davu-netide	Fatty acids	Fatty acids	Estro-gens	Estro-gens	Minocy-cline	Minocy-cline	Mino-cycline	Minocy-cline	Mino-cycline	Mino-cycline	NAC	NAC	Statin	Vareni-cline	Vareni-cline
Study	*Laan et al. (2010)*	*Javitt et al. (2012)*	*Fenton et al. (2001)*	*Emsley et al. (2014)*	*Kulkarni et al. (2016)*	*Weiser et al. (2017)*	*Chaudhry et al. (2012)*	*Deakin et al. (2018)*	*Levkot-vitz et al. (2010)*	*Liu et al. (2014)*	*Weiser et al. (in press)*	*Kelly et al. (2015)*	*Breier et al. (2018)*	*Sepeh-rmanesh et al. (2018)*	*Vin-cenzi et al. (2014)*	*Hong et al. (2011)*	*Smith et al. (2016)*
Attention/vigi-lance	–	–	–	–	–	–	–	n/a	–	+	–	–	–	n/a	–	–	–
Communica-tion	n/a	–	n/a	n/a	n/a	n/a	n/a	n/a	n/a	n/a	n/a	n/a	n/a	n/a	n/a	n/a	n/a
Comprehen-sion/planning	n/a	–	n/a	n/a	n/a	n/a	n/a	n/a	n/a	n/a	n/a	n/a	n/a	n/a	n/a	n/a	n/a
Executive functions	n/a	n/a	n/a	n/a	n/a	–	–	n/a	+	–	–	n/a	–	n/a	n/a	n/a	n/a
Financial Skills	n/a	–	n/a	n/a	n/a	n/a	n/a	n/a	n/a	n/a	n/a	n/a	n/a	n/a	n/a	n/a	n/a
Fine locomo-tor skills	–	n/a	n/a	n/a	n/a	n/a	n/a	n/a	n/a	–	n/a	n/a	n/a	n/a	n/a	n/a	n/a
Household management	n/a	–	n/a	n/a	n/a	n/a	n/a	n/a	n/a	n/a	n/a	n/a	n/a	n/a	n/a	n/a	n/a
IQ	n/a	n/a	n/a	n/a	n/a	n/a	n/a	–	n/a	n/a	n/a	n/a	n/a	n/a	n/a	n/a	n/a
Language	n/a	n/a	–	n/a	–	n/a	n/a	n/a	n/a	n/a	n/a	n/a	n/a	n/a	n/a	n/a	n/a
Medication management	n/a	–	n/a	n/a	n/a	n/a	n/a	n/a	n/a	n/a	n/a	n/a	n/a	n/a	n/a	n/a	n/a
Memory	–	n/a	n/a	n/a	n/a	n/a	n/a	n/a	n/a	n/a	n/a	n/a	n/a	n/a	n/a	n/a	n/a
Memory (delayed memory)	n/a	n/a	–	n/a	–	n/a	n/a	n/a	n/a	n/a	n/a	n/a	n/a	n/a	n/a	n/a	n/a
Memory (immediate memory)	n/a	n/a	–	n/a	–	n/a	n/a	n/a	n/a	n/a	n/a	n/a	n/a	n/a	n/a	n/a	n/a

(continued)

Table 22.3 (continued)

	Aspirin	Davunetide	Fatty acids	Fatty acids	Estrogens	Estrogens	Minocycline	Minocycline	Minocycline	Minocycline	Minocycline	Minocycline	NAC	NAC	Statin	Varenicline	Varenicline
Memory (verbal memory)	n/a	n/a	n/a	n/a	n/a	–	n/a	n/a	n/a	n/a	–	n/a	–	n/a	n/a	n/a	n/a
Memory (visuospatial memory)	n/a	n/a	n/a	n/a	n/a	n/a	–	n/a	+	n/a	n/a	n/a	n/a	n/a	n/a	n/a	n/a
Memory (working memory)	n/a	–	n/a	–	n/a	–	n/a	n/a	n/a	–	–	–	–	n/a	–	n/a	–
Motor speed	n/a	n/a	n/a	n/a	n/a	–	n/a	n/a	n/a	n/a	–	n/a	–	n/a	n/a	n/a	n/a
Problem solving	n/a	n/a	n/a	–	n/a	n/a	n/a	n/a	n/a	–	n/a	–	n/a	n/a	–	n/a	–
Processing speed	n/a	–	n/a	–	n/a	n/a	n/a	–	n/a	–	n/a	–	n/a	n/a	n/a	–	–
Psychomotor skills	–	n/a	n/a	n/a	n/a	n/a	n/a	n/a	n/a	–	n/a	n/a	n/a	n/a	n/a	n/a	n/a
Psychomotor speed	n/a	n/a	n/a	n/a	n/a	n/a	–	n/a	–	n/a	n/a	n/a	n/a	n/a	n/a	n/a	n/a
Reasoning/ problem-solving	n/a	–	n/a	n/a	n/a	n/a	n/a	n/a	n/a	n/a	n/a	n/a	n/a	n/a	n/a	n/a	n/a
Social cognition	n/a	–	n/a	–	n/a	n/a	n/a	n/a	n/a	n/a	n/a	–	n/a	n/a	–	n/a	–
Transportation	n/a	–	n/a	n/a	n/a	n/a	n/a	n/a	n/a	n/a	n/a	n/a	n/a	n/a	n/a	n/a	n/a
Verbal fluency	n/a	n/a	n/a	n/a	n/a	–	n/a	n/a	n/a	–	–	n/a	–	n/a	n/a	n/a	n/a
Verbal learning	n/a	–	n/a	–	n/a	n/a	n/a	n/a	n/a	–	n/a	–	n/a	n/a	–	n/a	–

Visual learning	n/a	–	n/a	–	n/a	n/a	n/a	n/a	n/a	–	n/a	–	n/a	n/ε	–	n/a	–
Visuospatial/ constructional	n/a	n/a	–	n/a	–	n/a	n/a	n/a	n/a	–	n/a	n/a	n/a	n/a	n/a	n/a	n/a
Cognitive tests used	RAVLT; HQ-CPT; PPT; TMT	UPSA; MCCB	RBANS	MCCB	RBANS	BACS	CANTAB	Wechsler Adult Intelligence Scale III	CANTAB	MCCB; WCST	BACS	MATRICS/ MCCB	BACS	MMSE; DSFBT; DSST; SCWT	MATRICS; UPSA-B	MCCB	MCCB

BACS brief assessment of cognition in schizophrenia, *CANTAB*, Cambridge neuropsychological test automated battery, *DGSBT* digit span forward and backward test, *DSST* digit symbol substitution test, *HQ-CPT* HQ continuous performance test, *IQ* intelligence quotient, *MCCB* MATRICS (measurement and treatment research to improve cognition in schizophrenia) consensus cognitive battery, *MMSE* mini-mental state examination, *n/a* not available, *NAC* *N*-acetylcysteine, *PPT* Purdue pegboard test, *RAVLT* Rey auditory verbal learning test, *RBANS* repeatable battery for the assessment of neuropsychological status; *SCWT* Stroop color-word test, *TMT* trail making test, *UPSA* University of California, San Diego Performance-Based Skills Assessment, *WCST* brief Wisconsin card sorting test, + positive significant effects on improving cognition (p-value < 0.05), – no significant effects on improving cognition

Cognitive domains were not subdivided

	NAC
Study	*Sepehrmanesh et al. (2018)*
MMSE (visuospatial/language/attention/concentration/memory recall/orientation)[a]	+
The digit span test, backward (verbal ability/memory short term)[a]	+
The digit span test, forward (verbal ability/memory short term)[a]	+
The digit symbol substitution test (brain damage/dementia/age/depression)[a]	+
The stroop test (processing speed/executive functions/working memory/cognitive development)[a]	+

+ positive significant effects on improving cognition (p-value < 0.05), *NAC N*-acetylcysteine
[a]Cognitive domains were not subdivided

dextromethorphan, melatonin, pioglitazone, piracetam, and WSE no data on cognitive effects were reported.

22.3 Discussion

The results of aspirin, fatty acids, estrogens, minocycline, and NAC showed significantly better results than placebo meta-analysis of at least two studies [19], while pioglitazone, piracetam, and WSE were significant in single studies.

22.3.1 Effects on Symptom Severity of Specific Components

Fatty acids as augmentation therapy for patients with schizophrenia showed borderline significant effects on decreasing symptom severity in the current study. However, the included studies showed great heterogeneity in the specific methods of additional treatment. Researchers investigated the addition of different fatty acids (i.e. EPA or DHA) or a combination of fatty acids (i.e. EPA and DHA combined). Moreover, three research groups added antioxidants to the fatty acid treatment regime [29, 31, 32]. Considering fatty acids augmentation (without antioxidants), the results showed a negative association, but this result was greatly influenced by a very substantial outlier [29]. Excluding, this outlier showed a positive significant association. Furthermore, FEP patients might benefit the most from treatment with fatty acids compared with patients with a longer illness duration.

In summary, based on the available data, a clear statement about the efficacy of fatty acids, either alone or in combination with antioxidants cannot be made yet. Possibly, fatty acids can be beneficial, but the field is still investigating what specific combination of fatty acids is efficacious, and whether or not antioxidants are beneficial. Further research is warranted before a clear recommendation can be made.

Estrogen augmentation therapy for schizophrenia patients showed beneficial effects for a relatively short duration of treatment (starting at 4 weeks). Estrogens act in different ways in the brain and may cause their beneficial effects by mechanisms that are not related to inflammation (e.g., by affecting angiotensin and neurotransmission) [83, 84].

Minocycline has strong inhibitory effects on microglia cell activation and may, therefore, be expected to have potential as augmentation therapy for schizophrenia [85]. Microglia activation plays an important role during brain development, but excessive microglia activation is also considered a hallmark of neuro-inflammation [85]. However, it should be noted that a large negative study provided almost 22% of the total amount of patients [58]. Deakin and colleagues investigated first-episode patients with an illness duration shorter than 5 years. Minocycline seems to have beneficial effects on improving negative symptoms in schizophrenia We noted that the study population studied by Deakin and colleagues had relatively low baseline levels of PANSS negative symptoms (+/− 17) compared with other studies investigating early-phase schizophrenia patients (>22).

NAC has clear anti-inflammatory and immune modulating actions. All five studies included in this meta-analysis showed beneficial effects on improving symptom severity. Only one study restricted inclusion to FEP patients and yielded the largest beneficial effects on symptom severity [72].

22.3.2 Side Effects

Of the five agents that showed positive results in at least two studies, aspirin use increases the risk of gastrointestinal bleeding and should, therefore, be combined with gastric protection. This serious side effect does not happen infrequently and, therefore, should be considered and monitored. On the other hand, aspirin also possesses cardioprotective properties, which can be beneficial in schizophrenia patients with metabolic syndrome.

Estrogens are not safe for a longer treatment duration than 1 to 2 months unless combined with progesterone. Estrogens such as raloxiphene are sometimes accompanied with hot flashes and gastrointestinal problems. There are potential risks for the occurrence of thromboembolic events and fatal stroke in women with or at increased risk for cardiovascular disease. Therefore, clinical risk for thromboembolic events should be evaluated and monitored during treatment [86, 87].

Fatty acids are usually well tolerated. There are some reported side effects during administration such as gastrointestinal effects (e.g., constipation or diarrhea) and infection (e.g., upper respiratory infection). The omega-3 fatty acid and antioxidant combination might be beneficial [29, 88].

NAC is a well-tolerated drug that can also be administered during pregnancy. NAC has other beneficial effects in schizophrenia, such as attenuating addiction [89]. For minocycline, in the published studies, no serious adverse events were observed in the treatment groups.

22.3.3 Limitations

An important limitation is that many anti-inflammatory augmentation treatment strategies have not been sufficiently investigated. Components with strong anti-inflammatory potency, such as glucocorticosteroids, have not been applied yet to patients with schizophrenia. Most studies did not stratify schizophrenia patients in subgroups of illness duration. Especially important with respect to personalized medicine efforts, there was insufficient description of signs of inflammation before the start of anti-inflammatory therapy. For designing future research it would be interesting to investigate whether signs of (low-grade) inflammation before the start of the trials would influence the outcome and degree of inflammation. There is increasing evidence from the biomarker research field that cytokine alterations are already present from disease-onset [90–92]. It is paramount for further trials to stratify patients according to the presence of immune alterations and to investigate which inflammatory subtypes would benefit the most from anti-inflammatory therapy. This opens up the way for personalized medicine based on inflammatory markers.

22.4 Conclusion

The anti-inflammatory medications minocycline, fatty acids, aspirin, estrogens, and NAC improved symptom severity in patients with schizophrenia. Generally, greater beneficial results are reported in early-psychosis studies. Studies investigating the effects on cognitive functions are scarce. Taken together, there is evidence for efficacy of some anti-inflammatory agents on symptom severity in schizophrenia, which could confirm the immune hypothesis in schizophrenia, but the field needs larger studies aimed at investigating the effects on negative and cognitive symptoms in patients groups stratified for the presence of immune abnormalities at baseline.

References

1. Debnath M, Cannon DM, Venkatasubramanian G. Variation in the major histocompatibility complex [MHC] gene family in schizophrenia: associations and functional implications. Prog Neuro-Psychopharmacol Biol Psychiatry. 2013;42:49–62.
2. Mokhtari R, Lachman HM. The major histocompatibility complex (MHC) in schizophrenia: a review. J Clin Cell Immunol. 2016;7
3. Takao K, Kobayashi K, Hagihara H, Ohira K, Shoji H, Hattori S, Koshimizu H, Umemori J, Toyama K, Nakamura HK, Kuroiwa M, Maeda J, Atsuzawa K, Esaki K, Yamaguchi S, Furuya S, Takagi T, Walton NM, Hayashi N, Suzuki H, Higuchi M, Usuda N, Suhara T, Nishi A, Matsumoto M, Ishii S, Miyakawa T. Deficiency of schnurri-2, an MHC enhancer binding protein, induces mild chronic inflammation in the brain and confers molecular, neuronal, and behavioral phenotypes related to schizophrenia. Neuropsychopharmacology. 2013;38:1409–25.
4. Sekar A, Bialas AR, de Rivera H, Davis A, Hammond TR, Kamitaki N, Tooley K, Presumey J, Baum M, Van Doren V, Genovese G, Rose SA, Handsaker RE, Daly MJ, Carroll MC, Stevens

B, McCarroll SA. Schizophrenia risk from complex variation of complement component 4. Nature. 2016;530:177–83.
5. Brown AS, Derkits EJ. Prenatal infection and schizophrenia: a review of epidemiologic and translational studies. Am J Psychiatry. 2010;167:261–80.
6. Fineberg AM, Ellman LM. Inflammatory cytokines and neurological and neurocognitive alterations in the course of schizophrenia. Biol Psychiatry. 2013;73:951–66.
7. Nimgaonkar VL, Prasad KM, Chowdari KV, Severance EG, Yolken RH. The complement system: a gateway to gene-environment interactions in schizophrenia pathogenesis. Mol Psychiatry. 2017;22:1554–61.
8. Presumey J, Bialas AR, Carroll MC. Complement system in neural synapse elimination in development and disease. Adv Immunol. 2017;135:53–79.
9. Muller N, Dursun SM. Schizophrenia genes, epigenetics and psychoneuroimmunology therapeutics: all make sense now? J Psychopharmacol (Oxford, England). 2011;25:713–4.
10. Muller N, Schwarz M. Schizophrenia as an inflammation-mediated dysbalance of glutamatergic neurotransmission. Neurotox Res. 2006;10:131–48.
11. Schizophrenia Working Group of the Psychiatric Genomics C, Ripke S, Neale BM, Corvin A, Walters JTR, Farh K-H, Holmans PA, Lee P, Bulik-Sullivan B, Collier DA, Huang H, Pers TH, Agartz I, Agerbo E, Albus M, Alexander M, Amin F, Bacanu SA, Begemann M, Belliveau RA Jr, Bene J, Bergen SE, Bevilacqua E, Bigdeli TB, Black DW, Bruggeman R, Buccola NG, Buckner RL, Byerley W, Cahn W, Cai G, Campion D, Cantor RM, Carr VJ, Carrera N, Catts SV, Chambert KD, Chan RCK, Chen RYL, Chen EYH, Cheng W, Cheung EFC, Ann Chong S, Robert Cloninger C, Cohen D, Cohen N, Cormican P, Craddock N, Crowley JJ, Curtis D, Davidson M, Davis KL, Degenhardt F, Del Favero J, Demontis D, Dikeos D, Dinan T, Djurovic S, Donohoe G, Drapeau E, Duan J, Dudbridge F, Durmishi N, Eichhammer P, Eriksson J, Escott-Price V, Essioux L, Fanous AH, Farrell MS, Frank J, Franke L, Freedman R, Freimer NB, Friedl M, Friedman JI, Fromer M, Genovese G, Georgieva L, Giegling I, Giusti-Rodríguez P, Godard S, Goldstein JI, Golimbet V, Gopal S, Gratten J, de Haan L, Hammer C, Hamshere ML, Hansen M, Hansen T, Haroutunian V, Hartmann AM, Henskens FA, Herms S, Hirschhorn JN, Hoffmann P, Hofman A, Hollegaard MV, Hougaard DM, Ikeda M, Joa I, Julià A, Kahn RS, Kalaydjieva L, Karachanak-Yankova S, Karjalainen J, Kavanagh D, Keller MC, Kennedy JL, Khrunin A, Kim Y, Klovins J, Knowles JA, Konte B, Kucinskas V, Ausrele Kucinskiene Z, Kuzelova-Ptackova H, Kähler AK, Laurent C, Lee Chee Keong J, Hong Lee S, Legge SE, Lerer B, Li M, Li T, Liang K-Y, Lieberman J, Limborska S, Loughland CM, Lubinski J, Lönnqvist J, Macek M Jr, Magnusson PKE, Maher BS, Maier W, Mallet J, Marsal S, Mattheisen M, Mattingsdal M, McCarley RW, McDonald C, McIntosh AM, Meier S, Meijer CJ, Melegh B, Melle I, Mesholam-Gately RI, Metspalu A, Michie PT, Milani L, Milanova V, Mokrab Y, Morris DW, Mors O, Murphy KC, Murray RM, Myin-Germeys I, Müller-Myhsok B, Nelis M, Nenadic I, Nertney DA, Nestadt G, Nicodemus KK, Nikitina-Zake L, Nisenbaum L, Nordin A, O'Callaghan E, O'Dushlaine C, O'Neill FA, Oh S-Y, Olincy A, Olsen L, Van Os J, Pantelis C, Papadimitriou GN, Papiol S, Parkhomenko E, Pato MT, Paunio T, Pejovic-Milovancevic M, Perkins DO, Pietiläinen O, Pimm J, Pocklington AJ, Powell J, Price A, Pulver AE, Purcell SM, Quested D, Rasmussen HB, Reichenberg A, Reimers MA, Richards AL, Roffman JL, Roussos P, Ruderfer DM, Salomaa V, Sanders AR, Schall U, Schubert CR, Schulze TG, Schwab SG, Scolnick EM, Scott RJ, Seidman LJ, Shi J, Sigurdsson E, Silagadze T, Silverman JM, Sim K, Slominsky P, Smoller JW, So H-C, Spencer CA, Stahl EA, Stefansson H, Steinberg S, Stogmann E, Straub RE, Strengman E, Strohmaier J, Scott Stroup T, Subramaniam M, Suvisaari J, Svrakic DM, Szatkiewicz JP, Söderman E, Thirumalai S, Toncheva D, Tosato S, Veijola J, Waddington J, Walsh D, Wang D, Wang Q, Webb BT, Weiser M, Wildenauer DB, Williams NM, Williams S, Witt SH, Wolen AR, Wong EHM, Wormley BK, Simon Xi H, Zai CC, Zheng X, Zimprich F, Wray NR, Stefansson K, Visscher PM, Trust Case-Control Consortium W, Adolfsson R, Andreassen OA, Blackwood DHR, Bramon E, Buxbaum JD, Børglum AD, Cichon S, Darvasi A, Domenici E, Ehrenreich H, Esko T, Gejman PV, Gill M, Gurling H, Hultman CM, Iwata N, Jablensky AV, Jönsson EG, Kendler KS, Kirov G, Knight J, Lencz T, Levinson DF, Li QS, Liu J, Malhotra AK, McCarroll SA, McQuillin A,

Moran JL, Mortensen PB, Mowry BJ, Nöthen MM, Ophoff RA, Owen MJ, Palotie A, Pato CN, Petryshen TL, Posthuma D, Rietschel M, Riley BP, Rujescu D, Sham PC, Sklar P, St Clair D, Weinberger DR, Wendland JR, Werge T, Daly MJ, Sullivan PF, O'Donovan MC. Biological insights from 108 schizophrenia-associated genetic loci. Nature. 2014;511:421.

12. Liu F, Zhang B, Xie L, Ruan Y, Xu X, Zeng Y, Messina L, Zhao J, Fan X. Changes in plasma levels of nitric oxide metabolites and negative symptoms after 16-week minocycline treatment in patients with schizophrenia. Schizophr Res. 2018;199:390–4.
13. Man L, Lv X, Du XD, Yin G, Zhu X, Zhang Y, Soares JC, Yang XN, Chen X, Zhang XY. Cognitive impairments and low BDNF serum levels in first-episode drug-naive patients with schizophrenia. Psychiatry Res. 2018;263:1–6.
14. Misiak B, Stanczykiewicz B, Kotowicz K, Rybakowski JK, Samochowiec J, Frydecka D. Cytokines and C-reactive protein alterations with respect to cognitive impairment in schizophrenia and bipolar disorder: a systematic review. Schizophr Res. 2018;192:16–29.
15. Cai HQ, Catts VS, Webster MJ, Galletly C, Liu D, O'Donnell M, Weickert TW, Weickert CS. Increased macrophages and changed brain endothelial cell gene expression in the frontal cortex of people with schizophrenia displaying inflammation. Mol Psychiatry. 2020;25(4):761–75.
16. Chew LJ, Fusar-Poli P, Schmitz T. Oligodendroglial alterations and the role of microglia in white matter injury: relevance to schizophrenia. Dev Neurosci. 2013;35:102–29.
17. Sommer IE, van Westrhenen R, Begemann MJ, de Witte LD, Leucht S, Kahn RS. Efficacy of anti-inflammatory agents to improve symptoms in patients with schizophrenia: an update. Schizophr Bull. 2014;40:181–91.
18. Sellgren CM, Gracias J, Watmuff B, Biag JD, Thanos JM, Whittredge PB, Fu T, Worringer K, Brown HE, Wang J, Kaykas A, Karmacharya R, Goold CP, Sheridan SD, Perlis RH. Increased synapse elimination by microglia in schizophrenia patient-derived models of synaptic pruning. Nat Neurosci. 2019;22(3):374–85.
19. Cakici N, Van Beveren NJM, Judge-Hundal G, Koola MM, Sommer IEC. An update on the efficacy of anti-inflammatory agents for patients with schizophrenia: a meta-analysis. Psychol Med. 2019;49:2307–19.
20. Roth GJ, Majerus PW. The mechanism of the effect of aspirin on human platelets. I Acetylation of a particulate fraction protein. J Clin Investig. 1975;56:624–32.
21. Vane JR, Bakhle YS, Botting RM. Cyclooxygenases 1 and 2. Annu Rev Pharmacol Toxicol. 1998;38:97–120.
22. Nye EJ, Hockings GI, Grice JE, Torpy DJ, Walters MM, Crosbie GV, Wagenaar M, Cooper M, Jackson RV. Aspirin inhibits vasopressin-induced hypothalamic-pituitary-adrenal activity in normal humans. J Clin Endocrinol Metab. 1997;82:812–7.
23. Vasovic V, Banic B, Jakovljevic V, Tomic Z, Milic-Djordjevic V. Effect of aminophylline on aspirin penetration into the central nervous system in rats. Eur J Drug Metab Pharmacokinet. 2008;33:23–30.
24. Laan W, Grobbee DE, Selten JP, Heijnen CJ, Kahn RS, Burger H. Adjuvant aspirin therapy reduces symptoms of schizophrenia spectrum disorders: results from a randomized, double-blind, placebo-controlled trial. J Clin Psychiatry. 2010;71:520–7.
25. Weiser M, Burshtein S, Fodoreanu L. A randomized trial administering aspirin, minocycline or pramipexole vs placebo as add-on to antipsychotics in patients with schizophrenia or schizoaffective disorder [abstract]. Neuropsychopharmacology. 2012;38:S351.
26. Calder PC. Mechanisms of action of (n-3) fatty acids. J Nutrit. 2012;142:592s–9s.
27. Solfrizzi V, Frisardi V, Capurso C, D'Introno A, Colacicco AM, Vendemiale G, Capurso A, Panza F. Dietary fatty acids in dementia and predementia syndromes: epidemiological evidence and possible underlying mechanisms. Ageing Res Rev. 2010;9:184–99.
28. Glantz LA, Lewis DA. Decreased dendritic spine density on prefrontal cortical pyramidal neurons in schizophrenia. Arch Gen Psychiatry. 2000;57:65–73.
29. Bentsen H, Osnes K, Refsum H, Solberg DK, Bohmer T. A randomized placebo-controlled trial of an omega-3 fatty acid and vitamins E+C in schizophrenia. Transl Psychiatry. 2013;3:e335.

30. Berger GE, Proffitt TM, McConchie M, Yuen H, Wood SJ, Amminger GP, Brewer W, McGorry PD. Ethyl-eicosapentaenoic acid in first-episode psychosis: a randomized, placebo-controlled trial. J Clin Psychiatry. 2007;68:1867–75.
31. Boskovic M, Vovk T, Koprivsek J, Plesnicar BK, Grabnar I. Vitamin E and essential polyunsaturated fatty acids supplementation in schizophrenia patients treated with haloperidol. Nutr Neurosci. 2016;19:156–61.
32. Emsley R, Chiliza B, Asmal L, du Plessis S, Phahladira L, van Niekerk E, van Rensburg SJ, Harvey BH. A randomized, controlled trial of omega-3 fatty acids plus an antioxidant for relapse prevention after antipsychotic discontinuation in first-episode schizophrenia. Schizophr Res. 2014;158:230–5.
33. Emsley R, Myburgh C, Oosthuizen P, van Rensburg SJ. Randomized, placebo-controlled study of ethyl-eicosapentaenoic acid as supplemental treatment in schizophrenia. Am J Psychiatry. 2002;159:1596–8.
34. Emsley R, Niehaus DJ, Koen L, Oosthuizen PP, Turner HJ, Carey P, van Rensburg SJ, Maritz JS, Murck H. The effects of eicosapentaenoic acid in tardive dyskinesia: a randomized, placebo-controlled trial. Schizophr Res. 2006;84:112–20.
35. Fenton WS, Dickerson F, Boronow J, Hibbeln JR, Knable M. A placebo-controlled trial of omega-3 fatty acid (ethyl eicosapentaenoic acid) supplementation for residual symptoms and cognitive impairment in schizophrenia. Am J Psychiatry. 2001;158:2071–4.
36. Jamilian H, Solhi H, Jamilian M. Randomized, placebo-controlled clinical trial of omega-3 as supplemental treatment in schizophrenia. Global J Health Sci. 2014;6:103–8.
37. Pawelczyk T, Grancow-Grabka M, Kotlicka-Antczak M, Trafalska E, Pawelczyk A. A randomized controlled study of the efficacy of six-month supplementation with concentrated fish oil rich in omega-3 polyunsaturated fatty acids in first episode schizophrenia. J Psychiatr Res. 2016;73:34–44.
38. Peet M, Brind J, Ramchand CN, Shah S, Vankar GK. Two double-blind placebo-controlled pilot studies of eicosapentaenoic acid in the treatment of schizophrenia. Schizophr Res. 2001;49:243–51.
39. Peet M, Horrobin DF. A dose-ranging exploratory study of the effects of ethyl-eicosapentaenoate in patients with persistent schizophrenic symptoms. J Psychiatr Res. 2002;36:7–18.
40. Medina-Estrada I, Alva-Murillo N, Lopez-Meza JE, Ochoa-Zarzosa A. Immunomodulatory effects of 17beta-estradiol on epithelial cells during bacterial infections. J Immunol Res. 2018;2018:6098961.
41. Liu X, Fan XL, Zhao Y, Luo GR, Li XP, Li R, Le WD. Estrogen provides neuroprotection against activated microglia-induced dopaminergic neuronal injury through both estrogen receptor-alpha and estrogen receptor-beta in microglia. J Neurosci Res. 2005;81:653–65.
42. Akhondzadeh S, Nejatisafa AA, Amini H, Mohammadi MR, Larijani B, Kashani L, Raisi F, Kamalipour A. Adjunctive estrogen treatment in women with chronic schizophrenia: a double-blind, randomized, and placebo-controlled trial. Prog Neuro-Psychopharmacol Biol Psychiatry. 2003;27:1007–12.
43. Ghafari E, Fararouie M, Shirazi HG, Farhangfar A, Ghaderi F, Mohammadi A. Combination of estrogen and antipsychotics in the treatment of women with chronic schizophrenia: a double-blind, randomized, placebo-controlled clinical trial. Clin Schizophr Relat Psychoses. 2013;6:172–6.
44. Khodaie-Ardakani MR, Khosravi M, Zarinfard R, Nejati S, Mohsenian A, Tabrizi M, Akhondzadeh S. A placebo-controlled study of raloxifene added to risperidone in men with chronic schizophrenia. Acta Med Iran. 2015;53:337–45.
45. Kianimehr G, Fatehi F, Hashempoor S, Khodaei-Ardakani MR, Rezaei F, Nazari A, Kashani L, Akhondzadeh S. Raloxifene adjunctive therapy for postmenopausal women suffering from chronic schizophrenia: a randomized double-blind and placebo controlled trial. Daru. 2014;22:55.
46. Kulkarni J, de Castella A, Fitzgerald PB, Gurvich CT, Bailey M, Bartholomeusz C, Burger H. Estrogen in severe mental illness: a potential new treatment approach. Arch Gen Psychiatry. 2008;65:955–60.

47. Kulkarni J, de Castella A, Headey B, Marston N, Sinclair K, Lee S, Gurvich C, Fitzgerald PB, Burger H. Estrogens and men with schizophrenia: is there a case for adjunctive therapy? Schizophr Res. 2011;125:278–83.
48. Kulkarni J, Gavrilidis E, Gwini SM, Worsley R, Grigg J, Warren A, Gurvich C, Gilbert H, Berk M, Davis SR. Effect of adjunctive Raloxifene therapy on severity of refractory schizophrenia in women: a randomized clinical trial. JAMA Psychiat. 2016;73:947–54.
49. Kulkarni J, Riedel A, de Castella AR, Fitzgerald PB, Rolfe TJ, Taffe J, Burger H. Estrogen - a potential treatment for schizophrenia. Schizophr Res. 2001;48:137–44.
50. Louza MR, Marques AP, Elkis H, Bassitt D, Diegoli M, Gattaz WF. Conjugated estrogens as adjuvant therapy in the treatment of acute schizophrenia: a double-blind study. Schizophr Res. 2004;66:97–100.
51. Usall J, Huerta-Ramos E, Labad J, Cobo J, Nunez C, Creus M, Pares GG, Cuadras D, Franco J, Miquel E, Reyes JC, Roca M. Raloxifene as an adjunctive treatment for postmenopausal women with schizophrenia: a 24-week double-blind, randomized, parallel, placebo-controlled trial. Schizophr Bull. 2016;42:309–17.
52. Weiser M, Levi L, Burshtein S, Hagin M, Matei VP, Podea D, Miclutia I, Tiugan A, Pacala B, Grecu IG, Noy A, Zamora D, Davis JM. Raloxifene plus antipsychotics versus placebo plus antipsychotics in severely ill decompensated postmenopausal women with schizophrenia or schizoaffective disorder: a randomized controlled trial. J Clin Psychiatry. 2017;78: e758–65.
53. Favero G, Franceschetti L, Bonomini F, Rodella LF, Rezzani R. Melatonin as an anti-inflammatory agent modulating inflammasome activation. Int J Endocrinol. 2017;2017:1835195.
54. Modabbernia A, Heidari P, Soleimani R, Sobhani A, Roshan ZA, Taslimi S, Ashrafi M, Modabbernia MJ. Melatonin for prevention of metabolic side-effects of olanzapine in patients with first-episode schizophrenia: randomized double-blind placebo-controlled study. J Psychiatr Res. 2014;53:133–40.
55. Watabe M, Kato TA, Monji A, Horikawa H, Kanba S. Does minocycline, an antibiotic with inhibitory effects on microglial activation, sharpen a sense of trust in social interaction? Psychopharmacology. 2012;220:551–7.
56. Chaudhry IB, Hallak J, Husain N, Minhas F, Stirling J, Richardson P, Dursun S, Dunn G, Deakin B. Minocycline benefits negative symptoms in early schizophrenia: a randomised double-blind placebo-controlled clinical trial in patients on standard treatment. J Psychopharmacol (Oxford, England). 2012;26:1185–93.
57. Chaves C, Marque CR, Maia-de-Oliveira JP, Wichert-Ana L, Ferrari TB, Santos AC, Araujo D, Machado-de-Sousa JP, Bressan RA, Elkis H, Crippa JA, Guimaraes FS, Zuardi AW, Baker GB, Dursun SM, Hallak JE. Effects of minocycline add-on treatment on brain morphometry and cerebral perfusion in recent-onset schizophrenia. Schizophr Res. 2015;161:439–45.
58. Deakin B, Suckling J, Barnes TRE, Byrne K, Chaudhry IB, Dazzan P, Drake RJ, Giordano A, Husain N, Jones PB, Joyce E, Knox E, Krynicki C, Lawrie SM, Lewis S, Lisiecka-Ford DM, Nikkheslat N, Pariante CM, Smallman R, Watson A, Williams SCR, Upthegrove R, Dunn G. The benefit of minocycline on negative symptoms of schizophrenia in patients with recent-onset psychosis (BeneMin): a randomised, double-blind, placebo-controlled trial. Lancet Psychiatry. 2018;5:885–94.
59. Ghanizadeh A, Dehbozorgi S, OmraniSigaroodi M, Rezaei Z. Minocycline as add-on treatment decreases the negative symptoms of schizophrenia; a randomized placebo-controlled clinical trial. Recent Patents Inflamm Allergy Drug Discov. 2014;8:211–5.
60. Kelly DL, Sullivan KM, McEvoy JP, McMahon RP, Wehring HJ, Gold JM, Liu F, Warfel D, Vyas G, Richardson CM, Fischer BA, Keller WR, Koola MM, Feldman SM, Russ JC, Keefe RS, Osing J, Hubzin L, August S, Walker TM, Buchanan RW. Adjunctive minocycline in clozapine-treated schizophrenia patients with persistent symptoms. J Clin Psychopharmacol. 2015;35:374–81.
61. Khodaie-Ardakani MR, Mirshafiee O, Farokhnia M, Tajdini M, Hosseini SM, Modabbernia A, Rezaei F, Salehi B, Yekehtaz H, Ashrafi M, Tabrizi M, Akhondzadeh S. Minocycline add-on to

risperidone for treatment of negative symptoms in patients with stable schizophrenia: randomized double-blind placebo-controlled study. Psychiatry Res. 2014;215:540–6.
62. Levkovitz Y, Mendlovich S, Riwkes S, Braw Y, Levkovitch-Verbin H, Gal G, Fennig S, Treves I, Kron S. A double-blind, randomized study of minocycline for the treatment of negative and cognitive symptoms in early-phase schizophrenia. J Clin Psychiatry. 2010;71:138–49.
63. Liu F, Guo X, Wu R, Ou J, Zheng Y, Zhang B, Xie L, Zhang L, Yang L, Yang S, Yang J, Ruan Y, Zeng Y, Xu X, Zhao J. Minocycline supplementation for treatment of negative symptoms in early-phase schizophrenia: a double blind, randomized, controlled trial. Schizophr Res. 2014;153:169–76.
64. Weiser M, Levi L, Burshtein S, Chirita R, Cirjaliu D, Gonen I, Yolken R, Davidson M, Zamora D, Davis JM. The effect of minocycline on symptoms in schizophrenia: results from a randomized controlled trial. Schizophr Res. 2018;206:325–32.
65. Zhang L, Zheng H, Wu R, Zhu F, Kosten TR, Zhang XY, Zhao J. Minocycline adjunctive treatment to risperidone for negative symptoms in schizophrenia: association with pro-inflammatory cytokine levels. Prog Neuro-Psychopharmacol Biol Psychiatry. 2018;85:69–76.
66. Palacio JR, Markert UR, Martinez P. Anti-inflammatory properties of N-acetylcysteine on lipopolysaccharide-activated macrophages. Inflamm Res. 2011;60:695–704.
67. Farr SA, Poon HF, Dogrukol-Ak D, Drake J, Banks WA, Eyerman E, Butterfield DA, Morley JE. The antioxidants alpha-lipoic acid and N-acetylcysteine reverse memory impairment and brain oxidative stress in aged SAMP8 mice. J Neurochem. 2003;84:1173–83.
68. Berk M, Copolov D, Dean O, Lu K, Jeavons S, Schapkaitz I, Anderson-Hunt M, Judd F, Katz F, Katz P, Ording-Jespersen S, Little J, Conus P, Cuenod M, Do KQ, Bush AI. N-acetyl cysteine as a glutathione precursor for schizophrenia—a double-blind, randomized, placebo-controlled trial. Biol Psychiatry. 2008;64:361–8.
69. Breier A, Liffick E, Hummer TA, Vohs JL, Yang Z, Mehdiyoun NF, Visco AC, Metzler E, Zhang Y, Francis MM. Effects of 12-month, double-blind N-acetyl cysteine on symptoms, cognition and brain morphology in early phase schizophrenia spectrum disorders. Schizophr Res. 2018;199:395–402.
70. Farokhnia M, Azarkolah A, Adinehfar F, Khodaie-Ardakani MR, Hosseini SM, Yekehtaz H, Tabrizi M, Rezaei F, Salehi B, Sadeghi SM, Moghadam M, Gharibi F, Mirshafiee O, Akhondzadeh S. N-acetylcysteine as an adjunct to risperidone for treatment of negative symptoms in patients with chronic schizophrenia: a randomized, double-blind, placebo-controlled study. Clin Neuropharmacol. 2013;36:185–92.
71. Sepehrmanesh Z, Heidary M, Akasheh N, Akbari H, Heidary M. Therapeutic effect of adjunctive N-acetyl cysteine (NAC) on symptoms of chronic schizophrenia: a double-blind, randomized clinical trial. Prog Neuro-Psychopharmacol Biol Psychiatry. 2018;82:289–96.
72. Zhang J-H, Chen B, Jian-Rui L. Treatment effect of risperidone alone and combined with N-acetly-cysteine for first-episode schizophenic patients [Chinese article]. J Clin Psychiatry. 2015;25:394–6.
73. Iranpour N, Zandifar A, Farokhnia M, Goguol A, Yekehtaz H, Khodaie-Ardakani MR, Salehi B, Esalatmanesh S, Zeionoddini A, Mohammadinejad P, Zeinoddini A, Akhondzadeh S. The effects of pioglitazone adjuvant therapy on negative symptoms of patients with chronic schizophrenia: a double-blind and placebo-controlled trial. Hum Psychopharmacol. 2016;31:103–12.
74. Grommes C, Karlo JC, Caprariello A, Blankenship D, Dechant A, Landreth GE. The PPARgamma agonist pioglitazone crosses the blood-brain barrier and reduces tumor growth in a human xenograft model. Cancer Chemother Pharmacol. 2013;71:929–36.
75. Brust P. Reversal of scopolamine-induced alterations of choline transport across the blood-brain barrier by the nootropics piracetam and pramiracetam. Arzneimittelforschung. 1989;39:1220–2.
76. Noorbala AA, Akhondzadeh S, Davari-Ashtiani R, Amini-Nooshabadi H. Piracetam in the treatment of schizophrenia: implications for the glutamate hypothesis of schizophrenia. J Clin Pharm Ther. 1999;24:369–74.

77. Khan B, Ahmad SF, Bani S, Kaul A, Suri KA, Satti NK, Athar M, Qazi GN. Augmentation and proliferation of T lymphocytes and Th-1 cytokines by Withania somnifera in stressed mice. Int Immunopharmacol. 2006;6:1394–403.
78. Mulabagal V, Subbaraju GV, Rao CV, Sivaramakrishna C, Dewitt DL, Holmes D, Sung B, Aggarwal BB, Tsay HS, Nair MG. Withanolide sulfoxide from Aswagandha roots inhibits nuclear transcription factor-kappa-B, cyclooxygenase and tumor cell proliferation. Phytother Res. 2009;23:987–92.
79. Chengappa KNR, Brar JS, Gannon JM, Schlicht PJ. Adjunctive use of a standardized extract of Withania somnifera (Ashwagandha) to treat symptom exacerbation in schizophrenia: a randomized, double-blind, placebo-controlled study. J Clin Psychiatry. 2018;79
80. Kumar G, Patnaik R. Exploring neuroprotective potential of Withania somnifera phytochemicals by inhibition of GluN2B-containing NMDA receptors: an in silico study. Med Hypotheses. 2016;92:35–43.
81. Howes OD, McCutcheon R. Inflammation and the neural diathesis-stress hypothesis of schizophrenia: a reconceptualization. Transl Psychiatry. 2017;7:e1024. https://doi.org/10.1038/tp.2016.278. PMID: 28170004; PMCID: PMC5438023.
82. Kahn RS, Keefe RS. Schizophrenia is a cognitive illness: time for a change in focus. JAMA Psychiat. 2013;70:1107–12.
83. O'Dell JR, Haire CE, Palmer W, Drymalski W, Wees S, Blakely K, Churchill M, Eckhoff PJ, Weaver A, Doud D, Erikson N, Dietz F, Olson R, Maloley P, Klassen LW, Moore GF. Treatment of early rheumatoid arthritis with minocycline or placebo: results of a randomized, double-blind, placebo-controlled trial. Arthritis Rheum. 1997;40:842–8.
84. Sanchez MG, Morissette M, Di Paolo T. Effect of a chronic treatment with 17beta-estradiol on striatal dopamine neurotransmission and the Akt/GSK3 signaling pathway in the brain of ovariectomized monkeys. Psychoneuroendocrinology. 2012;37:280–91.
85. Inta D, Lang UE, Borgwardt S, Meyer-Lindenberg A, Gass P. Microglia activation and schizophrenia: lessons from the effects of minocycline on postnatal neurogenesis, neuronal survival and synaptic pruning. Schizophr Bull. 2017;43:493–6.
86. Adomaityte J, Farooq M, Qayyum R. Effect of raloxifene therapy on venous thromboembolism in postmenopausal women. A meta-analysis. Thromb Haemost. 2008;99:338–42.
87. Barrett-Connor E, Mosca L, Collins P, Geiger MJ, Grady D, Kornitzer M, McNabb MA, Wenger NK. Effects of raloxifene on cardiovascular events and breast cancer in postmenopausal women. N Engl J Med. 2006;355:125–37.
88. Bentsen H, Landro NI. Neurocognitive effects of an omega-3 fatty acid and vitamins E+C in schizophrenia: a randomised controlled trial. Prostaglandins Leukot Essent Fatty Acids. 2018;136:57–66.
89. Gipson CD. Treating addiction: unraveling the relationship between N-acetylcysteine, glial glutamate transport, and behavior. Biol Psychiatry. 2016;80:e11–2.
90. Schwarz E, van Beveren NJ, Ramsey J, Leweke FM, Rothermundt M, Bogerts B, Steiner J, Guest PC, Bahn S. Identification of subgroups of schizophrenia patients with changes in either immune or growth factor and hormonal pathways. Schizophr Bull. 2014;40:787–95.
91. Upthegrove R, Manzanares-Teson N, Barnes NM. Cytokine function in medication-naive first episode psychosis: a systematic review and meta-analysis. Schizophr Res. 2014;155:101–8.
92. van Beveren NJ, Schwarz E, Noll R, Guest PC, Meijer C, de Haan L, Bahn S. Evidence for disturbed insulin and growth hormone signaling as potential risk factors in the development of schizophrenia. Transl Psychiatry. 2014;4:e430.

Immunomodulation of Resistant Depression

23

Djamila Bennabi and Emmanuel Haffen

23.1 Introduction

Depressive disorders are a severe and impairing psychiatric illness, directly accounting for 4.4% of disease burden worldwide and 7.2% in the European Union [1]. Major depressive disorder (MDD) is a predominantly recurrent disorder, as 50–80% of patients who have received psychiatric care for an episode of major depression have at least one more episode and a median of four episodes in a lifetime. In addition to frequent psychiatric comorbidity, co-occurring medical conditions are also common, leading to greater severity, disability and poorer treatment response [2, 3]. Moreover, approximately 20–30% of patients with MDD develop a chronic course of their disease, resulting in decreased quality of life and increased care utilisation and costs [2, 3]. Despite the progress in pharmacopoeia, it has been estimated that more than one-third of MDD patients do not respond satisfactorily to initial and subsequent antidepressant treatments, including combinations of pharmacotherapy and psychotherapy [4, 5]. Treatment-resistant depression (TRD), defined as the failure of at least two attempts of antidepressant treatment administered sequentially at an adequate dose and duration, increases the burden of the disease and the resulting costs [6]. Several factors have been related to a poor response to antidepressant treatment, including psychosocial factors, severity and duration of the current depressive episode, psychiatric and somatic comorbidities and biological factors [7–9]. Taken together, all these considerations underlie the particular relevance for

D. Bennabi
Service de Psychiatrie, CIC-1431 INSERM, CHU de Besançon, Besançon cedex, France
e-mail: djamila.bennabi@univ-fcomte.fr

E. Haffen (✉)
Integrative Research Laboratory in Neurosciences and Psychology Cognitive - UR LINC, UFC, UBFC, Besançon, France
e-mail: emmanuel.haffen@univ-fcomte.fr

M. Berk et al. (eds.), *Immuno-Psychiatry*, https://doi.org/10.1007/978-3-030-71229-7_23

the determination of contributing factors and the necessity of implementation of alternative therapeutic options.

The involvement of inflammatory processes and brain-immune interactions in the pathogenesis, course and treatment of MDD has received increased attention over the last 20 years [10, 11]. Elevations in proinflammatory mediators have been repeatedly shown to produce effects on key processes such as impairment of hippocampal (HC) neuroplasticity, induction of glucocorticoid insensitivity of the hypothalamic-pituitary-adrenal axis (HPA), increase of oxidative stress in the HC, reduction of serotonin levels and creation of neurotoxic serotonergic metabolites (i.e., 3-hydroxykynurenine and quinolinic acid) [12]. Activation of astrocytes and microglial cells and disruption of the blood-brain barrier have similarly been implicated in the pathophysiology of depression through anti-neuroplastic, pro-oxidative and pro-inflammatory effects [13, 14]. The role of inflammation has also been emphasised in TRD. Especially, preliminary evidence indicates that treatment resistance could imply dysregulated inflammatory activity and that high inflammation might be a predictor of poor clinical response to pharmacological treatment. Moreover, levels of inflammation might be modifiable with antidepressant treatment and some types of anti-inflammatory treatments can produce antidepressant effects in depressed patients with peripheral blood evidence of inflammation [15–17]. Accordingly, a neuroimmune model of depression has been proposed and immunomodulatory therapies have been studied in patients with MDD.

23.2 Inflammation, Resistance and Prediction of Outcome

Evidence indicates that treatment resistance might be associated with dysregulated inflammatory activity. A broad inflammatory state, including high levels of Th1 and Th2 cytokines and chemokines, has been reported in TRD in comparison to non-TRD patients and healthy controls [17, 18]. This immune dysregulation is thought to represent a common link between treatment resistance and other core elements of TRD, such as physical illness or poor physical health [19, 20], chronicity and/or recurrence of depressive illness [19], cognitive impairment [21] or early life trauma [17, 22]. It has also been proposed that the multiple effects of inflammation on neurotransmission and neurogenesis may in part serve to explain the resistance to antidepressants in patients with increased inflammation.

Exploring the unique immune-modulatory effects of antidepressant classes is critical to further developing innovative treatment approaches. Antidepressants, especially selective serotonin reuptake inhibitors (SSRIs), are now considered to exert some of their neurobiological effects via the immune system [23]. The most prominent effects of antidepressants comprised a decline in blood levels of IL-1β, IL-6 and (partially) TNF-α [16, 23]. For example, a meta-analysis of 22 studies indicated that SSRIs may reduce the level of IL-1β, IL6 and TNF-α, without reducing cytokine levels [23]. It has been suggested that while noradrenalin reuptake inhibitor antidepressants suppress Th1-type cytokines and shift the balance towards humoral immunity, SSRIs reduce the production of Th2-type cytokines and shift the balance towards a cellular immune response. The immunomodulatory effects of conventional antidepressants might also implicate other cell populations including a transient increase in the circulating T cell population, an increased circulating B cell population, and an increased number of NK cells [24, 25].

Concerning the question as to whether inflammatory marker levels at baseline may predict treatment outcome, a data trend towards a relationship between the grade of inflammation, the antidepressant applied and the therapeutic outcome has been observed. High baseline levels of IL-12p70, IL-6, IL-8 and TNF-α have been associated with poorer treatment outcomes in samples of TRD patients [12, 16]. Moreover, elevated post-treatment C-reactive protein (CRP), IL-6 and monocyte chemoattractant protein-4 (MCP4) predicted poorer long-term and physical health outcomes in depressed patients [17, 26]. An open-label trial by Uher and colleagues [27] demonstrated that the CRP level at baseline differentially predicted treatment outcome with escitalopram and nortriptyline, with a better response to escitalopram in those patients with low levels of CRP (<1 mg/L) and a better response to nortriptyline when serum levels of CRP were higher. A direct comparison of immune effects of SSRIs and SNRIs conducted by Yoshimura demonstrated that plasma IL-6 level, but not plasma TNF-α level, was higher in SSRI-refractory than SSRI-responsive depressed patients, and higher in SNRI-refractory than SNRI-responsive depressed patients [28].

23.3 Immunomodulatory Strategies in Treatment-Resistant Depression

23.3.1 Cytokine Inhibitors

Treatments with monoclonal antibodies represent a promising therapeutic approach in TRD, though associated with the risk of potentially serious side effects [15]. An interesting study conducted by Raison and colleagues suggests that TNF-α antagonists may hold promise for the treatment of resistant depression in individuals with elevated peripheral inflammatory activity [29]. In this double-blind, placebo-controlled trial testing infliximab, 60 medically healthy adults with TRD were randomised to either receive three infusions of infliximab (5 mg/kg) or three saline infusions at baseline, week 2 and week 6. Although there was no significant difference in change in depressive symptoms between treatment groups, an exploratory analysis focusing on patients with a baseline CRP concentration greater than 5 mg/L revealed a treatment response (50% reduction in HAM-D score) of 62% in infliximab-treated patients versus 33% in placebo group [29]. Conversely, in patients with CRP <5 mg/L, the treatment response was 41% for the infliximab group and 57% for the placebo group. For patients with a baseline CRP >5 mg/L, the effect size observed was 0.41, which is in line with the efficacy of standard antidepressants compared to placebo. Nevertheless, because the test of the a priori hypothesis in this study was negative, the question has remained as to whether targeting TNF-α via large molecules introduced in the periphery alone can produce an antidepressant effect, or whether therapies that reduce TNF-α signalling must instead directly engage targets in the CNS [30].

It is also suggested that reducing the levels of TNF-α improves sleep alterations in a subset of patients. In 36 patients with TRD, Weinberger and colleagues measured sleep parameters at baseline and 2 weeks after three infusions (week 8) of either the TNF-α antagonist infliximab (n = 19) or placebo (n = 17); the authors observed an increase in sleep efficiency in infliximab-treated patients with high inflammation (CRP >5 mg/L) (n = 9) [31]. Like infliximab, etanercept is another TNF-α antagonist that may even be useful as a monotherapy for depression. However, its application as monotherapy in two patients suffering from TRD revealed equivocal antidepressant effects [32]. Notwithstanding, a meta-analysis of seven randomised controlled trials (RCTs) showed a significant antidepressant effect of anti-cytokine treatments in 2370 patients with chronic inflammatory conditions with a small-to-moderate size effect [33]. These results suggest that anti-cytokine drugs may be particularly effective in TRD patients with increased inflammation.

23.3.2 Non-steroidal Anti-Inflammatory Drugs (NSAIDs)

The targeting of inflammatory signalling pathways has also been suggested as an interesting strategy to improve the responsiveness of unipolar depressive patients. The administration of pharmacological agents that inhibit cyclo-oxygenase (COX), the enzyme that converts arachidonic acid into prostaglandin, is the most common approach in this regard. Prostaglandins have been shown to be increased in depression and are known to exert an important role in the inflammatory response. A meta-analysis of 14 studies conducted by Köhler and colleagues emphasised the antidepressant properties of the selective COX-2 inhibitor celecoxib in monotherapy on remission and response, without increased risks of adverse effects [34]. Augmentation with COX-2 inhibitors has been studied in MDD with promising results. To date, celecoxib at a daily dose of 400 mg/day as an add-on therapy to antidepressants was found to improve depressive outcomes in three RCTs (compared to reboxetine 4 mg/day, and fluoxetine 40 mg/day, sertraline 200 mg/day; N = 40 for each RCT) [35–37]. Interestingly, in the study by Müller and colleagues, the ratio of kynurenine to tryptophan, which reflects the activity of the pro-inflammatory cytokine-driven enzyme Indoleamine 2,3-Dioxygenase (IDO), predicted the antidepressant response to celecoxib [37].

A pharmacovigilance study (n = 1528) reported a positive association between chronic exposure to NSAIDs (excluding COX-2 inhibitors and salicylates) and poorer antidepressant outcomes after adjustment for comorbidities and sociodemographic variables [38]. Interestingly, resistance to antidepressant treatment was not related to the use of COX-2 inhibitors and salicylates alone. It was stressed that authors were not able to adjust the association with medical conditions and suggested avoiding classical NSAIDs in patients with depression and to prefer other inflammatory mechanism-related actions such as COX-2 inhibitors and salicylates among these patients. Based on these data, it seems that an add-on strategy with NSAIDs might be a good strategy in MDD, even though additional studies with larger sample size effects including the measurement of immunological biomarkers are necessary in TRD patients.

23.3.3 Minocycline

Minocycline, a tetracycline derivative, has effects on multiple interacting systems that are thought to be involved in the pathophysiology of depression due to its anti-inflammatory, anti-oxidant and anti-apoptotic effects, as well as on the modulation of glutamate and monoamine neurotransmission [39, 40]. Studies in animal models have shown that minocycline administration decreases glutamate-induced neurotoxicity and has antidepressant-like properties [41]. There is also some preliminary evidence suggesting that minocycline augmentation of antidepressant treatment is effective in psychotic unipolar depression [42]. In a multi-site, 12-week, double-blind, placebo-controlled, pilot trial, Husain and colleagues examined the efficacy of minocycline (200 mg daily) as an adjunct to treatment as usual (TAU) in 41 patients with treatment-resistant MDD [43]. A large improvement in depressive symptoms was observed in the minocycline group compared to the placebo group, with an effect size of 1.21. Although these results seem promising, studies with larger sample sizes and longer follow-up periods are required before minocycline can be recommended for routine clinical use. Moreover, the measurement of inflammatory cytokines such as IL-6 and TNF-α, amongst others, is necessary to determine the association between changes in inflammatory biomarkers and improvement in depressive symptoms.

23.3.4 Ketamine

The *N*-methyl-D-aspartate (NMDA) receptor antagonist ketamine has rapid antidepressant effects, with potential application in TRD and suicidal ideation. Assumed modes of action range from the inhibition of NMDA receptors, activation of AMPA (α-amino-3-hydroxy-5-methyl-4-isoxazolepropionic acid) receptors and molecular signalling through mTOR (the mammalian target of rapamycin), which result in enhanced expression of hippocampal brain-derived neurotrophic factor (BDNF) and increased synaptogenesis. Further anti-inflammatory properties have been found, i.e. reduced release of pro-inflammatory cytokines like TNF-α and IL-6 in TRD. Especially, Park and colleagues observed that baseline cytokine levels and changes in the cytokine levels, including IL-6 and TNF-α, at 230 min after ketamine infusion were not related to a positive antidepressant response in TRD [44]. Kiraly and colleagues obtained similar results in 33 patients suffering from TRD, despite a significant decrease in the levels of IL-6 and IL-1α compared to baseline values [45]. These findings support the idea that ketamine rapidly modulates proinflammatory cytokines, but that this modulation is not the primary mechanism involved in its rapid antidepressant effects in TRD [44].

23.3.5 Non-pharmacological Anti-inflammatory Strategies

Some non-pharmacological treatments used in TRD in monotherapy or as add-on strategies have demonstrated anti-inflammatory effects. Electroconvulsive therapy (ECT) is recognised as an effective strategy in the treatment of TRD, even though the cerebral mechanisms underlying its effects remain unclear. Mounting evidence from both animals and human studies suggest that ECT influences the immuno-inflammatory cascade that is activated during MDD [46]. An acute and transient immune activation with an increase of pro-inflammatory cytokines has been reported immediately following an ECT session, whereas repetitive ECT treatment results in long-term down-regulation of immune activation. ECT has been found to increase lipopolysaccharide-stimulated production of pro-inflammatory IL-6 and TNF-α, whereas cytokines with anti-inflammatory properties IL-4 and IL-10 were unaffected [47]. After an initial increase in these levels, repeated ECT led to a normalisation of TNF-α levels in depressed patients. Nevertheless, it is unclear whether such a normalisation results from a direct suppressive effect of the treatment on the immune system or whether it is merely secondary to clinical remission [48]. Inflammatory processes have also been implicated in the action of deep brain stimulation (DBS), as the positive effects have been linked to regional inflammation, which was temporally correlated with elevations in glial fibrillary acidic protein (GFAP) immunoreactivity [49]. Interestingly, this study suggested that the use of anti-inflammatory drugs after electrode implantation may attenuate the early anti-depressive response in DBS patients.

Transcranial direct current stimulation (tDCS) has also been explored as a non-pharmacological treatment for depression. While data for TRD are unavailable, Brunoni and colleagues observed in 236 depressed patients that plasma levels of nerve growth factor predicted early depression improvement for tDCS versus escitalopram, while other biomarkers (i.e. IL-1ß, IL-6, IL-8, IL-10, IL-12p70, IL-18, IL-33, TNF-α), and its soluble receptors sTNFr1 and sTNFr2) did not significantly predict treatment improvement [50].

Other non-pharmacological therapeutic approaches, such as exercise and mind-body therapies (MBTs) have been described as able to regulate emotional and affective response to stress and therefore influence the immune system in MDD. MBTs may lead to a decrease in CRP levels [51], and regular endurance exercise has been found to decrease inflammatory markers, mainly CRP [52] with further effects on tryptophan availability, thereby influencing the kynurenine pathway [53]. In addition, high baseline levels of TNF-α have been found to predict better outcomes with exercise treatment as opposed to antidepressant medications, for which high TNF-α is linked to a poor response [54]. Harley and colleagues [55] pooled an antidepressant randomised controlled trial (RCT) and a psychological intervention RCT for MDD and reported that elevated CRP predicted a greater non-response to interpersonal psychotherapy or cognitive behavioural therapy (CBT) but a good response to nortriptyline or fluoxetine.

23.4 Discussion

Mounting evidence has demonstrated that immune processes, both within the central nervous system and the periphery of the body, play a central role in the pathogenesis, course and treatment of depression. Immunomodulatory therapies represent one of the most interesting therapeutic alternatives in MDD, especially for patients with an immunological deregulation profile and/or treatment resistance to conventional therapy. Heightened inflammation has been associated with a poor response to psychological intervention [55], a good response to anti-inflammatory agents [29, 56] and a poorer response to antidepressants, albeit with mixed findings [16]. However, there is currently insufficient evidence to support a personalised treatment selection strategy based on inflammatory markers and to recommend the clinical use of any particular agent in TRD. Firstly, current studies are limited by small sample sizes, poorly defined illness durations or variation in the definition of TRD, which makes it impossible to provide recommendations on the routine clinical use of immunomodulatory therapies. Secondly, many of the factors often present in TRD complicate the interpretation of the inflammation literature, including the intake of multiple medications, prolonged illnesses and comorbidities. Thirdly, the immune mechanism leading to pro-inflammatory activation in MD, and possibly to resistance, remain unclear and need to be elucidated.

Due to the paucity of research focusing specifically on well-established TRD, a better characterisation of immunological dysregulation in these patients is necessary. Immune analyses, conducted at baseline and at the end of each line of treatment, could help to stratify patient groups based on their immune profile and to tailor treatment selection.

Other agents with anti-inflammatory activity are promising approaches in the field of MDD. Supplemental polyunsaturated fatty acids (PUFAs), nutraceuticals like zinc and omega-3 fatty acids or curcumin have been shown to have beneficial effects on depression due to their ability to modulate immunity [57]. Statins [58] and the antidiabetic drug pioglitazone [59] have all been proposed as agents with supposed antidepressant and anti-inflammatory properties.

More research is also needed to identify specific treatment strategies via targeted modulation of the gut microbiome, in line with recent data showing therapeutic benefits of supplementing with probiotics containing *Lactobacillus* and *Bifidobacterium* [60, 61]. The range of antidepressants may increase in the future if promising initial data on other drug targets such as toll-like receptor inhibitors or glycogen synthase kinase-3 inhibitors are verified in upcoming clinical trials [15].

23.5 Conclusion

While the currently published evidence strongly advocates for the development of novel pharmacological and behavioural strategies that target the immune system, prospective studies on the efficacy of anti-inflammatory treatment that combines the evaluation of depressive symptoms with the quantification of inflammatory biomarkers are needed before these alternative approaches can be applied in clinical practice. Well-designed clinical trials are still required in order to better identify the most appropriate strategies in TRD. The implementation of such variables in clinical practice could assist in guiding optimal care targeting specific vulnerable subgroups and planning short- and long-term treatments through relevant staging models.

References

1. Murray CJL, Vos T, Lozano R, Naghavi M, Flaxman AD, Michaud C, Ezzati M, et al. Disability-adjusted life years (DALYs) for 291 diseases and injuries in 21 regions, 1990-2010: a systematic analysis for the global burden of disease study 2010. Lancet (London, England). 2012;380(9859):2197–223. https://doi.org/10.1016/S0140-6736(12)61689-4.
2. Gilmer WS, Trivedi MH, Rush AJ, Wisniewski SR, Luther J, Howland RH, Yohanna D, Khan A, Alpert J. Factors associated with chronic depressive episodes: a preliminary report from the STAR-D project. Acta Psychiatr Scand. 2005;112(6):425–33. https://doi.org/10.1111/j.1600-0447.2005.00633.x.
3. Murphy JA, Byrne GJ. Prevalence and correlates of the proposed DSM-5 diagnosis of chronic depressive disorder. J Affect Disord. 2012;139(2):172–80. https://doi.org/10.1016/j.jad.2012.01.033.
4. Rush AJ, Trivedi MH, Wisniewski SR, Nierenberg AA, Stewart JW, Warden D, Niederehe G, et al. Acute and longer-term outcomes in depressed outpatients requiring one or several treatment steps: a STAR*D report. Am J Psychiatry. 2006;163(11):1905–17. https://doi.org/10.1176/ajp.2006.163.11.1905.
5. Trivedi MH, John Rush A, Wisniewski SR, Nierenberg AA, Warden D, Ritz L, Norquist G, et al. Evaluation of outcomes with citalopram for depression using measurement-based care in STAR*D: implications for clinical practice. Am J Psychiatry. 2006;163(1):28–40. https://doi.org/10.1176/appi.ajp.163.1.28.
6. Brown S, Rittenbach K, Cheung S, McKean G, MacMaster FP, Clement F. Current and common definitions of treatment-resistant depression: findings from a systematic review and qualitative interviews. Can J Psychiatry. 2019;64(6):380–7. https://doi.org/10.1177/0706743719828965.
7. Balestri M, Calati R, Souery D, Kautzky A, Kasper S, Montgomery S, Zohar J, Mendlewicz J, Serretti A. Socio-demographic and clinical predictors of treatment resistant depression: a prospective European multicenter study. J Affect Disord. 2016;189:224–32. https://doi.org/10.1016/j.jad.2015.09.033.
8. Bennabi D, Aouizerate B, El-Hage W, Doumy O, Moliere F, Courtet P, Nieto I, et al. Risk factors for treatment resistance in unipolar depression: a systematic review. J Affect Disord. 2015;171:137–41. https://doi.org/10.1016/j.jad.2014.09.020.
9. Souery D, Oswald P, Massat I, Bailer U, Bollen J, Demyttenaere K, Kasper S, et al. Clinical factors associated with treatment resistance in major depressive disorder: results from a European multicenter study. J Clin Psychiatry. 2007;68(7):1062–70.
10. Dowlati Y, Herrmann N, Swardfager W, Liu H, Sham L, Reim EK, Lanctôt KL. A meta-analysis of cytokines in major depression. Biol Psychiatry. 2010;67(5):446–57. https://doi.org/10.1016/j.biopsych.2009.09.033.

11. Miller AH, Maletic V, Raison CL. Inflammation and its discontents: the role of cytokines in the pathophysiology of major depression. Biol Psychiatry. 2009;65(9):732–41. https://doi.org/10.1016/j.biopsych.2008.11.029.
12. Eyre HA, Lavretsky H, Kartika J, Qassim A, Baune BT. Modulatory effects of antidepressant classes on the innate and adaptive immune system in depression. Pharmacopsychiatry. 2016;49(3):85–96. https://doi.org/10.1055/s-0042-103159.
13. Eyre HA, Stuart MJ, Baune BT. A phase-specific neuroimmune model of clinical depression. Progress Neuro-Psychopharmacol Biol Psychiatry. 2014;54:265–74. https://doi.org/10.1016/j.pnpbp.2014.06.011.
14. Setiawan E, Wilson AA, Mizrahi R, Rusjan PM, Miler L, Rajkowska G, Suridjan I, et al. Role of translocator protein density, a marker of neuroinflammation, in the brain during major depressive episodes. JAMA Psychiat. 2015;72(3):268–75. https://doi.org/10.1001/jamapsychiatry.2014.2427.
15. Schmidt FM, Kirkby KC, Lichtblau N. Inflammation and immune regulation as potential drug targets in antidepressant treatment. Curr Neuropharmacol. 2016;14(7):674–87. https://doi.org/10.2174/1570159X14666160115130414.
16. Strawbridge R, Arnone D, Danese A, Papadopoulos A, Herane Vives A, Cleare AJ. Inflammation and clinical response to treatment in depression: a meta-analysis. Eur Neuropsychopharmacol. 2015;25(10):1532–43. https://doi.org/10.1016/j.euroneuro.2015.06.007.
17. Strawbridge R, Hodsoll J, Powell TR, Hotopf M, Hatch SL, Breen G, Cleare AJ. Inflammatory profiles of severe treatment-resistant depression. J Affect Disord. 2019;246:42–51. https://doi.org/10.1016/j.jad.2018.12.037.
18. Chamberlain SR, Cavanagh J, de Boer P, Mondelli V, Jones DNC, Drevets WC, Cowen PJ, et al. Treatment-resistant depression and peripheral C-reactive protein. Br J Psychiatry. 2019;214(1):11–9. https://doi.org/10.1192/bjp.2018.66.
19. Duivis HE, de Jonge P, Penninx BW, Na BY, Cohen BE, Whooley MA. Depressive symptoms, health behaviors, and subsequent inflammation in patients with coronary heart disease: prospective findings from the heart and soul study. Am J Psychiatry. 2011;168(9):913–20. https://doi.org/10.1176/appi.ajp.2011.10081163.
20. Maes M, Kubera M, Obuchowiczwa E, Goehler L, Brzeszcz J. Depression's multiple comorbidities explained by (neuro)inflammatory and oxidative & nitrosative stress pathways. Neuro Endocrinol Lett. 2011;32(1):7–24.
21. Allison DJ, Ditor DS. The common inflammatory etiology of depression and cognitive impairment: a therapeutic target. J Neuroinflamm. 2014;11:151. https://doi.org/10.1186/s12974-014-0151-1.
22. Danese A, McEwen BS. Adverse childhood experiences, allostasis, allostatic load, and age-related disease. Physiol Behav. 2012;106(1):29–39. https://doi.org/10.1016/j.physbeh.2011.08.019.
23. Hannestad J, DellaGioia N, Bloch M. The effect of antidepressant medication treatment on serum levels of inflammatory cytokines: a meta-analysis. Neuropsychopharmacology. 2011;36(12):2452–9. https://doi.org/10.1038/npp.2011.132.
24. Frank MG, Hendricks SE, Burke WJ, Johnson DR. Clinical response augments NK cell activity independent of treatment modality: a randomized double-blind placebo controlled antidepressant trial. Psychol Med. 2004;34(3):491–8.
25. Ravindran AV, Griffiths J, Merali Z, Anisman H. Lymphocyte subsets associated with major depression and dysthymia: modification by antidepressant treatment. Psychosom Med. 1995;57(6):555–63.
26. Ladwig K-H, Marten-Mittag B, Löwel H, Döring A, Koenig W, MONICA-KORA Augsburg Cohort Study 1984-1998. C-reactive protein, depressed mood, and the prediction of coronary heart disease in initially healthy men: results from the MONICA-KORA Augsburg cohort study 1984-1998. Eur Heart J. 2005;26(23):2537–42. https://doi.org/10.1093/eurheartj/ehi456.
27. Uher R, Tansey KE, Dew T, Maier W, Mors O, Hauser J, Dernovsek MZ, et al. An inflammatory biomarker as a differential predictor of outcome of depression treatment with escitalo-

pram and nortriptyline. Am J Psychiatry. 2014;171(12):1278–86. https://doi.org/10.1176/appi.ajp.2014.14010094.
28. Yoshimura R, Hori H, Ikenouchi-Sugita A, Umene-Nakano W, Ueda N, Nakamura J. Higher plasma interleukin-6 (IL-6) level is associated with SSRI- or SNRI-refractory depression. Prog Neuro-Psychopharmacol Biol Psychiatry. 2009;33(4):722–6. https://doi.org/10.1016/j.pnpbp.2009.03.020.
29. Raison CL, Rutherford RE, Woolwine BJ, Shuo C, Schettler P, Drake DF, Haroon E, Miller AH. A randomized controlled trial of the tumor necrosis factor antagonist infliximab for treatment-resistant depression: the role of baseline inflammatory biomarkers. JAMA Psychiat. 2013;70(1):31–41. https://doi.org/10.1001/2013.jamapsychiatry.4.
30. Bhattacharya A, Derecki NC, Lovenberg TW, Drevets WC. Role of neuro-immunological factors in the pathophysiology of mood disorders. Psychopharmacology. 2016;233(9):1623–36. https://doi.org/10.1007/s00213-016-4214-0.
31. Weinberger JF, Raison CL, Rye DB, Montague AR, Woolwine BJ, Felger JC, Haroon E, Miller AH. Inhibition of tumor necrosis factor improves sleep continuity in patients with treatment resistant depression and high inflammation. Brain Behav Immun. 2015;47:193–200. https://doi.org/10.1016/j.bbi.2014.12.016.
32. Schmidt FM, Kirkby KC, Himmerich H. The TNF-alpha inhibitor Etanercept as monotherapy in treatment-resistant depression - report of two cases. Psychiatr Danub. 2014;26(3):288–90.
33. Kappelmann N, Lewis G, Dantzer R, Jones PB, Khandaker GM. Antidepressant activity of anti-cytokine treatment: a systematic review and meta-analysis of clinical trials of chronic inflammatory conditions. Mol Psychiatry. 2018;23(2):335–43. https://doi.org/10.1038/mp.2016.167.
34. Köhler O, Benros ME, Nordentoft M, Farkouh ME, Iyengar RL, Mors O, Krogh J. Effect of anti-inflammatory treatment on depression, depressive symptoms, and adverse effects: a systematic review and meta-analysis of randomized clinical trials. JAMA Psychiat. 2014;71(12):1381–91. https://doi.org/10.1001/jamapsychiatry.2014.1611.
35. Abbasi S-H, Hosseini F, Modabbernia A, Ashrafi M, Akhondzadeh S. Effect of celecoxib add-on treatment on symptoms and serum IL-6 concentrations in patients with major depressive disorder: randomized double-blind placebo-controlled study. J Affect Disord. 2012;141(2–3):308–14. https://doi.org/10.1016/j.jad.2012.03.033.
36. Akhondzadeh S, Jafari S, Raisi F, Nasehi AA, Ghoreishi A, Salehi B, Mohebbi-Rasa S, Raznahan M, Kamalipour A. Clinical trial of adjunctive celecoxib treatment in patients with major depression: a double blind and placebo controlled trial. Depress Anxiety. 2009;26(7):607–11. https://doi.org/10.1002/da.20589.
37. Müller N, Schwarz MJ, Dehning S, Douhe A, Cerovecki A, Goldstein-Müller B, Spellmann I, et al. The cyclooxygenase-2 inhibitor celecoxib has therapeutic effects in major depression: results of a double-blind, randomized, placebo controlled, add-on pilot study to reboxetine. Mol Psychiatry. 2006;11(7):680–4. https://doi.org/10.1038/sj.mp.4001805.
38. Gallagher PJ, Castro V, Fava M, Weilburg JB, Murphy SN, Gainer VS, Churchill SE, et al. Antidepressant response in patients with major depression exposed to NSAIDs: a pharmacovigilance study. Am J Psychiatry. 2012;169(10):1065–72. https://doi.org/10.1176/appi.ajp.2012.11091325.
39. Hashimoto K, Ishima T. A novel target of action of minocycline in NGF-induced neurite outgrowth in PC12 cells: translation initiation [corrected] factor EIF4AI. PLoS One. 2010;5(11):e15430. https://doi.org/10.1371/journal.pone.0015430.
40. Soczynska JK, Mansur RB, Brietzke E, Swardfager W, Kennedy SH, Woldeyohannes HO, Powell AM, Manierka MS, McIntyre RS. Novel therapeutic targets in depression: minocycline as a candidate treatment. Behav Brain Res. 2012;235(2):302–17. https://doi.org/10.1016/j.bbr.2012.07.026.
41. Arakawa S, Shirayama Y, Fujita Y, Ishima T, Mao H, Muneoka K, Iyo M, Hashimoto K. Minocycline produced antidepressant-like effects on the learned helplessness rats with alterations in levels of monoamine in the amygdala and no changes in BDNF levels in the hippo-

campus at baseline. Pharmacol Biochem Behav. 2012;100(3):601–6. https://doi.org/10.1016/j.pbb.2011.09.008.
42. Miyaoka T, Wake R, Furuya M, Liaury K, Ieda M, Kawakami K, Tsuchie K, et al. Minocycline as adjunctive therapy for patients with unipolar psychotic depression: an open-label study. Prog Neuro-Psychopharmacol Biol Psychiatry. 2012;37(2):222–6. https://doi.org/10.1016/j.pnpbp.2012.02.002.
43. Husain MI, Chaudhry IB, Husain N, Khoso AB, Rahman RR, Hamirani MM, Hodsoll J, Qurashi I, Deakin JF, Young AH. Minocycline as an adjunct for treatment-resistant depressive symptoms: a pilot randomised placebo-controlled trial. J Psychopharmacol (Oxford, England). 2017a;31(9):1166–75. https://doi.org/10.1177/0269881117724352.
44. Park M, Newman LE, Gold PW, Luckenbaugh DA, Yuan P, Machado-Vieira R, Zarate CA. Change in cytokine levels is not associated with rapid antidepressant response to ketamine in treatment-resistant depression. J Psychiatr Res. 2017;84:113–8. https://doi.org/10.1016/j.jpsychires.2016.09.025.
45. Kiraly DD, Horn SR, Van Dam NT, Costi S, Schwartz J, Kim-Schulze S, Patel M, et al. Altered peripheral immune profiles in treatment-resistant depression: response to ketamine and prediction of treatment outcome. Transl Psychiatry. 2017;7(3):e1065. https://doi.org/10.1038/tp.2017.31.
46. Guloksuz S, Rutten BPF, Arts B, van Os J, Kenis G. The immune system and electroconvulsive therapy for depression. J ECT. 2014;30(2):132–7. https://doi.org/10.1097/YCT.0000000000000127.
47. Yrondi A, Sporer M, Péran P, Schmitt L, Arbus C, Sauvaget A. Electroconvulsive therapy, depression, the immune system and inflammation: a systematic review. Brain Stimul. 2018;11(1):29–51. https://doi.org/10.1016/j.brs.2017.10.013.
48. van Buel EM, Patas K, Peters M, Bosker FJ, Eisel ULM, Klein HC. Immune and neurotrophin stimulation by electroconvulsive therapy: is some inflammation needed after all? Transl Psychiatry. 2015;5:e609. https://doi.org/10.1038/tp.2015.100.
49. Perez-Caballero L, Pérez-Egea R, Romero-Grimaldi C, Puigdemont D, Molet J, Caso J-R, Mico J-A, Pérez V, Leza J-C, Berrocoso E. Early responses to deep brain stimulation in depression are modulated by anti-inflammatory drugs. Mol Psychiatry. 2014;19(5):607–14. https://doi.org/10.1038/mp.2013.63.
50. Brunoni AR, Padberg F, Vieira ELM, Teixeira AL, Carvalho AF, Lotufo PA, Gattaz WF, Benseñor IM. Plasma biomarkers in a placebo-controlled trial comparing TDCS and escitalopram efficacy in major depression. Prog Neuro-Psychopharmacol Biol Psychiatry. 2018;86:211–7. https://doi.org/10.1016/j.pnpbp.2018.06.003.
51. Morgan N, Irwin MR, Chung M, Wang C. The effects of mind-body therapies on the immune system: meta-analysis. PloS One. 2014;9(7):e100903. https://doi.org/10.1371/journal.pone.0100903.
52. Haaland DA, Sabljic TF, Baribeau DA, Mukovozov IM, Hart LE. Is regular exercise a friend or foe of the aging immune system? A systematic review. Clin J Sport Med. 2008;18(6):539–48. https://doi.org/10.1097/JSM.0b013e3181865eec.
53. Badawy AA-B. Tryptophan availability for kynurenine pathway metabolism across the life span: control mechanisms and focus on aging, exercise, diet and nutritional supplements. Neuropharmacology. 2017;112(Pt B):248–63. https://doi.org/10.1016/j.neuropharm.2015.11.015.
54. Rethorst CD, Toups MS, Greer TL, Nakonezny PA, Carmody TJ, Grannemann BD, Huebinger RM, Barber RC, Trivedi MH. Pro-inflammatory cytokines as predictors of antidepressant effects of exercise in major depressive disorder. Mol Psychiatry. 2013;18(10):1119–24. https://doi.org/10.1038/mp.2012.125.
55. Harley J, Luty S, Carter J, Mulder R, Joyce P. Elevated C-reactive protein in depression: a predictor of good long-term outcome with antidepressants and poor outcome with psychotherapy. J Psychopharmacol (Oxford, England). 2010;24(4):625–6. https://doi.org/10.1177/0269881109102770.

56. Husain MI, Strawbridge R, Stokes PR, Young AH. Anti-inflammatory treatments for mood disorders: systematic review and meta-analysis. J Psychopharmacol (Oxford, England). 2017b;31(9):1137–48. https://doi.org/10.1177/0269881117725711.
57. Sublette ME, Galfalvy HC, Hibbeln JR, Keilp JG, Malone KM, Oquendo MA, Mann JJ. Polyunsaturated fatty acid associations with dopaminergic indices in major depressive disorder. Int J Neuropsychopharmacol. 2014;17(3):383–91. https://doi.org/10.1017/S1461145713001399.
58. Kim S-W, Kang H-J, Jhon M, Kim J-W, Lee J-Y, Walker AJ, Agustini B, Kim J-M, Berk M. Statins and inflammation: new therapeutic opportunities in psychiatry. Front Psychiatry. 2019;10:103. https://doi.org/10.3389/fpsyt.2019.00103.
59. Colle R, de Larminat D, Rotenberg S, Hozer F, Hardy P, Verstuyft C, Fève B, Corruble E. Pioglitazone could induce remission in major depression: a meta-analysis. Neuropsychiatr Dis Treat. 2017;13:9–16. https://doi.org/10.2147/NDT.S121149.
60. Huang R, Wang K, Jianan H. Effect of probiotics on depression: a systematic review and meta-analysis of randomized controlled trials. Nutrients. 2016;8(8):483. https://doi.org/10.3390/nu8080483.
61. Valles-Colomer M, Falony G, Darzi Y, Tigchelaar EF, Wang J, Tito RY, Schiweck C, et al. The neuroactive potential of the human gut microbiota in quality of life and depression. Nat Microbiol. 2019;4(4):623–32. https://doi.org/10.1038/s41564-018-0337-x.

Diet, Immune System, and Psychiatric Disorders

24

Jane Pei-Chen Chang and Kuan-Pin Su

24.1 Introduction: The Era of Nutritional Psychiatry

Nutritional psychiatry is an emerging field that holds promise to reduce the burden carried by psychiatric disorders. Nutritional psychiatry emerged in the past two decades and has been formally supported by the International Society of Nutritional Psychiatric Research (ISNPR) in 2015 as a new field of research focused on developing a comprehensive, cohesive, scientifically rigorous evidence base to support a shift in thinking around the role of diet and nutrition in mental health [1]. Recent research evidence supports the notion of nutritional psychiatry, where higher intakes of a "healthy" diet (i.e. fruit, vegetables, fish, and whole grains) were associated with a reduced likelihood of depression (OR: 0.84; 95% CI: 0.76, 0.92) [2]. Moreover, cross-sectional, prospective observational studies and meta-analyses reported inverse associations between adherence to healthy dietary patterns and reduced risk for or likelihood of mental health disturbances in both youth and adults [2, 3]. In addition, new studies have focused on the understanding of the biological pathways that mediate the observed relationships between diets, nutrition, and

J. P.-C. Chang
Mind-Body Interface Laboratory (MBI-Lab) and Department of Psychiatry, China Medical University Hospital, Taichung, Taiwan

College of Medicine, China Medical University, Taichung, Taiwan

Institute of Psychiatry, Psychology and Neuroscience, King's College London, London, UK

K.-P. Su (✉)
Mind-Body Interface Laboratory (MBI-Lab) and Department of Psychiatry, China Medical University Hospital, Taichung, Taiwan

College of Medicine, China Medical University, Taichung, Taiwan

Institute of Psychiatry, Psychology and Neuroscience, King's College London, London, UK

An-Nan Hospital, China Medical University, Tainan, Taiwan

M. Berk et al. (eds.), *Immuno-Psychiatry*, https://doi.org/10.1007/978-3-030-71229-7_24

mental health. These are pointing to the immune system and the gut-brain axis (GBA) as the key targets for nutritional interventions in mental health.

Major depressive disorder (MDD) and attention deficit hyperactivity disorder (ADHD) are two common psychiatric disorders seen in adults and children. Both disorders not only cause disability and mortality to the affected individual but also affect their family members and have a great impact on the society as a whole. Depression is estimated to affect 350 million people, and on average about 1 in 20 people report having an episode of depression in the previous year [4]. MDD has been predicted by World Health Organization (WHO) to be one of the leading causes of disability by 2030. Although there are more than 50 kinds of antidepressant available, only less than one-third of people recovered with the first selected serotonin-reuptake inhibitor (SSRI), the first-line treatment in MDD, in the largest study of MDD conducted in the United States [5]. Recent studies supported that nutritional supplementation may offer another treatment option for MDD, with evidence for omega-3 polyunsaturated fatty acids (n-3 PUFAs) [6–9] and probiotics [10, 11].

ADHD, a common neurodevelopmental disorder with a prevalence rate of 5–10% [12], has as a high comorbidity with other psychiatric disorders, including conduct disorders [13], mood disorders [13], anxiety disorders, and substance use disorders [14]. If left untreated, it can have a great impact on the society, where there would be more absenteeism at work, more motor vehicle accidents, more substance use problems, and lower economic growth [15]. Despite the efficacy of pharmacotherapy in children with ADHD, around 60–80%, about 20–40% of patients with ADHD either respond poorly to the current medications available or suffer from medication side effects [16]. On the other hand, studies have pointed to nutritional interventions, such as n-3 PUFAs [17, 18] and probiotics [19, 20], as potential treatment options in children with ADHD.

In this chapter, we discuss the research evidence supporting nutritional supplements in MDD and ADHD, focusing on n-3 PUFAs and probiotics in the context of inflammatory regulation.

24.2 Omega-3 Polyunsaturated Fatty Acids (N-3 PUFAs)

There are two main types of PUFAs in the human body, the omega-6 polyunsaturated fatty acids (n-6 PUFAs) from the cis-linoleic acid (LA, 18:2n-6) and the omega-3 PUFAs (n-3 PUFAs) from the α-linolenic acid (ALA, 18:3n-3). N-3 and n-6 PUFAs are important constituents of all cell membranes; they are called the essential fatty acids (EFAs), because they are crucial for the survival for the humans and mammals but cannot be synthesized within the body [21]. EFAs can only be obtained from diets [21]. The PUFAs appear to be biologically active, and some of their functions require their conversion into metabolites including eicosanoids. Linoleic acid can be converted to gamma-linolenic acid (GLA, 18:3n-6) and GLA can be elongated to form dihomo-GLA (20:3n-6), which is the precursor of the prostaglandin (PG)-1 s. Dihomo-GLA can also be converted to arachidonic acid

(AA, 20:4n-6), which is the precursor of the PG-2 s, thromboxanes (Txs), and the Leukotriene (LT)-4 s. On the other hand, ALA can be converted to eicosapentaenoic acid (EPA; 20:5n-3), and EPA forms the precursor of PG-3 s and LT-5 s. In addition, EPA can be converted to docosahexaenoic acid (DHA; 22:6n-3). Both PGs and LTs are highly biologically active, have immunoregulatory action, and are known to be involved in the pathophysiology of inflammation-associated disorders, such as atherosclerosis, asthma, cardiovascular diseases, cerebrovascular diseases, inflammatory bowel syndrome, neurological diseases, and metabolic syndrome [21, 22].

Several lines of evidence support the importance of n-3 PUFAs in brain disorders [7, 8, 23]. DHA and EPA are both essential for the brain and the body, and the deficiency of both may impair brain development and contribute to the development of several brain disorders such as depression. For example, deficiency of DHA has been associated with neuronal membrane instability and dysfunctional transmission of serotonin, norepinephrine, and dopamine [24, 25], which might be connected to the etiology of the mood and cognitive dysfunction of depression. In addition, clinical trials showed that n-3 PUFAs helped to improve and prevent symptoms of depression [7–9, 25, 26] and cognitive function in mild cognitive impairment [27].

24.2.1 N-3 PUFAs and Inflammation

EPA is important in balancing the immune functions and physical health by reducing membrane AA (a n-6 PUFAs) and prostaglandin E2 (PGE2) synthesis [28], and might be associated with medical comorbidity and somatic symptoms in depression [29]. EPA and DHA have been shown to increase anti-inflammatory actions via inhibition of free radical generation and oxidant stress [21], and to regulate neurotransmitter and immune functions via the modulation of lipid rafts signalling platforms on the cell membrane [30]. In cellular experiments, we reported that both EPA and DHA reduced expressions of tumour necrosis factor (TNF)-α, interleukin (IL)-6, nitric oxide synthase, and cyclo-oxygenase-2, induced by interferon (IFN)-γ, and induced upregulation of heme oxygenase-1 (HO-1) in BV-2 microglia. In addition, EPA and DHA caused AKT and extracellular-regulated kinase (ERK) activation, which could be attenuated by phosphoinositide-3 (PI-3) kinase/AKT and mitogen-activated protein kinase (MEK)/ERK inhibitors. EPA and DHA also increased IkB kinase (IKK)α/β phosphorylation, IκB α phosphorylation, and IκB α degradation, while both nuclear factor (NF)-κB and IκB protease inhibitors could inhibit DHA-induced HO-1 expressions [31]. Moreover, a recent animal study further showed that n-3-deficient diet exacerbated inflammation in an animal model of maternal immune activation, where the pregnant mice were injected with lipopolysaccharide (LPS) to induce inflammation reaction. This induced spatial memory deficits in the adult offspring; while the adult offspring of the mice fed with n-3-balanced diet during gestation had no memory deficits [32].

One of the hypothesized mechanisms underlying PUFAs' psychotrophic effects is their anti-inflammatory action [33]. Moreover, n-3 PUFAs have been found to have beneficial effects in cytokine-induced behavioral changes in animal models of depression [34, 35]. Of particular relevance, our previous study demonstrated that lower n-3 PUFA levels in the peripheral blood are associated with an increased risk of developing IFN-α-induced depression over the following weeks [36]. In addition, we conducted a 2-week, double-blind, RCT, to test the effects of n-3 PUFA supplementation in the prevention of IFN-α-induced depression. We found that the incident rates of IFN-α-induced depression were significantly lower in EPA-, but not in DHA- or placebo-treated patients [8]. This study further confirms the notion that n-3 PUFAs may be effective antidepressants in the context of depression associated with inflammation.

24.2.2 N-3 PUFAs in Depression

Epidemiological studies have observed that societies with high consumption of n-3 PUFAs appear to have lower prevalence rates of depression [37]. Case-controlled studies revealed lower levels of n-3 PUFAs in patients with depression [38]. N-3 PUFAs concentration has been shown to become increasingly suboptimal toward the clinical spectrum of depressive symptoms [39], and its level is significantly negatively correlated with the severity of depressive symptoms [40]. N-3 PUFAs effectively treated depressive disorders in recent studies and some studies have shown EPA alone [41] or a combination of EPA and DHA [9, 25] had positive effects for patients with MDD. N-3 PUFAs improved the 4-month course of illness in patients with bipolar disorder in a preliminary trial [42], and in the further analysis and of the preliminary trial found that n-3 PUFAS are more beneficial in the depressive phase than in the manic phase in patients with bipolar I disorder [29, 43]. In fact, n-3 PUFAs have been found to have antidepressant effects in several placebo-controlled trials [6, 26].

To translate numerous supportive evidence from RCTs and meta-analyses of n-3 PUFAs' antidepressant effects, the sub-committee of the International Society for Nutritional Psychiatry Research (ISNPR) organized an expert panel and conducted a literature review and a Delphi-process to develop a consensus-based practice guideline for clinical use of n-3 PUFAs in MDD [44]. The key practice guidelines include not only the formulation and dosage but also the agreement on using n-3 PUFAs in MDD treatment for pregnant women [45–48], children, and the elderly, and prevention in high-risk populations [49].

24.2.3 N-3 PUFAs in ADHD

Deficiency in n-3 PUFAs has recently been investigated as a potential pathogenetic mechanism in ADHD [50]. In epidemiological studies, children of mothers who have lower seafood intake during pregnancy are at risk of suboptimal outcomes for prosocial behaviors, fine motor coordination, verbal communication, and social development [23]. Moreover, we have shown that children with ADHD have greater severity of EFA deficiency, a clinical syndrome associated with insufficient fatty acid levels and comprising symptoms such as dry and scaly skin, eczema, and dry eyes [51]. In addition, EFA dietary deficiency in children with ADHD correlates negatively with plasma DHA levels [50], and a recent case-control study showed that EFA deficiency positively correlates with ADHD symptoms [51]. In terms of PUFAs levels, lower red blood cells (RBCs) PUFAs [50] and a higher n-6/n-3 ratio [52] have been reported in ADHD, and lower n-3 PUFAs levels are positively associated with the severity of ADHD symptoms in children [52, 53]. A recent meta-analysis also showed that children with ADHD had lower blood levels of DHA, EPA, and total n-3 PUFAs when compared with typically developing (TD) children [17].

Of note, single nucleotide polymorphisms (SNPs) of the FADS1 and FADS2 (fatty acid desaturase) genes, which code for the enzymes, delta-5 desaturase and delta-6 desaturase, responsible for the metabolism of PUFAs, are associated with ADHD [54]. ADHD has been associated with SNP rs498793 in the FADS2 gene, while the two SNPs rs174545 and rs174548 in the FADS1 gene were nominally associated with ADHD in the prenatal alcohol-exposed group of children [54].

Meta-analyses further showed positive effects of n-3 PUFAs on ADHD clinical symptoms [17, 55–59] and cognitive symptoms [17]. In addition, a recent meta-analysis also showed that n-3 PUFAs supplementation with EPA $\geq$ 500 mg/d improved clinical hyperactivity/impulsivity symptoms [17]. In addition, due to its safety profile and anti-inflammatory effects, n-3 PUFAs have been of great interest as a potential treatment for ADHD. Moreover, a previous study examining 10 ADHD clinical trials with 699 children with ADHD (predominantly males, 60–87%) showed that a high dose of EPA (1–2 g) supplementation was required to show significant improvement of clinical symptoms in ADHD [60].

The findings from clinical trials of n-3 PUFAs in children with ADHD have been controversial. Some clinical trials with n-3 PUFAs supplementation in ADHD have shown improvement in clinical symptoms [61–63] and cognitive performances [64–66]. Moreover, most of the trials used DHA as the main component of the n-3 PUFAs [63, 64, 66], or used a rather low combined dosage of DHA and EPA (<500 mg/d) [61, 65]. On the other hand, we recently showed that a high EPA dosage of 1200 mg/d improved cognitive function (focused attention and vigilance) in children with ADHD with a low EPA level (*more inflamed*), but did not improve cognitive function in those children with normal or high EPA level [9]. This further implies that subtyping ADHD with inflammation status or endogenous n-3 PUFAs level may contribute to the personalized medicine in ADHD with n-3 PUFAs as treatment; where endogenous n-3 PUFAs levels and inflammation status can be used as a treatment response predictor of n-3 PUFAs in ADHD.

24.3 Gut-Brain Axis (GBA), Probiotics, and Inflammation

Dysregulation of the gut-brain axis (GBA) has been suggested to be associated with inflammation observed in both MDD and ADHD. The GBA is the bidirectional communication system that allows gastrointestinal (GI) microbes to communicate with the brain [67]. GI microbes help protect against GI pathogens and exert neuroactive properties to influence the brain [68], and can communicate with the brain through a variety of routes, including activation of the vagus nerve, production of short-chain fatty acids (SCFAs), and cytokines [69]. There are more than a 1000 different species in the GI tract [70] and their composition can be affected by genetics [71], disease, medication [72], and age [73]. A high variability of GI microbes is important in that they may be able to stop the growth of pathogenic bacteria [74], strengthen GI permeability to prevent systemic inflammation, and allow normal physiological functioning in other organs, especially the brain [69]. Moreover, healthy microbial composition in the GI tract is crucial for human neurodevelopment at the age of 2–3 years [75], since GI microbes affect both the function and maturation of immune cells, which further affect neurodevelopment. An animal study showed that introducing microbiota to germ-free (GF) mice helped reverse impaired maturation of microglia [76]. Findings from preclinical studies further suggested that the vagus nerve may be the key communication route between GI microbes and the brain: (1) post-vagotomy was associated with elimination of central effects of *Lactobacillus rhamnosus* [77] and (2) humans who received a vagotomy at an early age have a decreased risk of certain neurologic disorders [78]. Moreover, GI microbes may regulate central neurotransmitters indirectly, since they produce neurotransmitters that affect the brain functions via enteric nervous system. GI microbes are also capable of producing neurotransmitters that are associated with brain function, for example, Lactobacillus and Bifidobacterium spp. can produce γ-aminobutyric acid (GABA), while *Bifidobacterium infantis* has been associated with plasma tryptophan levels, which may influence central serotonin transmission [79]. Escherichia, Bacillus, and Saccharomyces spp. produce noradrenaline; Candida, Streptococcus, Escherichia, and Enterococcus spp. produce serotonin; Bacillus produce dopamine; and Lactobacillus produce acetylcholine [80, 81].

SCFAs are essential metabolic products produced by GI microbes from polysaccharides that cannot be properly digested by the GI system. Bacetroides spp. and Clostridiae spp. are two of the important microbes that are associated with production of SCFAs. SCFAs act on leukocytes and endothelial cells through at least two mechanisms: activation of G-protein-coupled receptors (GPCRs: GPR41 and GPR43) and inhibition of histone deacetylase (HDAC). SCFAs regulate several leukocyte functions including production of cytokines, TNF-α, IL-2, IL-6, and IL-10, eicosanoids, and chemokines. SCFAs affect not only the immune system but also the CNS [76]; they may also affect the brain through GPCRs sparsely located in the brain.

GBA also use cytokines as another mean of communication to relay messages from the GI to the brain [82]. Cytokines from GI can travel to the brain via bloodstream, but under normal healthy circumstances, these cytokines are blocked from entering the brain by the blood-brain barriers (BBB). However, more evidence has shown that the cytokines can cross BBB and affect the brain where the BBB is deficient, such as the hypothalamus. For example, cytokines including IL-1 and IL-6 have been shown to activate the hypothalamus-pituitary-adrenal (HPA) axis and influence the release of cortisol, which may then affect GABA and result in gut dysbiosis, which is the imbalance between protective and pathogenic microbes in the GI. Moreover, an animal study showed that stress changes the gut barrier function and allows LPS and other molecules to reach the bloodstream, and result in the production of inflammatory cytokines [83]. Another animal study showed that early stressors such as maternal separation alter behavioral phenotype and decrease GI microbiota diversity [84]. Gut dysbiosis and HPA axis dysregulation have both been suggested to play a role in the pathogenesis of both MDD [85, 86] and ADHD [87, 88].

Probiotics, on the other hand, are live microorganisms that claim to provide health benefits by restoring GI microbes, reverse dysbiosis, and improve the dysregulation of GBA. Recent studies have supported the effect of probiotics not only in physical disorders but also in psychiatric disorders.

24.3.1 GBA and Probiotics in MDD

A growing body of literature suggested that a dysfunctional GBA may contribute to the pathophysiology of depression. Gut dysbiosis has been suggested to lead to depression-like behavior. Administration of antibiotics in mice was shown to lead to gut dysbiosis, depression-like behavior, and altered neuronal hippocampal signaling. This phenotype is reversible after administration of probiotic treatment with *Lactobacillus casei* [89]. Some studies [90, 91] further showed that transplanting GI microbiota from humans with depression to germ-free or microbiota-deficient rodents induces a depression-like phenotype, including anhedonia and anxiety-like behaviors. However, such behavioral changes were not observed in mice receiving microbiota transplantation from healthy controls. Moreover, sequencing the fecal microbiota of patients with depression and healthy controls further showed that several genera were different between the two groups [92]. The depression group had higher levels of Enterobacteriaceae and Alistipes, and lower levels of Faecalibacterium [92]. Depression has also been associated with higher levels of Anaerostipes, Blautia, Clostridium, Klebsiella, Lachnospiraceae incertae sedis, Parabacteroides, Parasutterella, Phascolarctobacterium, and Streptococcus and lower levels of Bifidobacterium, Dialister, Escherichia/Shigella, Faecalibacterium, and Ruminococcus [93]. Although no consensus has emerged from existing human studies of depression and gut microbiota concerning which bacterial taxa are most relevant to depression, studying microbial functioning in depression may be more productive than a purely taxonomic approach [93].

Alternatively, intervention with probiotics has shown improvement in depression symptoms [86]. Depression and anxiety symptom severity were negatively associated with GI microbiota diversity in psychiatric inpatients [94]. Moreover,

GI microbiota diversity early in the course of hospitalization was able to predict depression remission at discharge [94].

24.3.2 GBA and Probiotics in ADHD

Several conditions associated with the risk of ADHD have been associated with gut dysbiosis. These conditions included (1) maternal prenatal stress, (2) the delivery mode of caesarean section (CS), (3) preterm birth, (4) not breast feeding, and (5) comorbidity with allergic disorders [95]. Maternal prenatal stress and preterm birth were associated with decreased lactobacillus [95], on the other hand, lactobacillus has been shown to protect the CNS, and has been associated with breast feeding [96]. Furthermore, CS, especially emergent CS, has been associated with a decrease in Bifidobacterium [97], which is important to assist with the encoding of CDT (cyclohexadienyl dehyratase); CDT is important for the synthesis of phenylalanine, the precursor of tyrosine. Tyrosine is metabolized to dopamine, one of the key neurotransmitters in the pathophysiology of ADHD [98]. CDT was negatively associated with reward anticipation, where decreased CDT leads to high phenylalanine, abnormal dopamine, and a reduced reward response, one of the hallmarks of ADHD [98]. ADHD was associated with a decrease in Faecalibacterium [99], while a decrease in Faecalibacterium has been associated with increased ADHD symptoms and allergic conditions [95]. Furthermore, a decreased microbial diversity (alpha diversity) has also been reported in ADHD [100], which may contribute to a "leaky gut" and low-grade systemic inflammation reported in ADHD.

GI microbes may also affect the brain via activation of the vagus nerve and alteration of the ANS. On the other hand, alteration of the ANS has also been reported in ADHD [101]. For example, low heart rate variability, reduced cardiac-linked parasympathetic activity associated with relative sympathetic dominance, has been suggested as a possible noninvasive marker for prefrontal hypoactivity in ADHD [102]. In sum, GI microbiota may play an important role in ADHD by altering the ANS and affecting the synthesis and metabolism of neurotransmitters associated with ADHD, including dopamine, serotonin, norepinephrine, and GABA [103].

Several studies with nutritional supplementation, including probiotics and n-3 PUFAs, showed advantageous effects in children with ADHD. A 10- week pilot study of broad spectrum of micronutrients increased the GI microbial diversity and increased Bifidobacterium abundance, which is associated with a decrease in clinical ADHD symptoms [104]. Furthermore, Lactobacillus administered to mothers prenatally (4 weeks before delivery) or postnatally (6 weeks, if they breastfed) or to the children, helped prevent the development of ADHD and autism spectrum disorder (ASD) in the children at the age of 13 [20]. Studies with n-3 PUFAs supplementation in healthy volunteers also showed an increase in Bifidobacterium and Lactobacillus [105], which are both neuroprotective. This may further offer some explanation for the treatment effects of n-3 PUFAs in ADHD.

24.4 Conclusion

Nutritional psychiatry is an emerging field that focuses on how diet and nutrition can transform the therapeutic strategies in psychiatric disorders. Epidemiological studies, case-control studies, and clinical studies have supported N-3 PUFAs and probiotics as potential treatment options for both MDD and ADHD via immunoregulation and restoration of the gut dysbiosis. However, more studies will be needed to provide more evidence for the personalized medicine approach of nutritional interventions in psychiatric disorders.

Acknowledgement The authors of this work were supported by the following grants: MOST 106-2314-B-039-027-MY3, 108-2320-B-039-048, 108-2813-C-039-133-B and 108-2314-B-039-016 from the Ministry of Science and Technology, Taiwan; NHRI-EX108-10528NI from the National Health Research Institutes, Taiwan; MYRG2018-00242-ICMS from University of Macau, China; CMRC-CMA-3 from Higher Education Sprout Project by the Ministry of Education (MOE), Taiwan; CMU108-SR-106 from the China Medical University, Taichung, Taiwan; and CRS-108-048, DMR-108-216 and DMR-109-102 from the China Medical University Hospital, Taichung, Taiwan.

References

1. Sarris J, Logan AC, Akbaraly TN, Paul Amminger G, Balanza-Martinez V, Freeman MP, et al. International Society for Nutritional Psychiatry Research consensus position statement: nutritional medicine in modern psychiatry. World Psychiatry. 2015;14(3):370–1. https://doi.org/10.1002/wps.20223.
2. Lai JS, Hiles S, Bisquera A, Hure AJ, McEvoy M, Attia J. A systematic review and meta-analysis of dietary patterns and depression in community-dwelling adults. Am J Clin Nutr. 2014;99(1):181–97. https://doi.org/10.3945/ajcn.113.069880.
3. Psaltopoulou T, Sergentanis TN, Panagiotakos DB, Sergentanis IN, Kosti R, Scarmeas N. Mediterranean diet, stroke, cognitive impairment, and depression: a meta-analysis. Ann Neurol. 2013;74(4):580–91. https://doi.org/10.1002/ana.23944.
4. WFMH. Depression: A Global Crisis: World Federation of Mental Health 2012.
5. Rush AJ. STAR*D: what have we learned? Am J Psychiatry. 2007;164(2):201–4.
6. Lin PY, Mischoulon D, Freeman MP, Matsuoka Y, Hibbeln J, Belmaker RH, et al. Are omega-3 fatty acids antidepressants or just mood-improving agents? The effect depends upon diagnosis, supplement preparation, and severity of depression. Mol Psychiatry. 2012;17(12):1161–3.; author reply 3-7. https://doi.org/10.1038/mp.2012.111.
7. Su KP, Huang SY, Chiu TH, Huang KC, Huang CL, Chang HC, et al. Omega-3 fatty acids for major depressive disorder during pregnancy: results from a randomized, double-blind, placebo-controlled trial. J Clin Psychiatry. 2008;69(4):644–51.
8. Su KP, Lai HC, Yang HT, Su WP, Peng CY, Chang JP, et al. Omega-3 fatty acids in the prevention of interferon-alpha-induced depression: results from a randomized, controlled trial. Biol Psychiatry. 2014;76(7):559–66. https://doi.org/10.1016/j.biopsych.2014.01.008.
9. Chang JP, Chang SS, Yang HT, Chen HT, Chien YC, Yang B, et al. Omega-3 polyunsaturated fatty acids in cardiovascular diseases comorbid major depressive disorder - results from a randomized controlled trial. Brain Behav Immun. 2020;85:14–20.
10. Akkasheh G, Kashani-Poor Z, Tajabadi-Ebrahimi M, Jafari P, Akbari H, Taghizadeh M, et al. Clinical and metabolic response to probiotic administration in patients with major depressive disorder: a randomized, double-blind, placebo-controlled trial. Nutrition. 2016;32(3):315–20. https://doi.org/10.1016/j.nut.2015.09.003.

11. Miyaoka T, Kanayama M, Wake R, Hashioka S, Hayashida M, Nagahama M, et al. Clostridium butyricum MIYAIRI 588 as adjunctive therapy for treatment-resistant major depressive disorder: a prospective open-label trial. Clin Neuropharmacol. 2018;41(5):151–5. https://doi.org/10.1097/WNF.0000000000000299.
12. Biederman J, Faraone SV. Attention-deficit hyperactivity disorder. Lancet. 2005;366(9481):237–48.
13. Biederman J, Newcorn J, Sprich S. Comorbidity of attention deficit hyperactivity disorder with conduct, depressive, anxiety, and other disorders. Am J Psychiatry. 1991;148(5):564–77. https://doi.org/10.1176/ajp.148.5.564.
14. Wilens TE, Biederman J. Alcohol, drugs, and attention-deficit/hyperactivity disorder: a model for the study of addictions in youth. J Psychopharmacol. 2006;20(4):580–8.
15. Volkow ND, Swanson JM. Clinical practice: adult attention deficit-hyperactivity disorder. N Engl J Med. 2013;369(20):1935–44. https://doi.org/10.1056/NEJMcp1212625.
16. Childress AC, Sallee FR. Attention-deficit/hyperactivity disorder with inadequate response to stimulants: approaches to management. CNS Drugs. 2014;28(2):121–9. https://doi.org/10.1007/s40263-013-0130-6.
17. Chang JP, Su KP, Mondelli V, Pariante CM. Omega-3 polyunsaturated fatty acids in youths with attention deficit hyperactivity disorder: a systematic review and meta-analysis of clinical trials and biological studies. Neuropsychopharmacology. 2018;43(3):534–45. https://doi.org/10.1038/npp.2017.160.
18. Chang JP, Su KP, Mondelli V, Satyanarayanan SK, Yang HT, Chiang YJ, et al. High-dose eicosapentaenoic acid (EPA) improves attention and vigilance in children and adolescents with attention deficit hyperactivity disorder (ADHD) and low endogenous EPA levels. Transl Psychiatry. 2019;9(1):303. https://doi.org/10.1038/s41398-019-0633-0.
19. Rianda D, Agustina R, Setiawan EA, Manikam NRM. Effect of probiotic supplementation on cognitive function in children and adolescents: a systematic review of randomised trials. Benefic Microbes. 2019;10(8):873–82. https://doi.org/10.3920/BM2019.0068.
20. Partty A, Kalliomaki M, Wacklin P, Salminen S, Isolauri E. A possible link between early probiotic intervention and the risk of neuropsychiatric disorders later in childhood: a randomized trial. Pediatr Res. 2015;77(6):823–8. https://doi.org/10.1038/pr.2015.51.
21. Das UN. Essential fatty acids: biochemistry, physiology and pathology. Biotechnol J. 2006;1(4):420–39. https://doi.org/10.1002/biot.200600012.
22. Connor WE. Importance of n-3 fatty acids in health and disease. Am J Clin Nutr. 2000;71(1 Suppl):171S–5S. https://doi.org/10.1093/ajcn/71.1.171S.
23. Hibbeln JR, Davis JM, Steer C, Emmett P, Rogers I, Williams C, et al. Maternal seafood consumption in pregnancy and neurodevelopmental outcomes in childhood (ALSPAC study): an observational cohort study. Lancet. 2007;369(9561):578–85. https://doi.org/10.1016/S0140-6736(07)60277-3.
24. Chalon S. Omega-3 fatty acids and monoamine neurotransmission. Prostaglandins Leukot Essent Fatty Acids. 2006;75(4–5):259–69. https://doi.org/10.1016/j.plefa.2006.07.005.
25. Su KP, Huang SY, Chiu CC, Shen WW. Omega-3 fatty acids in major depressive disorder. A preliminary double-blind, placebo-controlled trial. Eur Neuropsychopharmacol. 2003;13(4):267–71.
26. Lin PY, Su KP. A meta-analytic review of double-blind, placebo-controlled trials of antidepressant efficacy of omega-3 fatty acids. J Clin Psychiatry. 2007;68(7):1056–61.
27. Chiu CC, Su KP, Cheng TC, Liu HC, Chang CJ, Dewey ME, et al. The effects of omega-3 fatty acids monotherapy in Alzheimer's disease and mild cognitive impairment: a preliminary randomized double-blind placebo-controlled study. Prog Neuro-Psychopharmacol Biol Psychiatry. 2008;32(6):1538–44. https://doi.org/10.1016/j.pnpbp.2008.05.015.
28. Farooqui AA, Ong WY, Horrocks LA. Inhibitors of brain phospholipase A(2) activity: their neuropharmacological effects and therapeutic importance for the treatment of neurologic disorders. Pharmacol Rev. 2006;58(3):591–620. https://doi.org/10.1124/pr.58.3.7.

29. Su KP. Biological mechanism of antidepressant effect of omega-3 fatty acids: how does fish oil act as a 'mind-body interface'? Neurosignals. 2009;17(2):144–52. https://doi.org/10.1159/000198167.
30. Chang JP, Su KP. The lipid raft hypothesis: the relation among omega-3 fatty acids, depression, and cardiovascular diseases. Taiwanese J Psychiatry. 2010;24(3):168–80.
31. Lu DY, Tsao YY, Leung YM, Su KP. Docosahexaenoic acid suppresses neuroinflammatory responses and induces Heme oxygenase-1 expression in BV-2 microglia: implications of antidepressant effects for omega-3 fatty acids. Neuropsychopharmacology. 2010;35(11):2238–48.
32. Labrousse VF, Leyrolle Q, Amadieu C, Aubert A, Sere A, Coutureau E, et al. Dietary omega-3 deficiency exacerbates inflammation and reveals spatial memory deficits in mice exposed to lipopolysaccharide during gestation. Brain Behav Immun. 2018;73:427–40. https://doi.org/10.1016/j.bbi.2018.06.004.
33. Su KP. Biological mechanism of antidepressant effect of omega-3 fatty acids: how does fish oil act as a 'mind-body interface'? Neurosignals. 2009;17(2):144–52.
34. Song C, Phillips AG, Leonard BE, Horrobin DF. Ethyl-eicosapentaenoic acid ingestion prevents corticosterone-mediated memory impairment induced by central administration of interleukin-1beta in rats. Mol Psychiatry. 2004;9(6):630–8.
35. Song C, Leonard BE, Horrobin DF. Dietary ethyl-eicosapentaenoic acid but not soybean oil reverses central interleukin-1-induced changes in behavior, corticosterone and immune response in rats. Stress. 2004;7(1):43–54.
36. Su KP, Huang SY, Peng CY, Lai HC, Huang CL, Chen YC, et al. Phospholipase A2 and cyclooxygenase 2 genes influence the risk of interferon-alpha-induced depression by regulating polyunsaturated fatty acids levels. Biol Psychiatry. 2010;67(6):550–7.
37. Hibbeln JR, Nieminen LR, Blasbalg TL, Riggs JA, Lands WE. Healthy intakes of n-3 and n-6 fatty acids: estimations considering worldwide diversity. Am J Clin Nutr. 2006;83(6 Suppl):1483S–93S. https://doi.org/10.1093/ajcn/83.6.1483S.
38. Peet M, Murphy B, Shay J, Horrobin D. Depletion of omega-3 fatty acid levels in red blood cell membranes of depressive patients. Biol Psychiatry. 1998;43(5):315–9.
39. Schiepers OJ, de Groot RH, Jolles J, van Boxtel MP. Plasma phospholipid fatty acid status and depressive symptoms: association only present in the clinical range. J Affect Disord. 2009;118(1–3):209–14. https://doi.org/10.1016/j.jad.2009.01.025.
40. Edwards R, Peet M, Shay J, Horrobin D. Omega-3 polyunsaturated fatty acid levels in the diet and in red blood cell membranes of depressed patients. J Affect Disord. 1998;48(2–3):149–55.
41. Peet M, Horrobin DF. A dose-ranging study of the effects of ethyl-eicosapentaenoate in patients with ongoing depression despite apparently adequate treatment with standard drugs. Arch Gen Psychiatry. 2002;59(10):913–9.
42. Stoll AL, Severus WE, Freeman MP, Rueter S, Zboyan HA, Diamond E, et al. Omega 3 fatty acids in bipolar disorder: a preliminary double-blind, placebo-controlled trial. Arch Gen Psychiatry. 1999;56(5):407–12. https://doi.org/10.1001/archpsyc.56.5.407.
43. Chiu CC, Huang SY, Chen CC, Su KP. Omega-3 fatty acids are more beneficial in the depressive phase than in the manic phase in patients with bipolar I disorder. J Clin Psychiatry. 2005;66(12):1613–4. https://doi.org/10.4088/jcp.v66n1219b.
44. Guu TW, Mischoulon D, Sarris J, Hibbeln J, McNamara RK, Hamazaki K, et al. International society for nutritional psychiatry research practice guidelines for omega-3 fatty acids in the treatment of major depressive disorder. Psychother Psychosom. 2019;88(5):263–73. https://doi.org/10.1159/000502652.
45. Nishi D, Su KP, Usuda K, Chang JP, Chiang YJ, Chen HT, et al. The efficacy of Omega-3 fatty acids for depressive symptoms among pregnant women in Japan and Taiwan: a randomized, double-blind, placebo-controlled trial (SYNCHRO; NCT01948596). Psychother Psychosom. 2019;88(2):122–4. https://doi.org/10.1159/000495296.
46. Nishi D, Su KP, Usuda K, Chang JP, Hamazaki K, Ishima T, et al. Plasma estradiol levels and antidepressant effects of omega-3 fatty acids in pregnant women. Brain Behav Immun. 2019; https://doi.org/10.1016/j.bbi.2019.02.014.

47. Nishi D, Su KP, Usuda K, Chiang YJ, Guu TW, Hamazaki K, et al. Omega-3 fatty acid supplementation for expectant mothers with depressive symptoms in Japan and Taiwan: an open-label trial. Psychiatry Clin Neurosci. 2016;70(6):253–4. https://doi.org/10.1111/pcn.12388.
48. Su KP, Huang SY, Chiu TH, Huang KC, Huang CL, Chang HC, et al. Omega-3 fatty acids for major depressive disorder during pregnancy: results from a randomized, double-blind, placebo-controlled trial. J Clin Psychiatry. 2008;69(4):644–51.
49. Su KP. Personalize medicine with omega-3 fatty acids for depression in pregnant women and children, and depression associated with inflammation. J Clin Psychiatry. 2015;76(11):e1476–7.
50. Stevens LJ, Zentall SS, Deck JL, Abate ML, Watkins BA, Lipp SR, et al. Essential fatty-acid metabolism in boys with attention-deficit hyperactivity disorder. Am J Clin Nutr. 1995;62(4):761–8.
51. Chang JP, Jingling L, Huang YT, Lu YJ, Su KP. Delay aversion, temporal processing, and N-3 fatty acids intake in children with attention- deficit/hyperactivity disorder (ADHD). Clin Psychol Sci. 2016;4(6):1094–103. https://doi.org/10.1177/2167702616637820.
52. Stevens L, Zhang W, Peck L, Kuczek T, Grevstad N, Mahon A, et al. EFA supplementation in children with inattention, hyperactivity, and other disruptive behaviors. Lipids. 2003;38(10):1007–21. https://doi.org/10.1007/s11745-006-1155-0.
53. Colter AL, Cutler C, Meckling KA. Fatty acid status and behavioural symptoms of attention deficit hyperactivity disorder in adolescents: a case-control study. Nutr J. 2008;7 https://doi.org/10.1186/1475-2891-7-8.
54. Brookes KJ, Chen W, Xu X, Taylor E, Asherson P. Association of fatty acid desaturase genes with attention-deficit/hyperactivity disorder. Biol Psychiatry. 2006;60(10):1053–61. https://doi.org/10.1016/j.biopsych.2006.04.025.
55. Cooper RE, Tye C, Kuntsi J, Vassos E, Asherson P. Omega-3 polyunsaturated fatty acid supplementation and cognition: a systematic review and meta-analysis. J Psychopharmacol. 2015;29(7):753–63. https://doi.org/10.1177/0269881115587958.
56. Gillies D, Sinn J, Lad SS, Leach MJ, Ross MJ. Polyunsaturated fatty acids (PUFA) for attention deficit hyperactivity disorder (ADHD) in children and adolescents. Cochrane Database Syst Rev. 2012;7:CD007986. https://doi.org/10.1002/14651858.CD007986.pub2.
57. Hawkey E, Nigg JT. Omega-3 fatty acid and ADHD: blood level analysis and meta-analytic extension of supplementation trials. Clin Psychol Rev. 2014;34(6):496–505. https://doi.org/10.1016/j.cpr.2014.05.005.
58. Puri BK, Martins JG. Which polyunsaturated fatty acids are active in children with attention-deficit hyperactivity disorder receiving PUFA supplementation? A fatty acid validated meta-regression analysis of randomized controlled trials. Prostaglandins Leukot Essent Fatty Acids. 2014;90(5):179–89. https://doi.org/10.1016/j.plefa.2014.01.004.
59. Sonuga-Barke EJ, Brandeis D, Cortese S, Daley D, Ferrin M, Holtmann M, et al. Nonpharmacological interventions for ADHD: systematic review and meta-analyses of randomized controlled trials of dietary and psychological treatments. Am J Psychiatry. 2013;170(3):275–89. https://doi.org/10.1176/appi.ajp.2012.12070991.
60. Bloch MH, Qawasmi A. Omega-3 fatty acid supplementation for the treatment of children with attention-deficit/hyperactivity disorder symptomatology: systematic review and meta-analysis. J Am Acad Child Adolesc Psychiatry. 2011;50(10):991–1000. https://doi.org/10.1016/j.jaac.2011.06.008.
61. Manor I, Magen A, Keidar D, Rosen S, Tasker H, Cohen T, et al. The effect of phosphatidylserine containing Omega3 fatty-acids on attention-deficit hyperactivity disorder symptoms in children: a double-blind placebo-controlled trial, followed by an open-label extension. Eur Psychiatry. 2012;27(5):335–42.
62. Perera H, Jeewandara KC, Seneviratne S, Guruge C. Combined omega3 and omega6 supplementation in children with attention-deficit hyperactivity disorder (ADHD) refractory to methylphenidate treatment: a double-blind, placebo-controlled study. J Child Neurol. 2012;27(6):747–53.
63. Richardson AJ, Puri BK. A randomized double-blind, placebo-controlled study of the effects of supplementation with highly unsaturated fatty acids on ADHD-related symptoms in

children with specific learning difficulties. Prog Neuro-Psychopharmacol Biol Psychiatry. 2002;26(2):233–9.
64. Sinn N, Bryan J, Wilson C. Cognitive effects of polyunsaturated fatty acids in children with attention deficit hyperactivity disorder symptoms: a randomised controlled trial. Prostaglandins Leukot Essent Fatty Acids. 2008;78(4–5):311–26.
65. Vaisman N, Kaysar N, Zaruk-Adasha Y, Pelled D, Brichon G, Zwingelstein G, et al. Correlation between changes in blood fatty acid composition and visual sustained attention performance in children with inattention: effect of dietary n-3 fatty acids containing phospholipids. Am J Clin Nutr. 2008;87(5):1170–80.
66. Voigt RG, Llorente AM, Jensen CL, Fraley JK, Berretta MC, Heird WC. A randomized, double-blind, placebo controlled trial of docosahexaenoic acid supplementation in children with attention-deficit/hyperactivity disorder. J Pediatr. 2001;139(2):189–96.
67. Rhee SH, Pothoulakis C, Mayer EA. Principles and clinical implications of the brain-gut-enteric microbiota axis. Nat Rev Gastroenterol Hepatol. 2009;6(5):306–14. https://doi.org/10.1038/nrgastro.2009.35.
68. Baumler AJ, Sperandio V. Interactions between the microbiota and pathogenic bacteria in the gut. Nature. 2016;535(7610):85–93. https://doi.org/10.1038/nature18849.
69. Dinan TG, Cryan JF. The microbiome-gut-brain axis in health and disease. Gastroenterol Clin N Am. 2017;46(1):77–89. https://doi.org/10.1016/j.gtc.2016.09.007.
70. Douglas-Escobar M, Elliott E, Neu J. Effect of intestinal microbial ecology on the developing brain. JAMA Pediatr. 2013;167(4):374–9. https://doi.org/10.1001/jamapediatrics.2013.497.
71. Goodrich JK, Waters JL, Poole AC, Sutter JL, Koren O, Blekhman R, et al. Human genetics shape the gut microbiome. Cell. 2014;159(4):789–99. https://doi.org/10.1016/j.cell.2014.09.053.
72. Dethlefsen L, Relman DA. Incomplete recovery and individualized responses of the human distal gut microbiota to repeated antibiotic perturbation. Proc Natl Acad Sci U S A. 2011;108(Suppl 1):4554–61. https://doi.org/10.1073/pnas.1000087107.
73. Buie T. Potential etiologic factors of microbiome disruption in autism. Clin Ther. 2015;37(5):976–83. https://doi.org/10.1016/j.clinthera.2015.04.001.
74. Gagliardi A, Totino V, Cacciotti F, Iebba V, Neroni B, Bonfiglio G, et al. Rebuilding the gut microbiota ecosystem. Int J Environ Res Public Health. 2018;15(8):1679. https://doi.org/10.3390/ijerph15081679.
75. Mohajeri MH, La Fata G, Steinert RE, Weber P. Relationship between the gut microbiome and brain function. Nutr Rev. 2018;76(7):481–96. https://doi.org/10.1093/nutrit/nuy009.
76. Erny D, Hrabe de Angelis AL, Jaitin D, Wieghofer P, Staszewski O, David E, et al. Host microbiota constantly control maturation and function of microglia in the CNS. Nat Neurosci. 2015;18(7):965–77. https://doi.org/10.1038/nn.4030.
77. Bravo JA, Forsythe P, Chew MV, Escaravage E, Savignac HM, Dinan TG, et al. Ingestion of Lactobacillus strain regulates emotional behavior and central GABA receptor expression in a mouse via the vagus nerve. Proc Natl Acad Sci U S A. 2011;108(38):16050–5. https://doi.org/10.1073/pnas.1102999108.
78. Svensson E, Horvath-Puho E, Thomsen RW, Djurhuus JC, Pedersen L, Borghammer P, et al. Vagotomy and subsequent risk of Parkinson's disease. Ann Neurol. 2015;78(4):522–9. https://doi.org/10.1002/ana.24448.
79. Desbonnet L, Garrett L, Clarke G, Kiely B, Cryan JF, Dinan TG. Effects of the probiotic Bifidobacterium infantis in the maternal separation model of depression. Neuroscience. 2010;170(4):1179–88. https://doi.org/10.1016/j.neuroscience.2010.08.005.
80. Lyte M. Microbial endocrinology in the microbiome-gut-brain axis: how bacterial production and utilization of neurochemicals influence behavior. PLoS Pathog. 2013;9(11):e1003726. https://doi.org/10.1371/journal.ppat.1003726.
81. Lyte M. Microbial endocrinology and the microbiota-gut-brain axis. Adv Exp Med Biol. 2014;817:3–24. https://doi.org/10.1007/978-1-4939-0897-4_1.
82. El Aidy S, Dinan TG, Cryan JF. Immune modulation of the brain-gut-microbe axis. Front Microbiol. 2014;5:146. https://doi.org/10.3389/fmicb.2014.00146.

83. Kelly JR, Kennedy PJ, Cryan JF, Dinan TG, Clarke G, Hyland NP. Breaking down the barriers: the gut microbiome, intestinal permeability and stress-related psychiatric disorders. Front Cell Neurosci. 2015;9:392. https://doi.org/10.3389/fncel.2015.00392.
84. O'Mahony SM, Marchesi JR, Scully P, Codling C, Ceolho AM, Quigley EM, et al. Early life stress alters behavior, immunity, and microbiota in rats: implications for irritable bowel syndrome and psychiatric illnesses. Biol Psychiatry. 2009;65(3):263–7. https://doi.org/10.1016/j.biopsych.2008.06.026.
85. Pariante CM. Why are depressed patients inflamed? A reflection on 20 years of research on depression, glucocorticoid resistance and inflammation. Eur Neuropsychopharmacol. 2017;27(6):554–9. https://doi.org/10.1016/j.euroneuro.2017.04.001.
86. Sanada K, Nakajima S, Kurokawa S, Barcelo-Soler A, Ikuse D, Hirata A, et al. Gut microbiota and major depressive disorder: a systematic review and meta-analysis. J Affect Disord. 2020;266:1–13. https://doi.org/10.1016/j.jad.2020.01.102.
87. Pinto R, Rijsdijk F, Ouellet-Morin I, Asherson P, McLoughlin G, Kuntsi J. The aetiological association between the dynamics of cortisol productivity and ADHD. J Neural Transm (Vienna). 2016;123(8):991–1000. https://doi.org/10.1007/s00702-016-1534-5.
88. Cenit MC, Nuevo IC, Codoner-Franch P, Dinan TG, Sanz Y. Gut microbiota and attention deficit hyperactivity disorder: new perspectives for a challenging condition. Eur Child Adolesc Psychiatry. 2017;26(9):1081–92. https://doi.org/10.1007/s00787-017-0969-z.
89. Guida F, Turco F, Iannotta M, De Gregorio D, Palumbo I, Sarnelli G, et al. Antibiotic-induced microbiota perturbation causes gut endocannabinoidome changes, hippocampal neuroglial reorganization and depression in mice. Brain Behav Immun. 2018;67:230–45. https://doi.org/10.1016/j.bbi.2017.09.001.
90. Kelly JR, Borre Y, O'Brien C, Patterson E, El Aidy S, Deane J, et al. Transferring the blues: depression-associated gut microbiota induces neurobehavioural changes in the rat. J Psychiatr Res. 2016;82:109–18. https://doi.org/10.1016/j.jpsychires.2016.07.019.
91. Zheng P, Zeng B, Zhou C, Liu M, Fang Z, Xu X, et al. Gut microbiome remodeling induces depressive-like behaviors through a pathway mediated by the host's metabolism. Mol Psychiatry. 2016;21(6):786–96. https://doi.org/10.1038/mp.2016.44.
92. Jiang H, Ling Z, Zhang Y, Mao H, Ma Z, Yin Y, et al. Altered fecal microbiota composition in patients with major depressive disorder. Brain Behav Immun. 2015;48:186–94. https://doi.org/10.1016/j.bbi.2015.03.016.
93. Cheung SG, Goldenthal AR, Uhlemann AC, Mann JJ, Miller JM, Sublette ME. Systematic review of gut microbiota and major depression. Front Psych. 2019;10:34. https://doi.org/10.3389/fpsyt.2019.00034.
94. Madan A, Thompson D, Fowler JC, Ajami NJ, Salas R, Frueh BC, et al. The gut microbiota is associated with psychiatric symptom severity and treatment outcome among individuals with serious mental illness. J Affect Disord. 2020;264:98–106. https://doi.org/10.1016/j.jad.2019.12.020.
95. Bull-Larsen S, Mohajeri MH. The potential influence of the bacterial microbiome on the development and progression of ADHD. Nutrients. 2019;11(11):2805. https://doi.org/10.3390/nu11112805.
96. Bezirtzoglou E, Tsiotsias A, Welling GW. Microbiota profile in feces of breast- and formula-fed newborns by using fluorescence in situ hybridization (FISH). Anaerobe. 2011;17(6):478–82. https://doi.org/10.1016/j.anaerobe.2011.03.009.
97. Penders J, Thijs C, Vink C, Stelma FF, Snijders B, Kummeling I, et al. Factors influencing the composition of the intestinal microbiota in early infancy. Pediatrics. 2006;118(2):511–21. https://doi.org/10.1542/peds.2005-2824.
98. Aarts E, Ederveen THA, Naaijen J, Zwiers MP, Boekhorst J, Timmerman HM, et al. Gut microbiome in ADHD and its relation to neural reward anticipation. PLoS One. 2017;12(9):e0183509. https://doi.org/10.1371/journal.pone.0183509.
99. Jiang HY, Zhou YY, Zhou GL, Li YC, Yuan J, Li XH, et al. Gut microbiota profiles in treatment-naive children with attention deficit hyperactivity disorder. Behav Brain Res. 2018;347:408–13. https://doi.org/10.1016/j.bbr.2018.03.036.

100. Prehn-Kristensen A, Zimmermann A, Tittmann L, Lieb W, Schreiber S, Baving L, et al. Reduced microbiome alpha diversity in young patients with ADHD. PLoS One. 2018;13(7):e0200728. https://doi.org/10.1371/journal.pone.0200728.
101. Negrao BL, Bipath P, van der Westhuizen D, Viljoen M. Autonomic correlates at rest and during evoked attention in children with attention-deficit/hyperactivity disorder and effects of methylphenidate. Neuropsychobiology. 2011;63(2):82–91. https://doi.org/10.1159/000317548.
102. Sekaninova N, Mestanik M, Mestanikova A, Hamrakova A, Tonhajzerova I. Novel approach to evaluate central autonomic regulation in attention deficit/hyperactivity disorder (ADHD). Physiol Res. 2019;68(4):531–45. https://doi.org/10.33549/physiolres.934160.
103. Dam SA, Mostert JC, Szopinska-Tokov JW, Bloemendaal M, Amato M, Arias-Vasquez A. The role of the gut-brain axis in attention-deficit/hyperactivity disorder. Gastroenterol Clin N Am. 2019;48(3):407–31. https://doi.org/10.1016/j.gtc.2019.05.001.
104. Stevens AJ, Purcell RV, Darling KA, Eggleston MJF, Kennedy MA, Rucklidge JJ. Human gut microbiome changes during a 10 week randomised control trial for micronutrient supplementation in children with attention deficit hyperactivity disorder. Sci Rep. 2019;9(1):10128. https://doi.org/10.1038/s41598-019-46146-3.
105. Watson H, Mitra S, Croden FC, Taylor M, Wood HM, Perry SL, et al. A randomised trial of the effect of omega-3 polyunsaturated fatty acid supplements on the human intestinal microbiota. Gut. 2018;67(11):1974–83. https://doi.org/10.1136/gutjnl-2017-314968.

Dietary Inflammation and Mental Health 25

Scott Teasdale, Hajara Abdus Samad, Joseph Firth, and Wolfgang Marx

25.1 Introduction

Extensive peer-reviewed literature clearly and consistently highlights the importance of nutrition across the lifespan for general well-being and the prevention and treatment of specific disease states. Unfortunately, only a small percent of people are following recommended dietary guidelines and recommendations. Dietary-related risk factors are increasingly driving ill-health. The Global Burden of Disease Series consistently lists child and maternal malnutrition and dietary risks (a collective of risks from excessive or inadequate food and nutrient intakes) as two primary drivers of disease and ill-health [1]. Globally in 2017, dietary factors were the leading risk factors for death (10.9 million deaths) and second leading risk factor for disability-adjusted life-years (DALYs) (255 million DALYs). High intake of sodium (three million deaths), low intake of wholegrains (three million deaths), low intake of fruits (two million deaths), low intakes of nuts and seeds (two million deaths), diets low in vegetables (1.5 million deaths), and low in seafood omega-3 fatty acids (1.5 million deaths) were the leading dietary risk factors for mortality [2].

In developed countries, dietary risks are directly implicated in the development of obesity, cardiovascular disease, diabetes and other endocrine disorders, and cancer. In low-to-middle-income countries, child and maternal malnutrition supersedes the typical dietary risks of developed countries and is driving the greatest burden of disease. Low levels of resources, suboptimal agricultural techniques, and an arid

S. Teasdale
Faculty of Medicine, School of Psychiatry, UNSW Sydney, Sydney, NSW, Australia

H. A. Samad · W. Marx (✉)
Food & Mood Centre, IMPACT—The Institute for Mental and Physical Health and Clinical Translation, School of Medicine, Barwon Health, Deakin University, Geelong, Australia
e-mail: wolf.marx@deakin.edu.au

J. Firth
Division of Psychology and Mental Health, University of Manchester, Manchester, UK

M. Berk et al. (eds.), *Immuno-Psychiatry*, https://doi.org/10.1007/978-3-030-71229-7_25

landscape significantly contribute to food insecurity in these regions. Interestingly, the prevalence of preventable chronic diseases typically seen in developed countries is rising, with the increasing availability of energy-dense, low-nutrient processed foods a likely driving factor [1].

Evidence supports a plant-based approach to eating for both environmental and health benefits [3]. Definitions for plant-based eating differ. However, they generally include higher amounts of vegetables, fruit, wholegrains, nuts and seeds, some fish and seafood, and beneficial oils such as extra virgin olive oil. This approach also emphasizes a reduced consumption of meat and dairy products, and limiting highly processed foods, which are limited in beneficial nutrients and generally high in added sugar and fats. It is well established that food intake and body weight are inherently linked; however, the importance of diet quality can often be overlooked. A 2017 meta-analysis pooled hazard ratios for all-cause mortality and found people who maintained a higher-diet quality over the 12-year period had a 9–14% lower risk of death from any cause [4]. Large-scale, international changes to food policy and the food environment are needed improve dietary intake.

The impact of nutrition on brain function, mental health and as a potential treatment for common mental illness has previously been under-explored. The emerging field of nutritional psychiatry is showing promise, particularly in the fields of general mental health and common mental illness, with consistent evidence from large epidemiological studies confirming a relationship between diet quality and domains of mental health, and more recently RCTs showing a causal relationship for improvements in diet quality and improvements in symptoms for people living with major depressive disorder [5, 8]. The pathways thought to be mediating this include, but are not limited to, inflammation and the gut microbiome, both of which are linked to physical health domains including chronic disease [7]. This further drives the idea that mental health and physical health are interrelated and should be treated as such. This chapter reviews the current evidence and future application of nutritional psychiatry.

25.2 The Role of Diet-Induced Inflammation in Mental Health

Diet-induced inflammation may explain the inverse relationship between poor diet quality and mental disorders. Associations between habitual diet quality and systemic inflammation has been revealed by population-based studies. For example, a cross-sectional study conducted on healthy women (The Nurses' Health Study) demonstrated that consumption of western dietary pattern was highly correlated with inflammatory markers such as C-reactive protein (CRP), interleukin 6 (IL-6) in plasma [6]. Conversely, the same study reported that a prudent dietary pattern, high in fruits, vegetables, fish, poultry, and whole grains, was associated with reduced levels of plasma inflammatory markers [6]. The ATTICA study reported similar findings, with adherence to a Mediterranean style diet being associated with lower levels of plasma inflammatory and coagulation markers [7].

Clinical trial data also support the role of diet quality in inflammation. For example, in a randomized control trial, healthy men who consumed 8 servings/d of vegetables and fruits had significantly reduced plasma CRP concentrations compared to those consuming 2 serving/d [8]. Hyperlipidemic adults who received a diet enriched with soy proteins, viscous fibre, and almonds reported lower levels of CRP markers compared to those who received a diet low in saturated fat or the same diet with statins [9]. Also, a randomized cross-over trial in 50 men showed that consumption of trans-fatty acids increased plasma CRP concentrations [10].

The growing evidence for diet-induced inflammation has led to the development of the Dietary Inflammatory Index (DII®) [11], a literature-derived dietary pattern based on the inflammatory potential of individual diet components. The DII scores has been validated against a number of different inflammatory markers (IL-1β, IL-4, IL-6, IL- 10, TNF-α, and CRP). Recently, the DII tool was modified to correct limitations related to generalizability, resulting in a tool that provides an estimate of the inflammatory potential of an individual's diet from up to 45 individual food parameters [11].

The DII has been widely used to measure the impact of dietary inflammation on a range of health outcomes including mental disorders [7800]. A large study based on the UK Biobank data ($n = 69{,}843$) showed that a more pro-inflammatory dietary pattern was more common in individuals with mental disorders (e.g. schizophrenia, bipolar disorder, and MDD), which persisted after adjusting for confounders (age, sex, total energy intake) [12]. Akbaraley et al. used the DII scores to determine the inflammatory potential of diet and showed that for each increment of 1 standard deviation of DII scores, the recurrent odds for depression increased by 66% in women [13]. Another meta-analysis investigated the influence of various a priori dietary patterns on depression in 41 prospective and cross-sectional studies. The Mediterranean diet, the Healthy Eating Index (HEI) and Alternative HEI (AHEI), the Dietary Approaches to Stop Hypertension (DASH) diet, and the Dietary Inflammatory Index were the dietary patterns considered for this analysis. Both the Mediterranean diet and a lower score of Dietary Inflammatory Index (i.e. a more anti-inflammatory dietary pattern) was associated with lower risk of depression both in the prospective and cross-sectional study designs [14].

25.3 Specific Anti-inflammatory Nutrients in Mental Health

Food contains important individual nutrients that are essential for the development and functioning of the brain. This includes nutrients such as omega −3/6 fatty acids, vitamins (e.g. E, C, and B vitamins), and minerals (e.g. zinc, magnesium, copper). These nutrients as well as bioactive plant compounds such as polyphenols (e.g. anthocyanins, flavonoids) possess many important functions to brain health including the modulation of pathways that can damage the brain by reducing inflammation and oxidative stress.

The second largest proportion of lipids in humans are found in the central nervous system (CNS). The brain constitutes polyunsaturated fatty acids (PUFA) in the form of omega-3 and omega-6 fatty acids. Omega-3 fatty acids and their metabolites are important signaling molecules in the process of regulating inflammation and neuroinflammation via inhibition of multiple inflammatory processes such as leucocyte chemotaxis and adhesion molecule expression as well as via the production of anti-inflammatory compounds such as resolvins, protectins, and maresins [15]. There are multiple lines of evidence demonstrating the association between the dietary intake of omega-3 fatty acids and neuropsychiatric pathologies, in particular depression and anxiety [19–21]. Pre-clinical studies have showed that deprivation of omega-3 fatty acids can induce depression-like behaviours in animal models [19, 20]. Additionally, there is a substantial body of evidence from human trials showing that omega-3 fatty acids are useful as adjunctive treatments for depression [17], particularly formulations high in eicosapentaenoic acid (rather than docosahexaenoic acid) [17].

Oxidative stress is implicated in the pathophysiology of both neurodegenerative and psychiatric disorders [21]. An imbalance of cellular redox potential and the body's oxidative stress defensive mechanisms lead to an excessive concentration of free radicals/reactive oxygen species (ROS), which possess detrimental effects including the upregulation of inflammatory pathways and is also implicated in neurological and psychiatric disorders [22]. Polyphenols in foods such as colourful fruits, vegetables, spices, teas, and wines are promising free radical scavengers that demonstrate antioxidant and anti-inflammatory properties [23]. The potential of polyphenols to enhance cognitive process via modulating extracellular signaling pathways and protection against ROS-derived lipid peroxidation and neuroinflammation have been shown in rats [24]. Berries, red wine, and peanuts are abundant source of resveratrol, a non-flavonoid polyphenol, and intake of these elements has been demonstrated to act against Abeta-induced toxicity and attenuate degeneration of memory and Abeta pathology in rats [25]. In humans, consuming polyphenol-rich foods or supplements has demonstrated positive implications in improving mood although there is limited evidence and methodological inconsistencies [26, 27].

Finally, minerals (e.g. zinc, copper) in diet also play a critical role in the etiology of mental disorders, especially depression and anxiety [28]. Minerals are vital for neurotransmission (e.g. glutamatergic system and monoaminergic system), oxidative stress pathways, and immune functioning [29, 30]. Ample evidence demonstrates that lack of these minerals is associated with psychiatric disorders. For instance, dietary zinc is inversely associated with risk of depression [31]. Depressed subjects had lower blood levels of zinc compared to healthy subjects and intervention studies have shown that zinc supplementation may be an effective intervention for depression [29, 30].

25.4 The Role of the Diet-Gut-Brain Axis in Inflammation

A potential pathway whereby dietary intake may modulate inflammation and mental health is via the significant influence of dietary components on gut microbiota composition [7900]. Rapidly expanding evidence highlights the gut-brain axis as a promising target for the treatment and management of mental illness and its role in neuropsychiatric disorders [32]. The gut brain-brain axis comprises the central nervous system, neuroendocrine and neuroimmune system, sympathetic and parasympathetic parts of the autonomic nervous system, enteric nervous system, and the gut microbiota [33]. Studies from germ-free rodents, antibiotics, probiotics, gastrointestinal infection, and fecal microbiota transplant studies [38–40] suggest that the gut microbiota modulates brain function and mental health through the gut-brain axis and this is mediated via several mechanistic pathways such as altering the immunc and inflammatory system, hypothalamic-pituitary-adrenalin axis (HPA), tryptophan metabolism, production of bacterial metabolites, and through the vagus nerve [37]. Gut microbiota also interacts with the innate and humoral immune system and may therefore perform immunomodulatory functions [38]. Evidence shows that the gut microbiota triggers the stress response system of the brain and, vice versa, stressful conditions can alter the gut microbiota in a bidirectional fashion [33].

Growing evidence suggest that psychological stress can weaken the GI epithelia and increase intestinal permeability [39]. The GI epithelial integrity is essential in order to prevent food substances in the lumen from reaching the circulation and bacterial translocation [40]. Increased intestinal permeability facilitates the passage of bacteria and endotoxins such as lipopolysaccharides (LPS) to the peripheral circulation [41] and triggers the innate immune system, which in turn exacerbates the production of pro-inflammatory cytokine and heighten chronic neuroinflammation [42]. Moreover, elevated concentration of serum IgM, and IgA, against LPS of enterobacteria was found in patients with MDD compared to subjects without MDD [39].

Multiple dietary components can influence the gut microbiota including fibre, fat (including omega-3 fatty acids, and saturated fat), and polyphenols. Pre-clinical data report that high fat diet can unfavourably modify the gut microbial composition by creating a shift in the bacterial phyla [43]. Diets high in saturated fats and low in fibre may facilitate intestinal permeability, thereby triggering inflammation [44]. Further, animal models suggest that administering a diet with a higher proportion of fat can increase brain inflammation, reduce brain-derived neurotrophic factors (BNDF), and impede cognition [45].

Increasing intake of prebiotic fibre has been shown to restore the microbiota composition and rectify the immune imbalance caused by a high fat diet [46]. Consumption of fermented foods favourably influences the gut by reinstating a healthy gut microbiome, attenuating inflammation, and improving the gut barrier [47]. Producing short chain fatty (SCFA) acids is one way how the gut microbiota regulates inflammation. Acetate, butyrate, and propionate are the key SCFAs that result from the bacterial fermentation in the hind gut. These molecules act as inflammation regulators in addition to serving as energy substrates for colonocytes [48, 49]. At the cellular level, the inflammatory response is driven by the activation of nuclear factor kappa-B (NFκB) and subsequent transcription of pro-inflammatory cytokines [49]. Pre-clinical evidence shows SCFA, especially butyrate, can attenuate transcription of NFκB and the production of pro-inflammatory factors such as NFκB and may strengthen the gut epithelial integrity. This is imperative in terms of suppressing bacterial translocation and thereby attenuating inflammation [50]. Similar to studies that have investigated dietary fibre, a recent animal study demonstrated that anthocyanins, a particular class of polyphenols, could prevent dysbiosis caused by a high-fat diet and that the changes in gut bacterial genera caused by the polyphenols were correlated with anti-neuroinflammatory properties [51]. Furthermore, the anti-neuroinflammatory effect of polyphenols was associated with modulation of gut-mediated metabolites within the kynurenine pathway, a pathway implicated in the severity of depressive symptoms [51, 52].

25.5 Obesity and Inflammation in Mental Illness

In addition to the direct role of diet-induced inflammation in mental illness, diet-induced inflammation may also indirectly affect mental illness by driving obesity [53]. Multiple lines of evidence suggest that obesity is a pro-inflammatory state. Population-based studies have shown that people with obesity had elevated circulatory levels of pro-inflammatory and pro-coagulant proteins [58–60]. Adipose tissue upregulates inflammatory molecules including IL-6, MCP-1, iNOS, MMPs, and lipocalin [57]. Altered adipocyte function, leptin, hypothalamic pituitary adrenal (HPA) axis dysfunction, oxidative stress, and inflammation are speculated to play synergistic role in obesity-associated inflammation, diet-induced inflammation, and neuropsychiatric disorders [58]. A meta-analysis of 17 studies showed a positive association between obesity and depression in the general population with a pronounced link in women [55]. Intervention trials have demonstrated that weight-reduction reduces circulating inflammatory markers and depressive symptoms. For example, a group of women who were under a calorie restriction diet experienced reduction in adipose tissue along with reduced circulatory TNFa, IL-6, IL-8 and leptin [56]. Furthermore, the recent RAINBOW randomized controlled trial, reported that the subjects in the collaborative treatment arm that incorporated weight-loss dietary counselling, problem-solving therapy, and antidepressant medication as per need reported statistically significant attenuation in body mass index and depressive symptoms compared to the subjects in the usual care arm [59].

25.6 Putting Theory into Practice: Dietary Interventions in Mental Healthcare

There is a role for diet interventions in reducing low-grade inflammation. A systematic review and meta-analysis exploring the effects of different dietary approaches on inflammatory markers in people with the metabolic syndrome found positive effects on immune function [60]. Specifically, a low-fat diet lowered CRP greater than control; however, through sensitivity analysis it was assumed that this effect was dependent on weight-loss [60]. Low-carbohydrate diets achieved weight-loss and reductions as insulin; however, there was no significant change in CRP (based on limited studies) [60]. The assumption of weight-loss playing a key role into the reduction in pro-inflammatory markers is supported by a review specifically assessing weight-loss interventions [61]. A separate meta-analysis of 28 RCTs found that neither glycaemic load nor glycaemic index had an effect on a range of pro-inflammatory biomarkers [62], suggesting that diet-induced inflammation is not due to concentration changes of glucose in the blood.

Over the last two-decades, there has been a shift away from focusing on nutrients to focusing on foods and overall dietary patterns. Two of the most researched dietary patterns for health benefits are the Nordic and Mediterranean dietary patterns. Adherence to the traditional Nordic diet has an inverse relationship with high-sensitivity and C-reactive protein [63]. Subsequent intervention studies found that a healthy diet may reduce low-grade inflammation; however, higher quality RCTs are yet to confirm this [63]. Meta-analysis of 17 RCTs found strong evidence that adherence to the Mediterranean dietary pattern reduces inflammation and improves endothelial function [64].

Intervention trials have also explored effects directly on symptoms of common mental illness. A 2019 systematic review and meta-analysis of RCTs explored the efficacy of dietary interventions as adjunctive treatment in depression and anxiety [65]. Dietary interventions were shown to have a small, significant effect on depressive symptoms and no effect on anxiety symptoms (with limited data). The SMILES trial was the only RCT included in the review to test whether improving diet will reduce symptoms of depression in people with clinical depression as a primary outcome [66]. The individualized three-month intervention based on a modified Mediterranean diet reduced symptoms of depression greater than the social support group, with 32.3% ($n = 10$) meeting remission criteria in the diet intervention compared to 8.0% ($n = 2$) in the social support group. Importantly, improvements in diet quality correlated with reductions in depressive symptoms [67]. Two further RCTs have replicated the impact of dietary intervention of symptoms of people experiencing clinical depression. Both support the hypothesis that improvements in diet lead to reductions in depressive symptoms in people with clinical depression [68, 69]. The HELFIMED trial [68], a three-month group intervention based on the Mediterranean dietary pattern, combined with fish oil supplementation, had results remarkably similar to the SMILES trial. These positive results were maintained at six-month follow-up. The most recent RCT included a brief (3-week) dietary intervention for young adults meeting criteria for clinical depression [69]. The intervention arm had significant reductions in depressive symptoms, whereas the habitual diet group had no significant changes in depressive symptoms. Importantly, changes in certain food intakes explained some of the variance for depression outcomes. Furthermore, the reductions in depressive symptoms were maintained at three-months follow-up. Despite cohort studies demonstrating clear links between diet, inflammation and mental illness, none of the above RCTs have shown that the causal relationship between diet and depression is due to reductions in inflammation [70]. It should also be noted that despite there being a focus on the Mediterranean dietary pattern in these trials, it is possible that other traditional dietary patterns, known for general health benefits, could also reduce depressive symptoms.

To examine the top tier evidence for the benefits and safety of nutrient supplementation in people with mental disorders, a 2019 meta-review [17] brought together the data from 33 meta-analyses of RCTs; which in total contained studies of over 10,000 individuals with mental illness, randomized to nutrient supplement treatment vs. placebo-controlled conditions. This meta-review found no evidence for any nutrients as a 'standalone' treatment for any disorder, as most were trialed as 'add-on' (or 'adjunctive') treatments to psychiatric medications. Nonetheless, all nutrient supplements were found to be safe and there was no indication of serious adverse effects or contraindications with psychiatric medications. In terms of benefits as adjunctive treatments, the majority of the evidence favoured omega-3 supplements for people with major depression. Although effect sizes were mostly small from omega-3s, there was some evidence that omega-3 supplements containing higher doses of eicosapentaenoic acid had more substantial benefits for depression. Furthermore, the review also found some emerging evidence for L-methylfolate (the most bioactive form of Folate, i.e. Vitamin B9) for major depression and schizophrenia, along with several benefits from *N*-acetylcysteine (an antioxidant amino acid) emerging across multiple different conditions—again when used as an adjunctive treatment. Beyond these few options, however, there was very little evidence to support the use of other vitamins, minerals, or amino acids in the treatment of mental illness.

The focus of dietary interventions in severe mental illness has been on cardiometabolic outcomes, given the stark physical health inequalities. While this is true for all mental disorders, those with severe mental illness experience the greatest physical health disparities. The impact of symptoms, cognitive impairments, social and financial constraints, and medication side effects has led to unacceptable levels of obesity, diabetes, cardiovascular disease, and early death. A meta-analysis of RCTs incorporating dietary interventions found positive effects on cardiometabolic outcomes (weight, waist circumference, blood glucose) [71]. Subgroup analysis and meta-regression analysis found much stronger effects for interventions that were (i) delivered by dietitians and (ii) delivered early in the course of antipsychotic treatment as a preventative measure. These concepts have formed part of the recommendations in the Lancet Commission into protecting the physical health of people with mental illness [72]. These concepts have successfully been translated into routine care in a mental health service, demonstrating acceptability and effectiveness for people in the early stages on psychosis [77–80]. The benefit of specific dietary patterns and delivering dietary interventions on mental health domains for people experiencing severe mental illness is currently unknown, and are limited to animal studies and case reports.

25.7 Conclusion

The current food environment is driving high rates of preventable chronic disease. Further, there is a clear link between suboptimal dietary intake and poorer mental health, particularly depressive symptoms. This is thought to be mediated, at least in part, through the gut microbiome and diet-induced inflammation. The field of nutritional psychiatry is commencing its transition from research to clinical practice. Diet modification is emerging as a promising adjunctive treatment for people with MDD. Alongside this, there is also evidence to support the use of high EPA omega 3. Diet modification for symptom reduction in other mental disorders is unclear; however, transition to a traditional dietary pattern can assist in protecting the physical health of people at high risk for cardiometabolic complications.

References

1. GBD 2017 Risk Factor Collaborators. Global, regional, and national comparative risk assessment of 84 behavioural, environmental and occupational, and metabolic risks or clusters of risks for 195 countries and territories, 1990–2017: a systematic analysis for the Global Burden of Disease Study 2017. Lancet. 2018;392:1923–94.
2. Afshin A, Sur PJ, Fay KA, Cornaby L, Ferrara G, Salama JS, et al. Health effects of dietary risks in 195 countries, 1990–2017: a systematic analysis for the global burden of disease study 2017. Lancet. 2019;393(10184):1958–72.
3. Willett W, Rockström J, Loken B, Springmann M, Lang T, Vermeulen S, et al. Food in the anthropocene: the EAT–lancet commission on healthy diets from sustainable food systems. Lancet. 2019;393(10170):447–92.
4. Sotos-Prieto M, Bhupathiraju SN, Mattei J, Fung TT, Li Y, Pan A, et al. Association of changes in diet quality with total and cause-specific mortality. N Engl J Med. 2017;377(2):143–53.
5. Jacka FN. Nutritional psychiatry: where to next? EBioMedicine. 2017;17:24–9.
6. Firth J, Solmi M, Wootton RE, Vancampfort D, Schuch FB, Hoare E, et al. A meta-review of "lifestyle psychiatry": the role of exercise, smoking, diet and sleep in the prevention and treatment of mental disorders. World Psychiatry. 2020;19(3):360–80. https://doi.org/10.1002/wps.20773. PMID: 32931092. PMCID: PMC7491615.
7. Marx W, Lane M, Hockey M, Aslam H, Berk M, Walder K, et al. Diet and depression: exploring the biological mechanisms of action. Mol Psychiatry. 2021;26(1):134–50. https://doi.org/10.1038/s41380-020-00925-x. PMID: 33144709.
8. Lopez-Garcia E, Schulze MB, Fung TT, Meigs JB, Rifai N, Manson JE, et al. Major dietary patterns are related to plasma concentrations of markers of inflammation and endothelial dysfunction. Am J Clin Nutr. 2004;80(4):1029–35.
9. Chrysohoou C, Panagiotakos DB, Pitsavos C, Das UN, Stefanadis C. Adherence to the Mediterranean diet attenuates inflammation and coagulation process in healthy adults: the ATTICA study. J Am Coll Cardiol. 2004;44(1):152–8.
10. Watzl B, Kulling SE, Möseneder J, Barth SW, Bub A. A 4-wk intervention with high intake of carotenoid-rich vegetables and fruit reduces plasma C-reactive protein in healthy, nonsmoking men. Am J Clin Nutr. 2005;82(5):1052–8.
11. Jenkins DJ, Kendall CW, Marchie A, Faulkner DA, Wong JM, de Souza R, et al. Effects of a dietary portfolio of cholesterol-lowering foods vs lovastatin on serum lipids and C-reactive protein. JAMA. 2003;290(4):502–10.
12. Baer DJ, Judd JT, Clevidence BA, Tracy RP. Dietary fatty acids affect plasma markers of inflammation in healthy men fed controlled diets: a randomized crossover study. Am J Clin Nutr. 2004;79(6):969–73.
13. Hébert JR, Shivappa N, Wirth MD, Hussey JR, Hurley TG. Perspective: the dietary inflammatory index (DII)—lessons learned, improvements made, and future directions. Adv Nutr. 2019;10(2):185–95.
14. Marx W, Veronese N, Kelly JT, Smith L, Hockey M, Collins S, et al. The dietary inflammatory index and human health: an umbrella review of meta-analyses of observational studies. Adv Nutr. 2021;nmab037. https://doi.org/10.1093/advances/nmab037. PMID: 33873204.

15. Firth J, Stubbs B, Teasdale SB, Ward PB, Veronese N, Shivappa N, et al. Diet as a hot topic in psychiatry: a population-scale study of nutritional intake and inflammatory potential in severe mental illness. World Psychiatry. 2018;17(3):365.
16. Akbaraly TN, Kerleau C, Wyart M, Chevallier N, Ndiaye L, Shivappa N, et al. Dietary inflammatory index and recurrence of depressive symptoms: results from the Whitehall II study. Clin Psychol Sci. 2016;4(6):1125–34.
17. Lassale C, Batty GD, Baghdadli A, Jacka F, Sánchez-Villegas A, Kivimäki M, et al. Healthy dietary indices and risk of depressive outcomes: a systematic review and meta-analysis of observational studies. Mol Psychiatry. 2018;24:965–86.
18. Calder PC. Omega-3 fatty acids and inflammatory processes: from molecules to man. Biochem Soc Trans. 2017;45(5):1105–15.
19. Larrieu T, Layé S. Food for mood: relevance of nutritional omega-3 fatty acids for depression and anxiety. Front Physiol. 2018;9:1047.
20. Firth J, Teasdale SB, Allott K, Siskind D, Marx W, Cotter J, et al. The efficacy and safety of nutrient supplements in the treatment of mental disorders: a meta-review of meta-analyses of randomized controlled trials. World Psychiatry. 2019;18(3):308–24.
21. Guu T-W, Mischoulon D, Sarris J, Hibbeln J, McNamara RK, Hamazaki K, et al. International society for nutritional psychiatry research practice guidelines for omega-3 fatty acids in the treatment of major depressive disorder. Psychother Psychosom. 2019;88:263–73.
22. Takeuchi T, Iwanaga M, Harada E. Possible regulatory mechanism of DHA-induced anti-stress reaction in rats. Brain Res. 2003;964(1):136–43.
23. Delion S, Chalon S, Hérault J, Guilloteau D, Besnard J-C, Durand G. Chronic dietary α-linolenic acid deficiency alters dopaminergic and serotoninergic neurotransmission in rats. J Nutr. 1994;124(12):2466–76.
24. Moylan S, Berk M, Dean OM, Samuni Y, Williams LJ, O'Neil A, et al. Oxidative & nitrosative stress in depression: why so much stress? Neurosci Biobehav Rev. 2014;45:46–62.
25. Berk M, Williams LJ, Jacka FN, O'Neil A, Pasco JA, Moylan S, et al. So depression is an inflammatory disease, but where does the inflammation come from? BMC Med. 2013;11:200.
26. Gomez-Pinilla F, Nguyen TT. Natural mood foods: the actions of polyphenols against psychiatric and cognitive disorders. Nutr Neurosci. 2012;15(3):127–33.
27. Williams CM, El Mohsen MA, Vauzour D, Rendeiro C, Butler LT, Ellis JA, et al. Blueberry-induced changes in spatial working memory correlate with changes in hippocampal CREB phosphorylation and brain-derived neurotrophic factor (BDNF) levels. Free Radic Biol Med. 2008;45(3):295–305.
28. Rossi L, Mazzitelli S, Arciello M, Capo C, Rotilio G. Benefits from dietary polyphenols for brain aging and Alzheimer's disease. Neurochem Res. 2008;33(12):2390–400.
29. Travica N, D'Cunha NM, Naumovski N, Kent K, Mellor DD, Firth J, et al. The effect of blueberry interventions on cognitive performance and mood: a systematic review of randomized controlled trials. Brain Behav Immun. 2020;85:96–105.
30. Marx W, Kelly JT, Marshall S, Cutajar J, Annois B, Pipingas A, et al. Effect of resveratrol supplementation on cognitive performance and mood in adults: a systematic literature review and meta-analysis of randomized controlled trials. Nutr Rev. 2018;76(6):432–43.
31. Nakamura M, Miura A, Nagahata T, Shibata Y, Okada E, Ojima T. Low zinc, copper, and manganese intake is associated with depression and anxiety symptoms in the Japanese working population: findings from the eating habit and well-being study. Nutrients. 2019;11(4):847.
32. Młyniec K, Gaweł M, Doboszewska U, Starowicz G, Pytka K, Davies CL, et al. Essential elements in depression and anxiety. Part II Pharmacol Rep. 2015;67(2):187–94.
33. Młyniec K, Davies CL, de Agüero Sánchez IG, Pytka K, Budziszewska B, Nowak G. Essential elements in depression and anxiety. Part I Pharmacol Rep. 2014;66(4):534–44.
34. Vashum KP, McEvoy M, Milton AH, McElduff P, Hure A, Byles J, et al. Dietary zinc is associated with a lower incidence of depression: findings from two Australian cohorts. J Affect Disord. 2014;166:249–57.
35. Berding K, Vlckova K, Marx W, Schellekens H, Stanton C, Clarke G, et al. Diet and the microbiota-gut-brain axis: sowing the seeds of good mental health. Adv Nutr. 2021;nmaa181. https://doi.org/10.1093/advances/nmaa181. PMID: 33693453.

36. Long-Smith C, O'Riordan KJ, Clarke G, Stanton C, Dinan TG, Cryan JF. Microbiota-gut-brain axis: new therapeutic opportunities. Ann Rev Pharmacol Toxicol. 2019;60:477–502.
37. Dinan TG, Cryan JF. Regulation of the stress response by the gut microbiota: implications for psychoneuroendocrinology. Psychoneuroendocrinology. 2012;37(9):1369–78.
38. Cryan JF, Dinan TG. Gut microbiota: microbiota and neuroimmune signalling—Metchnikoff to microglia. Nat Rev Gastroenterol Hepatol. 2015;12(9):494.
39. Dinan TG, Cryan JF. Melancholic microbes: a link between gut microbiota and depression? Neurogastroenterol Motil. 2013;25(9):713–9.
40. Mayer EA, Knight R, Mazmanian SK, Cryan JF, Tillisch K. Gut microbes and the brain: paradigm shift in neuroscience. J Neurosci. 2014;34(46):15490–6.
41. Kelly JR, Clarke G, Cryan JF, Dinan TG. Brain-gut-microbiota axis: challenges for translation in psychiatry. Ann Epidemiol. 2016;26(5):366–72.
42. Foster JA, Neufeld K-AM. Gut–brain axis: how the microbiome influences anxiety and depression. Trends Neurosci. 2013;36(5):305–12.
43. Kelly JR, Kennedy PJ, Cryan JF, Dinan TG, Clarke G, Hyland NP. Breaking down the barriers: the gut microbiome, intestinal permeability and stress-related psychiatric disorders. Front Cell Neurosci. 2015;9:392.
44. Conlon MA, Bird AR. The impact of diet and lifestyle on gut microbiota and human health. Nutrients. 2014;7(1):17–44.
45. Leclercq S, Matamoros S, Cani PD, Neyrinck AM, Jamar F, Stärkel P, et al. Intestinal permeability, gut-bacterial dysbiosis, and behavioral markers of alcohol-dependence severity. Proc Natl Acad Sci. 2014;111(42):E4485–E93.
46. Slyepchenko A, Maes M, Jacka FN, Köhler CA, Barichello T, McIntyre RS, et al. Gut microbiota, bacterial translocation, and interactions with diet: pathophysiological links between major depressive disorder and non-communicable medical comorbidities. Psychother Psychosom. 2017;86(1):31–46.
47. Candido TLN, Alfenas RDCG, Bressan J. Dysbiosis and metabolic endotoxemia induced by high-fat diet. Nutr Hosp. 2018;35:1432–40.
48. Araújo JR, Tomas J, Brenner C, Sansonetti PJ. Impact of high-fat diet on the intestinal microbiota and small intestinal physiology before and after the onset of obesity. Biochimie. 2017;141:97–106.
49. Pistell PJ, Morrison CD, Gupta S, Knight AG, Keller JN, Ingram DK, et al. Cognitive impairment following high fat diet consumption is associated with brain inflammation. J Neuroimmunol. 2010;219(1–2):25–32.
50. Delzenne NM, Neyrinck AM, Cani PD. Modulation of the gut microbiota by nutrients with prebiotic properties: consequences for host health in the context of obesity and metabolic syndrome. Microb Cell Fact. 2011;10(1):1–1.
51. Aslam H, Green J, Jacka FN, Collier F, Berk M, Pasco J, et al. Fermented foods, the gut and mental health: a mechanistic overview with implications for depression and anxiety. Nutr Neurosci. 2018:1–13.
52. Vinolo MA, Rodrigues HG, Nachbar RT, Curi R. Regulation of inflammation by short chain fatty acids. Nutrients. 2011;3(10):858–76.
53. Vinolo M, Rodrigues H, Nachbar R, Curi R. Modulation of inflammatory and immune responses by short-chain fatty acids. . Diet, Immunity and Inflammation. Elsevier; 2013. p. 435–58.
54. Peng L, Li Z-R, Green RS, Holzman IR, Lin J. Butyrate enhances the intestinal barrier by facilitating tight junction assembly via activation of AMP-activated protein kinase in Caco-2 cell monolayers. J Nutr. 2009;139(9):1619–25.
55. Marques C, Fernandes I, Meireles M, Faria A, Spencer JPE, Mateus N, et al. Gut microbiota modulation accounts for the neuroprotective properties of anthocyanins. Sci Rep. 2018;8(1):11341.
56. Ogyu K, Kubo K, Noda Y, Iwata Y, Tsugawa S, Omura Y, et al. Kynurenine pathway in depression: a systematic review and meta-analysis. Neurosci Biobehav Rev. 2018;90:16–25.

57. Ferrante A Jr. Obesity-induced inflammation: a metabolic dialogue in the language of inflammation. J Intern Med. 2007;262(4):408–14.
58. Ouchi N, Kihara S, Funahashi T, Matsuzawa Y, Walsh K. Obesity, adiponectin and vascular inflammatory disease. Curr Opin Lipidol. 2003;14(6):561–6.
59. De Wit L, Luppino F, van Straten A, Penninx B, Zitman F, Cuijpers P. Depression and obesity: a meta-analysis of community-based studies. Psychiatry Res. 2010;178(2):230–5.
60. Arvidsson E, Viguerie N, Andersson I, Verdich C, Langin D, Arner P. Effects of different hypocaloric diets on protein secretion from adipose tissue of obese women. Diabetes. 2004;53(8):1966–71.
61. Hotamisligil GS, Peraldi P, Budavari A, Ellis R, White MF, Spiegelman BM. IRS-1-mediated inhibition of insulin receptor tyrosine kinase activity in TNF-α-and obesity-induced insulin resistance. Science. 1996;271(5249):665–70.
62. Cuijpers P, Berking M, Andersson G, Quigley L, Kleiboer A, Dobson KS. A meta-analysis of cognitive-behavioural therapy for adult depression, alone and in comparison with other treatments. Can J Psychiatry. 2013;58(7):376–85.
63. Ma J, Rosas LG, Lv N, Xiao L, Snowden MB, Venditti EM, et al. Effect of integrated behavioral weight loss treatment and problem-solving therapy on body mass index and depressive symptoms among patients with obesity and depression: the RAINBOW randomized clinical trial. JAMA. 2019;321(9):869–79.
64. Steckhan N, Hohmann C-D, Kessler C, Dobos G, Michalsen A, Cramer H. Effects of different dietary approaches on inflammatory markers in patients with metabolic syndrome: a systematic review and meta-analysis. Nutrition. 2016;32(3):338–48.
65. Forsythe LK, Wallace JMW, Livingstone MBE. Obesity and inflammation: the effects of weight loss. Nutr Res Rev. 2008;21(2):117–33.
66. Milajerdi A, Saneei P, Larijani B, Esmaillzadeh A. The effect of dietary glycemic index and glycemic load on inflammatory biomarkers: a systematic review and meta-analysis of randomized clinical trials. Am J Clin Nutr. 2018;107(4):593–606.
67. Lankinen M, Uusitupa M, Schwab U. Nordic diet and inflammation—a review of observational and intervention studies. Nutrients. 2019;11(6):1369.
68. Schwingshackl L, Hoffmann G. Mediterranean dietary pattern, inflammation and endothelial function: a systematic review and meta-analysis of intervention trials. Nutr Metab Cardiovasc Dis. 2014;24(9):929–39.
69. Firth J, Marx W, Dash S, Carney R, Teasdale SB, Solmi M, et al. The effects of dietary improvement on symptoms of depression and anxiety: a meta-analysis of randomized controlled trials. Psychosom Med. 2019;81(3):265.
70. Jacka FN, O'Neil A, Opie R, Itsiopoulos C, Cotton S, Mohebbi M, et al. A randomised controlled trial of dietary improvement for adults with major depression (the 'SMILES'trial). BMC Med. 2017;15(1):23.
71. Opie RS, O'Neil A, Jacka FN, Pizzinga J, Itsiopoulos C. A modified Mediterranean dietary intervention for adults with major depression: dietary protocol and feasibility data from the SMILES trial. Nutr Neurosci. 2017;21:487–501.
72. Parletta N. A Mediterranean-style dietary intervention supplemented with fish oil improves diet and mental health in people with depression: a 6-month randomized controlled trial (HELFIMED). Nutr Neurosci. 2017;22:474–87.
73. Francis H, Stevenson R, Chambers J, Gupta D, Newey B, Lim C. A brief diet intervention can reduce symptoms of depression in young adults – a randomised controlled trial. PLoS One. 2019;14:e0222768.
74. Firth J, Veronese N, Cotter J, Shivappa N, Hebert J, Ee C, et al. What is the role of dietary inflammation in severe mental illness? A review of observational and experimental findings. Front Psych. 2019;10:350.
75. Teasdale SB, Ward PB, Rosenbaum S, Samaras K, Stubbs B. Solving a weighty problem: systematic review and meta-analysis of nutrition interventions in severe mental illness. Br J Psychiatry. 2016;210:110–8.

76. Firth J, Siddiqi N, Koyanagi A, Siskind D, Rosenbaum S, Galletly C, et al. The lancet psychiatry commission: a blueprint for protecting physical health in people with mental illness. Lancet Psychiatry. 2019;6(8):675–712.
77. Curtis J, Watkins A, Rosenbaum S, Teasdale S, Kalucy M, Samaras K, et al. Evaluating an individualized lifestyle and life skills intervention to prevent antipsychotic-induced weight gain in first-episode psychosis. Early Interv Psychiatry. 2016;10(3):267–76.
78. Curtis J, Watkins A, Teasdale S, Lederman O, Kalucy M, Lappin J, et al. 2 year follow-up: still keeping the body in mind. Aust N Z J Psychiatry. 2018;52:602–3.
79. Teasdale S, Ward P, Rosenbaum S, Watkins A, Curtis J, Kalucy M, et al. A nutrition intervention is effective in improving dietary components linked to cardiometabolic risk in youth with first-episode psychosis. Br J Nutr. 2016;115(11):1987.
80. Teasdale SB, Rosenbaum S, Watkins A, Curtis J, Kalucy M, Samaras K, et al. Preventing antipsychotic-induced weight gain in first-episode psychosis: transitioning dietitians into routine care. Nutr Diete. 2015;73:303–4.

Exercise and Inflammation

26

Kandola Aaron and Stubbs Brendon

26.1 Introduction

As demonstrated throughout this book, the relevance of inflammation is increasingly being recognised in psychiatry. Evidence is also emerging that physical activity and exercise have anti-inflammatory properties and represent promising new forms of treatment for a range of psychiatric conditions, including depression [1].

Physical activity refers to any movement of skeletal muscles that requires energy expenditure [2]. Data from prospective cohort studies suggest that higher levels of physical activity is associated with a reduced risk of depression [3] and physical inactivity is associated with a greater risk of depression [4, 5]. Exercise is a structured form of physical activity aimed at improving or maintaining at least one component of physical fitness [2]. Several systematic reviews have found that exercise can treat the symptoms of depression with a moderate to large effect size [1, 6].

People with depression have elevated levels of pro-inflammatory markers, such as interleukin (IL)-6 and tumour necrosis factor alpha (TNF-α) [7], which may contribute to onset and progression of symptoms [8]. Some of the anti-depressant effects of exercise may be attributable to their capacity to ameliorate this inflammation [10].

K. Aaron (✉)
Division of Psychiatry, University College London, London, UK

Institute of Mental Health, University College London, London, UK
e-mail: a.kandola.18@ucl.ac.uk

S. Brendon
Department of Psychological Medicine, Institute of Psychiatry, Psychology, and Neuroscience, King's College London, London, UK

Physiotherapy Department, South London and Maudsley National Health Services Foundation Trust, London, UK
e-mail: brendon.stubbs@kcl.ac.uk

M. Berk et al. (eds.), *Immuno-Psychiatry*, https://doi.org/10.1007/978-3-030-71229-7_26

This chapter provides an overview (1) of the role of exercise in maintaining low inflammatory profile, (2) the role of exercise in reducing inflammation in clinical populations, (3) the potential and evidence for exercise in reducing inflammation in people with depression and (4) Clinical implications and future research.

It is worth noting that there are several different types of exercise that modulate different types of physical fitness. For example, aerobic exercise involves the use of large muscle groups in dynamic activities that improve the function of the cardiovascular system, such as running or cycling [9]. Resistance training is designed to increase musculature and strength and derives energy from glycolysis and stored phosphocreatine, such as weightlifting. Different types of exercise elicit different biological mechanisms and are likely to have different inflammatory profiles [11]. In this chapter, we primarily discuss research on aerobic exercise, but studies using resistance exercise will also be included where relevant.

26.2 The Role of Exercise in Maintaining a Low Inflammatory Profile

In non-clinical populations, systematic reviews have found that higher physical activity levels and exercise training are associated with lower circulating levels of inflammatory markers including C reactive protein (CRP) [12]. Several prospective cohort studies have found that low physical activity levels over a 10-year period are associated with higher circulating levels of inflammatory markers including C-reactive protein (CRP), interleukin (IL)-6, fibrinogen and adiponectin [13, 14]. Conversely, high physical activity levels are associated with reductions in CRP and IL-6 [15]. Cross-sectional studies in healthy populations have also found higher physical activity level to be associated with lower concentrations of inflammatory markers including CRP, IL-6, fibrinogen and TNF-α [16–20].

Evidence suggests that physical activity and exercise are associated with lower basal levels of inflammation. Several mechanisms may underlie these effects. Since the discovery that muscles can synthesize and release cytokines, known as myokines, their actions during acute bouts of exercise are thought to play an important role in the long-term anti-inflammatory effects of exercise training [21].

When considering exercise as an intervention, the largest meta-analysis in this area contains data from 7487 mostly healthy participants across 160 randomised controlled trials (RCTs) investigating aerobic and resistance exercise training programmes [22]. The authors found that exercise training over a median of 12 weeks (ranging from 2 weeks to 2 years) led to lower levels of pro-inflammatory markers IL-18, leptin, fibrinogen and angiotensin II. Another systematic review that included a subgroup analysis of 19 trials in healthy participants found exercise to be associated with lower levels of leptin [23]. Several large-scale RCTs in healthy populations have failed to find any anti-inflammatory effects of exercise training (e.g. [24–27]), but this is likely due to differences in study design, demographics, exercise protocol or modality and inflammatory markers assessed [27].

During acute bouts of exercise, significant changes are seen in levels of IL-6, a myokine involved in a range of metabolic processes including fat oxidation and lipolysis [28]. One meta-analysis found that between 30 to 60 minutes of moderate to high intensity exercise was sufficient to cause a 145% increase in IL-6 [29]. In most cases, IL-6 is preceded by an increase in pro-inflammatory factors, such as TNF-α [30]. But the muscular release of IL-6 in response to exercise is unique in that it does not involve elevations of TNF-α and is instead followed by an elevation of anti-inflammatory markers such as IL-10 and the IL-1 receptor antagonist (IL-1ra) [31–33]. These factors are released by monocytes and macrophages and inhibit the production of pro-inflammatory cytokines including IL-1β, IL-1α and TNF-α [34, 35]. While IL-6 peaks at the end of an exercise session, IL-1r continues to increase for several hours post-exercise [33], extending the anti-inflammatory window of acute exercise.

Acute exercise also activates the hypothalamic-pituitary-adrenal (HPA) axis and the sympathetic nervous system (SNS) via neuronal signalling from the motor cortex [36]. This leads to further anti-inflammatory action through hormonal changes. The adrenal gland and medulla trigger the release of adrenaline and cortisol, which further inhibit TNF-α production by monocytes and increase IL-10 release [33, 37]. In one study mimicking the effects of exercise, the elevations in cortisol also led to elevations in circulating immune-protective neutrophils and a reduction in the number of lymphocytes [33].

Muscle contractions during acute bouts of exercise essentially elicit an initial inflammatory spike that triggers several counteractive responses to create an anti-inflammatory environment mediated by myokines [38]. Repeated bouts of exercise stimulate a homeostatic adjustment to the various anti-inflammatory pathways activated through acute exercise, thereby extending its effects.

Another important anti-inflammatory pathway of exercise training relates to changes in adipose tissue. Both acute and regular exercise generally reduce adipose tissue, particularly around visceral organs, such as the liver [39]. For example, one study found that reducing participants' daily steps from 10,000 to 1500 led to a significant increase in visceral fat without changes in total fat [40]. Through the activation of multiple pathways, the accumulation of adipose tissue can create chronic systemic inflammation through the release of pro-inflammatory adipokines (cytokines that are released by adipose tissue), such as IL-6, IL-18, TNF-α, leptin, resistin, angiopoietin-like protein 2 (ANGPTL2) and nicotinamide phosphoribosyltransferase (NAMPT) [41]. The extent to which metabolic dysfunction is present with the accumulation of adipose tissue will determine the degree of systemic inflammation. By counteracting the accumulation of adipose tissue, regular exercise can prevent or limit the presence of this source of chronic systemic inflammation.

It is possible that this process is still partially mediated by myokines, such as IL-15 [38]. IL-15 is protective against the accumulation of adipose tissue [42, 43] and present in higher concentrations in trained human muscle [44]. The increase in IL-15 can also stimulate the secretion of adiponectin [43], a cytokine that produces anti-inflammatory effects through insulin sensitization [45]. Longer term exercise (>6 months) causes higher basal levels of adiponectin in blood plasma in overweight men and women [46]. In healthy women, a 10-week training programme produced increases in serum adiponectin and retinol-binding protein-4 (RBP4), which increased insulin sensitivity [45].

Some studies have found similar reductions in inflammatory markers related to metabolism that are independent of weight-loss [47]. Beyond reducing the amount of adipose tissue, animal models suggest exercise may even modulate the inflammatory properties of adipose tissue [36]. The immune cell profile of adipose tissue can change depending on its composition of pro-inflammatory M1 macrophage cells to anti-inflammatory M2 macrophage cells [48]. Several animal studies have found that exercise training can reduce levels of pro-inflammatory cytokines through reducing M1 macrophage adipose tissue content [49, 50]. There is some support for this in humans, but the research is limited [34].

Exercise training can also induce lasting alterations in toll-like receptor (TLR)-dependent inflammation. TLRs are proteins that upregulate the release of pro-inflammatory cytokines in response to pathogens via monocytes and play an important role in mediating the immune system [51, 52]. In one study with young and older healthy participants, a 12-week endurance and resistance training programme led to lower basal levels of IL-6 and a significant reduction in TLR4 expression on cluster of differentiation 14 (CD14) monocyte cells [53]. Similar studies in healthy participants have also found exercise training to reduce TLR4 expression [54–56]. Animal models have also demonstrated that exercise training can modulate TLR4 expression on cells other than monocytes, including in skeletal muscles and adipose tissue [57]. Such findings suggest that exercise training could have a broad, systemic anti-inflammatory effect through TLR modulation, but more human work is needed in this area.

Through a series of interacting pathways, exercise training can help to create an anti-inflammatory environment in the body. Some key mechanisms underlying these effects relate to the actions of myokines, the modulation of adipose tissue, TLRs and monocytes. Several other potential anti-inflammatory mechanisms of exercise are also being established, such as the upregulation of heat shock proteins [58].

26.3 The Role of Exercise in Reducing Inflammation amongst Clinical Populations

Given its anti-inflammatory properties, exercise could be a useful clinical tool for reducing inflammation in clinical populations. Several meta-analyses in people with cardiovascular disease found that exercise interventions can reduce concentrations of CRP, IL-6, fibrinogen and vascular cell adhesion molecule 1 [59, 60]. Meta-analyses of trials in overweight or obese individuals have found exercise training may reduce serum concentrations of leptin, CRP (non-significant trend $p = 0.07$; [61]) and increased the anti-inflammatory marker adiponectin [62], independent of weight-loss [63]. One review found that combining aerobic and resistance training was more effective at reducing leptin than aerobic exercise alone

[63]. Meta-analyses in people with pre-diabetes and type 2 diabetes found that exercise can reduce CRP, leptin and IL-6, but had no effect, or increased adiponectin [64, 65]. In people recovering from cancer, meta-analyses have found that exercise can reduce IL-2, IL-6, IL-8 and TNF-α [66]. Finally, other meta-analyses that mostly include from people with cardiovascular disease, type 2 diabetes, overweight and obesity have also found that exercise interventions reduce CRP, IL-18, leptin, fibrinogen and angiotensin II and increase adiponectin across all population groups [22, 23, 67, 68]).

There is good evidence to suggest that exercise can be useful in reducing inflammation across a wide range of conditions [69]. As in research on healthy participants, there are still inconsistencies in the literature. For example, a recent systematic review of 11 studies in people with type 2 diabetes found exercise had no effect on CRP [70]. In a meta-analysis of inflammatory rheumatic disease trials, exercise improved disease progression and joint damage, but no changes in CRP [71]. An earlier meta-analysis that found no significant effect of exercise on CRP did find that exercise decreased body fat in healthy adults [72]. Both rheumatic disease progression and adiposity are intrinsically linked with inflammation [41, 73]. It stands to reason that significant changes in these factors would influence inflammatory profiles and may be represented by variance in other inflammatory markers not measured in these studies.

26.4 The Potential for Exercise to Reduce Inflammation in People with Depression

A growing body of evidence exists to suggest that there may be an inflammatory component to some cases of depression [74], which is associated higher levels of pro-inflammatory markers, such as IL-1, IL-6, TNF-α and CRP [7, 75–77]. As exercise can reduce the circulation of these pro-inflammatory markers, it could be a useful method of treating inflammation in people with depression. People with depression are also more likely to have greater amounts of adipose tissue exasperating the inflammation [78]. Through also reducing adipose tissue [39], exercise may indirectly attenuate inflammation further.

While several systematic reviews have found exercise interventions can effectively reduce depressive symptoms [1, 6, 79], it is unclear if this co-occurs with a reduction in inflammation. Few interventional exercise studies have attempted to measure inflammatory markers in people with depression. One systematic review [80] of the biological mechanisms associated with exercise in people with depression found just three studies measured inflammatory markers [81–83]. However, none of these studies found that exercise elicited any significant changes in inflammatory markers. In one of the studies, changes in IL-β and higher baseline levels of TNF-α were associated with greater improvements in depressive symptoms following the exercise intervention [83].

Other, more recent findings have been promising. In one RCT, people with depression were assigned to a cognitive behavioural therapy (CBT) group, and CBT with exercise (CBTe) group and a waitlist control (WL) for 16 weeks [84]. 30 matched controls were also included at baseline to make immunological comparisons. Participants with depression had elevated CRP, neutrophil and monocyte counts, and lower IL-10 than controls. Following the intervention, the CBTe group had significantly higher IL-10 than the other groups, but no other inflammatory changes were found. In a 12-week trial, 116 people with depression were assigned three 60-minute exercise sessions each week [85]. Blood samples were taken before and after the trial to measure IL-6 concentrations. After the intervention, there was a significant reduction in IL-6 concentrations, which coincided with reductions in depression severity. Exercise trials in people without depression have found that exercise can reduce depressive symptoms that correlate with reductions in TNF-α, CRP, IL-6 and IL-8 markers [86, 87]. However, high-intensity exercises such as interval training can cause increases in TNF-α and IL-6 [87].

Currently, very few exercise trials take blood samples pre- and post-intervention for measuring inflammatory markers [80]. The lack of research in this area makes it difficult to determine whether exercise can reduce inflammation in people with depression. However, recent findings have been promising.

26.5 Clinical Implications and Future Research

Exercise has the potential to treat and prevent inflammation across a range of different populations and conditions. The transdiagnostic utility of exercise is recognised in a recent paper reviewing the evidence for prescribing exercise in the treatment of 26 different conditions [69]. Similar benefits have been reported across a range of mental disorders [88, 89]. There are few adverse side effects associated with exercise, it can be administered in low-resource settings and is accessible to most people [90]. Exercise also has a range of benefits that extend beyond its direct effects on reducing inflammation and symptoms, such as improving sleep [91] or enhancing quality of life in people with chronic health conditions [92]. As a result, the inclusion of exercise as a transdiagnostic clinical tool is a safe and broadly beneficial method of reducing inflammation.

However, unlike most pharmaceutical agents, there is a lack of consensus over the correct 'dose' of exercise. Dose could refer to the frequency, duration, intensity or modality of exercise. It is unclear whether aerobic or resistance training is most suitable for treating inflammation and both are likely to have different inflammatory profiles [11]. For example, aerobic exercise is more effective at reducing adipose tissue than resistance training [93] and may be more effective at targeting inflammation caused by adipokines. In people with type 2 diabetes, some studies suggest that resistance exercise does not decrease the circulation of inflammatory markers (e.g. [65]), while others suggest it does [94, 95]. But in one of these studies, aerobic exercise was found to be superior at decreasing circulating adipokines [95]. In two studies comparing both types of exercise in healthy participants, one found that resistance training increased CRP levels while aerobic training did not [96] and the other found aerobic, not resistance training reduced CRP, IL-18 and IL-6 [86]. One study combined aerobic and resistance exercise over a 24-week period and found healthy participants had lower CRP, leptin and resistin post-intervention [97]. Such conflicting findings highlight a need for more studies that make direct comparisons between these exercise modalities to determine the most effective at reducing inflammation in different populations and conditions.

It will also be important to consider the duration and intensity of exercise sessions. Some studies have found high-intensity interval training (HIIT) to be superior to moderate intensity continuous training in reducing inflammation [98], some have found HIIT to increase inflammation [87] and others have found no correlation between intensity and inflammation [22, 65]. Exercise duration is the biggest determinant of myokine response [99], which explains around 50% of the variance in plasma IL-6 and IL-10 following exercise [31, 100]. One meta-analysis of type 2 diabetes trials found that the most effective exercise protocols for reducing IL-6 had longer durations and larger numbers of sessions [65]. Another meta-analysis of trials in various health conditions found no effect of different intensity [22]. It is possible that different durations and intensities are appropriate for different population groups or conditions, which may underlie some of these conflicting findings.

However, it is possible for more extreme durations and intensities of exercise to be harmful. More extreme forms of exercise can cause muscle damage and systemic endotoxemia [99]. Following an acute bout of strenuous exercise, a temporary immunosuppressant period follows [101, 102].

For example, studies have found that long distance endurance events, such as triathlons, marathons (42 km), ultra-marathons (200 km) or spartathalons (246 km) can produce acute elevations of inflammatory markers including CRP, IL-1, IL-6, IL-8 and IL-10 [103–107]. One study found elevations in CRP lasting for 6 days after the event [105]. These negative effects are more pronounced in non-athletes performing strenuous exercise [108]. Similar elevations in inflammatory markers were not found with acute, strenuous resistance training [109], which could be related to the shorter exercise duration period.

Over time, the immunosuppressant effects of strenuous exercise may increase the risk of disease. Several studies have found that elite athletes have a greater risk of upper respiratory tract infection and this is likely to be partially due to the immunosuppressant effects of strenuous exercise [110, 111]. But it is important to note that these effects are only seen with extreme forms of exercise and are far outweighed by the vast health benefits of exercise more broadly [36]. It would be beneficial for future research to determine the point at which exercise can become harmful in terms of its intensity, duration, or overall lifetime exposure. This information will be important in ensuring that exercise-based treatments are as safe as possible.

26.6 Conclusion

Through several interconnected pathways, both acute exercise and exercise training can produce anti-inflammatory effects. It is possible for exercise to be used to maintain a low inflammatory profile in non-clinical population groups via mechanisms that include the modulation of myokine activity, adipose tissue, TLRs and monocytes. These anti-inflammatory effects may extend to the treatment of people with inflammatory conditions.

Depression is increasingly considered to have an inflammatory component and several trials have shown that exercise can treat depressive symptoms. It is possible that the anti-inflammatory effects of exercise represent one pathway through which exercise reduces depressive symptoms. However, there has been little research that directly assesses the capacity for exercise to influence levels of inflammation in people with depression. Given the wider utility of exercise in the treatment of depression, more research in this area would be beneficial for establishing factors such as the optimal dose of exercise.

References

1. Schuch FB, Vancampfort D, Richards J, Rosenbaum S, Ward PB, Stubbs B. Exercise as a treatment for depression: A meta-analysis adjusting for publication bias. J Psychiatr Res. 2016a;77:42–51.
2. Caspersen CJ, Powell KE, Christenson GM. Physical activity, exercise, and physical fitness: definitions and distinctions for health-related research. Public Health Rep. 1985; 100(2):126.
3. Schuch FB, Vancampfort D, Firth J, Rosenbaum S, Ward PB, Silva ES, et al. Physical activity and incident depression: a meta-analysis of prospective cohort studies. Am J Psychiatry. 2018;175(7):631–48.
4. Mammen G, Faulkner G. Physical activity and the prevention of depression: a systematic review of prospective studies. Am J Prev Med [Internet]. 2013;45(5):649–57.
5. Teychenne M, Ball K, Salmon J. Sedentary behavior and depression among adults: A review. Int J Behav Med [Internet]. 2010;17(4):246–54.
6. Kvam S, Kleppe CL, Nordhus IH, Hovland A. Exercise as a treatment for depression: a meta-analysis. J Affect Disord. 2016;202:67–86. https://doi.org/10.1016/J.JAD.2016.03.063.
7. Köhler CA, Freitas TH, Maes M, de Andrade NQ, Liu CS, Fernandes BS, et al. Peripheral cytokine and chemokine alterations in depression: a meta-analysis of 82 studies. Acta Psychiatr Scand. 2017;135(5):373–87. https://doi.org/10.1111/acps.12698.
8. Dantzer R, O'Connor JC, Freund GG, Johnson RW, Kelley KW. From inflammation to sickness and depression: when the immune system subjugates the brain. Nat Rev Neurosci [Internet]. 2008;9(1):46–56.
9. Howley ET. Type of activity: resistance, aerobic and leisure versus occupational physical activity. Med Sci Sports Exerc. 2001;33(6):S364–9.
10. Eyre HA, Papps E, Baune BT. Treating Depression and Depression-Like Behavior with Physical Activity: An Immune Perspective. Front Psychiatry [Internet]. 2013;4:3.
11. Strasser B, Arvandi M, Siebert U. Resistance training, visceral obesity and inflammatory response: a review of the evidence. Obes Rev. 2012;13(7):578–91.
12. Kasapis C, Thompson PD. The effects of physical activity on serum C-reactive protein and inflammatory markers: a systematic review. J Am Coll Cardiol. 2005;45(10):1563–9.
13. Hamer M, Sabia S, Batty GD, Shipley MJ, Tabák AG, Singh-Manoux A, Kivimaki M. Physical activity and inflammatory markers over 10 years: follow-up in men and women from the Whitehall II cohort study. Circulation. 2012;126(8):928–33.
14. Rana JS, Arsenault BJ, Després JP, Côté M, Talmud PJ, Ninio E, et al. Inflammatory biomarkers, physical activity, waist circumference, and risk of future coronary heart disease in healthy men and women. Eur Heart J. 2009;32(3):336–44.

15. Hamer M, Molloy GJ, de Oliveira C, Demakakos P. Leisure time physical activity, risk of depressive symptoms, and inflammatory mediators: The English Longitudinal Study of Ageing. Psychoneuroendocrinology [Internet]. 2009;34(7):1050–5.
16. Bergström G, Behre CJ, Schmidt C. Moderate intensities of leisure-time physical activity are associated with lower levels of high-sensitivity C-reactive protein in healthy middle-aged men. Angiology. 2012;63(6):412–5.
17. Borodulin K, Laatikainen T, Salomaa V, Jousilahti P. Associations of leisure time physical activity, self-rated physical fitness, and estimated aerobic fitness with serum C-reactive protein among 3803 adults. Atherosclerosis. 2006;185(2):381–7.
18. Colbert LH, Visser M, Simonsick EM, Tracy RP, Newman AB, Kritchevsky SB, et al. Physical activity, exercise, and inflammatory markers in older adults: findings from the health, aging and body composition study. J Am Geriatr Soc. 2004;52(7):1098–104.
19. Gomez-Marcos MA, Recio-Rodríguez JI, Patino-Alonso MC, Martinez-Vizcaino V, Martin-Borras C, de-la-Cal-dela-Fuente A, et al. Relationship between physical activity and plasma fibrinogen concentrations in adults without chronic diseases. PLoS One. 2014;9(2):e87954.
20. Yu Z, Ye X, Wang J, Qi Q, Franco OH, Rennie KL, et al. Associations of physical activity with inflammatory factors, adipocytokines, and metabolic syndrome in middle-aged and older Chinese people. 2009.
21. Pedersen BK. Exercise-induced myokines and their role in chronic diseases. Brain Behav Immun [Internet]. 2011:811–6.
22. Lin X, Zhang X, Guo J, Roberts CK, McKenzie S, Wu W, et al. Effects of exercise training on cardiorespiratory fitness and biomarkers of cardiometabolic health: a systematic review and meta-analysis of randomized controlled trials. J Am Heart Assoc. 2015;4(7) https://doi.org/10.1161/JAHA.115.002014.
23. Fedewa MV, Hathaway ED, Ward-Ritacco CL, Williams TD, Dobbs WC. The effect of chronic exercise training on leptin: a systematic review and meta-analysis of randomized controlled trials. Sports Med. 2018;48(6):1437–50.
24. Church TS, Earnest CP, Thompson AM, Priest E, Rodarte RQ, Sanders T, et al. Exercise without weight loss does not reduce C-reactive protein: the INFLAME study. Med Sci Sports Exerc. 2010;42(4):708.
25. Conroy SM, Courneya KS, Brenner DR, Shaw E, O'Reilly R, Yasui Y, et al. Impact of aerobic exercise on levels of IL-4 and IL-10: results from two randomized intervention trials. Cancer Med. 2016;5(9):2385–97.
26. Lakka TA, Lakka HM, Rankinen T, Leon AS, Rao DC, Skinner JS, et al. Effect of exercise training on plasma levels of C-reactive protein in healthy adults: the HERITAGE family study. Eur Heart J. 2005;26(19):2018–25.
27. Sloan RP, Shapiro PA, McKinley PS, Bartels M, Shimbo D, Lauriola V, et al. Aerobic exercise training and inducible inflammation: results of a randomized controlled trial in healthy, young adults. J Am Heart Assoc. 2018;7(17):e010201. https://doi.org/10.1161/JAHA.118.010201.
28. Febbraio MA, Pedersen BK. Muscle-derived interleukin-6: mechanisms for activation and possible biological roles. FASEB J. 2002;16(11):1335–47. https://doi.org/10.1096/fj.01-0876rev.
29. Brown WMC, Davison GW, McClean CM, Murphy MH. A systematic review of the acute effects of exercise on immune and inflammatory indices in untrained adults. Sports Med Open. 2015;1(1):35. https://doi.org/10.1186/s40798-015-0032-x.
30. Pedersen BK, Febbraio MA. Muscle as an Endocrine Organ: Focus on Muscle-Derived Interleukin-6. Physiol Rev [Internet]. 2008;88(4):1379–406.
31. Cabral-Santos C, de Lima Junior EA, Fernandes IM, Pinto RZ, Rosa-Neto JC, Bishop NC, Lira FS. Interleukin-10 responses from acute exercise in healthy subjects: a systematic review. J Cell Physiol. 2019;234(7):9956–65. https://doi.org/10.1002/jcp.27920.
32. Pedersen BK, Fischer CP. Physiological roles of muscle-derived interleukin-6 in response to exercise. Curr Opin Clin Nutr Metab Care. 2007;10(3):265–71. https://doi.org/10.1097/MCO.0b013e3280ebb5b3.

33. Steensberg A, Fischer CP, Keller C, Møller K, Pedersen BK. IL-6 enhances plasma IL-1ra, IL-10, and cortisol in humans. Am J Physiol Endocrinol Metab. 2003;285(2):E433–7. https://doi.org/10.1152/ajpendo.00074.2003.
34. Lancaster GI, Febbraio MA. The immunomodulating role of exercise in metabolic disease. Trends Immunol. 2014;35(6):262–9. https://doi.org/10.1016/J.IT.2014.02.008.
35. Pedersen M, Bruunsgaard H, Weis N, Hendel HW, Andreassen BU, Eldrup E, et al. Circulating levels of TNF-alpha and IL-6-relation to truncal fat mass and muscle mass in healthy elderly individuals and in patients with type-2 diabetes. Mech Ageing Dev. 2003;124(4):495–502. https://doi.org/10.1016/S0047-6374(03)00027-7.
36. Gleeson M, Bishop NC, Stensel DJ, Lindley MR, Mastana SS, Nimmo MA. The anti-inflammatory effects of exercise: mechanisms and implications for the prevention and treatment of disease. Nat Rev Immunol. 2011;11(9):607–15. https://doi.org/10.1038/nri3041.
37. van der Poll T, Coyle SM, Barbosa K, Braxton CC, Lowry SF. Epinephrine inhibits tumor necrosis factor-alpha and potentiates interleukin 10 production during human endotoxemia. J Clin Investig. 1996a;97(3):713–9. https://doi.org/10.1172/JCI118469.
38. Pedersen BK. Anti-inflammatory effects of exercise: role in diabetes and cardiovascular disease. Eur J Clin Investig. 2017;47(8):600–11. https://doi.org/10.1111/eci.12781.
39. Thompson D, Karpe F, Lafontan M, Frayn K. Physical activity and exercise in the regulation of human adipose tissue physiology. Physiol Rev. 2012;92(1):157–91. https://doi.org/10.1152/physrev.00012.2011.
40. Olsen RH, Krogh-Madsen R, Thomsen C, Booth FW, Pedersen BK. Metabolic responses to reduced daily steps in healthy nonexercising men. JAMA. 2008;299(11):1261. https://doi.org/10.1001/jama.299.11.1259.
41. Ouchi N, Parker JL, Lugus JJ, Walsh K. Adipokines in inflammation and metabolic disease. Nat Rev Immunol [Internet]. 2011;11(2):85–97.
42. Nielsen AR, Hojman P, Erikstrup C, Fischer CP, Plomgaard P, Mounier R, et al. Association between Interleukin-15 and obesity: Interleukin-15 as a potential regulator of fat mass. J Clin Endocrinol Metabol. 2008;93(11):4486–93. https://doi.org/10.1210/jc.2007-2561.
43. Quinn L, Straitbodey L, Anderson B, Argiles J, Havel P. Interleukin-15 stimulates adiponectin secretion by 3T3-L1 adipocytes: evidence for a skeletal muscle-to-fat signaling pathway. Cell Biol Int. 2005;29(6):449–57. https://doi.org/10.1016/j.cellbi.2005.02.005.
44. Rinnov A, Yfanti C, Nielsen S, Åkerström TCA, Peijs L, Zankari A, et al. Endurance training enhances skeletal muscle interleukin-15 in human male subjects. Endocrine. 2014;45(2):271–8. https://doi.org/10.1007/s12020-013-9969-z.
45. Lim S, Choi SH, Jeong I-K, Kim JH, Moon MK, Park KS, et al. Insulin-sensitizing effects of exercise on adiponectin and retinol-binding protein-4 concentrations in young and middle-aged women. J Clin Endocrinol Metabol. 2008;93(6):2263–8. https://doi.org/10.1210/jc.2007-2028.
46. Mujumdar PP, Duerksen-Hughes PJ, Firek AF, Hessinger DA. Long-term, progressive, aerobic training increases adiponectin in middle-aged, overweight, untrained males and females. Scand J Clin Lab Invest. 2011;71(2):101–7. https://doi.org/10.3109/00365513.2011.554995.
47. Balducci S, Zanuso S, Nicolucci A, Fernando F, Cavallo S, Cardelli P, et al. Anti-inflammatory effect of exercise training in subjects with type 2 diabetes and the metabolic syndrome is dependent on exercise modalities and independent of weight loss. Nutr Metab Cardiovasc Dis. 2010;20(8):608–17. https://doi.org/10.1016/j.numecd.2009.04.015.
48. Osborn O, Olefsky JM. The cellular and signaling networks linking the immune system and metabolism in disease. Nat Med. 2012;18(3):363–74. https://doi.org/10.1038/nm.2627.
49. Kawanishi N, Mizokami T, Yano H, Suzuki K. Exercise attenuates M1 macrophages and CD8+ T cells in the adipose tissue of obese mice. Med Sci Sports Exerc. 2013;45(9):1684–93. https://doi.org/10.1249/MSS.0b013e31828ff9c6.
50. Kawanishi N, Yano H, Yokogawa Y, Suzuki K. Exercise training inhibits inflammation in adipose tissue via both suppression of macrophage infiltration and acceleration of phenotypic switching from M1 to M2 macrophages in high-fat-diet-induced obese mice. Exerc Immunol Rev. 2010;16:105–18.

51. Akira S, Uematsu S, Takeuchi O. Pathogen recognition and innate immunity. Cell. 2006;124(4):783–801. https://doi.org/10.1016/j.cell.2006.02.015.
52. Takeda K, Akira S. Toll-like receptors in innate immunity. Int Immunol. 2004;17(1):1–14. https://doi.org/10.1093/intimm/dxh186.
53. Stewart LK, Flynn MG, Campbell WW, Craig BA, Robinson JP, McFarlin BK, et al. Influence of exercise training and age on CD14+ cell-surface expression of toll-like receptor 2 and 4. Brain Behav Immun. 2005;19(5):389–97.
54. Flynn MG, McFarlin BK, Phillips MD, Stewart LK, Timmerman KL. Toll-like receptor 4 and CD14 mRNA expression are lower in resistive exercise-trained elderly women. J Appl Physiol. 2003;95(5):1833–42. https://doi.org/10.1152/japplphysiol.00359.2003.
55. McFarlin BK, Flynn MG, Campbell WW, Stewart LK, Timmerman KL. TLR4 is lower in resistance-trained older women and related to inflammatory cytokines. Med Sci Sports Exerc. 2004;36(11):1876–83.
56. Timmerman KL, Flynn MG, Coen PM, Markofski MM, Pence BD. Exercise training-induced lowering of inflammatory (CD14+CD16+) monocytes: a role in the anti-inflammatory influence of exercise? J Leukoc Biol. 2008;84(5):1271–8. https://doi.org/10.1189/jlb.0408244.
57. Oliveira AG, Carvalho BM, Tobar N, Ropelle ER, Pauli JR, Bagarolli RA, et al. Physical exercise reduces circulating lipopolysaccharide and TLR4 activation and improves insulin signaling in tissues of DIO rats. Diabetes. 2011;60(3):784–96. https://doi.org/10.2337/db09-1907.
58. Henstridge DC, Febbraio MA, Hargreaves M. Heat shock proteins and exercise adaptations. Our knowledge thus far and the road still ahead. J Appl Physiol. 2016;120(6):683–91. https://doi.org/10.1152/japplphysiol.00811.2015.
59. Hammonds TL, Gathright EC, Goldstein CM, Penn MS, Hughes JW. Effects of exercise on c-reactive protein in healthy patients and in patients with heart disease: A meta-analysis. Heart Lung. 2016;45(3):273–82.
60. Swardfager W, Herrmann N, Cornish S, Mazereeuw G, Marzolini S, Sham L, Lanctôt KL. Exercise intervention and inflammatory markers in coronary artery disease: a meta-analysis. Am Heart J. 2012;163(4):666–676.e3. https://doi.org/10.1016/J.AHJ.2011.12.017.
61. García-Hermoso A, Sánchez-López M, Escalante Y, Saavedra JM, Martínez-Vizcaíno V. Exercise-based interventions and C-reactive protein in overweight and obese youths: a meta-analysis of randomized controlled trials. Pediatr Res. 2016;79(4):522.
62. Yu N, Ruan Y, Gao X, Sun J. Systematic review and meta-analysis of randomized, controlled trials on the effect of exercise on serum leptin and adiponectin in overweight and obese individuals. Horm Metab Res. 2017;49(03):164–73.
63. Rostás I, Pótó L, Mátrai P, Hegyi P, Tenk J, Garami A, et al. In middle-aged and old obese patients, training intervention reduces leptin level: a meta-analysis. PLoS One. 2017;12(8):e0182801.
64. Becic T, Studenik C, Hoffmann G. Exercise increases adiponectin and reduces leptin levels in prediabetic and diabetic individuals: systematic review and meta-analysis of randomized controlled trials. Med Sci. 2018;6(4):97.
65. Hayashino Y, Jackson JL, Hirata T, Fukumori N, Nakamura F, Fukuhara S, et al. Effects of exercise on C-reactive protein, inflammatory cytokine and adipokine in patients with type 2 diabetes: a meta-analysis of randomized controlled trials. Metabolism. 2014;63(3):431–40. https://doi.org/10.1016/J.METABOL.2013.08.018.
66. Meneses-Echávez JF, Correa-Bautista JE, González-Jiménez E, Río-Valle JS, Elkins MR, Lobelo F, Ramírez-Vélez R. The effect of exercise training on mediators of inflammation in breast cancer survivors: a systematic review with meta-analysis. Cancer Epidemiol Prevent Biomarkers. 2016;25(7):1009–17.
67. Fedewa MV, Hathaway ED, Ward-Ritacco CL. Effect of exercise training on C reactive protein: a systematic review and meta-analysis of randomised and nonrandomised controlled trials. Br J Sports Med [Internet]. 2017;51(8):670–6.

68. Simpson KA, Singh MAF. Effects of exercise on adiponectin: a systematic review. Obesity. 2008;16(2):241–56.
69. Pedersen BK, Saltin B. Exercise as medicine - evidence for prescribing exercise as therapy in 26 different chronic diseases. Scand J Med Sci Sports. 2015;25:1–72. https://doi.org/10.1111/sms.12581.
70. Melo LC, Dativo-Medeiros J, Menezes-Silva CE, Barbosa FT, Sousa-Rodrigues CFD, Rabelo LA. Physical exercise on inflammatory markers in type 2 diabetes patients: a systematic review of randomized controlled trials. Oxid Med Cell Longevity. 2017;2017
71. Sveaas SH, Smedslund G, Hagen KB, Dagfinrud H. Effect of cardiorespiratory and strength exercises on disease activity in patients with inflammatory rheumatic diseases: a systematic review and meta-analysis. Br J Sports Med. 2017;51(14):1065–72.
72. Kelley GA, Kelley KS. Effects of aerobic exercise on C-reactive protein, body composition, and maximum oxygen consumption in adults: a meta-analysis of randomized controlled trials. Metabolism. 2006;55(11):1500–7. https://doi.org/10.1016/J.METABOL.2006.06.021.
73. Dinarello CA, Simon A, van der Meer JWM. Treating inflammation by blocking interleukin-1 in a broad spectrum of diseases. Nat Rev Drug Discov. 2012;11(8):633–52. https://doi.org/10.1038/nrd3800.
74. Miller AH, Maletic V, Raison CL. Inflammation and its discontents: the role of cytokines in the pathophysiology of major depression. Biol Psychiatry. 2009;65(9):732–41.
75. Dowlati Y, Herrmann N, Swardfager W, Liu H, Sham L, Reim EK, Lanctôt KL. A meta-analysis of cytokines in major depression. Biol Psychiatry. 2010;67(5):446–57.
76. Howren MB, Lamkin DM, Suls J. Associations of depression with C-reactive protein, IL-1, and IL-6: a meta-analysis. Psychosom Med. 2009;71(2):171–86.
77. Valkanova V, Ebmeier KP, Allan CL. CRP, IL-6 and depression: A systematic review and meta-analysis of longitudinal studies. J Affect Disord. 2013;150(3):736–44. https://doi.org/10.1016/j.jad.2013.06.004.
78. Capuron L, Lasselin J, Castanon N. Role of adiposity-driven inflammation in depressive morbidity. Neuropsychopharmacology. 2017;42(1):115–28. https://doi.org/10.1038/npp.2016.123.
79. Cooney GM, Dwan K, Greig CA, Lawlor DA, Rimer J, Waugh FR, et al. Exercise for depression. Cochrane Database Syst Rev. 2013;9
80. Schuch FB, Deslandes AC, Stubbs B, Gosmann NP, da Silva CTB, de Almeida Fleck MP. Neurobiological effects of exercise on major depressive disorder: a systematic review. Neurosci Biobehav Rev. 2016b;61:1–11. https://doi.org/10.1016/J.NEUBIOREV.2015.11.012.
81. Hennings A, Schwarz MJ, Riemer S, Stapf TM, Selberdinger VB, Rief W. Exercise affects symptom severity but not biological measures in depression and somatization–results on IL-6, neopterin, tryptophan, kynurenine and 5-HIAA. Psychiatry Res. 2013;210(3):925–33.
82. Krogh J, Videbech P, Thomsen C, Gluud C, Nordentoft M. DEMO-II Trial. Aerobic exercise versus stretching exercise in patients with major depression—a randomised clinical trial. PLoS One. 2012;7(10):e48316.
83. Rethorst CD, Toups MS, Greer TL, Nakonezny PA, Carmody TJ, Grannemann BD, et al. Pro-inflammatory cytokines as predictors of antidepressant effects of exercise in major depressive disorder. Mol Psychiatry. 2013;18(10):1119–24.
84. Euteneuer F, Dannehl K, del Rey A, Engler H, Schedlowski M, Rief W. Immunological effects of behavioral activation with exercise in major depression: an exploratory randomized controlled trial. Transl Psychiatry. 2017;7(5):e1132. https://doi.org/10.1038/tp.2017.76.
85. Lavebratt C, Herring MP, Liu JJ, Wei YB, Bossoli D, Hallgren M, Forsell Y. Interleukin-6 and depressive symptom severity in response to physical exercise. Psychiatry Res. 2017;252:270–6. https://doi.org/10.1016/j.psychres.2017.03.012.
86. Kohut ML, McCann DA, Russell DW, Konopka DN, Cunnick JE, Franke WD, et al. Aerobic exercise, but not flexibility/resistance exercise, reduces serum IL-18, CRP, and IL-6 independent of β-blockers, BMI, and psychosocial factors in older adults. Brain Behav Immun. 2006;20(3):201–9. https://doi.org/10.1016/J.BBI.2005.12.002.

87. Paolucci EM, Loukov D, Bowdish DM, Heisz JJ. Exercise reduces depression and inflammation but intensity matters. Biol Psychol. 2018;133:79–84.
88. Ashdown-Franks G, Sabiston CM, Stubbs B. The evidence for physical activity in the management of major mental illnesses: a concise overview to inform busy clinicians' practice and guide policy. Curr Opin Psychiatry. 2019;
89. Kandola A, Vancampfort D, Herring M, Rebar A, Hallgren M, Firth J, Stubbs B. Moving to beat anxiety: epidemiology and therapeutic issues with physical activity for anxiety. Curr Psychiatry Rep. 2018;20(8) https://doi.org/10.1007/s11920-018-0923-x.
90. Stubbs B, Vancampfort D, Hallgren M, Firth J, Veronese N, Solmi M, et al. EPA guidance on physical activity as a treatment for severe mental illness: a meta-review of the evidence and position statement from the European Psychiatric Association (EPA), supported by the International Organization of Physical Therapists in Mental Health (IOPTMH). Eur Psychiatry. 2018;54:124–44.
91. Kelley GA, Kelley KS. Exercise and sleep: a systematic review of previous meta-analyses. J Evid Based Med. 2017;10(1):26–36.
92. Buffart LM, Kalter J, Sweegers MG, Courneya KS, Newton RU, Aaronson NK, et al. Effects and moderators of exercise on quality of life and physical function in patients with cancer: an individual patient data meta-analysis of 34 RCTs. Cancer Treat Rev. 2017;52: 91–104.
93. Ismail I, Keating SE, Baker MK, Johnson NA. A systematic review and meta-analysis of the effect of aerobic vs. resistance exercise training on visceral fat. Obes Rev. 2012;13(1): 68–91.
94. Jorge MLMP, de Oliveira VN, Resende NM, Paraiso LF, Calixto A, Diniz ALD, et al. The effects of aerobic, resistance, and combined exercise on metabolic control, inflammatory markers, adipocytokines, and muscle insulin signaling in patients with type 2 diabetes mellitus. Metabolism. 2011;60(9):1244–52.
95. Kadoglou NPE, Fotiadis G, Kapelouzou A, Kostakis A, Liapis CD, Vrabas IS. The differential anti-inflammatory effects of exercise modalities and their association with early carotid atherosclerosis progression in patients with type 2 diabetes. Diabet Med. 2013;30(2): e41–50.
96. Donges CE, Duffield R, Drinkwater EJ. Effects of resistance or aerobic exercise training on interleukin-6, C-reactive protein, and body composition. Med Sci Sports Exerc. 2010;42(2):304–13. https://doi.org/10.1249/MSS.0b013e3181b117ca.
97. Ihalainen JK, Schumann M, Eklund D, Hämäläinen M, Moilanen E, Paulsen G, et al. Combined aerobic and resistance training decreases inflammation markers in healthy men. Scand J Med Sci Sports. 2018;28(1):40–7. https://doi.org/10.1111/sms.12906.
98. Ramos JS, Dalleck LC, Tjonna AE, Beetham KS, Coombes JS. The impact of high-intensity interval training versus moderate-intensity continuous training on vascular function: a systematic review and meta-analysis. Sports Med. 2015;45(5):679–92.
99. Ostrowski K, Rohde T, Asp S, Schjerling P, Pedersen BK. Pro- and anti-inflammatory cytokine balance in strenuous exercise in humans. J Physiol. 1999;515(1):287–91. https://doi.org/10.1111/j.1469-7793.1999.287ad.x.
100. Fischer CP. Interleukin-6 in acute exercise and training: what is the biological relevance? Exerc Immunol Rev. 2006;12:6–33.
101. Steensberg A, Febbraio MA, Osada T, Schjerling P, van Hall G, Saltin B, Pedersen BK. Interleukin-6 production in contracting human skeletal muscle is influenced by pre-exercise muscle glycogen content. J Physiol. 2001a;537(2):633–9. https://doi.org/10.1111/j.1469-7793.2001.00633.x.
102. Steensberg A, Toft AD, Bruunsgaard H, Sandmand M, Halkjær-Kristensen J, Pedersen BK. Strenuous exercise decreases the percentage of type 1 T cells in the circulation. J Appl Physiol. 2001b;91(4):1708–12. https://doi.org/10.1152/jappl.2001.91.4.1708.
103. Gomez-Merino D, Drogou C, Guezennec CY, Burnat P, Bourrilhon C, Tomaszewski A, et al. Comparison of systemic cytokine responses after a long distance triathlon and a

100-km run: relationship to metabolic and inflammatory processes. Eur Cytokine Netw. 2006;17(2):117–24.
104. Goussetis E, Spiropoulos A, Tsironi M, Skenderi K, Margeli A, Graphakos S, et al. Spartathlon, a 246 kilometer foot race: effects of acute inflammation induced by prolonged exercise on circulating progenitor reparative cells. Blood Cell Mol Dis. 2009;42(3):294–9. https://doi.org/10.1016/j.bcmd.2009.01.003.
105. Kim HJ, Lee YH, Kim CK. Changes in serum cartilage oligomeric matrix protein (COMP), plasma CPK and plasma hs-CRP in relation to running distance in a marathon (42.195 km) and an ultra-marathon (200 km) race. Eur J Appl Physiol. 2009;105(5):765–70. https://doi.org/10.1007/s00421-008-0961-x.
106. Suzuki K, Peake J, Nosaka K, Okutsu M, Abbiss CR, Surriano R, et al. Changes in markers of muscle damage, inflammation and HSP70 after an ironman triathlon race. Eur J Appl Physiol. 2006;98(6):525–34. https://doi.org/10.1007/s00421-006-0296-4.
107. Takayama F, Aoyagi A, Takahashi K, Nabekura Y. Relationship between oxygen cost and C-reactive protein response to marathon running in college recreational runners. Open Access J Sports Med. 2018;9:261–8. https://doi.org/10.2147/OAJSM.S183274.
108. Andersson J, Jansson J-H, Hellsten G, Nilsson TK, Hallmans G, Boman K. Effects of heavy endurance physical exercise on inflammatory markers in non-athletes. Atherosclerosis. 2010;209(2):601–5. https://doi.org/10.1016/j.atherosclerosis.2009.10.025.
109. Uchida MC, Nosaka K, Ugrinowitsch C, Yamashita A, Martins E, Moriscot AS, Aoki MS. Effect of bench press exercise intensity on muscle soreness and inflammatory mediators. J Sports Sci. 2009;27(5):499–507. https://doi.org/10.1080/02640410802632144.
110. Gleeson M, Bishop NC. URI in Athletes. Exerc Sport Sci Rev. 2013;41(3):148–53. https://doi.org/10.1097/JES.0b013e3182956ead.
111. Walsh NP, Gleeson M, Shephard RJ, Gleeson M, Woods JA, Bishop NC, et al. (2011). Position Statement Part one: Immune function and exercise CONSENSUS STATEMENT. http://eir--isei.de/2011/eir-2011-006-article.pdf

GPSR Compliance

The European Union's (EU) General Product Safety Regulation (GPSR) is a set of rules that requires consumer products to be safe and our obligations to ensure this.

If you have any concerns about our products, you can contact us on ProductSafety@springernature.com

In case Publisher is established outside the EU, the EU authorized representative is:

Springer Nature Customer Service Center GmbH
Europaplatz 3
69115 Heidelberg, Germany

Batch number: 10732031

Printed by Printforce, the Netherlands